HEALTH ECONOMICS AND FINANCING

HEALTH ECONOMICS AND FINANCING

Fourth Edition

Thomas E. Getzen
Temple University

JOHN WILEY & SONS, INC.

—to Karen, Matt, Zoa, and Kayla

Publisher	George Hoffman
Associate Publisher	Judith Joseph
Associate Editor	Jennifer Manias
Editorial Assistant	Emily McGee
Associate Director of Marketing	Amy Scholz
Assistant Marketing Manager	Diane Mars
Marketing Assistant	Laura Finley
Senior Media Editor	Greg Chaput
Production Manager	Janis Soo
Assistant Production Editor	Song Yee Lyn
Production Assistant	Mary Alma
Designer	Wendy Lai
Cover Photo Credits	© Andy Brown/Alamy

This book was set in Minion by Aptara, Inc., and printed and bound by Hamilton Printing Company. The cover was printed by Hamilton Printing Company.

This book is printed on acid free paper. ∞

Library of Congress Cataloging-in-Publication Data

Getzen, Thomas E.
    Health economics and financing / Thomas E. Getzen. – 4th ed.
        p. cm.
    Includes index.
    ISBN 978-0-470-46901-9 (cloth)
    1. Medical economics.   2. Medical care, Cost of.   3. Flow of Funds.   I. Title.
    RA410.G48 2011
    338.4'33621–dc22

                            2009033765

Printed in the United States of America
10 9 8 7 6 5 4 3

BRIEF CONTENTS

Preface   xxi

Acknowledgments   xxiii

About the Author   xxiii

Foreword   xxv

1   **Choices: Money, Medicine, and Health**   1

2   **Demand and Supply**   26

3   **Cost-Benefit and Cost-Effectiveness Analysis**   48

4   **Health Insurance: Financing Medical Care**   79

5   **Insurance Contracts and Managed Care**   108

6   **Physicians**   135

7   **Medical Education, Organization, and Business Practices**   157

8   **Hospitals**   184

9   **Management and Regulation of Hospital Costs**   206

10   **Long-Term Care**   224

11   **Pharmaceuticals**   248

12   **Capital Financing and Ownership of Health Care Providers**   275

13   **Macroeconomics of Medical Care**   305

14   **The Role of Government**   333

15   **Public Goods and Public Health**   354

16   **History, Demography, and the Growth of Modern Medicine**   373

17 **International Comparisons of Health and Health Expenditures** 399

18 **Value for Money in the Future of Health Care** 429

Glossary 447

Index 457

CONTENTS

Preface   xxi

Acknowledgments   xxiii

About the Author   xxiii

Foreword   xxv

1   Choices: Money, Medicine, and Health   1

Questions   1

1.1   WHAT IS ECONOMICS?   2
Terms of Trade   2
Can We Pay Somebody to Care?   3
Financing Health Care   4
Value   5

1.2   THE FLOW OF FUNDS   5
Health Care Spending in the United States   6
Sources of Financing   8
Health Care Providers: The Uses of Funds   10

1.3   ECONOMIC PRINCIPLES AS CONCEPTUAL TOOLS   11
Scarcity (Budget Constraints)   11
Opportunity Cost   11
Willingness to Pay   12
Trade   12
Money Flows in a Circle   12
Maximization: Marginal Costs and Marginal Benefits   12
Choice: Are Benefits Greater than Costs?   12
Investment   13
Contracts: Complex Exchanges to Deal with Timing
and Risk   13
Organizations Adapt and Evolve   14

1.4   HEALTH ECONOMICS: WHAT MAKES MEDICINE
DIFFERENT?   14
Illness Is Contingent, Urgent, Uncertain   14
Health Is Priceless   15

Health Affects the Value of All Other Goods 15

Having More Does Not Reduce the Value of Health 15

Dynamic Change, Driven by Research and Technology 15

Differences over Time and Place Are Larger than the Choices Patients Face 16

Quality, Not Quantity 16

Quality Is Hard to Measure, and Not Additive 16

Individual Choices: Lifestyle Matters More than Medicine 17

Health Risks Are More Public than Private 17

Personal Tastes and Preferences Are Secondary 17

1.5 RESEARCH, TEACHING, AND CHARITY: SHIFTING OVERHEAD 17

1.6 EQUITY AND DISTRIBUTION 18

1.7 WHOSE CHOICES: PERSONAL, GROUP, OR PUBLIC? 19

1.8 SOCIAL SCIENCE AND RATIONAL CHOICE THEORY 21

Suggestions for Further Reading 22

Summary 22

Problems 23

Endnotes 24

2 Demand and Supply 26

Questions 26

2.1 THE DEMAND CURVE 26

The Diamonds–Water Paradox: An Example of Marginal Analysis 27

Consumer Surplus: Marginal versus Average Value of Medicine 28

Ceteris Paribus 30

Individual, Firm, and Market Demand Curves 30

2.2 THE SUPPLY CURVE 30

Marginal Revenue 31

2.3 PRICE SENSITIVITY 32

Price Elasticity and Marginal Revenue 33

Price Discrimination 34

2.4 IS MONEY THE ONLY PRICE? 35

The Labor–Leisure Choice 36

2.5 INPUTS AND PRODUCTION FUNCTIONS 37

Marginal Productivity 37

Production Functions 37

2.6   MARKETS: THE INTERSECTION OF DEMAND AND SUPPLY   38

2.7   NEED VERSUS DEMAND   39

2.8   THE PRODUCTION OF HEALTH   40

How Much Is a Doctor Visit Worth?   41

The Demand for Medical Care Is *Derived* Demand   41

The Demand for Health: What Makes Medical
Care Different   42

2.9   EFFICIENCY   42

Suggestions for Further Reading   44

Summary   44

Problems   46

Endnotes   47

3   Cost-Benefit and Cost-Effectiveness Analysis   48

Questions   48

3.1   COST-BENEFIT ANALYSIS IS ABOUT MAKING CHOICES   49

An Everyday Example: Knee Injury   49

Stepwise Choices: Yes or No? How Much?   52

Calculating Marginal and Average Costs   53

Defining Marginal: What Is the Decision?   54

Opportunity Cost: Looking at Alternatives   57

Expected Value   58

3.2   MAXIMIZATION: FINDING THE OPTIMUM   59

Declining Marginal Benefits   60

Optimization: Maximum Net Benefits   60

Why Marginals Are "the Max," and Averages Are Misleading   61

3.3   MEASURING BENEFITS   62

Health   62

Productivity   63

Reductions in Future Medical Costs   63

3.4   MEASURING COSTS   64

Medical Care and Administration: Charges versus Costs   64

Follow-up and Treatment   64

Time and Pain of Patient and Family   65

Provider Time and Inconvenience   65

3.5   EVIDENCE-BASED MEDICINE   65

3.6   THE VALUE OF LIFE   66

3.7   QUALITY-ADJUSTED LIFE YEARS (QALYs)   68

Discounting Over Time   69

QALY League Tables   69

3.8 PERSPECTIVES: PATIENT, PAYER, GOVERNMENT, PROVIDER, SOCIETY 71

Distribution: Whose Costs and Whose Benefits? 71

CBA Is a Limited Perspective 72

CBA and Public Policy Decision Making 72

Suggestions for Further Reading 72

Summary 73

Problems 74

Endnotes 76

4 Health Insurance: Financing Medical Care 79

Questions 79

4.1 METHODS FOR COVERING RISKS 80

Savings 80

Family and Friends 80

Charity 80

Private Market Insurance Contracts 81

Social Insurance 82

Strengths and Weaknesses of Different Forms of Risk Spreading 82

4.2 INSURANCE: THIRD-PARTY PAYMENT 83

Why Third-Party Payment? 84

Variability 85

Third-Party Transactions 86

Who Pays? How Much? 87

How Are Benefits Determined? 88

4.3 RISK AVERSION 88

4.4 ADVERSE SELECTION 90

4.5 MORAL HAZARD 92

Welfare Losses Due to Moral Hazard 94

4.6 TAX BENEFITS 95

4.7 EFFECTS OF HEALTH INSURANCE ON LABOR MARKETS 96

4.8 HISTORY OF HEALTH INSURANCE 97

4.9 FINANCING HEALTH CARE: INSURANCE AS A FUNDING MECHANISM 100

Entitlements: Open or Closed Financing? 100

Suggestions for Further Reading 101

Summary 102

Problems 103

Endnotes 105

5   Insurance Contracts and Managed Care   108

Questions   **108**

5.1   **TYPES OF INSURANCE PLANS   108**
Medicare   **109**
Employer-Based Group Health Insurance   **109**
Self-Paid Private Insurance   **112**
Medicaid   **112**
Other Government Programs and Charity   **112**
The Uninsured   **112**
State Children's Health Insurance Program   **113**

5.2   **HSAs, MEDICAL SAVINGS ACCOUNTS, AND HIGH-DEDUCTIBLE "CONSUMER-DRIVEN HEALTH PLANS"   113**
Defined Contribution Health Plans   **114**
High-Deductible Insurance   **115**

5.3   **A RANGE OF RISK BEARING: FIXED PREMIUMS, ADMINISTERED SERVICES ONLY, AND SELF-INSURANCE   116**
The Underwriting Cycle   **117**
ERISA, Taxes, and Mandated Benefits   **118**

5.4   **MANAGED CARE PLANS   119**
Why *Managed* Care?   **119**
Management: The Distinctive Feature of Managed Care   **120**
Contractual Reforms to Reduce Costs   **121**
A Fourth Way: Reforming the Organization to Reduce Cost   **122**
Medical Loss Ratios   **123**

5.5   **THE RANGE OF MANAGED CARE PLANS   124**
Provider Networks   **124**
Gatekeeping   **125**
Capitation   **125**
Withholds   **127**
Utilization Review   **127**

5.6   **MANAGED COMPETITION AND THE FEHBP   128**

5.7   **INCENTIVES—TO PATIENTS, TO PAYERS, AND TO PROVIDERS   128**

Suggestions for Further Reading   **129**
Summary   **130**
Problems   **131**
Endnotes   **133**

6 Physicians 135

Questions 135

6.1 FINANCING PHYSICIAN SERVICES: REVENUES 135
Copays, Assignment, and Balance Billing 139
Physician Payment in Managed Care Plans 140
Incentives: Why Differences in the Type of
Payment Matter 141
A Progression: From Prices to Reimbursement
Mechanisms 141

6.2 PHYSICIAN INCOMES 142

6.3 PHYSICIAN FINANCING: EXPENSES 143
Physician Practice Expenses 143
The Labor–Leisure Choice 144
The Doctor's Workshop and Unpaid Hospital Inputs 145
Malpractice 146

6.4 THE TRANSACTION BETWEEN DOCTOR AND PATIENT 146
Asymmetric Information 147
Agency: Whose Choices? 147

6.5 UNCERTAINTY 148

6.6 LICENSURE: QUALITY OR PROFITS? 148
How Does Licensure Increase Physician Profits? 149
Supply and Demand Response in Licensed versus
Unlicensed Professions 150
How Does Licensure Improve Quality? 151
A Test of the Quality Hypothesis: Strong versus
Weak Licensure 152

Suggestions for Further Reading 153
Summary 153
Problems 154
Endnotes 155

7 Medical Education, Organization, and Business Practices 157

Questions 157

7.1 MEDICAL EDUCATION 157

7.2 THE ORIGINS OF LICENSURE AND LINKAGE TO
MEDICAL EDUCATION 158
AMA Controls over Physician Supply, 1930–1965 159
Breaking the Contract: The Great Medical Student Expansion
of 1970–1980 161

Building Pressure: Fixed Domestic Graduation
Rates 1980–2008   **162**

7.3   ADJUSTING PHYSICIAN SUPPLY   162

The Flow of New Entrants and the Stock of Physicians   **162**

Immigration of International Medical Graduates   **163**

Growth in Non-M.D. Physicians   **163**

Balancing Supply and Incomes: Tracing the Past and Projecting
the Future   **164**

**7.4   GROUP PRACTICE: HOW ORGANIZATION AND TECHNOLOGY
AFFECT TRANSACTIONS   165**

7.5   KICKBACKS, SELF-DEALING, AND SIDE PAYMENTS   167

7.6   PRICE DISCRIMINATION   169

7.7   PRACTICE VARIATIONS   171

**7.8   INSURANCE, PRICE COMPETITION, AND THE STRUCTURE OF
MEDICAL MARKETS   174**

7.9   CHOICES *BY* AND *FOR* PHYSICIANS   176

Suggestions for Further Reading   **176**

Summary   **177**

Problems   **178**

Endnotes   **182**

8   Hospitals   184

Questions   **184**

**8.1   FROM CHARITABLE INSTITUTIONS TO CORPORATE CHAINS:
DEVELOPMENT OF THE MODERN HOSPITAL   184**

8.2   HOSPITAL FINANCING: REVENUES   186

Sources of Revenues   **186**

8.3   HOSPITAL FINANCING: EXPENSES   192

8.4   FINANCIAL MANAGEMENT AND COST SHIFTING   192

8.5   HOW DO HOSPITALS COMPETE?   196

Competing for Patients   **196**

Competing for Physicians   **197**

Competing for Contracts   **197**

Measuring Competitive Success   **198**

Measuring the Competitiveness of Markets   **199**

**8.6   ORGANIZATION: WHO CONTROLS THE HOSPITAL AND
FOR WHAT ENDS?   199**

Suggestions for Further Reading   **201**

Summary   **201**

Problems   **202**

Endnotes   **204**

9 Management and Regulation of Hospital Costs 206

Questions 206

9.1 WHY DO SOME HOSPITALS COST MORE THAN OTHERS? 206

9.2 HOW MANAGEMENT CONTROLS COSTS 207

Short-Run versus Long-Run Cost Functions 207

Uncertainty and Budgeting 209

9.3 CONFLICT BETWEEN ECONOMIC THEORY AND ACCOUNTING MEASURES OF PER UNIT COST 211

Timing 211

Whose Costs? 213

9.4 ECONOMIES OF SCALE 214

The Hospital Is a Multiproduct Firm 215

Contracting Out 215

9.5 QUALITY AND COST 215

Technology: Cutting Costs or Enhancing Quality? 215

Improved Efficiency May Raise Total Spending 216

9.6 CONTROLLING HOSPITAL COSTS THROUGH REGULATION 217

Suggestions for Further Reading 220

Summary 220

Problems 221

Endnotes 223

10 Long-Term Care 224

Questions 224

10.1 DEVELOPMENT OF THE LONG-TERM CARE MARKET 225

10.2 DEFINING LTC: TYPES OF CARE 227

10.3 MEDICAID: NURSING HOMES AS A TWO-PART MARKET 229

10.4 CERTIFICATE OF NEED: WHOSE NEEDS? 232

Money and Quality 232

Competing for Certificates of Need, Not for Patients 232

Evidence on the Effects of CON 233

10.5 CASE-MIX REIMBURSEMENT 234

10.6 SUBSTITUTION 235

10.7 FINANCIAL REIMBURSEMENT CYCLES 237

10.8 THE EFFECTS OF AGING ON COST AND UTILIZATION 239

Age and Health Care Spending 239

Defining Boundaries: Is Long-Term Care "Medical"? 240

LTC Insurance **241**

Continuing Care Retirement Communities and the Wealthy
Elderly **242**

Suggestions for Further Reading **243**

Summary **244**

Problems **245**

Endnotes **246**

11 Pharmaceuticals **248**

Questions **248**

11.1   PHARMACEUTICAL REVENUES: SOURCES OF FINANCING **249**

Inpatient Pharmaceuticals **251**

11.2   USES OF FUNDS **251**

Retail Pharmacies **252**

Wholesalers **253**

Insurance Companies and PBMs **253**

Pharmaceutical Firms **253**

Cost Structure **255**

11.3   HISTORY AND REGULATION OF PHARMACEUTICALS **255**

11.4   RESEARCH AND DEVELOPMENT **259**

11.5   PHARMACOECONOMICS AND TECHNOLOGY
ASSESSMENT **261**

11.6   INDUSTRY STRUCTURE AND COMPETITION **262**

Medicare D: An Experiment in Rational Choice **263**

Market Segmentation: Types of Buyers **264**

Contractual Responses to Pharmacy Benefits Management **264**

Value and Cost **265**

The Role of Middlemen: Distribution versus Marketing **266**

Research Productivity **268**

11.7   TRENDS: FORM FOLLOWS FUNCTION (AND MONEY) **270**

Suggestions for Further Reading **270**

Summary **271**

Problems **272**

Endnotes **273**

12 Capital Financing and Ownership of Health Care Providers **275**

Questions **275**

12.1   WHAT IS CAPITAL FINANCING? **275**

12.2   VALUE AND RATE OF RETURN **276**

The Time Value of Money   **276**

Interest Rates and Present Value   **277**

IRR: The Internal Rate of Return   **278**

Human Capital: Medical Education as an Investment   **280**

Risk   **281**

Valuing Assets   **283**

12.3   UNCORRELATED (INDEPENDENT) AND CORRELATED (SYSTEM) RISKS   284

Which Is Riskier: Nursing Homes or Drug Companies?   **285**

Assessing Business Risk   **285**

12.4   OWNERSHIP AND AGENCY   287

Equity and Debt   **287**

Who Owns the Business? Who Owns the Patient? Agency Issues   **288**

The Role of Financial Intermediaries   **289**

Health Insurers as Financial Intermediaries   **290**

12.5   CAPITAL FINANCING: HOSPITALS   290

12.6   HMO OWNERSHIP AND CAPITAL MARKETS: SUCCESS AND FAILURE   293

Business Risks for an HMO   **293**

Kaiser Health Plan: The Evolution of an HMO   **294**

GHA: A Consumer Co-op Gets Bought Out by a Franchise Chain   **296**

12.7   CORPORATE ADVANTAGE   297

U.S. Healthcare: A Profitable Growth Company   **298**

Suggestions for Further Reading   **300**

Summary   **300**

Problems   **302**

Endnotes   **303**

13   Macroeconomics of Medical Care   305

Questions   **305**

13.1   WHAT IS MACRO?   305

Micro and Macro Perspectives on Spending   **306**

13.2   THE CONSUMPTION FUNCTION   307

The Permanent Income Hypothesis   **309**

Shared Income   **310**

Public and Private Decisions   **311**

Budget Constraints: Borders that Matter   **312**

13.3 **ADJUSTING TO CHANGE: DYNAMICS** 312

Permanent Income and Adjustment of Health Spending
to GDP 314

Adjustment to Inflation 315

Adjustment to GDP: Rates of Change and Time Series
Analysis 318

13.4 **FORECASTING FUTURE HEALTH EXPENDITURES** 319

13.5 **COST CONTROLS: SPENDING GAPS AND THE PUSH
TO REGULATE** 320

Capacity Constraints and Budget Constraints 322

13.6 **WORKFORCE DYNAMICS: "SPENDING" IS MOSTLY LABOR** 323

Employment 323

Wages 327

Suggestions for Further Reading 328

Summary 328

Problems 329

Endnotes 331

14 The Role of Government 333

Questions 333

14.1 **GOVERNMENT HEALTH FINANCING** 333

14.2 **THE ROLES OF GOVERNMENT** 335

Government Is Necessary, Even for Private Exchange 335

Efficiency of Markets under Conditions of
Perfect Competition 336

Government in a Mixed Economy 337

14.3 **LAW AND ORDER** 337

14.4 **PUBLIC GOODS AND EXTERNALITIES** 338

Externalities 339

The Coase Theorem: Transaction Costs and Property Rights 339

Politicians: Entrepreneurs Who Try to Get Votes 340

14.5 **MARKET FAILURE** 341

Monopoly 341

Paternalism 342

14.6 **REDISTRIBUTION AND CARE OF THE POOR** 343

Medicaid and Medicare: Dependency or Rights? 343

14.7 **HOW GOVERNMENT WORKS** 344

The Voluntary Sector 345

Government as the Citizen's Agent 346

Winners and Losers 348

14.8 PROS AND CONS OF REGULATION AND COMPETITION 348

Suggestions for Further Reading 350

Summary 350

Problems 351

Endnotes 352

15 Public Goods and Public Health 354

Questions 354

15.1 CHARACTERISTICS OF PUBLIC GOODS 354

Privatizing Public Goods 355

Social Costs Depend on the Number of People 356

Insurance Makes Any Good More Public 356

15.2 INFORMATION 357

Rational Consumer Ignorance 358

Milk or Bread: Which Is More Public? 358

15.3 THE THEORY OF PURE PUBLIC GOODS 359

Public Goods Make Most People Better Off, but Few Happy 361

15.4 INFECTIOUS DISEASE EXTERNALITIES 363

Epidemics 363

HIV/AIDS 364

The Sanitary Revolution: A Moral Campaign for
Public Health 365

Formation of the U.S. Public Health Service 366

15.5 SEX, DRUGS, AND WAR: PUBLIC HEALTH IN ACTION 366

Who Counts as a Citizen? Abortion and Other Dilemmas 367

Addiction 368

War and Public Health 369

Suggestions for Further Reading 370

Summary 370

Problems 371

Endnotes 371

16 History, Demography, and the Growth of Modern Medicine 373

Questions 373

16.1 ECONOMIC GROWTH HAS DETERMINED THE SHAPE OF HEALTH CARE 373

16.2 BIRTH RATES, DEATH RATES, AND POPULATION GROWTH 374

16.3 THE STONE AGE 374

16.4 THE AGRICULTURAL AGE 375

Investment and Trade 376

Civilization, War, and Government 376

The Decline of Civilizations Leads to
Population Declines 377

The Plague 378

Food Supply Determines Population 378

The Rise of Economics 378

The Malthusian Hypothesis 379

16.5 THE INDUSTRIAL AGE 380

Why Malthus Was Wrong 381

Demographic Transition 382

Demographic Change, Income Distribution, and the Rise of the
Middle Classes 383

16.6 THE INFORMATION AGE 384

16.7 INCOME AND HEALTH 385

16.8 REDUCING UNCERTAINTY: THE VALUE OF LIFE AND
ECONOMIC SECURITY 387

The Value of Risk Reduction 388

Social Security and Health Insurance 389

16.9 THE RISE OF MODERN MEDICINE 389

Preconditions for Change 390

The Growth of Medical Science and Technology 390

Did Better Medical Care Increase Life Expectancy? 392

Suggestions for Further Reading 393

Summary 393

Problems 395

Endnotes 396

17 **International Comparisons of Health and
Health Expenditures** 399

Questions 339

17.1 WIDE DIFFERENCES AMONG NATIONS 399

Size of the Market 401

17.2 MICRO VERSUS MACRO ALLOCATION: HEALTH AS A NATIONAL
LUXURY GOOD 402

17.3 CAUSALITY: DOES MORE SPENDING IMPROVE HEALTH? 404

17.4 LOW-INCOME COUNTRIES 405

Sudan 406

Health Care in Kenya 408

17.5 MIDDLE-INCOME COUNTRIES 409

The Health Care System of Mexico 410

Poland 411

17.6 HIGH-INCOME COUNTRIES 413

Japan 413

The Health System in Germany 417

The Expensive Exception: The United States 421

17.7 INTERNATIONAL TRADE IN HEALTH CARE 422

People and Ideas 422

Services 423

Equipment 423

Pharmaceuticals 423

Suggestions for Further Reading 425

Summary 425

Problems 426

Endnotes 426

18 Value for Money in the Future of Health Care 429

Questions 429

18.1 FORCING THE QUESTION: WHO GETS HEALTHY AND WHO GETS PAID? 429

18.2 SPENDING MONEY OR PRODUCING HEALTH? 431

18.3 DYNAMIC EFFICIENCY 432

18.4 DISTRIBUTION, DISTRIBUTION, DISTRIBUTION 434

18.5 PATH DEPENDENCE AND THE POSSIBILITIES FOR REFORM 435

How Did We Get Here? 435

What Did Medicine Miss? 436

What Went Wrong? Notable Failures and Unresolved Dilemmas 436

18.6 THE PATH FORWARD: STEP BY STEP 439

What Might Work? 439

18.7 THE SHAPE OF HEALTH CARE SPENDING TO COME 441

18.8 THE LONG RUN: 2050 AND BEYOND 442

Suggestions for Further Reading 443

Summary 443

Problems 444

Endnotes 445

Glossary 447

Index 457

PREFACE

Health Economics and Financing is a primer for the economic analysis of medical markets. Its intended audiences are students of medicine, public health, policy, and administration who wish to engage the central economic issues of their field without prolonged preparatory work; beginning students in economics who wish to study an applied area in detail without recourse to extensive mathematical manipulation; and more advanced students in economics who may be familiar with analytical techniques but lack knowledge of the many institutional features that make the study of health and health care so unique and rewarding.[*] This book draws upon the work of many scholars, but in keeping with its design as a primer for introducing students to the principles and concepts of health economics rather than its literature and research methods, the use of attribution, footnotes, and references is purposely limited. Suggestions for additional reading and more advanced source materials and databases are listed at the end of each chapter and are available on the text Web site at www.wiley.com/college/getzen or from the author at getzen@temple.edu.

The first eleven chapters use a flow of funds approach to investigate the sources and uses of financing and to explore the incentives and organizational structure of the health care system. Transactions between patients and physicians (and others) are examined to see how profits are made, costs covered, contracts written (or implied) and regulations formed. The long-term consequences of exchanging services for money in a particular way are revealed by exploring the historical development of those distinctive features that characterize the industrial organization of health care: licensure, third-party insurance, nonprofit hospitals, and government regulation. The last seven chapters take a wider macroeconomic perspective in order to explore the dynamics of change within the health care system and to explicitly consider determinants of national health spending and the role of governments in public and private health.

The introductory chapter lays out the overall flow of funds, schematically presents the complexity of medical care transactions, and introduces the basic principles that form the toolkit for economic analysis. Chapter 2 examines the economic concept of demand and compares it to the medical concept of need. Chapter 3 applies the basic principles of supply and demand, marginalism and equilibrium, using a cost-benefit approach in a clinical context. The more detailed investigation of medical care organization begins in Chapters 4 and 5 on insurance and third-party reimbursement, which has become the dominant source of funds in medical care. The physician—the patient's agent and a central player in all medical care transactions—is the subject of the next two chapters. Chapters 8 and 9 cover the reimbursement, regulation, and cost structure of hospitals. Nursing homes, long-term care, and the effects of aging on medical costs are covered in Chapter 10. In Chapter 11,

---

[*] The special features, which make medical care so interesting as a subject for economic analysis, also tend to make the application of simple models difficult or implausible. Those students who have the desire and opportunity to do so are well advised to get a firm grasp of basic principles using a text such as Heyne's *The Economic Way of Thinking* or Samuelson's *Economics* before attempting to grapple with the complexities and ambiguities of medical care.

pharmaceuticals provide an exemplar of the modern "information economy," where the fixed costs of research and marketing outweigh the cost of production and where competition relies on continuous innovation. Then, in Chapter 12, the means and consequences of access to capital for health care providers are briefly reviewed, with particular attention to the implication of nonprofit status and ownership structure.

In order to understand the interactions between the parts, it is necessary to place health care in a macroeconomic context that includes redistribution, taxation, inflation, and growth. The dynamics of national health expenditure are presented in Chapter 13 as an application of the permanent income hypothesis. Chapter 14 explores the role of government, and Chapter 15 examines public goods as particular forms of market failure that requires intervention. The economic history of health is traced in Chapter 16, drawing on the contributions of demography and the cliometric work of Fogel and North. Chapter 17 provides international comparisons of health and medical care expenditures, taking Kenya, Sudan, Mexico, Poland, Germany, and Japan as illustrative examples. A final chapter addresses the probable trends in health care spending, suggesting that the primary barrier to increased effectiveness and efficiency is poor allocation and problems of effective political alignment.

Health economics is fascinating to study, but it is not easily summarized or readily captured in neat equations. In part, that is because the study of health economics is relatively new and still in the process of refinement, but primarily it is because the transactions made by doctors and hospitals are not simple, and cut to the heart of what it means to be human. What is the value of life? Who pays the price of pain, and what does it mean to trust a surgeon who profits because of a crisis? Since most medical care is funded through taxes and insurance, there is no direct linkage between the amount paid and the resources used in treatment. As a consequence, "prices" become more ambiguous and are often of less immediate relevance to the trading parties than ongoing relationships of trust and professional behavior. It is important to understand how economic forces continue to operate when markets are indirect and inefficient, and how other organizing principles (professionalism, licensure, agency, regulation) act as substitutes for prices. Although most of the special features of medical markets are there to make people better off, they have also been shaped by those groups who had the power to modify the rules in their own interest, subject to the controls of economic and political competition. Tracing the economic rationale and development of medical care organization, and making those forces more clearly visible and amenable to analysis, is the purpose of this book.

CHANGES FOR THE FOURTH EDITION

As this preface is written (June 2009) the United States *appears* to be standing on the cusp of a major change in health care and medical financing—but such moments have come and gone before. The potential for change, and the well-grounded expectation that any changes will grow out of what has come before (a process known as "path dependence") is addressed in a newly revised Chapter 18. While forecasts of the future are necessarily somewhat speculative, this chapter does offer students and instructors some chance to step back and think about (a) some general policy principles and (b) the practical aspects of forecasting in an economy for which change is constant. It may also provide a brief introduction to behavioral economics, the dynamics of technological change, the expansion of welfare to include "happiness" and alternative valuations of "GDP," disequilibrium, and some other issues that are now at the forefront of contemporary economics research. Most students need to obtain a set of skills, an economic toolkit, in order to work. This fourth edition continues to emphasize basic "principles" material (opportunity cost, scarcity, demand, marginal revenue, value, fundamental theory of exchange) in Chapters 1 and 2. For classes emphasizing economic evaluation, a more detailed quantitative and diagrammatic presentation can be quite useful. For general classes directed toward clinicians, administrators, or policy makers, it can be a bit too long and dry, severely taxing their enthusiasm for health economics before they have fully worked through the mechanics of determining the marginal rate of technical substitution. I usually find time to review this material in most classes by adjusting the length of the presentation and the number of illustrative examples to the extent of familiarity within that particular class setting. Teaching notes, presentation slides, and problem sets for all chapters can be found online at http://www.wiley.com/college/getzen. WWW references are used throughout the text to provide access to constantly updated material. There are links to a variety of major sources of health economics data and commentary such as the NCHS, WHO, OECD, CDC, CMS, GAO, and others. Your comments and queries are welcome. For adopting professors, online help, answers to all problems, and chapter teaching guidelines are available through the text Web site, and also through email at getzen@temple.edu.

ACKNOWLEDGMENTS

The writing of this book incurred intellectual and personal debts sufficient to preclude any complete listing of those who have contributed. My family and extended family (Rufus and Beverley Getzen, Sydney White, Bill W.) come first. My initial research on these topics began at the University of Washington, with the assistance of Yoram Barzel, Gardner Brown, Steve Shortell, Bill Richardson, and Mike Morrisey, and while working under Gordon Bergey, who was an exemplar of the concerned physician and administrator. I am indebted to the efforts of Joe Newhouse, Mark Pauly, Tony Culyer, Morris Barer, Mike Drummond, Bill Swan, and others who have done so much to build the field and create a rigorous body of literature in health economics, and I thank them for their service to *i*HEA. Patrick Bernet of Florida Atlantic University created and revised the Instructor's Manual and Laura Shinn, Ph.D. (candidate) of Chestnut Hill College created the new Test Bank. David Barton Smith, Bill Aaronson, Chuck Hall, Jackie Zinn, and other colleagues at Temple have shaped the health economics course as it was taught. Alan Maynard sheltered and inspired me during my sabbatical at York during which the first edition was begun, Richard "Buz" Cooper at LDI schooled me on workforce projections, and Uwe Reinhardt kept me informed, amused, and concerned at Princeton during some revisions. The numerous reviewers over four editions have provided invaluable feedback and suggestions. The usual and heartfelt disclaimer applies: all remaining errors are mine.

ABOUT THE AUTHOR

Thomas E. Getzen is Professor of Risk, Insurance, and Health Management at Temple University and the founder and Executive Director of *i*HEA, the International Health Economics Association. After receiving an undergraduate degree in literature from Yale University, he worked for the U.S.P.H.S. Centers for Disease Control Venereal Disease program in New York and Los Angeles, and then obtained an MHA degree in Medical Care Organization and Ph.D. in Economics from the University of Washington. Dr. Getzen's main research contributions have been in the areas of contracting, price indexes, and forecasting of health care spending. His consulting work has included employee benefit negotiations, projections of health care cost trends and premiums, laboratory diagnostics, risk assessment, and capital financing for managed care. Dr. Getzen has been a visiting professor at the University of Toronto, the Center for Health and Wellbeing of the Woodrow Wilson School at Princeton University, the Wharton School at the University of Pennsylvania, and the University of York (U.K.). He has served on the boards of Covenant House, a local community health center in northwest Philadelphia, MSI, a venture-capital financed managed behavioral health care corporation, and CHE, a multi-institutional health provider system with over 60 hospitals and nursing homes. Dr. Getzen has written more than 80 papers in the field and serves on the editorial board of the journal *Health Economics*.

FOREWORD

Public policy in almost any field depends on specific knowledge of the field, but it usually also depends (or should depend) on general principles of economics. For example, the building of a bridge requires knowledge of engineering, to know what is feasible; it requires knowledge of traffic patterns; and it requires knowledge of economic principles, to see whether the traffic that will use the bridge and the value of the time saving to that traffic will justify the costs imposed by the engineering requirements. So, too, there is a need of economic analysis to help in the construction of a system of health care. First of all, indeed, we must know what medical care can do, and how much in the way of skilled professionals, other workers, machinery, and buildings it takes to achieve any given level of medical care. But second, we must analyze how the payment mechanisms to compensate for these supplies affect the delivery of medical care.

Medical care is indeed a more complex economic problem than bridge-building. Like some other professions but unlike many other goods and even services, it is difficult for the consumer (here the patient) to evaluate the quality of the services received. Much depends on the self-control and reliability of the individual practitioner, the supplying group, and the medical profession as a whole, in ways that the patient cannot readily check. Then, too, the service provided is needed only at unpredictable intervals, but it frequently is very important when it is needed. Further, the costs, a reflection of the resources used, are very uncertain and can be very high. All these reasons lead to the use of some form of insurance, a natural economic institution for improving everyone's welfare. But insurance reduces the incentive of an individual patient or physician to seek the most economical means of treatment. As a result, new institutions and regulations develop to overcome this "moral hazard," as it has been termed—institutions such as health maintenance organizations, managed care by insurance companies, and regulations such as those that govern Medicare expenditures. The standard paradigms of economics have been enriched to discuss problems such as this.

The difficulties of quality evaluation and moral hazard are special cases of a more general phenomenon, differences in information between the two sides of a transaction. These differences, though not confined to medical practice, are especially important there, and have further consequences beyond those already noted, as in the need for licensing physicians or the specially important role of nonprofit institutions.

The economic problems of allocating resources to medical care have long been a major part of government economic policy, more in other countries than in the United States. The steady rise in the expenditures on medical care, outstripping the rise in national income by a considerable margin, has brought these issues to the fore of public attention. Equally important has been the increase of explicit consideration of costs within the medical profession; the historically unwelcome trade-off between costs and treatment has come forcibly to the fore. The need for good education and good texts has become acute, and Professor Getzen's book is a welcome attempt to meet this strongly felt need.

Kenneth J. Arrow

CHAPTER 1

CHOICES: MONEY, MEDICINE, AND HEALTH

QUESTIONS

1. Why does health care cost so much?
2. Does everyone get the same kind of care?
3. Who decides: the patient, the doctor, the hospital, or the government?
4. Do some people pay more (or less) than their fair share?
5. Who is made better off: the surgeon or the patient?
6. Are there futures contracts in health care?
7. Is health scarce?
8. Who pays when you skip a workout to watch television?
9. Why is health care bought and sold differently from other goods and services?

Should I return to the doctor since the medicine they gave me yesterday does not seem to be working? Which seriously ill patient will get the kidney transplant? Is it worth extending the Supplemental Children's Health Insurance Program (SCHIP) legislation to cover legal immigrants? Questions like these are dealt with every day in peoples' homes, in hospitals, and in the halls of Congress. They are the subject of health economics, along with more mundane decisions that cumulatively have an even greater impact on your personal health: how much exercise to get, the value of reducing cholesterol in your diet, whether to study until 3 A.M. or get a good night's sleep, and so on.

Economics is sometimes described as the "theory of choice," and health economics is about the choices people make with regard to health, choices medical providers make in order to care for people and earn money, and choices made collectively (by Congress, community groups, or professional associations). What does it mean to make a choice? It means making a decision that what is given up is not as valuable as what you get. If I choose to go back to the doctor I saw yesterday, it will take time and money to do so. If an organization chooses patient A to receive the kidney transplant, the potential therapeutic benefits to (and insurance payments from) patient B must be given up. If Congress extends SCHIP, then it will have to cut some other program, raise taxes, or run a temporary deficit and borrow money.

Making a choice means deciding that what you give up, the **opportunity cost**, is not worth as much to you as what you get. Doctors and hospitals make similar decisions, determining whether or not what they will get is worth more to them than the services they have to provide in order to get paid. When a patient and a medical provider agree to a transaction, making a trade that exchanges money for services, both have decided that it will make them better off.

1.1 WHAT IS ECONOMICS?

Trade, "making a buck," is the quintessential economic activity. Its focal point is the market, the place where buyers and sellers exchange dollars for goods and services. Without buyers and sellers there would be no economy—no rich surgeons, no insurance companies, no hospital billing departments (or textbook royalties for health economists). To say that there would be no rich surgeons is not a statement of envy but one of fact. Without an advanced economy, a person could not spend 15 years studying and practicing eye surgery, and hence could not provide a highly specialized form of labor that is so much more valuable than digging ditches; therefore, patients could not reap the benefits of so much knowledge and training.

For a surgeon to be a seller, the patient must be a buyer. They both must agree on a price so that an exchange can occur. The surgeon would probably prefer that the price be higher and the patient would probably prefer that it be lower, but both must be satisfied in order for a trade to take place. As economists, we can observe that since a transaction took place, there must have been mutual agreement that made both the buyer and the seller better off. If the surgeon would rather have watched television than perform another operation, she would have turned down the case. If the patient would rather have saved the money, or gone to a different surgeon, he could have done so. The insight that both parties must be benefiting if they freely agreed to make a trade is central to an economic vision of the world, and is known as the *fundamental theorem of exchange*.

FUNDAMENTAL THEOREM OF EXCHANGE

The foundation of market economics is that trade makes both parties better off. People make a deal because they expect it will provide more satisfaction than not making the deal. The surgeon and the patient expect to gain from trade—the surgeon by receiving money and gratitude, and the patient by being healed. It may turn out that the patient dies and the surgeon gets sued for malpractice, but both made the transaction with the expectation that they would become better off. Trade does not take advantage of people so that one party is made better off at the expense of the other (that is stealing). Trade takes advantage of differences in skills, endowments, and tastes so that people can make exchanges that are mutually advantageous.

Terms of Trade

The "terms of trade" specify what the buyer is to give to the seller and what the seller is to give to the buyer in return. When you buy a common item in a store, such as aspirin, a simple price of $1.29 per bottle of 50 may tell you everything you need to know about the transaction. For services, and for medical care in particular, the transaction is apt to be much more complex. For example, consider the transaction for an operation to implant an artificial intra-ocular lens (IOL) in a patient's eye to replace the natural lens that has become clouded by cataracts. The patient is to pay a $200 deposit up front and $800 more within 30 days after the surgery is completed and all sutures are removed. Reduced to its most simple element, the terms of trade in this exchange can be expressed as a monetary price of $1,000 for the IOL implant. Yet much more than the $1,000 is being agreed to in this transaction. The physician agrees to provide not just any artificial lens, but to choose the correct one, continuously monitor the quality of the operation, and control adverse reactions to postoperative medications. The patient agrees to make payment in two parts, with a time limit, and may assume that the operation will be redone without further charges if the first attempt is not satisfactory. Many of the agreed-upon conditions (that the physician is licensed, will use only qualified assistants, will not try to boost the bill needlessly to increase her fees, and will keep the patient informed of any possible adverse consequences, and that the patient will wear bandages as long as necessary and not go skydiving) will never be specified explicitly unless some disagreement and subsequent legal action force the doctor and patient into court.

In the simplified neoclassical model of perfectly competitive behavior with which most textbooks begin, price is the only term that matters in a transaction and both the buyer and seller are "price takers." That is, there are so many buyers that whether one person buys or not has little influence on the price in the market; therefore, buyers must "take" the price as given. Similarly, there are so many firms selling the same product that no single firm can affect prices; hence, all firms must take the price as given. This uncomplicated model of perfectly competitive behavior is not too distant from reality when you buy a bottle of aspirin. The model works reasonably well for most of the purchases made by consumers, and thus can be used to frame the analysis of the economy as a whole. However, buying a bottle of aspirin is not representative of most medical decisions, and an elementary model does not capture many of the essentials when life and death decisions are being made by doctors in the operating room. No one needs a prescription to rent a DVD. You don't have to have insurance or sign a consent form to have your car's fuel pump worked on, and almost anyone can cut your hair without a license. Treating disease requires knowledge and entails risks that are quite special—forcing a patient to trust the judgment of the surgeon and leading to special forms of economic organization and contracts in medicine (professional licensure, hospital staff bylaws, regulatory review). Studying such adaptations reveals the potential of economics as a discipline in a way that the analysis of more standard markets cannot.

Can We Pay Somebody to Care?

Doctors and nurses want to care for patients. Given a chance, they will make extraordinary efforts on your behalf. Medicine is as much about caring as it is about curing. Does paying somebody make them care for you? Probably not. However, not paying people can make it impossible for them to care for you. If doctors and nurses had to find another way to make a living and pay the bills, then they could not spend their time looking after your health.

Do your friends expect to be paid because they care for you? Not precisely, but they do expect to be paid back in kind, by your caring for them. If you treat your friends as if you did not care, eventually you will not have any friends. Parents are a bit more understanding, but in part that is because they know that however ungrateful you may be for their help, you will probably be willing to put up with your own ungrateful kids (their grandchildren) someday. Medical professionals are even more compassionate. They work for many hours even when a case is nearly hopeless, knowing they will not get additional pay for all the extra effort. However, as professionals, they can expect respect, and a reasonable income. The development of medicine as a **profession** (see Chapter 7), dedicated to science and caring, is a great social innovation—one of the adaptations of economic organization mentioned above. Sometimes it is only the professionalism of the helpers that keeps someone who is poor and sick from being left all alone to deal with an illness.

Doctors work on your behalf. Most important, to an economist, it is doctors who decide what medicine is right or wrong, not you. Although patients do ultimately have the right to make their own decisions, in practice, those decisions are made largely by the professionals who take care of them. In the operating room, it is not the patient who decides, but the surgeon (in some ways, it is a bit like a family, where the parents make decisions on behalf of their children). In basic trades, all that is required is that a buyer and a seller agree on a price. In medicine, the buyer/seller distinction is not clear. Is the doctor the one who is "buying" the surgery, or the one selling it? A medical "trade" is made on the patient's behalf by someone who cares about them, not by the patient acting on their own. The situation is complex and involves a set of professional expectations and external forces (quality regulations, consent forms, insurance) as well as the patient's illness or their personal tastes and preferences. Caring, from an economic point of view, means making decisions for someone else—to help them, rather than just to help yourself.

Financing Health Care

What does it mean "to finance" something—a house, a car, your education? When you finance a car, you have to make payments over many months. To buy a house, you go to a bank for a loan, which is then usually bundled with other mortgages by Fannie Mae or some other financial entity and sold to many investors. Financing your education often means making tuition payments over time, taking out student loans, getting money from parents, and maybe a scholarship from the university. If it is a public university, taxpayers are usually covering a large part of the costs. At a private college, donations and income from the endowment are used to supplement student fees (and indirectly subsidized by tax breaks). Financing means that many parties are involved, not just the buyer and the seller. Frequently there are *financial intermediaries*, like banks, that help to make the transaction possible by providing guarantees over time and spreading the risks across many investors. For student loans, Sallie Mae (the Student National Loan Agency) is the financial intermediary making loans possible with the backing of the federal government, which is the largest intermediary of all and makes possible the whole banking system as well as all the subsidies from taxpayers for national defense, schools, and health care.

The development of medicine as a caring profession is sort of primitive financial intermediation—those who can afford to, pay more, so that those who can't pay still get professional care. With transplants and therapies costing hundreds of thousands of dollars, professional goodwill and charity alone are hardly sufficient, so there are public and private insurance plans pooling funds and sharing risks across millions of people that provide most of the financing for health care (see Chapters 4 and 5). Looking into the funding of research provides additional insight. The people who benefit from medical research are not usually the people who pay for it. A study of brain function or cell structure will do nothing for a patient in the hospital today, and not much for the foundation that donated money or the taxpayers funding a research grant. Tomorrow's miracle drugs are paid for by adding overhead into the price of today's pharmaceuticals (see Chapter 11), and advances in surgical technique by adding overhead into the price of an operation. The basic discoveries that make all of this new technology possible are funded by federal grants and other forms of taxpayer support, with benefits coming far into the future, if at all. Only sometimes do the efforts succeed, and those few successes must provide sufficient rewards to make the overall returns on a risky investment worthwhile.

The two core concepts of financial analysis are **timing** and **risk**. Something that cannot be used until far into the future is not worth as much as something you could start using today (time discounting, or present value—see Chapter 3 and Chapter 12). Uncertainty also makes a thing less valuable (risk adjustment or discounting). Often, the longer you have to wait for something, the more risky it is, so its value is discounted both for time and risk. Discounting for the future and for uncertainty are some of the factors that make it hard to get college sophomores to spend less to save for retirement, or to stop eating French fries so that they can be healthier when they are in their 50s, or for a soldier being sent to war to give up smoking. In health care the benefits are almost never immediate or certain and thus must be discounted, and are almost always financed by others rather than paid for directly, so that the patient almost never stops to compare costs and benefits before going to the doctor. The fundamental theorem of exchange, that two people are both made better off when they trade, becomes more complex and uncertain when there are thousands or millions of people involved in complex transactions with effects lasting for decades or generations.

Value

Why does health care cost so much? Because health is so precious that its value exceeds that of all the things we possess. What benefit do I get from spending my money on books or art or cars or clothes if I am dead? Sick and in pain, confronted with the possibility of death, people would be willing to spend almost any amount of money to get their health back. Health care costs so much because people are willing to pay so much for it. The many years a surgeon spends in training, the billions of dollars government spends on public health, and the comprehensive health insurance plans provided by employers are consequences of the value we as a society place on health care. They are effects, rather than causes. We are willing to spend so much on physician training, public health, and health insurance because what they produce is valuable to us. If we stopped caring about (or paying for) health, no new magnetic resonance imaging (MRI) scanners would be built, surgeons would stop spending years in training, and our taxes would go toward highways or national parks instead of AIDS and cancer research. Cows can get just as many diseases as humans do and we could put all those resources to work saving cows, but we don't. Cows, I am sure, would set priorities rather differently, but they are not paying the bills.

1.2   THE FLOW OF FUNDS

Goods and services are provided in a market economy only if the people who want them are willing to pay for them and if suppliers are willing to accept those payments in return. Exchange is based on voluntary agreement, so that trade between a buyer and seller occurs only when both parties believe that they will be made better off by trading (the fundamental theorem of exchange). In the simplest form of trade, consumers buy from businesses, exchanging money for goods and services in a two-party transaction.

Consumers make up the demand side of this simple service market, while firms make up the supply side (see Chapter 2). In legal terms, firms are contractual entities that can own, buy, and sell property, and pay taxes just as people do. To get the labor, land, and other inputs needed for production, the firm (the seller) in Figure 1.1 must also be a buyer, as shown in Figure 1.2. These secondary two-party transactions are characteristic of derived demand, purchases made as an intermediate step in production, rather than for final consumption. Firms are owned by individuals (or other firms) that provide the capital, labor, and organizational effort necessary to get them started and keep them running. Thus,

FIGURE 1.1   Two-Party Transaction

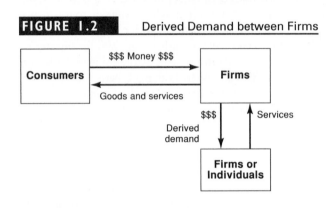

FIGURE 1.2   Derived Demand between Firms

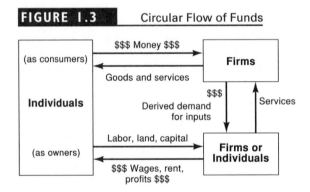

FIGURE 1.3   Circular Flow of Funds

every dollar that a consumer gives to a firm, whether used for wages, profits, or purchase of input from another firm, ultimately ends up in the hands of someone who wants to spend it. When workers or owners spend money, they become consumers, and therefore complete the circular flow of funds through the economy, as shown in Figure 1.3.

Health Care Spending in the United States

Medical care in the United States is a trillion-dollar business ($2,624,400,000,000), with an estimated average of $8,459 spent per person in 2010.[1] The 310 million citizens of the United States received services from more than 4,000 hospitals, 30,000 nursing homes, 800,000 physicians, 2.8 million registered nurses, and 9 million other health care workers. Financial flows, the major sources and uses of health care funding during 2010, are indicated in Table 1.1. Individuals paid $296 billion, or 11 percent of total funding; private (mostly employer-based) health insurance paid 34 percent; and government, the largest payer, paid 48 percent (20 percent Medicare, 16 percent Medicaid, 12 percent other government programs). The remaining 7 percent of total health care financing came from a variety of other

TABLE 1.1			U.S. Health Care Spending, 2010		
Uses of Funds	**Percentage of Total**	**Amount per Person**	**Sources of Funds**	**Percentage of Total**	**Amount per Person**
Hospital	32%	$2,674	Medicare	20%	$1,661
Physician	21%	1,778	*Paycheck deduction*		*1,079*
Dental	4%	343	Medicaid	16%	1,351
Other	6%	500	VA & DOD	3%	247
Nursing home	6%	487	Other govt	9%	771
Home health	3%	240	Total government	48%	
Drugs	10%	825			
Products	3%	216	Employer insurance	34%	2,874
Admin costs	7%	613	*Tax subsidy*		*956*
Public health	3%	246	Self-paid	11%	937
Research	2%	147	Charity, etc.	7%	618
Construction	5%	390			8,459

Based on a projected U.S. population of 310 million. *Source:* U.S. Office of the Actuary, National Health Projections,
http://www.cms.gov/NationalHealthExpendData/.

private sources (philanthropy, industrial clinics, interest, and rental income of providers). The largest use of funds was the $830 billion spent on hospital care, 32 percent of the total.

Figure 1.4 presents this information graphically, highlighting a simple yet important fact about financial balances: the "sources (in)" and "uses (out)" bars are of equal height. Every dollar spent by a patient, insurance company, or government is recorded as a cost but is also recorded as income to a physician, hospital, agency, administrator, or other health employee. Therefore the totals must be equal: financial flows in and out balance each other. The flow of money is circular. Money itself is only a way of keeping track of all the obligations within the economy. Every dollar spent by one person is, of necessity, a dollar of income for

FIGURE 1.4   U.S. Sources and Uses of Health Care Funds, 2010

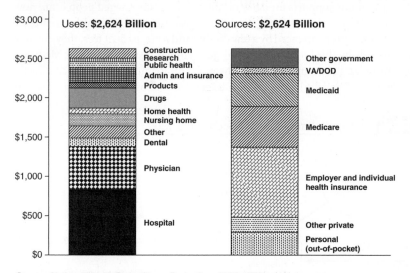

Source: National Health Expenditures Projections 2007–2017 <www.cms.gov>

TABLE 1.2	Sources of Financing 1929, 1970 and 2010		
	1929	**1970**	**2010**
Total health spending (millions)	$ 3,656	$ 74,894	$ 2,624,400
Adjusted for inflation (2010 dollars)	38,531	343,314	2,624,400
Per capita (adjusted)	317	1,632	8,459
As a percent of GDP	3.5%	7.2%	17.7%
percent paid by			
Self (out-of-pocket)	81%	33%	11%
Third parties	19%	67%	89%
Government	*13%*	*38%*	*48%*
Private insurance	*<1%*	*21%*	*34%*
Philanthropy, other	*6%*	*8%*	*7%*

someone else. Tracing the flow of funds through this complex system provides some sense of the forces that shape the economy.

Sources of Financing

Health care spending has grown enormously. In 2010, it accounted for more than 17 percent of the Gross Domestic Product (GDP) and 1 of every 10 employees in the labor force. That growth has been facilitated by the shift from individual payments to third-party financing. In 1929, 81 percent of medical expenditures were financed by individual out-of-pocket payments and only 19 percent from government and other third-party organizations (Table 1.2). By 2010, this ratio had been reversed, with individuals paying only 11 percent directly and the remaining 89 percent of financing coming from third-party transactions involving government, nonprofit organizations, and insurance.

All of the elements that characterized health care in 2010 were present in some form one hundred years ago, but their relative importance to the flow of funds has changed so much that the transactions look entirely different today.[2] Physicians, who in 1900 were tradespeople sometimes making do with partial payment in eggs or flour, have become highly paid and technologically sophisticated professionals who rarely talk to their patients about paying the bills. Hospitals, once minor supports for a few disabled and disadvantaged people, are now technological palaces of intensive treatment and the largest users of U.S. health care funds. Whereas in 1900 hospitals were financed by a few donors and some patient fees, they are now financed almost entirely by third parties: either by government insurance such as Medicare and Medicaid or by private insurance provided through employment or purchased directly by consumers (Figures 1.5 and 1.6). For every $100 spent in the hospital, less than 2 percent

FIGURE 1.5   Health Care Flow of Funds, circa 1900

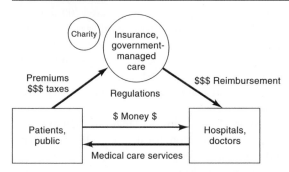

FIGURE 1.6   Health Care Flow of Funds, circa 2010

now comes from charitable donations. Even the 3 percent paid for by patients out-of-pocket does not really flow through a two-party transaction, because much of that 3 percent consists of copayments, deductibles, and other fees related to third-party insurance payments.

There are many reasons health care spending has grown rapidly. An increasingly wealthy population is willing to spend more on all goods and services. Extra spending on health care has a greater appeal after basic necessities such as food and housing are taken care of. Technological advances make modern medicine more desirable. An aging population favors health care over other goods. Insurance now finances more of the cost. Shifting the financial burden from individuals to third parties through insurance not only changed the way funds flowed, but also made more funds available, so that the health care system could grow rapidly and absorb an ever larger share of total economic output.

Such "cost-shifting" has made the financing system complex and opaque—almost no one knows who is paying for what.[3] Billed charges bear little resemblance to what is paid or what the provider receives, and provider revenues are usually identified not as "income" but as "reimbursement." Third-party payments are made with:

- Taxes paid to government agencies (Chapters 13 and 14)
- Employer and employee payments to commercial insurance companies (Chapters 4 and 5), and for-profit and nonprofit managed care firms, including health maintenance organizations (HMOs), preferred provider organizations (PPOs), and other organizations
- Philanthropic contributions to charities (Chapters 4 and 14)

Each of these major categories of third-party payments exists in endless variations. The details differ widely, but from a financial perspective they all have a similar purpose: pooling funds from many people to pay the bills of the few patients who need care.

Who gets care and what kind of care are decisions made according to embedded rules and the opinions of professionals who run the health care system. In each case, indirect third-party payment weakens the monetary linkage between buyer and seller that characterizes the direct two-party transactions typical in most other sectors of the economy. For most medical transactions, there is no exchange of money between the recipient of services and the provider. The patients (or their families) pay insurance premiums and taxes, and the doctors and hospitals are paid by the government and insurance companies. In the absence of a direct link between the amount paid and the resources used in treatment, "prices" become more ambiguous and less important to the transaction than ongoing relationships of trust and professional behavior. One of the purposes of this textbook is to explain how economic forces continue to operate when prices do not function in a normal way and how other organizing principles (professionalism, licensure, regulation) serve as replacements.

Health Care Providers: The Uses of Funds

Payments by patients, government, and insurance companies have increased 200-fold over the past sixty years; thus, payments received by doctors, hospitals, and other care providers have increased by the same amount. In general, both the public, as users of the system, and providers, as suppliers of care, have been happy with this large increase in spending. The public has gotten a health care system that is technologically advanced and responsive to their needs. Providers have gained glory in the fight against disease and substantial gains in income, making them eager to continue the struggle.

Part of the increase in health care spending from almost $4 billion in 1929 to $2,624 billion in 2010 is just an accounting fiction due to inflation, because $1 in 1929 is roughly the same as $11 in 2010. Also, some of the increase reflects a rise in the number of people who must be cared for. Yet even after adjusting for changes in population and inflation, real per capita spending has increased more than ten-fold since 1929. Some of this real increase in spending is due to a real increase in wages. As per capita incomes rise, workers expect more real goods and services per hour of work. Therefore, expenditures on labor-intensive services tend to rise more rapidly than expenditures on goods and capital-intensive commodities. Furthermore, the wages of health care workers have risen more rapidly than for other types of labor.[4] This probably reflects both the increased education of health professionals today and the increased demand for their services. Increases in the quantity of services provided account for some of the growth in total expenditures, but the medical services most commonly counted, number of days spent in the hospital and number of visits to physicians, have actually declined since 1970 (see Table 1.3).[5] However, nursing home days and number of prescriptions per person have increased substantially.

After taking all these factors into account—inflation, higher health care wages, and use of services—there still has been a tremendous increase in expenditures over the last forty years, more than 400 percent. How can spending increase so much more rapidly than the

TABLE 1.3	Changes in the Use of Health Care Funds over Eighty Years		
	1929	**1970**	**2010**
Spending per person (in 2010 dollars)	$317	$1,632	$8,459
Percent usage			
Hospital	23%	37%	32%
Physician	36	19	21
Dental	12	6	4
Drugs	18	7	10
Other	1	3	4
Nursing home	na	5	6
Home health	na	na	3
Products	3	6	3
Admin & insurance costs	3	4	7
Public health	3	2	3
Research	1	3	2
Construction	na	8	5
Total	*100%*	*100%*	*100%*
Hospital days per person	0.9	1.2	0.6
Hospital employees per patient	<0.5	2.9	8.4
Physician visits per person	2.6	5.0	4.0

increase in the number of services or in the wages of those who provide them? By increasing the **intensity and quality of services**. More tests are done for a patient in a modern intensive care unit during a single day than were done for a patient over the course of a month in his or her wooden bed in 1929. Many of those tests (MRIs, blood glucose, heart monitoring) were not available back then. The physician who drove to the patient's house and worked alone out of a black bag has been replaced by a team of therapists, technicians, and support staff assisting a group of physicians, many of whom are specialists using an array of medical equipment. Another factor that explains some of the growth in spending is that, as some common, acute (short-term) diseases have become curable or preventable, medical care is increasingly applied in cases of chronic diseases that were once considered hopeless. The shift from simple caring to technologically sophisticated curing is reflected by shifts in the categories of expenditure; more is going to institutional care in hospitals and nursing homes, while the share devoted to personal services by doctors has declined. The fraction of the health care dollar spent for manufactured goods such as drugs has also fallen, while the cost of labor-intensive services has risen.

1.3 ECONOMIC PRINCIPLES AS CONCEPTUAL TOOLS

Looking carefully at how people make deals with physicians, with hospitals, and with each other to improve their health is a natural approach to health economics. Simplified assumptions and abstractions are used to clarify the forces that lead to economic change. Tracing the flow of funds through the health care system makes it possible to apply principles of price theory to situations involving life and death, nonprofit organizations, professional licensure, addiction, and other issues. The powerful generalizations and concepts of microeconomics, macroeconomics, finance, and industrial organization allow us to see how medical transactions are like, and yet unlike, most of the rest of the economy. As a practical matter, it will be helpful if you already have a basic grasp of economic theory and applications. Reviewing a textbook like *Economics* by Samuelson and Nordhaus, *Principles of Economics* by Mankiw, *Microeconomics* by McConnell and Brue, or *The Economic Way of Thinking* by Heyne may prove useful. An instructor's manual for this textbook is available at www.wiley.com/college/getzen, and you are urged to check this site for current links, updates, and other material or to contact the author directly at **getzen@temple.edu**. Some of the most common principles used by economists as tools for understanding society and the decisions people make are listed below. Most of these will be evident to you based on your own experience or previous study.

Scarcity (Budget Constraints)

Why does a decision always involve giving something up? It is because reality imposes constraints or limits on what you can do. The most basic limit is time. You have only 24 hours per day and once your days are gone (due to death) you have no more life to use in production or consumption. Your income and your bank balance, the place you live, the things and friends you have, and even your credit rating all put limits on what you can do to make yourself better off. Economists call them "budget constraints." This term applies not only to money but also to time, things, relationships, and any other limited resource.

Opportunity Cost

The best measure of what something costs is what you have to give up to get it. The trip to Cancun might cost you $750 in savings; an extra weekend date might cost you an A as your grade falls to a B+ because you gave up study time. Conversely, you might say that the decision to be a grind and get an A cost you a date. It is the decision you make, not the price tag or money, that really determines the cost of something. The primary cost of attending this class is the time it takes (the fun you could have had and/or the money you could have earned), not the amount spent on tuition and books.

Willingness to Pay

The best measure for the value of what you get is your "willingness to pay"—the complement and mirror image of "opportunity cost." Value includes money, time, pleasure, relief from pain—all of those things that when given up are counted negatively as costs and when received are considered positively to be benefits. The only real difference between a "cost" and a "benefit" is the sign. Note however that *value* often differs depending on who gets and who gives, which is why trading can increase the total value to society even when all that happens is that some things (including dollars) are moved back and forth from one person to another.

Trade

People engage in trade, exchanging things, time, favors, money, and information, because it makes them better off. Both sides must benefit, or they would not agree to trade. This is the "fundamental theorem of exchange" and perhaps the most basic principle of economic reasoning.

Money Flows in a Circle

When someone buys something, the money spent must be received by someone else. The seller wants those dollars for what he or she, in turn, can buy. The dollar is almighty because it flows—because it can be changed into anything else—not because there is any inherent value in a wrinkled piece of paper. Circularity implies that every dollar of "cost" is also some provider's "income." Protecting income is one reason few cuts in spending are actually made in practice even though most doctors, hospitals, and insurance companies claim that they want to reduce costs.

Maximization: Marginal Costs and Marginal Benefits

Productive effort and exchange (trade) are ways people make themselves better off. What principle determines when to stop? When the incremental (marginal) benefits from the next step are outweighed by the incremental (marginal) costs. Each decision increment (read one more page, eat one more slice of pizza, play one more game) adds a little value (marginal benefit). Each step also takes a little more time or money (marginal cost). The real issue is not whether something (grades, food, playing time) is good, but whether you would be better off with more or less of it. As more and more is done a point is usually reached at which the benefits of each additional step become smaller and smaller (diminishing marginal returns), and the costs of each additional unit become greater. Maximum net benefits are obtained by pushing to the point at which rising marginal costs equal falling marginal benefits.

Choice: Are Benefits Greater than Costs?

Every decision involves a trade-off, giving something up to get something else, choosing the option that means more to you. This is obvious when you engage in trade with someone else. It is also true whenever you make a choice, even though you "trade" only with yourself (e.g., giving up a workout at the gym in order to study, passing up a new CD in order to buy dinner at a restaurant, giving up some of your savings in order to take a trip to Cancun). Economists assume that people tend to make choices that make them better off in a way they value (not necessarily financially). This is known as the "benefit-cost principle." In the abstract, economists assume that people behave perfectly rationally, precisely conforming to principles of maximization expressed mathematically in "rational choice theory." More realistically, we accept that people behave "sort of" rationally, not deviating too much from perfect rationality, but not exactly conforming to it or meeting that exact standard even in everyday affairs—smoking when they say they want to quit, failing to save enough for retirement, or morosely lamenting the sunk costs of the opportunity that they passed up when they decided to go to Cancun for a vacation (see "Social Science and Rational Choice Theory" below). With regard to health, it is useful to distinguish three somewhat different categories of individual choices:

- Lifestyle (smoking, exercise, child care)
- Risk Modification (statins, HBP medications, hospice, nursing home)
- Illness Treatment (what we usually mean by "medicine")

A person's health may be mostly determined over the long run by choice of lifestyle and risk modification, but most of the decisions and special institutional features studied by health economists arise in response to illness (see Section 1.4, "Health Economics: What Makes Medicine Different?"). These urgent needs are what drive medical care as a business.

Investment

Investment increases future productivity by diverting current output to infrastructure improvement rather than to immediate consumption. The economic approach to *human capital* uses concepts such as depreciation and rate of return to analyze going to school, having children, getting married, brushing teeth, and other activities that depend upon a long-run perspective. Taking time to exercise and giving up sweets are forms of investment. It is difficult to improve your health once it has deteriorated. Spending money on medicine once you are seriously ill is a little like spending money on your car after the engine has begun to burn oil; regular maintenance is a lot cheaper. How healthy you are when you get old depends not so much on the medical care you get then but on what you have done to and for your body over the years. Income at age 55 depends not on how hard you work then but on what you have done to advance in your career. Most readers of this textbook are studying now for a future reward: knowledge, grades, a degree, and enhanced earnings. Medical school is a form of investment, usually a very good one (see Chapters 7 and 12), as is the research done by pharmaceutical companies, using some current profits to discover new drug that will begin to sell in fifteen years (Chapter 11).

Contracts: Complex Exchanges to Deal with Timing and Risk

The seller must have faith that the money obtained in trade will have value. The buyer must have faith that the goods received are what they are supposed to be. Both buyer and seller must be able to trust each other. More complex transactions require more trust and external guarantees. Buying on credit or for future delivery (mail order, new custom home, knee surgery) creates potential problems and requires a financial intermediary, as does shared purchasing through insurance, cooperatives, or public funds. Acceptance of risk and uncertainties in value (a used car "as is," a share of stock in a start-up company, an experimental drug to treat your rash, trip insurance for your Cancun vacation) also force greater reliance on trust and contract specifications. Using a financial intermediary as a third party that handles the money (purchasing agent, insurance company) can make a transaction easier and safer, but it also makes transactions complex and vulnerable. Two of the parties may collude to take advantage of the third party. Often, tracing the flow of funds helps reveal the underlying economic forces at work, even if the contracts are confusing or people lie.

Organizations Adapt and Evolve

Organizations evolve to build trust and increase the efficiency of exchange. Laws, rules, political parties, mandatory labels, certified measures, corporate financial statements, clubs, professions, and nonprofit organizations are all in a sense market responses to market failure, as difficulties in making simple price transactions are resolved by more comprehensive contracts. Government is the most comprehensive of such social structures. Exchange and economic potential remain limited until a solid base of personal trust, laws, contractual organization (markets, firms, credit, regulations), and social structure evolves. The growth and output of a modern economy has more to do with the efficiency of organization than the endowment of natural resources, numbers of people, financial aid, or any other factor.[6]

1.4 HEALTH ECONOMICS: WHAT MAKES MEDICINE DIFFERENT?

Medicine is not all, or even mostly, about money. Science, caring, professionalism, and even religious concerns regarding birth and death are often more important than dollars. Economics gives one important and clear perspective, but it is a limited view, analogous to the kind of limited view that an X-ray provides of a person or that radiology provides for all of medicine. Just as radiology has been expanded to include sonograms, computed tomography (CT), positron-emission tomography (PET), MRI scans, and other forms of diagnostic imaging, economics has expanded to examine social relationships, behavioral response, politics, and the financing of technological advances. Yet, no matter how powerful economics is for analyzing decisions, it still remains just one piece of a larger picture. Most of medicine and health lies outside the scope of this textbook, but several attributes distinguish health care from most other commodities and help explain why medical markets have special features.

Illness Is Contingent, Urgent, Uncertain

Since the need for medical care is contingent, a person never knows when or if it will arise, or what treatment will be needed. Every patient coming through the clinic door may have a different illness. The routines developed for efficient manufacturing and standard service provision are difficult to apply when every case is different. Uncertain urgent needs mean that neither patient nor provider can really plan in advance. Perhaps even more unsettling is the reality that no one, even the most educated academic physician, knows for certain how well treatment will work in any particular patient—one can recover spectacularly while another dies on the same medicine. Although lifestyle and risk modification choices are seldom made in crisis mode, illness is different, striking suddenly with fear about unknown effects and uncertain outcomes. Hence it is not so much the desire for health but rather the response to illness that creates special features in medical markets—professional licensure, nonprofit providers, prescription drugs, pervasive regulation, and insurance.

Health Is Priceless

Death is the ultimate constraint. In a crisis, people will pay almost anything for medical care. The opportunity cost is too great to bargain over "how much?" when your life is at stake. Given time, you can get money, or you can spend your time meditating, hunting for berries in the woods, or writing poems in the sand. At least you are alive. If you have money, but no time left, the money is worthless. Once the sum total of all your hours is gone, there are no second chances, no credit advances—and no more decisions to make. While all economists acknowledge that scarcity is fundamentally defined by the consumer's lifetime, this awareness is more acute among health economists because the business of medical care centers on life and death decisions.

People do not want to make difficult decisions about trading off dollars for health. Indeed, it is often impossible to do so. This is one reason that virtually every modern economy offers medical care on demand and extensive programs of health insurance. Much of the struggle in health economics involves facing up to the inevitable trade-offs by stepping out of crisis mode and looking at the larger picture regarding costs and benefits. Life and death decisions are different from "what color?" or "how large?" When an event is identifiable as potentially life-threatening, it deserves special treatment. Even ordinary deaths are attended by distinctively solemn professionals: funeral directors, priests, rabbis, and ministers.

Health Affects the Value of All Other Goods

To use your money as a consumer you must have time. What modern medicine can do is prolong life and make it more productive. Health is irreplaceable, and any change in health can strongly affect the value of many other goods (pair of skis, steak dinner, trip to Cancun). My aging body cannot hear music or see a sunset the way it used to. A car can always be replaced if it cannot be repaired, but a human face or knee damaged in a crash may never be put right again. Health is more precious and time more limited than money. Better health can provide more enjoyment from each thing you buy, and also give you more days to enjoy the fruits of economic success.

Having More Does Not Reduce the Value of Health

The demand for medical care seems almost insatiable. Usually, the more you have of anything, the less it is worth to get a bit more. If I already have lots of food, how much do I care about one more pizza? With three cars in the garage, I will take a fourth, but it is not a priority. I am even starting to buy new computers with much less than the maximum processing capability. This principle of *diminishing marginal utility* is not so applicable to health: the value of a therapy that provides relief or a one percent reduction in mortality may be more and more valuable (rather than less) the healthier the person is.[7]

Dynamic Change, Driven by Research and Technology

Fortunately the science of medicine has developed rapidly over time so that cures are becoming ever more likely for many diseases. The cost of continually innovating and changing medical treatments and delivery systems is staggeringly high, yet the forgone opportunity cost of not innovating is much greater. What athlete injured today would wish to forgo arthroscopic knee surgery and accept a hot mustard plaster? Senior citizens may say they want to turn back the clock to the good old days, but any politician who threatens to take away Medicare, or even cut benefits slightly, gets defeated at the polls. The American public demands a modern, constantly updated health care system. Research into new therapies and new forms of organization is the force that has made it worth spending $2,624 billion today rather than the $4 billion spent when your grandfather was born.

Differences over Time and Place Are Larger than the Choices Patients Face

Heart surgery in 2009 was so much better than the kind practiced in 1969 that no one would choose the latter. Rich patients may fly from Guatemala to the United States for superior medical care, but few U.S. tourists would decide to have knee replacement surgery done in Guatemala while on vacation to save a few dollars.[8] Individual market choices for quality are important and persistent for goods such as clothing and housing, but medical care is more like the market for cell phones and video equipment, in which most people pay for what is newest.

Quality, Not Quantity

Patients always want the best. In choosing a surgeon, they look for someone who is well trained, perhaps even famous for a particular operation. They do not look for more scalpels, more hours, or a two-for-the-price-of-one deal. A patient usually consumes one and only one "unit" of care—an operation in this case—for each illness. The only trade-off made is in the quality of the procedure, not the quantity. Although in other kinds of markets getting "more" ounces or pounds or boxes or whatever is usually very important, in medical care it is quality that matters most.

Quality Is Hard to Measure, and Not Additive

Having budget decisions made over quality rather than quantity tends to complicate economic analysis. Price per unit may remain constant as the quantity increases or decreases, but any change in quality usually changes price. Quality cannot simply be added up or multiplied to arrive at a total spending limit the way quantity can. Although it is evident that the quality of medical care has increased over the last thirty years, it is not so clear whether quality has increased more than, less than, or approximately the same amount as the percentage increase in cost. Measures such as the consumer price index (CPI) attempt to deal with these issues, but there is no consensus on how accurate they are, or even on exactly what these measures should be. Can quality be measured by number of lives saved, number of lives saved per dollar spent, number of tests or services provided, level of physician knowledge (should this count if the patient dies), or patient satisfaction?

Historically, most quality measurement was done at the individual level: a procedure, a patient, or a physician. Was the surgery done properly, did the patient heal well and was he satisfied with the care he received, was the doctor adequately trained for the procedure with a certified supporting staff? Recently a more comprehensive statistical perspective has come to the fore. What percentage of patients suffer infections as a result of surgery? What percentage of patients require a second operation? How do these rates compare with surgeons and hospitals in other states or countries? These **population health** measures, which shift the focus from individual errors and competence to assessment of system performance, have been facilitated by the development of information technology, but have not yet begun to change the business of medicine or to substantially affect the way patients choose doctors and hospitals.

Individual Choices: Lifestyle Matters More than Medicine

To the extent that individual choices influence health, lifestyle matters more than medical purchases. It is not that medicine isn't important, but that most people will almost always pay for the important types of care, and most medical care provided in the United States is pretty good. The remaining marginal choices, Branch Creek Hospital versus University Hospital, generic naproxen sodium versus brand name Aleve, doctor at the local health department clinic versus specialist in private practice, will not have a major impact on death rates, although they may have a lot to do with personal satisfaction and the quality of the experience. Flying first class on a major carrier is more comfortable than flying cut rate in economy class, but safety (the likelihood of dying in a crash) is about the same. Similarly in medicine, the available choices in a generally high-quality and highly regulated system mean that "better" care often does not have a measurable impact on mortality.

Health Risks Are More Public than Private

The income you can expect to earn depends somewhat on your individual skills and effort, but depends even more upon when and where you were born—the society you live in. Imagine being a brilliant mathematician squatting in a Neanderthal cave, or a great salesman peddling fruit in Bangladesh. Compared with starting your life in Switzerland, being born in rural Sudan severely curtails both your earning power and your life expectancy.

Personal Tastes and Preferences Are Secondary

Almost everyone with a *Clostridium tetani* infection will want the same treatment, as will everyone who suffers a gastric aneurism. Individual differences matter much less than differences in disease. In most nonmedical markets, people want very different things even when their basic human needs are all pretty much the same. Shoppers in New York City buy medieval art, Darjeeling tea, kosher lamb, pistachio ice cream, and fresh apricots all at reasonable prices. One person gets red shoes with pointed toes while another buys white clogs, and both will try on several styles and sizes. In medical markets, it is the various kinds and severity of illness that matter, rather than personal tastes and preferences.

1.5   RESEARCH, TEACHING, AND CHARITY: SHIFTING OVERHEAD

Technology has been the driving force in the health care system—saving babies, extending lives, creating hospitals, linking medical records worldwide, and raising the American public's willingness to spend more than $2 trillion a year. Spending could probably be doubled without complaint if the research laboratories were to come up with a vaccine for AIDS, a cure for cancer, and a reversal of Alzheimer's disease. Medical discoveries often have been fortuitous outgrowths of other activities (Pasteur's discovery of bacteria grew out of an investigation into the causes of spoiled wine and beer) or the refinement of insights from patient care. Historically, what little direct funding there was for research came mostly from philanthropists. Today, taxpayers are the largest source of pure research funding through support of the National Institutes of Health and similar programs. However, a much larger portion of research financing is hidden in the cost of patient care, as the work of physicians to develop and refine new technologies is covered through reimbursement. The most prestigious hospitals and clinics are deemed superior because cutting-edge research and innovative therapies are first applied there. Being on the cutting edge is expensive, and charges for patient care at the top academic medical centers are as much as three times higher than those at local community hospitals (see Chapters 8 and 9).

Some of the extra costs borne by academic medical centers are due to educating new doctors and the social mission of providing service to the poor (who are conveniently helpful in providing training cases for the students). Advanced medical education is intensive, usually carried out in small groups or one-on-one encounters with specialists rather than large lectures. Such personalized attention is valuable but also costly. Service to the poor is socially rewarding but not financially remunerative. Clinic patients often do not have insurance and cannot pay, or they receive coverage under state Medicaid plans that pay much less than Medicare or private insurance (see Chapters 4 and 5).

Most of the costs of charity care, research, and teaching do not show up in the national health accounts because they are covered as part of patient care reimbursement. Similarly, most of the research and development (R&D) at pharmaceutical companies is buried as an overhead cost in the production of drugs. Even more hidden is the cost of administrative innovation. Developing new forms of contracting, such as HMOs, or new methods of delivering care, such as home health companies and life care communities, is very costly, largely because it is a trial-and-error process requiring many expensive failures before a better system can be found. Such organizational development is not usually even recognized as being research, and its cost is almost never tallied alongside the cost of laboratories and biomedical scientists.

Research, teaching, and care of the poor/uninsured are essential parts of modern medicine, but none of these vital services is fully compensated under the existing U.S. health care financing system. Instead, regular patients who have insurance or who can afford to pay more are overcharged to cover these uncompensated expenses—a process termed *cost-shifting* (see Chapters 8 and 9). This source of indirect funding is being undermined as budget crises and the growth of managed care (see Chapter 5) increase price competition in the hospital services market.

1.6 EQUITY AND DISTRIBUTION

Economists measure equity in terms of the *distribution* of money and goods within a society. A society in which the top decile (10 percent) of the population took 10 percent of the money and goods, the next decile also had 10 percent, and the bottom half of the families had exactly 50 percent, would be described as having no inequality (and does not exist). Conversely, a society in which just 2 percent of the people took 20 percent of all the income and goods would be relatively unequal (and many nations are far less equal than that).[9] Although most goods are distributed privately through markets to whoever can pay for them, anything considered vital to life and fundamental to human happiness (freedom, the right to vote, protection of the law, air and water) is usually made available to everyone by the government and paid for with taxes. One way of defining who belongs in a society and who is excluded is access to such services (see Chapters 14 and 15).

Medical care can be viewed as a matter of life and death or, in other circumstances, as just one of many goods that it would be better to have more of. Few societies would stand aside and watch someone die when vital medical intervention was easily available, yet the extent to which medical care is made dependent upon ability to pay varies widely (see Chapter 17). In Australia, Canada, Japan, and many European countries every citizen (and often noncitizens as well) have access to high-quality medical care at minimal or no charge regardless of income. In most poor developing countries, only very wealthy families can

TABLE 1.4	Annual Mortality Rate among Middle-Aged Men	
	Mortality Rate	
Income Category	**White**	**Black**
<$9,999	0.918%	1.234%
$10,000–$14,999	0.840%	1.123%
$15,000–$19,999	0.706%	0.899%
$20,000–$24,999	0.660%	0.867%
$25,000–$29,999	0.591%	0.603%
$30,000+	0.542%	****

Source: G. D. Smith et al., *American Journal of Public Health* 86 (1996): 486–504.

obtain good care. In the United States the picture is somewhat mixed. Everyone has access to high-quality medical care, but responsibility for payment can vary widely depending upon insurance status, and medical bills are a not-infrequent cause of personal bankruptcy.

Spending money on medical care is only one of many ways that the economy affects people's health. Economic prosperity enables people to have a better diet, to avoid hazardous jobs, and to clean up the environment, as well as to purchase more medical care.[10] A major benefit of higher incomes is education, which changes values and production possibilities in ways that are favorable to health. Chapter 16 provides a more detailed examination of the complex relationships between economic growth, income distribution, medical care, and health. An introductory example of some issues regarding distributional equity in health is provided in Table 1.4, which presents the results of research on 320,000 middle-aged men enrolled in a trial of cardiac risk reduction.[11] Income for this study is based not on individual wages but on the community in which the person lived (average per capita income of the zip code of residence). Reading down the columns, it becomes evident that men in poorer communities face a much higher risk of death each year, a finding that holds even as the groups are adjusted for age, unemployment, use of medical care, and other factors. Indeed, those living in areas with average incomes below $10,000 per year were twice as likely to die as those in areas with average incomes above $30,000 per year. Blacks were more likely to die than whites, largely because of living in lower income areas. Yet even after controlling for differences in income, black mortality is still significantly greater each year. Similar differences in morbidity and mortality rates by socioeconomic and ethnic grouping are observed among women, the elderly, and children.

Although insurance and government assistance has done much to equalize access to medical care, large disparities in actual health and life expectancy endure. Inequalities in health are found throughout the world. Countries such as Sweden and the United Kingdom, which have universal national health systems, also show substantial differences in mortality between groups, as do poorer countries such as Bangladesh and Ghana, where a national health infrastructure is almost nonexistent. Health economists are still working to understand the persistence of excess mortality among disadvantaged groups despite tremendous increases and redistribution in health care spending.

1.7 WHOSE CHOICES: PERSONAL, GROUP, OR PUBLIC?

A common quip from geneticists is: "Want to live longer? Choose better parents!" Superficially silly, from another perspective this statement is quite sensible. Parents not only determine your genetic makeup, they also determine your nutrition and lifestyle during your formative years, provide for your education, and are the basis for many of the work and health habits you carry into later life. Your "personal" choices are as much a reflection of what they wanted for you, and the expectations of the social group where you were born, as of any purely individual preferences or effort. Do you smoke cigarettes? Is that a personal choice or a result of your background and social group? (See the box "Do You Choose to Smoke?")

Choice occurs along a continuum from the purely *private* individual choices that do not involve anyone else, to those that are purely *public* that must be made collectively and affect everyone (Chapters 14 and 15). Interstate highways, the law, water supply, air quality standards, 911 emergency help systems, and the TC/IP protocol for the Internet are all examples of public goods. Every public choice represents a compromise since it includes many people who must all chose or agree to abide by the same decision. For many public goods, "quantity" is not very economically meaningful, but quality is. Air quality and pollution can be addressed through various improvements, each of which has a cost. Being universal does not exempt public goods from scarcity. Public funds, although much greater than those of any individual, are still subject to budget constraints. The price of better air must be paid by giving up some other public goods, or by all of us giving up some of our private goods by paying higher taxes.

DO YOU CHOOSE TO SMOKE? PERSONAL AND COLLECTIVE DECISIONS

Smoking is a personal choice. An individual's decision is influenced by inherent desires and genetic makeup, but is often even more strongly shaped by the decisions of others. If many of your friends gather and smoke on Friday nights, it is more likely that you will do so. If you know few people who smoke, and most of your friends speak disparagingly of those who do, then you are less likely to do so. When smoking is considered cool, sophisticated, and a sign of maturity, it is more desired than when it is considered a pathetic habit born out of ignorance. In the nineteenth century, smoking cigarettes was a form of "conspicuous consumption" by the wealthy—a way of showing that you had "money to burn." During the depression it was the Hollywood stars (and doctors) that smoked, rather than the poor, and cigarettes were accordingly considered a sign of glamour and sophistication. During the 1950s and 1960s scientific studies showed conclusively that cigarettes were harmful to health, and public opinion began to change. However, behavior and social norms changed only slowly. For many years after cigarettes were banned in hospitals, smoking was still allowed in airplanes, restaurants—and economics classes. Even in the 1970s it was inconceivable to professors that a university would try to regulate their behavior within their own personal offices, yet today most universities ban smoking from all buildings.

Peer pressure and the social norms created by group choices are powerful. Formal public choices such as a tax of $3 per pack, or a ban on smoking in bars and restaurants, may even have the force of law. Of course the choice of whether or not to smoke is a personal one, but group and public decisions set the context within which each individual choice is made, and may overwhelm individual tastes and preferences.

Smoking has been banned on airplanes, trains, and buses, and in office buildings of many firms, universities, and hospitals. Air quality has been improved without paying for pollution control equipment or raising taxes. Does this mean that these improvements in air quality came without a price tag or that no trade-offs had to be made? Of course not. Listen to the smokers gripe or to the complaints of nonsmoking libertarians who worry that the next distasteful behavior to be banned will be drinking, or sex, or gun ownership. While it does not appear that anything has been bought or sold, a transaction has in fact taken place. The opportunity cost of a smoke-free workplace was a discernible, but small, loss of personal liberty. This is the "price" of the gain in air quality. People have made it clear that this is a price they are willing to pay—and just as clear that some measures advocated by health advisors are too costly to be implemented. Even though such collective relationships are inherently complex, involving millions of people, the fundamentals of opportunity cost, budget constraints, and trade-offs still apply.

"Private" and "public" are polar concepts. Few goods are so purely private that they are entirely unregulated regarding safety, ingredients, and disposal, and few goods are so public that there are no differences among individuals regarding use or quality.[12] The economic organization of medical care clusters more services toward the public end than is immediately apparent. Even though each of us goes individually to the hospital emergency room, in a small city we must all go to the same emergency room and get pretty much the same quality of care. The mayor may get better service than a homeless person who is brought in off the street, but the mayor will be operated on by the same surgeon, will be cared for by the same nursing staff, and might end up in the same room as the homeless person. In a large city with many hospitals, there is somewhat more variation, but patients are rarely able to choose their surgeon, nursing staff, or room. Contrast that with the purchase of a coat, a birthday cake, or even a wheelchair, in which there are many more choices and much more individual control over quality. Financing systems also tend to make medical care a public good. All employees in a firm often have the same insurance plan. Therefore, the mail clerk and the executive vice president are equally valued customers of the hospital. In Chapters 4 and 5 we will examine how the pooling of funds into insurance for payment of medical expenses can distort choices and obscure budget constraints.

Connecting the public and private spheres are choices made as a group. An informal group (seniors at Hilltop High, friends of the band, libertarians) may exert a powerful social influence, but only formally constituted groups (corporations) that have legal status as fictitious collective "persons" can enter into contracts and create the circular flow of funds (opening a bank account, buying or selling a truckload of cigarettes, hiring an employee, getting sued). Physician groups, insurance plans, hospitals, and nurses unions are all corporate entities engaging in medical care. Of particular interest to health economists is why so many of the relevant organizations in medicine are different from those in other markets—licensed professions or nonprofit voluntary hospitals, for example.

1.8 SOCIAL SCIENCE AND RATIONAL CHOICE THEORY

Groups are a pervasive force because humans are *social* beings, working constantly to set up and maintain markets, clubs, governments, medical facilities, and other institutions. Economics, sociology, anthropology, and politics are often lumped together as "social sciences," but each emphasizes a different perspective to study interpersonal exchange. Economists look first and foremost at markets, and thus concentrate on the formal transactions between people and organizations using money. However, the economic principles developed in studying those transactions can also be used to study the family, group psychology, education, war, the behavior of birds, and health, even when no money is changing hands. The core conceptual tools of economic price theory—scarcity, investment, maximization, marginalism, equilibrium, cost-benefit—are expressed mathematically as "rational choice theory" and have been popularly applied to other areas, invigorating new fields of study such as sociobiology and neuroeconomics. "Rationality" in economics means that people make choices to make themselves better off (maximize utility, minimize risk) subject to constraints, and organizations make choices to meet their objectives (maximize profits, minimize cost, get elected). It does not mean that people are "perfectly rational" but that they tend to choose in ways that make them better off rather than worse. Rather like "natural selection" in biology, "rationality" is a concept that organizes and guides a field of study rather than a precisely specified term. Just as physics uses the equations of Newtonian mechanics to analyze motion, "rational choice theory" describes actions as if they occurred in a vacuum, without the complications and frictions of the real world. The equations tell us as much, and as little, as knowing that the force of gravity is 32 feet per second squared tells us about the trajectory of a home-run hit or a dancer leaping across the stage. Like gravity, economic rationality and self-interest is always there. It is not the whole story, though, and may sometimes miss the human meaning even as it calculates the path traced by the ball and the ballerina.

What makes "health" economics so special is the focus on humanity. Questions of life and death are as salient as buying and selling. It definitely matters that we are talking about *people* rather than things. Selling human tissue or attaching a patient to a ventilator is not the same as buying chicken fingers or attaching a car to a tow truck. "Behavioral economics" examines what it means that human beings rather than rational calculators are making these decisions, looking at "consistently irrational" behavior such as stock-market bubbles and why people's willingness to pay for X is often different from the amount they want to receive in compensation in order to give it up, or why a $1,500 bonus is spent differently than a $1,500 check from the insurance company. Just as the principles of economics have been used to study politics, mating behavior, and even baseball, the quirks of human psychology can be used to analyze the twists and turns in perception and monetary flows.[13]

The effects of medical care on the economy are as profound as the effects of economics on health. Not only has medicine led to better health, greater longevity, and increased productivity, it has also become one of the largest businesses in the world. Investments are made in hospital bonds and biotech stocks to make people better off monetarily, not just better off in terms of health. To those who directly or indirectly earn their living from medicine (physicians, nurses, hospital administrators, equipment vendors, and even health economists), the business aspects—the contracts that are used to allocate health services—are important. The invisible hand plays a role in creating a demand for health economics that is just as powerful, and more direct, than the desire to improve the standard of living and care for the sick.

SUGGESTIONS FOR FURTHER READING

Health United States, 2008. U.S. Department of Health and Human Services (annual publication), (http://www.cdc.gov/nchs/).

National Health Expenditures 1960–2007 and *National Health Expenditure Projections 2008–2018*, U.S.D.H.H.S., Centers for Medicare and Medicaid, National Health Accounts, (http://www.cms.hhs.gov/NationalHealthExpendData/).

Kaiser Family Foundation Health Policy Studies (www.kff.org).

Victor Fuchs, "Economics, Values and Health Care Reform," *American Economic Review* 86, no. 1 (1996): 1–24.

Paul Starr, *The Social Transformation of American Medicine* (New York: Basic Books, 1982).

SUMMARY

1.   **Trade** is not the goal of health care, it is the means. For people to get what they want from the system, exchanges between patients and providers must be made. **Health economics** is the study of how those transactions are made and of the bottom line results.

2.   The **terms of trade** are the specifics of a transaction. Only in a very simple exchange are all of the terms of trade captured in the money price. The **fundamental theorem of exchange** states that for a trade to take place, both the buyer and the seller must believe that it makes them better off.

3.   **Value** is not inherent in a good, but rather in the trading relationship. **Health care costs so much because people are willing to pay for it**. As a wealthy country, the United States was willing to spend more than 2.6 trillion dollars in 2010, $8,459 per person, supporting a dynamic and technologically sophisticated health care system.

4.   Health care costs have consistently **risen 2 to 5 percent more rapidly than incomes** and now account for more than **17 percent of GDP**. Costs are **unevenly distributed**. Seventy percent of total health care dollars are spent on the 10 percent of people who become most ill during a year. Due to the uncertain and uneven distribution of medical costs, most health care is financed by **third-party insurance** intermediaries, which pool and transfer funds. This system replaces the direct exchange of money for services between two parties (consumers and providers), which is common to most markets.

5.   Most choices in medicine are made by **professionals** such as doctors (rather than consumers), and these choices are mostly about quality (rather than price or quantity), making the economics of this special market more interesting and complex. **Physicians** account for about 0.6 percent of the U.S. labor force, about the same percentage as in 1880. However, the number of nurses and other health workers per physician has risen from 0.2 to 16. **Hospitals** (32 percent) are the largest users of health care funds.

6.   **Government** is the largest provider of health care funds (48 percent). Most **research** into new drugs and therapeutic techniques is financed directly by government or indirectly by cost-shifting overheads added to the prices of hospitals, drugs, and surgery. Although research is very expensive, the forgone **opportunity cost** of not innovating would be much greater. Research, health statistics, airline safety, environmental regulations, and malpractice laws are **public** goods and involve choices that must be made by society as a whole. Pooled financing through insurance can make medical care into a form of public good even though services are provided and consumed in private transactions between doctors and patients.

7.   Improvement in **health and longevity** has come mostly from **economic growth, more knowledge, social factors,** and inexpensive **public health** activities rather than the application of expensive medical technology. Insurance and government programs have greatly reduced disparities in the use of medical care between income groups, but **socioeconomic differentials in health status have persisted**. Residents of poor neighborhoods are twice as likely to die as are people of the same age and sex who live in wealthy neighborhoods.

PROBLEMS

1.   {*economic principles*} What is the opportunity cost of going to a doctor to be examined for skin cancer?

2.   {*economic principles*} What is the primary budget constraint facing an 84-year-old billionaire?

3.   {*planning resources per capita*} Using the data in *Health United States 2006* (http://www.cdc.gov/nchs/hus.htm), calculate the number of physicians, nurses, hospitals,

and nursing homes there would be in an average small town with 10,000 people (total U.S. population was approximately 300 million in 2006).

4.   {*local estimates*} Using the telephone book for your city, try to determine whether the number of physicians, nurses, hospitals, and nursing homes is greater than or less than the number you calculated for Problem 3. Why is it more difficult to estimate the number of physicians than the number of hospitals? Why is it so difficult to estimate the number of nurses?

5.   {*distribution of health expenditures*} Ranking everyone by the amount spent on medical care, 30 percent of the total (all expenditures for all people) is accounted for by the top 1 percent of patients. Take the overall average per capita personal health expenditure and determine how much on average is spent on each of these high-cost patients. The top half of the population accounts for 90 percent of total spending. What is the average amount spent on the remaining people in the bottom half of the distribution? Is the median (i.e., amount spent on the person who is at the middle of distribution, with half of all people spending more, and half of all people spending less) higher or lower than the mean?

6.   {*philanthropy, $ versus percent*} Has the dollar amount of charitable giving for health increased or decreased since 1929? Has the percentage of health expenditures paid for by charity increased or decreased?

7.   {*manpower*} Which has increased more rapidly since 1929: the number of physicians or the number of ancillary health workers? As medicine becomes more technologically advanced, which will grow faster: the number of more-skilled workers or the number of less-skilled workers?

8.   {*utilization*} Did people go to the doctor more often or less often in 2010 than in 1970? In 1929? Did they spend more or fewer days in the hospital? Why?

9.   {*causality*} Have health expenditures increased because the number of people employed in health care has increased, or has health employment increased because total health expenditures have increased?

10.   {*causality*} Would eliminating research reduce or increase the cost of U.S. health care?

11.   {*normative and positive judgments*} Are public choices better or worse than private choices?

12.   {*fieldwork*} Contact three people and find out how much they spent on health care last year. Try to estimate how much they spent out of their own pockets and how much was spent by their employers, insurance companies, or the government. Did the people with more serious health problems always end up spending more of their own money on health care? Did they personally end up paying a larger or smaller percentage of their total health bills out of pocket?

ENDNOTES

1.   National Health Care Expenditures Projections 2008–2018. U.S.D.H.H.S., Centers for Medicare and Medicaid, National Health Accounts (http://www.cms.hhs.gov/NationalHealthExpendData/), accessed March 28, 2009. The CMS Office of the Actuary is the source for all expenditure estimates in this and subsequent chapters, unless noted otherwise. The figure of $8,459 is an estimate for 2010 that includes research, construction, and other overhead as well as personal health expenditures.

2.   Committee on the Costs of Medical Care, *Medical Care for the American People* (Chicago: University of Chicago Press, 1932); Odin W. Anderson, *Health Services as a Growth Enterprise in the United States since 1875* (Ann Arbor, Mich.: Health Administration Press, 1990).

3. The distribution of costs across individuals can be measured only for personal health care costs that are billed to individuals, not for overhead items such as public health, construction, and insurance administration. Such overhead items make up about 15 percent of national health expenditures. Hence, the "personal health expenditures" account for only 85 percent of national health expenditures in Table 1.1 and elsewhere. In truth, even when charges are billed to an individual, many costs have overhead components and are difficult to assign unambiguously to a single person, although they are clearly concentrated on the most ill and not evenly distributed. Many economists would argue that costs are more concentrated than statistics indicate (see Figure 4.1 and Table 4.2) since hospitals and physicians typically overcharge the least complex patients to subsidize the most difficult and complex cases (see the discussion of "cost shifting" in Chapter 8).

4. Bureau of Labor Statistics, U.S. Department of Labor, *Employment and Earnings* (http://www.bls.gov). Bureau of Labor Statistics, U.S. Department of Labor, *Employment Cost Indexes and Levels, 1975–90*, Bulletin 2372, 1990.

5. U.S. Department of Health and Human Services, *Health United States 1975*, and *Health United States 2008* (http://www.cdc.gov/nchs/hus.htm). See also L. A. Green et al., "The Ecology of Medical Care Revisited," *New England Journal of Medicine* 344:26 (June 28, 2001): 2021–2025, which provides statistics indicating that the number of people experiencing symptoms, consulting physicians, and being admitted to the hospital was roughly constant from 1961 to 1996.

6. Compare Japan and Nigeria. One is a resource-poor island that has become one of the wealthiest societies in the world, while the other is a resource-rich nation that flounders to escape poverty. See Dani Rodrk, Arvind Subramanian, and Francesco Trebbi, "Institutions Rule: The Primacy of Institutions over Geography. . . ," *Journal of Economic Growth* 9(2):131–165, 2004.

7. Health affects the utility of all other goods and services. A kayak, a mountain bike, even a luxury car are not worth much if you are not healthy enough to use them. One way this is dealt with by economic theorists is to model utility with a multiplicative health variable rather than an additively separable term.

8. Theo Francis, "Medical Tourism is Still Small," *Wall Street Journal*, page D2, May 6, 2008.

9. Basic information about the distribution of wealth can be gleaned from standard sources such as the Census Bureau's *Current Population Survey* and the Federal Reserve Bank's *Survey of Income and Assets*. More refined measures of inequality commonly used by economists include the "Gini Coefficient" and the "Thiel Index."

10. Thomas McKeown, *The Modern Rise of Population* (London: Edwin Arnold, 1976); Massimo Livi-Bacci, *A Concise History of World Population*, trans. Carl Ipsen (Cambridge, Mass.: Blackwell, 1992). James P. Smith, "Healthy Bodies and Thick Wallets: The Dual Relationship Between Health and Economic Status," *Journal of Economic Perspectives* 13, no. 2 (Spring 1999): 145–166.

11. G. D. Smith, J. D. Neaton, D. Wentworth, R. Stamler, and J. Stamler, "Socioeconomic Differentials in Mortality Risk Among Men Screened for the Multiple Risk Factor Intervention Trial," *American Journal of Public Health* 86 (1986): 486–504.

12. Joseph E. Stiglitz, *The Economics of the Public Sector* (New York: W.W. Norton, 1986). See Chapter 15.

13. Richard Thaler and Cass Sunstein, *Nudge: Improving Decisions About Health, Wealth and Happiness* (New Haven, Conn.: Yale University Press, 2008); Michael M. Lewis, *Moneyball* (New York: W.W. Norton, 2003); Daniel Kahneman, Paul Slovic, and Amos Tversky, *Judgement Under Uncertainty: Heuristics and Biases* (New York: Cambridge University Press, 1982); Richard Frank, "Behavioral Economics and Health Economics," NBER working paper #10881, November 2004.

CHAPTER 2

DEMAND AND SUPPLY

QUESTIONS

1. Is price the only thing that matters? What is the difference between *price* and *value*?
2. What is the difference between Mr. Axel's **demand** for physical therapy, and his **need** for physical therapy?
3. Why would a life-saving cardiac drug cost less than one providing only temporary symptomatic relief?
4. Do buyers and sellers face the same demand curve?
5. Can better quality actually decrease demand?
6. Which is more sensitive to price changes—one person, one firm, or the whole market?
7. Do politicians face demand curves?
8. Is medical spending a luxury, with rich people spending much more than the poor?

The choices made by buyers constitute **demand**, while the choices made by sellers constitute **supply**. Most people are active on both sides, exchanging money for goods and services as demanders and exchanging labor and other assets for money as suppliers. Money is moved around continuously between people and organizations in the endless loop of linked transactions discussed as the *circular flow of funds* in Chapter 1. We are more apt to be most directly involved in health care on the demand side as patients, but to understand the system we must also analyze the supply side, made up of doctors (Chapters 6 and 7), hospitals (Chapters 8 and 9) nursing homes and other long term care providers (Chapter 10), and pharmaceuticals (Chapter 11), as well as the role of insurance companies as financial intermediaries (Chapters 4 and 5).

2.1 THE DEMAND CURVE

When a patient chooses to buy he or she becomes a part of demand. Wanting to buy (drugs, plastic surgery, artificial hip, etc.) but not doing so leaves that potential patient invisible, a part of *latent demand* that does not effectively participate in the market. That extra demand will be revealed if the price goes low enough. For example, consider the development of an artificial heart. If each heart costs $1 million, they would only be used in matters of life and

FIGURE 2.1   Demand Curve for Artificial Hearts

death. If further development reduced the cost of artificial hearts to $100,000 each, more people would get them (Figure 2.1). The artificial hearts would still be used only for people with serious illnesses, but they might be implanted long before a person's natural heart gave out. If the cost of making an artificial heart dropped to $100, one would be readily available to anyone who needed it. Consider what would happen if the cost of an artificial heart dropped to $10 and could be easily implanted during a 15-minute visit to the doctor. Some people who had never been ill but were just worried, or who thought that they were weak and wanted a supercharger to help them run faster, might have new hearts implanted.

The demand curve shows how many patients are willing to buy at the current price and also at other potential prices. Thus the demand curve can be used to calculate the total and incremental benefits of each additional artificial heart sold. At a price of $1 million, the artificial heart would be implanted in only two people who believed they would receive more than $1 million in benefits and were willing to pay that much. At a price of $100,000, the artificial heart would be implanted in 38 people, adding 36 people whose perceived benefit is less than $1 million but equal to or more than $100,000. At $60,000, the artificial heart would be implanted in one more person, whose marginal benefit falls between $100,000 and $60,000, and at a price of $20,000, it would be implanted in two more people whose incremental benefit falls between $60,000 and $20,000. If, due to insurance, the effective price were reduced to $0, then a total of 42 people would receive artificial hearts.

There are two important observations to note here. First, the demand curve is downward sloping because as price continues to be reduced, more and more people will buy (assuming all other conditions remain constant), a generalization known as the **law of demand**. Second, there is no such thing as "the value" of an artificial heart. Its value depends on how many are used. If only a few hearts were available across the United States, their value would be fantastically high, many millions of dollars each. Once many artificial hearts were sold, their value would drop, and eventually if a sufficiently large number (hundreds of thousands) were sold then the additional (marginal) value would be quite low.

The Diamonds–Water Paradox: An Example of Marginal Analysis

All ordinary economic goods show the same functional relationship between marginal benefit and quantity. The goods are extremely valuable when only a few units are available. They are of moderate value to a larger number of people, and each additional unit is of less and less value as more and more people receive them, with extra services being almost

FIGURE 2.2   The Diamonds–Water Paradox

worthless or even harmful. The founder of modern economics, Adam Smith, was intrigued by the following problem: If water, which is necessary for life itself, is so valuable, why does it cost so little, and why do diamonds, which are simply ornamental, cost so much? Although Smith was a brilliant economist, he was never able to explain this phenomenon. With the benefit of price theory using demand and supply curves, the situation is easily explained by making the distinction between marginal benefits and total benefits. The value of the first ounce of water is very high because it can save the life of a dehydrated person. The second ounce is worth less and the third still less. In many areas, water is so plentiful that there are literally millions of gallons available, and few people have to pay more than a few cents for a glass of water. The total benefit, the value indicated by the area under the entire demand curve, is very large. The marginal benefit, the value of one more glass of water at this point (price) on the demand curve, is very small.

For diamonds, the situation is quite different. The area under the demand curve (total benefit) is not large (I can live very well with no diamonds at all). However, diamonds are scarce enough that the incremental benefit from obtaining one more is still substantial. This is shown in Figure 2.2. Whether the purchase is a bottle of water or a diamond or surgery, the decision to purchase is a decision made at the margin. How much is it worth to pay for one more?

It is useful to keep the diamonds–water paradox in mind when analyzing health policy. Treatments that are highly beneficial to a few selected patients get supplied to so many people that the system is moved further and further down the marginal benefit curve, and eventually the bulk of the work is being done on patients for whom doctors can do little good. Efficiency in medical care is not just a matter of technical excellence and minimizing the cost of production. More often, efficiency depends on how much is produced and which patients get treated. Some of the nation's problems with the high cost of medical care come from using diamonds when a bandage around the finger would do just as well.

Consumer Surplus: Marginal versus Average Value of Medicine

The demand curve for artificial hearts described above can be used to illustrate the distinction between average and marginal value. With the price at $60,000 there are 39 hearts being bought (and sold). Anyone who values an artificial heart at $60,000 or more purchases one. What would be the incremental value of putting one additional heart on the market? Obviously something less than $60,000, since everyone who wants to pay that much already has done so. The demand curve in Figure 2.1 indicates that price will have to drop down to $50,000 in order to sell one more heart—that is, to have 40 people voluntarily purchasing artificial hearts at the market price. Thus the marginal value of that additional heart is about $50,000 in this particular market. Since the other 39 people were all willing to pay more than $50,000 they are receiving a consumer's surplus—extra value to them above and beyond what they had to pay. How much extra value? Well, two were willing to pay $1 million or more, the third was willing to pay almost that much ($975,000) and the next was willing to pay just a little bit less ($950,000) and so on, until we get to the 39th person who valued an artificial heart at $75,000, and finally to the last (marginal) buyer (the 40th), who was only willing to pay $50,000. All except the last receives a consumer surplus. How much consumer surplus? Adding up the value to each of the 40 people who are buying ($1,025,000 + 1,000,000 + 975,000 + 950,000... + 50,000) indicates that the total value to all 40 people is $21,500,000. The person valuing the heart at $950,000 received $950,000 − $50,000 = $900,000 in consumer surplus. The person who thought the benefit to them was worth $125,000 gets a consumer surplus of $75,000. The average value among the people who buy a heart is $21,500,000 ÷ 40 = $537,500, making the average consumer surplus $487,500 ($537,500 − $50,000). That shows what a tremendous value the introduction of artificial hearts brings to this market. Note that some people (those who value the benefits near $1 million) receive much more of the consumer surplus than others, and the marginal buyer (the 40th) who values the benefits at just $50,000 and pays $50,000 for the heart gets little or no consumer surplus.

The distinction between average and marginal value is crucial to an understanding of how markets work. This case is not atypical. The top value, and even the average value, of benefits usually greatly exceeds the costs and the marginal value of providing a few extra units of service. As we will see in Chapter 3 where cost-benefit methods are discussed in more detail, the total and average value of modern medical care (total benefits ÷ total number of people) is gigantic, yet the incremental benefits of providing treatment to a few more patients, or the incremental benefits of adding some more treatments to those already available, are often less than the cost.

Angioplasty and Aspirin   "Diamonds–water" pricing can be found in medical care as well. Angioplasty, the procedure in which a catheter is inserted through the major vein in the leg and up into the heart, can be used to diagnose and treat heart disease. The procedure is difficult and expensive, costing $5,000 to $25,000. Yet angioplasty works well only some of the time, provides only a temporary cure, and must often be repeated or followed up with major surgery. Research has shown that a low-dose aspirin tablet, taken daily, prevents many heart attacks, yet the price is minimal. Since firms can produce tons of aspirin for less than 1¢ per tablet, it remains by far the cheapest way to reduce cardiac mortality.

Perceptions: A Water–Water Paradox   Even water is not always priced the same. It may be available free from the tap or drinking fountains yet sell for two dollars or more in a store or restaurant. It is what buyers believe they are getting—not what they actually get—that counts here. Even though some people claim that bottled water is healthier, most biological analyses show little difference between it and tap water (much bottled water comes from the same source as tap water). Yet the two kinds of water are not the same if we perceive them differently. If you think that Evian water is more purified and you value purity, you will pay extra for it.

The dominance of perception is evident when examining treatment for breast cancer. For many years, even small lesions were removed using a radical mastectomy, in which all breast tissue, underlying muscle, and surrounding lymph nodes were removed. Subsequent research showed that much less invasive surgery (a lumpectomy) was usually just as effective, and often a patient could wait to see whether any surgery at all was necessary. The fact that millions of women had painful, disfiguring, and expensive radical mastectomies does not mean that they or their doctors were irrational, but rather that, at the moment they had to choose, they believed they were choosing the right treatment.[1]

Medicine always deals with uncertain outcomes. At the moment of decision, expectations are more important than results. People buy lottery tickets, go on dates, book vacations, buy stock, major in computer science, or make appointments for surgery based on what they expect to get, even though many times they will be disappointed. Similarly, the outcomes from chemotherapy, infertility treatment, and heart transplants are never certain. When the purchase decision is being made, it is the expected value, not realized value, that counts (see Chapters 3 and 4).

Ceteris Paribus

Expectation is just one of the factors that can affect demand. Income, population growth, taste (i.e., personal preferences), health status, the availability of other goods, thunderstorms, war, and a host of other factors can influence the quantity demanded even when price is held constant. Such factors, usually known as **demand shifters**, are, in turn, the subject of economic analysis. At this stage, it is necessary to limit our discussion so that the effects of price and price alone can be examined. We will make use of the notion of *ceteris paribus*, a Latin phrase that means "all other things held the same." This assumption—that all other factors besides the one under discussion are assumed to hold constant—is standard and usually unstated.

Individual, Firm, and Market Demand Curves

So far, we have been rather casual about exactly who is to be counted when constructing the demand curve. Economists define individual, firm, and market demand, with the distinction depending upon the decision being made. To determine how many times Alice Anderson will visit the doctor, we look only at Alice's behavior, her **individual demand**. To estimate the use of ambulance services in Lockport, Maine, we look only at people in the town and the surrounding area, not the entire state. To project how a change in the hospital deductible for Medicare will affect spending, it is necessary to look at the entire elderly population, some 35 million seniors. The **market demand** is the sum of all individuals in that market. The definition of "the market" depends entirely on the particular decision being made. It may correspond to a geographic area, a group of friends, or all the people who visit a particular Web site. If we count only how many units of service people will buy from a specific provider, then we analyze **firm demand**. At that point, however, we have moved beyond the discussion of consumer demand and on to the supply side.

2.2 THE SUPPLY CURVE

Just as market demand includes all individuals and organizations currently buying the specific good (artificial heart, aspirin, water), market supply includes all organizations that are currently selling that good or service to them. Since every unit that is bought must be sold, it is a tautological identity that quantity demanded equals quantity supplied. The market supply curve is usually upward sloping, with a higher price calling forth a higher quantity supplied. However, this may not be the case in some markets with substantial economies of scale (see Chapter 8). Whereas demand and willingness to pay depend upon the tastes and preferences of individuals, and may be highly variable, the standard economic analysis of supply assumes that a firm is interested in just one thing, *profit*, and that external constraints such as the cost of inputs and the technology of production largely determine the shape and position of the supply curve.

If there were only one pharmacy in Lockport, it would be a **monopolist** (sole seller) and the demand of the market as a whole would be the same as the demand for the firm. Suppose instead that there are four pharmacies in Lockport. What demand curve is relevant to them? The pharmacies are concerned with more than individual demand, since each of them has many customers. Yet none of them fills all the prescriptions in Lockport; therefore, a pharmacy's own business is not the same as market demand. Rather, each pharmacy can sell a greater or lesser fraction of all the drugs sold in town by changing prices. Economists say that the pharmacy "faces a **firm demand** curve" of potential customers (which is some fraction of the entire market). If one pharmacy's prices are much cheaper than the others, it will get the bulk of business. Conversely, even a pharmacy charging high prices will get some business from customers who live nearby, or if it is the only one open in the middle of the night.

Marginal Revenue

A firm's profits depend not on how many units are sold, but on the amount of money they bring in (revenue). In deciding whether to sell more, not only does price matter, but also important is how much price must be lowered to increase sales. If a pharmacy sells two bandages at $10 each, its total revenue is $2 \times \$10 = \$20$. Suppose that to sell three bandages under the same circumstances, the pharmacy would have to lower the price to $8. At the lower price, the pharmacy's total revenue will rise to $3 \times \$8 = \$24$. The gain in total sales is just $24 – $20, or $4. This is the **marginal revenue** of the third unit of sale. One way of looking at marginal revenue is that to increase sales, the $8 received from the additional unit sold is partially offset by the $2 price reduction (from $10 to $8) of the other two units, so that the net gain is just $4.

Suppose your cousin Bob is a star plastic surgeon, doing rhinoplasties (nose reconstructions) for $10,000 each. He has bragged to you that each operation takes him only 2 hours, and that if he lost money in the stock market, he could make it up by doing more noses. Knowing how little he needs the money, you suggest he help out Aunt Martha, who has been struggling to save enough to pay for a nose job. "Give Aunt Martha a deal," you say, "Do her nose for $4,000." Bob explains the realities of business to you. "I really want to help Aunt Martha, I really do. But I can't do her nose for $4,000. That will make me look like I'm cheating all my other patients. And you know Aunt Martha—she'll have to tell everyone what a deal she got. Every other patient is going to come after me for a cut-rate price. Pretty soon, I'm just a run of the mill guy who gets $5,000 per nose job. Given my expenses, I'd be lucky to be able to keep the yacht, much less the beach house. If I have to do her a favor, I'll just do it for free." The threat to Bob's income is not the loss on one operation. It is the way that a change in price affects all units sold. Without ever having taken an economics course, Bob is focused on the information relevant to his decision—marginal revenue. It is not how much Aunt Martha pays that matters, but rather how changing the price for her affects the revenues from all other patients.

It is total revenue and total cost, not the apparent "costs" and "charges" that appear on bills and accounting statements, that count. The way to maximize profits (*Total Revenues – Total Costs*) is to sell additional units as long as the marginal revenue is greater than the marginal cost. Once marginal revenue is less than marginal cost, the sale is a loser, even if the price is still above cost. The concept of marginal revenue takes a while to grasp but is essential for understanding business decisions. The relevant decision is about a bit more or a bit less, and how total revenue will change as a result: a decision *at the margin*.

2.3 PRICE SENSITIVITY

The distinctive feature of the economic approach to demand is the emphasis on *change*, rather than the amount. A measure is needed that focuses on movement and differences, on the sensitivity of the buying decision to an increase or decrease in price. Economists have borrowed a calculation from engineering, **elasticity**, to measure price sensitivity. A demand curve indicating that the quantity demanded will change a lot for any small change in price is said to be "price **elastic**." If the quantity demanded barely budges when the price rises, demand is said to be **inelastic**. More precisely, price elasticity is measured by the percentage change in quantity demanded for each 1 percent change in price.

$$Price\ Elasticity = \frac{\%\ Change\ in\ Quantity}{\%\ Change\ in\ Price}$$

The elasticity measure of price sensitivity can be used to investigate the similarities and differences in demand. If Alice's demand for Claritin is likely to decline by 25 percent if the price increases by 10 percent, then her elasticity is –2.5. If Alice's response is pretty much average, then even though we may be talking about thousands of prescriptions, the effect on the market as a whole will still be a 25 percent decline for a 10 percent price increase. That is, market price elasticity and average individual demand elasticity are the same, even though the total quantities are much different. This demonstrates one of the advantages of the elasticity measure—it is dimensionless. We could have measured quantity in terms of the number of pills or the number of bottles containing 50 doses for one person or for 10,000, and the percentage changes would still be the same.

What about the firm demand for Eastside Pharmacy in Lockport? Chances are, it will be more price sensitive than the individual or market demands. If Eastside Pharmacy raised prices, many customers would start buying from Central Pharmacy instead. Only if all four pharmacies in Lockport raised prices by 10 percent would it be likely that all four would experience a 25 percent decline in demand. Why is firm demand so much more price sensitive? Because the other firms in the market are good substitutes. The more substitutes available, the more price sensitive demand is.

SUBSTITUTES—ANOTHER WATER PARADOX

Why are there so few drinking fountains at sports arenas? By reducing the number of substitutes, soda vendors can increase demand and decrease the price sensitivity of consumers. Such attempts to shift demand are common in most commercial activity. At games, fans expect to pay more to eat and drink and park, and understand that such overcharges are part of the price they pay to see their team in action. Are there analogues in the medical arena? What does this behavior suggest about the enthusiasm of pharmacists to provide information about massage, chiropractic treatment, or herbs as alternatives to a prescription for back pain?

To see how substitution affects price sensitivity, consider what would happen if there were 10 percent increases not just in the price of Claritin, but also in the prices of all allergy medications. Alice would not be so quick to cut her purchases of Claritin, since all of her alternatives had also increased in price. Considering the range of substitution provides more insight into why so much medical care is price inelastic. If I think that a particular medication is best for me, or that my doctor is the only one who can understand my headaches—that there are no good substitutes for the care she provides—I am not likely to be very sensitive to price. On the other hand, if I consider all doctors and allergy medications to be pretty much the same, I will be quite happy to switch to save a few dollars.

The change in demand due to a change in price also depends on the amount of time available to find a substitute. Acute need (heart attack, stroke) makes it impossible to shop around for the best price in medical care. However, you might have a long time to look for a surgeon to operate on your sore knee or to find a nursing home for your grandfather. With an extended time horizon, demand is more sensitive to price.

Price Elasticity and Marginal Revenue

If the percentage change in price is equal to the percentage change in quantity, demand is said to be "unit elastic."[2] Such demand has a special property. If the price of drugs went up by 2 percent, causing the quantity of prescriptions filled to decline also by 2 percent, the total amount spent would remain unchanged (see Figure 2.3). Firms facing elastic demand find that revenues increase when prices are reduced to sell more units. Firms facing inelastic demand find that total revenue goes down when they reduce price to sell more units.

Most medical care is relatively insensitive to price. Pain, critical needs, fear of uncertainty, and the prevalence of insurance tend to attenuate the role of price in patient decision making. Note what happens to a firm selling more of an inelastic good. Since increasing the quantity sold by 2 percent requires a large decline in price, perhaps 10 percent, the firm will actually lose money. For example, a firm that lowers price from $99 to $90 will see a 2 percent increase in units sold from 300 to 306, but will find that total revenue declined from $29,700 to $27,540. If demand had been unit elastic so that quantity rose by 10 percent to 330, total revenue would have remained unchanged at $29,700. If demand were elastic, so that the 10 percent price reduction led to a 50 percent increase in quantity (from 300 to 450), then total revenue would rise from $29,700 to $40,500. Conversely, the firm facing inelastic demand that sells fewer units will be able to raise the price by a larger percentage and will actually

FIGURE 2.3 Effect of Reducing Price on Total Revenue: Elastic, Unitary, and Inelastic Demand

The area within the dashed lines shows total revenue (Price × Quantity) at price of $10, the shaded area shows total revenues at price of $5.

take in more, not less, total revenue for a smaller quantity sold. For example, if raising the price from $10 to $11 reduced sales only slightly, from 50 units to 48, the marginal revenue from raising the price and selling fewer units would be $(48 \times \$11) - (50 \times \$10) = +\$28$. To summarize, raising prices (and reducing quantity) increases total revenue if demand is inelastic, and decreases total revenue if demand is elastic. Since most hospitals face very inelastic demand, especially for emergency services, it follows that they are charging less than profit-maximizing prices. Why don't they charge more if it would increase profits? The reasons are many, ranging from a desire to help the poor to administrative controls over allowable changes. Also, the sensitivity to price change today is significantly less than the ultimate response to a price change in the long run (after people organize protests, build another hospital, or shift their business across town).

Some medical goods—especially those for which consumers have several choices and good information in advance of purchase, such as allergy medications—are price elastic. For these goods, firms would reduce total revenues if they raised prices. Thus, it is more likely that a medical provider facing elastic demand is behaving more like a standard profit-maximizing firm. However, price controls, informal norms about overcharging, and other deviations from perfect competition may still be significant even in the more price-sensitive medical markets.

Price Discrimination

A firm does not necessarily face the same price elasticity in each market in which it operates. Where should it try to raise prices? In the market that is least price sensitive. Consider a young radiologist, Dr. Almon, who is starting a practice in Los Angeles. He works at a posh Beverly Hills clinic on Tuesday and Thursday, seeing a few patients, and on Monday, Wednesday, and Friday in a crowded clinic in East L.A., seeing a multitude of patients. Initially, he charges $25 to read a routine X-ray in both places. He finds that raising prices to $35 makes little difference in Beverly Hills, but he loses half his clients in East L.A. He can increase the profits of his overall practice by raising prices in Beverly Hills to $45 and lowering prices to $20 in East L.A. He is just as busy as he was before, but he is making more money.

Charging different prices in different markets is a standard strategy used by both business and nonprofit organizations to increase revenues. The practice is known as "price discrimination." Hot dogs cost more in baseball parks, clothes cost less if you work in the store (being there gives you great information and increases price sensitivity, and you may get an employee discount), and scholarships reduce the price of a college education for students who have the most choices (athletes and scholars). Price discrimination is socially accepted and pervasive in medicine. The most common form, charging more to patients with higher incomes and/or better insurance, has the advantage of appearing socially beneficial and fair. Even the federal government practices price discrimination, making higher income states pay a higher proportion of Medicaid expenditures. It seems right to charge less to those who can afford less, but is it? Milk and bread are not sold at a discount to people with less money, so why should radiology or physical therapy be? One major reason is that any attempt to sell bread and milk cheaper would be undercut by **arbitrage** (see the glossary for a definition): rich people would drive to East L.A. for low-priced groceries.

Why is there no arbitrage between Beverly Hills and East L.A. for Dr. Almon's services? Some patients will switch clinics to obtain a lower price, but only a few. Service markets are much easier to separate for purposes of price discrimination than goods markets because patients actually have to show up at the office to receive services. First, they must find out that the price differential exists, and then they must be willing to incur the extra travel costs.

The profit-maximizing price for a monopolist to charge in a market depends on the price elasticity. Dr. Almon can charge more in Beverly Hills because his patients are less price sensitive there, not because they have higher incomes, can afford more, or deserve to pay more (even though these reasons may count for something as well). He will choose to set prices in each market relative to the price-elasticity demand among consumers there. Looking at Figure 2.3, he would raise prices in (c) where demand is inelastic, and reduce prices in (a) where demand is elastic. It would be a mistake to assume that rich people are always less price sensitive than poor people. For example, inner city patients often lack transportation, which makes it difficult to shop around for the best prices. Many pharmaceuticals are priced higher in low-mobility city neighborhoods than they are in suburbs, where patients can easily drive to several stores and price competition is intense.

Just as markets can be separated by distance, they can also be separated by time. All that is needed for price discrimination is that consumers not be able to arbitrage by easily transferring goods from a low-price period to a high-price period. Movies are cheaper in the afternoon because customers are more price sensitive then—and they cannot transfer the picture to view it later in the evening.[3] Dining out is often less expensive during the week than on Saturday night for the same reason. Computer makers routinely roll out the newest machines at a high price to pick up the dollars of customers who must have a new machine now, then gradually reduce prices. Many DVD and CD producers practice price discrimination over time in the same way. One interesting question is why some forms of temporal price discrimination are discouraged. For instance, it would be considered highly unethical for a doctor to charge a patient more during an emergency than for similar services on a routine visit, even though it is clear that patients are very price inelastic during a medical emergency.

The frequency with which price discrimination is practiced in medicine was one of the factors that first convinced economists that physicians had a substantial monopoly power even though there are many physicians competing for patients in every city. The evidence that physicians use monopoly power to increase their incomes is well established, but tells only a small part of the story since there is even more persuasive evidence that physicians do not behave as profit-maximizing monopolists. Charging lower prices in poor neighborhoods may help increase total revenues, but providing care for free (which many physicians routinely do) is altruistic behavior inconsistent with profit maximization. As noted above, physicians also tend not to exploit patients' willingness to pay more during medical emergencies. Even more interesting to many economists is the evidence that for much of the medical care provided in hospitals and doctors' offices every day, demand is inelastic, but prices do not rise. As demonstrated earlier, a profit-maximizing firm would keep raising prices in the face of inelastic demand until it reached an elastic portion higher up the demand curve. While demand and supply analysis can give us some insight into the economics of medicine, it does not account for many of the features that make medicine a notable profession with a special place in human society rather than just another way to make money.

2.4 IS MONEY THE ONLY PRICE?

What does it mean to pay for something? To a politician, it may mean losing some votes or giving up a pet project. To a student going out partying on Sunday night, it may mean a headache and a lower grade on Monday's exam. To someone who wants a driver's license, it may mean hours of anxiety. In each case, something has to be given up to get something else. Economists often use the term "price" to refer to all of the things one has to give up to get some desirable good in trade. For medical care, it is common to talk about time, pain, and risk of death as part of the price of treatment. The concept of a **time price** was developed in recognition that the time spent traveling to and from the hospital, in treatment, and confined to bed in recovery has an opportunity cost. At the margin, the cost of time is roughly equivalent to the time price, and so a net price of time + money can be calculated. Pain is far more difficult to value, since there is no objective measure for it. A monk and a businessman can go through identical operations, and one has much more pain than the other. Furthermore, even if the pain were in some technical sense the same, the two patients might value it differently. Some people can function well with a level of pain that would make others miserable. For hazardous procedures such as thoracic surgery and chemotherapy, it may not be pain but the risk of death due to therapy that is the most important cost associated with treatment.

Services can be allocated to patients through time, pain, and risk just as they can through money. In Canada, where patients do not pay directly for most doctors' services, waiting times have increased. By discouraging those who are not willing to spend time waiting for care, the number of patients treated is limited just as effectively as it is when price is used to discourage those who are not willing to pay money for care. An example of allocation by pain is provided by pain clinics that insist on screening patients with an uncomfortable diagnostic procedure known as an electromyelogram (EMG). Patients who are not willing to undergo an EMG cannot obtain clinic services.

A fundamental difference between a money price and a "time price" or a "pain price" is that the money is transferred to the other party in the transaction. If an arm brace costs $10, the store receives $10. In contrast, if a patient has to wait six extra hours in the waiting room, no one receives those six hours. If an EMG is painful, a patient's willingness to undergo it may convince the therapist that the patient needs services, but the pain does not yield pleasure to the therapist. The patient's time and pain is a personal cost that does not directly benefit the provider. While every dollar spent on medicine by one person is income to someone else, contributing to GDP, there is no "circular flow of time" or "circular flow of pain." Economists tend to favor money prices as a rationing mechanism because they entail fewer such "dead weight" costs (waste) that provide no revenue or benefit to the supplier.

The Labor–Leisure Choice

The main price of any activity, the most significant opportunity cost forgone, is time. Work confronts us directly with this choice: how much money versus how much time for everything else? That trade-off between time and money is known by economists as the "labor–leisure choice" and establishes the price of your time in monetary terms. That is, if you are willing to take on extra work at $20 per hour, then your leisure must be worth less than $20, and if you turn down extra hours of work at $15, it becomes clear that your extra leisure is worth more than $15 per hour. Suppose I offered you $100 per hour—would you take it? Probably you would, but eventually working more and more hours, even at $100, isn't worth it (an example of diminishing marginal utility). Thus there is no such thing as the value of your time in general, only "at the margin." Even at $1,500 per hour, you would eventually want to stop and enjoy all that money rather than just work more and more—after all, the purpose of money is to spend it and enjoy life.

For those who work on a fixed salary, the labor–leisure choice and the varying marginal value of time may not be so immediately apparent as it is to a self-employed businessperson, such as a physician (see Chapter 6). For physicians, every extra dollar means more time away from home and family, and striving for success can lead to significant stress.

2.5   INPUTS AND PRODUCTION FUNCTIONS

The economic concept of supply is always that of a **supply curve**, emphasizing change, focusing on how firms will vary the amount supplied as price increases or decreases. The supply curve also relies on the ceteris paribus assumption, implicitly holding many factors constant that are not being talked about. Just as the demand curve is a marginal benefit curve, showing how people in the market are willing to pay for one more unit of a good, under perfect competition *the supply curve is a marginal cost curve*, showing how much must be paid to induce firms in the market to supply one more unit.[4]

Marginal Productivity

The cost of each additional unit, and thus the supply curve, is determined by the technology available to the firm, its managerial expertise, and the price of the inputs (labor, machinery, chemicals) that are used in production. While a more complete discussion of supply and production is provided in any basic economics textbook, one basic result from the theory of production should be made evident here. A firm will use more of input A and less of input B if that enables it to make the same amount of goods and services at lower cost (or to produce more for the same total cost). Thus an input that costs twice as much should be twice as productive. More precisely:

$$\frac{\textbf{Price Input A}}{\textbf{Price Input B}} = \frac{\textit{Marginal } \textbf{Productivity of A}}{\textit{Marginal } \textbf{Productivity of B}}$$

Why marginal productivity? Because we are analyzing the trade-off between using a bit more of A and a bit less of B, or using a bit more B and bit less A—that is, a decision at the margin. For example, producing tablets of a drug requires the use of both labor and machinery. It is not possible to run the factory without any labor, and barely possible to make drugs with no machinery. The company will choose the combination of labor and machinery that allows them to produce tablets at least cost. If each machine costs $150,000 and each technician costs $50,000, then the trade-off is 3:1. One implication of the formula above is that if the price of labor increases, then the company will try to use more labor-saving machinery to cut costs. Conversely, in a low-wage country there will be lots of labor and fewer machines (or older, cheaper machinery that is less automated). Once again, we see the operation of the *law of diminishing marginal returns.*

Production Functions

A table or formula showing exactly how much is produced with any possible combination of inputs is called a **production function**. Often the full set of relationships is so complex that only a few basic results—such as the formula above—are important in practice. Yet the concept of a production function provides a way of thinking about the economics of the situation even when quantification is imprecise and uncertain. The basic principles involved help us to analyze behavior, even if there is no money involved. Consider an athlete training for the Olympics. She must spend time both lifting weights and running in order to get in shape. If running an hour more is twice as helpful as lifting an hour more, then she will do more running and less lifting until the law of diminishing returns equalizes the rewards from each activity. If the "price" of running increases (perhaps because of an injury or because the weather gets cold) then she will optimize her workouts by shifting some time from running to lifting. Athletes, architects, financial firms and drug manufacturers all try to do their best—and doing so leads them to show the kind of behavior that economics analyzes.

2.6 MARKETS: THE INTERSECTION OF DEMAND AND SUPPLY

Competitive **markets** use prices *to allocate* goods and services to consumers who want them the most (in monetary terms) and *to pay* suppliers for producing those goods and services. As noted above, most real markets, and virtually all medical markets, depart to some degree from the model of perfect competition. Nevertheless, it is a useful starting point for analyzing the underlying economic forces that shape human transactions even when time, pain, uncertainty, and tradition cause substantial deviations from the simple model.

In most competitive markets with which you are familiar, supply and demand are quite distinct, and the process of organization and maximization is straightforward. The firms set whatever price they choose, and consumers decide how much to buy. Firms experiment with different prices to maximize profits, just as consumers experiment with different patterns of consumption to maximize the benefits they can obtain within their budgets. Market price is the point at which all the stresses are met and balanced. The decision rule for a profit-maximizing firm is quite simple. Sell more (lower your price) if the marginal revenue (MR) obtained is greater than the marginal cost (MC) of providing the goods. The firm will continue to lower price until the gains from additional sales are offset by the costs—that is, until MR = MC. In a perfectly competitive market with lots of buyers and sellers and perfect information and price transparency, the market demand curve is the same as the marginal revenue curve, and the marginal cost curve is the same as the supply curve. An increase in demand (due to an increase in incomes, population, or the price of competing substitute services) shifts the demand curve outward and then the market price and quantity will both increase as in Figure 2.4a. A supply increase (due to an improvement in productive technology or a reduction in input prices) shifts the supply curve outward, and then the market quantity will increase while the price falls as in Figure 2.4b.

FIGURE 2.4   Shifting Demand and Supply

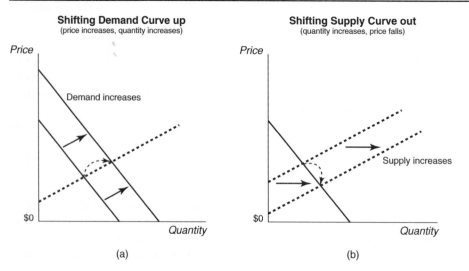

(a)   (b)

FIGURE 2.5   Fixed Supply and Fixed Demand

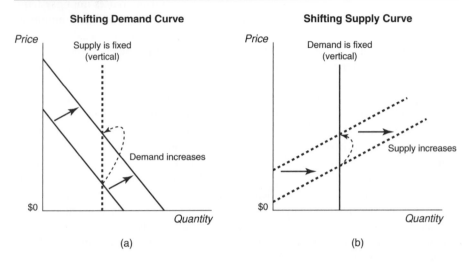

Shifting Demand Curve

Price

Supply is fixed
(vertical)

Demand increases

$0   Quantity

(a)

Shifting Supply Curve

Price

Demand is fixed
(vertical)

Supply increases

$0   Quantity

(b)

What would happen if the quantity supplied did not vary with price but were fixed? Then the supply "curve" would be a specific amount, as represented by the vertical line in Figure 2.5a. Since quantity is fixed by the vertical supply curve, only the demand curve can move, and all it can do is move price up and down. If, however, it was the quantity demanded that was fixed and not sensitive to price changes at all, then it would be said to be "perfectly inelastic" and the demand curve would be the vertical line in Figure 2.5b. Only the supply curve could move, and all it would do is to move price up and down without changing quantity. A totally inelastic vertical demand curve may seem to be an extreme case, but it corresponds rather closely to the concept of "medical need" (where treatment is determined totally by illness and prices are irrelevant). The other extreme case, a totally inelastic vertical supply curve demand curve, is fairly descriptive of the restricted entry into the profession controlled by licensure as discussed in Chapter 7.

2.7 NEED VERSUS DEMAND

Decisions regarding who gets what medical services, and when, are made mostly by doctors.[5] Doctors tend to consider medical decisions in terms of **need**. This perspective frames each decision as a response to a technical question regarding the level of service required to adequately treat the illness of a particular patient. Such a need-based medical perspective focuses on differences in health status and ignores the role of prices and incomes in allocating scarce resources. To concentrate on patient needs, physicians try not to think about who pays (employer, patient, taxpayer) and who gets paid (themselves, hospitals) so as not to be distracted by economic concerns. Their task is to operate within a given system to allocate resources and to advocate for patients. Because physicians are supposed to act in a patient's best interest, they try to behave as though prices are set anonymously by somebody else, as if the bills get paid to some agency unrelated to their personal incomes and as if insurance payments are really paid by some insurance company rather than taken out of wages.

For decisions regarding individual patients, a need-based medical perspective is suitable. Within the health care system, most physicians strive to do the best for their patients, not to change the system or help people they have never met. We do not ask doctors to determine what is best for taxpayers or employers or insurance companies, yet someone must address the question of financing. Economists are required to think about differences among systems: how choosing one set of insurance regulations means more children will get immunized but fewer elderly will receive home care, while another plan might protect accident victims, reduce taxes, or provide more incentives to work. The trade-offs between medical care and other goods, among different groups of patients and different types of care, are the issues that health economics is designed to address.

Although a *demand curve for medical care* is a concept that is awkward when applied to a specific individual who either is or is not sick, it is a tool that works well regarding groups of people or society as a whole. In large groups there is always a range of illnesses and a range of treatments available; therefore, the necessity for choices and balancing at the margin (i.e., an incremental adjustment of a little bit more or less) is obvious. Need and demand are different, yet complementary, perspectives on the complex set of human, financial, and scientific exchanges that constitute medicine. Done properly, the two perspectives can be combined to provide a fuller understanding of how the system works on different levels: the individual, the hospital, the company, the community, and society as a whole.

There is often an unnecessary and acrimonious division between economists and doctors in addressing medical care because the two are trying to answer different questions. For doctors, the question is: "If money is no problem, what should I do for *this patient*?" Economists, even health economists, have no particular skill at addressing such a question. They focus on a different issue: "Given that there is not enough for everyone to have all that they need, how can optimal decisions be made? Who should get treated? How should resources used for medical care vary across groups?" Doctors often think about the benefits of treatment in terms of the total or average, while economists focus on the margin: how much benefit would really come from treating a few more patients and what it would cost. It could be said that, to some extent, doctors ignore economics, whereas economists ignore medicine. Bringing the science of medicine together with the structure of economics is the interdisciplinary task of health economics.

2.8 THE PRODUCTION OF HEALTH

Epidemiologists joke that in order to live a long life, you should "choose good parents" to get healthy genes. From a population health perspective, it is also apparent that you should try to be born in the twentieth century rather than the nineteenth (or maybe in the twenty-second century if you have cancer or schizophrenia). It's probably better to be a statistician rather than a soldier, and to live in a healthy environment. Medical care is only one of many factors that determine health. However, it is the one that you have control over, that you can really choose to get when you want and need it most.

Determinants of Health

- Genetics
- Environment
- Childhood
- Nutrition/Lifestyle
- Medical care
- Biological limits

Thinking about the various determinants of health and reviewing the results of scientific studies make it apparent that medical care alone is not the most important factor.[6] A common estimate is that less than a quarter of the gain in life expectancy over the last 100 years is attributable to medical care, with improvements in public health, scientific knowledge, education, income per capita, and nutrition of relatively greater importance (see Chapter 16). This estimate understates the effect of medical *science*, since many improvements in nutrition, sanitation, and child rearing owe much to the discoveries made by doctors and physiologists. What is striking, though, is the extent of dependence on context (the place and time in which one is living) rather than personal choices, and that among those individual choices, the choice of which doctor or hospital to go to, or which drug to take, may be among the less important. If this is so, why is so much of health economics concerned with the business of medical care rather than other determinants of health?

How Much Is a Doctor Visit Worth?

From an economic perspective, the problem with using the environment, genetics, and the state of medical technology to modify health is that there is not much that you personally can do about them—they are not objects of choice, and hence are not analyzable as economic behavior. Even "lifestyle" is not much of a choice when the crucial medical decisions are being made. It does not really help to quit smoking, or eat more fruits and vegetables, the day after you have a heart attack or a stroke. Once an illness strikes, there is very little you can do—except go to the doctor and seek treatment.

How much is that treatment worth to you? It depends, and it does not depend very much upon how healthy you are. It does depend on how rich you are, because the more money you have, the less it matters if you have to pay $5,000 for treatment. It also depends on what your options are. If you can get free treatment through a Veterans Administration clinic, it may not be worth much to go to a private doctor. If just lying in bed and waiting will eventually allow you to get well, then it is only the time lost by being sick that makes it worthwhile to seek care. If the illness is life-threatening, treatment is worth a lot. Indeed, even if there is very little chance that some special new expensive drug will cure your cancer, you may quickly spend your life savings because it is the only chance you've got. The "opportunity cost" principle is at work here. The value of medical care depends in part on what you get from treatment, and on what you have to give up—what the best forgone alternative is.

The Demand for Medical Care Is *Derived* Demand

You get medical care only if you need it, if you think that doing so will improve your health. No one buys heart surgery, chemotherapy, or X-rays just because these are fun things to have or because the hospital is having a sale. As economists, you would say that the demand for medical care is **derived demand** and depends on the usefulness of the treatment in providing health. This is the case with most goods. A cast-iron skillet is bought not for the metal, but as a utensil for cooking food. Skis are bought for skiing, not to take up space in the closet. The business of health, the actual transactions observed—doctor visits, surgery, prescriptions—are in the derived realm of medical care, they are not direct trades for health itself. If we could simply buy health—adding to life expectancy the way one picks up a three-year guarantee on a new computer—then much of what makes health economics special would simply fade away.

Intermediate microeconomic theory courses build from an abstract base that begins with the ultimate source of demand, the utility function. Indifference curves, budget lines, and production functions are used to explore the mechanics of optimization. Such an approach is necessary for extending theory. It is possible to approach health economics in this way, but to do so is to risk losing track of all the structural features and organizational details that make medicine worthy of special study.

The Demand for Health: What Makes Medical Care Different

Most markets are driven by differences in consumer tastes and preferences. People buy red or black or blue shoes in all different sizes, music by Bono, Beethoven, or Tupac Shakur, and a great variety of books. If the price was right, you might even buy a shirt or a DVD that you were not all that sure you needed. Medical care is different. No one would get surgery unless they had suffered from progressive heart disease. Every patient may be different; but it is their illness rather than their preferences that distinguish them, and most patients with the same illness want the same medicine—not lots of variety to choose from. There is little individual variation in the "taste" for treatment.

When they are sick, patients expect to be cared for (which is hardly what they would expect from a visit to the mall), and they want someone to help them right now. At the moment of need, medical care is perhaps the only thing patients can buy to make themselves feel better. The other factors that determine health (genetics, lifestyle, accumulated exposure to pollutants, luck, nutritional history) cannot be purchased on demand. None of us can buy new parents. In the United States, however, most of us can buy the surgical care needed to mend and straighten a broken nose. In an emergency, we will spend a fortune on medical care that may or may not make a difference, but often we will not take the time to exercise, put down a pack of cigarettes, or buy low-dose aspirin for daily prevention. Life is the most important thing you have, and yet life-and-death decisions about yourself as a patient are largely made by a doctor, not by you. Furthermore, for the most part, someone else is paying the bill (see Chapters 4 and 5). These special features make medical care different enough that it is worthwhile to carefully study health economics. While the demand for medical care is derived demand, like that for many other goods, the derivation is not so straightforward as it is for batteries or a new printer.

Hospitals and doctors are often not allowed to set their own prices, but must accept prices that are set administratively by government or insurance companies. Patients buy what is needed (i.e., what providers think patients should buy) and do not pay any price directly, but rather pay some amount indirectly through taxes and premiums. The transactions are highly regulated, and some of the funding comes from grants and philanthropy rather than sales. This is so different from the model of perfect competition that legislators and actuaries want information that spells out what would happen if medical transactions were "normal." Chapter 3 provides cost-benefit and cost-effectiveness estimates that are used to derive the values that would be obtained ("shadow prices") and the decisions that would be made under regular economic principles (opportunity cost, marginalism, and so on). The practice of such methods of "economic evaluation" replicates on paper what a market would do if it existed, but with some of the rules changed: acting as if rich and poor had the same purchasing power, assuming that decisions are made in advance rather than at a time of crisis, and assuming that decisions are rationally based on medical evidence rather than on patient expectations and fears.

2.9 EFFICIENCY

Every economy must address certain basic questions: What should it produce? How? For whom? These are never purely technical questions, but at this stage, it is useful to concentrate on only partial answers—looking at the efficiency of production. Even if we assume away all conflict over values, distribution, and culture, the question of production efficiency can become very complicated. For the sake of clarity, the following discussion simplifies a complex interdependent process into a set of discrete steps (see Table 2.1).

TABLE 2.1	*Efficiency:* Steps in the Decision Process
How do we get the most out of these inputs?	*Supervisory efficiency*
What processes should be used?	*Technique efficiency*
What combination of inputs should be used?	*Cost minimization*
How much should be produced?	*Allocative efficiency (profit maximization)*
How should contracts be formed with customers and suppliers?	*Transaction efficiency*
How should production change over time?	*Dynamic efficiency*
What is best overall (externalities)?	*Social efficiency*

The first step, often forgotten, is *management*. Labor, capital, and other inputs do not produce anything unless effort is put into making them do so. If the machines or the workers are idle, if supplies are being pilfered, or if directions are not being followed, output falls. The second step concerns process—what *technology and techniques* to use. This decision depends not only on the state of knowledge at the time, but also on the price of labor, capital, and other inputs, as well as on external conditions. A "just-in-time" inventory system is not very efficient for a field hospital operating in the Cambodian jungle. Given adequate management and a choice of technology, the third step is the choice of the optimal combination of inputs to produce a specified level of output at the lowest cost. In many textbooks, the first two steps are called the **production function** and, in combination with input choice, are defined as **cost minimization**. Yet the production of output is not an end in itself.

What should that specified level of output be? The task of management is to provide benefits to customers and to satisfy salaried workers, unions, government, other interested parties, and vendors who supply inputs. Both demand- and supply-side considerations must enter into deciding how much to produce and how to distribute goods to consumers and income to producers. Jointly maximizing the total value of output is necessary to achieve *allocative efficiency*. In the abstract world of perfect competition, the optimum is identical to the profit-maximizing solution, in which marginal revenue equals marginal cost for all goods and services. In the real world, this is not always possible (see Chapter 14). We often care more about who gets care than about how much care is produced or about making it possible for the incomes of surgeons or pharmaceutical companies to rise.

Minimizing the cost of production and distributing output is not sufficient to guarantee efficiency. In health care, insurance, finance, and other complex systems, the costs of transacting and exchange are especially high and far exceed the direct costs of production. Salespeople, insurance agents, lawyers, clerks, computer programmers, and accountants are all components of *transaction costs*. Many of the chapters in this book address how an organization may be structured—through property rights, professional associations, and regulations—to economize on transaction costs and promote efficiency. Understanding *dynamic efficiency* (i.e., how to create technological and organizational change to improve economic efficiency in the future) is even more challenging. In his *History of Economic Analysis*, Joseph Schumpeter attributes growth in a mature market economy to a process of "creative destruction," yet little is known about how entrepreneurial renewal occurs, except that some current efficiency must be sacrificed.[7] A purely cost-minimizing organization is not likely to be the most creative. In order to make new discoveries, scientists need time to tinker undisturbed, whereas managers need free time to come up with ideas for new products and service delivery systems. Finally, the effects of economic decisions on everything else that matters must be factored in. The externalities and social costs of cloning, antibiotic use (and overuse), the creation of bacteria that excrete gold (yes, it is possible), muscle and brain enhancements, and the extension of life beyond 200 years cannot be taken lightly.

How can an organization lower costs? Why would it want to? Do not assume that more competition and greater efficiency are always good and desired by everyone. Competition is beneficial for the system as a whole, but for any given individual, more competition means more anxiety, more work, and a higher chance of failure. Greater efficiency comes at a cost to the individuals involved. First of all, change itself is difficult and often painful. Some workers will not be able to make the transition. Those who do must be willing to try harder, spend time learning new techniques, and make mistake after mistake in order to improve the process. All of the effort required to increase efficiency is clearly beneficial to the firm and to the economy, but it is worthwhile to the worker only to the extent that he or she shares in the benefits (e.g., through higher wages, greater job security, or more time off). If workers are paid by the hour regardless of the organization's output, why should they innovate or exert themselves? Capturing the benefits of increased productivity requires managers who know what gains are possible, an awareness of the costs to all of the people in the organization, and a willingness to share some of the gains with them.

SUGGESTIONS FOR FURTHER READING

Paul Heyne, *The Economic Way of Thinking* (Upper Saddle River, N.J.: Prentice Hall, 2002).
Joseph Newhouse, *Pricing the Priceless* (Cambridge, Mass.: MIT Press, 2002).
Thomas Rice, *The Economics of Health Reconsidered* (Chicago: Health Administration Press, 2002).

SUMMARY

1. The **law of demand** states that a rise in prices will, ceteris paribus (all other things being constant), cause the quantity purchased to fall. It is a reflection of the most fundamental trade-off a buyer must make, recognizing that having more of one good means having less of something else.

2. The concept of **need**, a professional assessment of the quantity of services required regardless of price or other trade-offs, is appropriate for individual decision making when price, cost, budget constraint, and other monetary factors have already been decided—for example, within a fully insured system. The concept of **demand**, a functional relationship (curve) showing how quantity changes as price changes, is more useful for decisions balancing the need for medical care with other goods, or allocating care among groups of people.

3. **Value** in trade is determined by supply and demand, not the inherent worth or usefulness of a medical treatment (the diamonds–water paradox).

4. The demand curve is a **marginal benefit** curve, tracing how much each additional unit of service is worth. Much of the total value of health care may lie in only a few units of service targeted to those most in need, with many subsequent services provided to a large number of people for little additional benefit. Some things that are essential to health (nutrition, exercise, preventive care) are plentiful and trade at a very low price in the market, whereas some services that make only a marginal contribution but are scarce (neurosurgery for someone who is already seriously ill) command a high price.

5. **Prices** arise from **transactions**, the actual exchange of money for service. Since most health care is funded by government or third-party insurance, there is no real price and therefore careful attention must be paid to the use of demand curve analysis, which depends on well-defined goods exchanged in markets that depend only on price.

6. The major **demand shifters** for most goods are income, prices of substitutes and complementary goods and services, population growth, and the catch-all term for

everything else, "taste." In medical care, **quality** and **illness status**, personal characteristics that would usually be lumped in with taste and not analyzed separately, are of greatest importance. In making a decision about value, **expectations** or perceptions, not actual results (which cannot be known in advance, or maybe ever) are what matter.

7. **Elasticities** measure the percentage change in one variable (quantity) with respect to the percentage change in another (price). Elasticities have the advantage of being dimensionless; they do not depend on units of measurement or the size of the market. Elasticity is virtually always larger the longer the **time allowed for adjustment**. The price elasticity facing a single firm, which has many other firms competing for the same customers, is much greater than the price elasticity of the market as a whole or of any individual consumer. A monopolist may use **price discrimination**, charging higher prices for the same good to consumers in the market with less price sensitivity (New York City versus Mexico City, insured versus uninsured, midnight versus daytime) to increase total revenues.

8. Empirical estimates of the **demand for medical care** usually show that it is quite **inelastic**, in the range of 0 to 0.5. However, elasticity is greater for items that are viewed as discretionary (dentistry, counseling) and less fully covered by insurance, and may well exceed 1.0 over the long period of time required to change health habits and beliefs.

9. **Marginal revenue**, the additional revenue that can be obtained by selling one more unit, is always less than average revenue (price), since a firm must reduce the price of goods to sell more. How much the price must be reduced depends on the elasticity of demand. A firm facing elastic demand that raises prices will see total revenues fall because the quantity demanded will fall by a larger percentage than the increase in price. A firm facing inelastic demand can raise prices and increase revenues because there will be only a small decrease in quantity sold.

10. The demand for medical care is **derived demand**. Even though other factors such as genetics, the environment, public health, lifestyle, and the state of technology are more important determinants of health, the only choice a patient can make at the time of need is whether or not to go to the hospital, and which one. For ordinary manufactured goods, supply and demand are clearly separated, with interaction occurring only through market forces. For health care, several factors make such a separation untenable: a strong physician–patient relationship of trust, the difficulty of making choices and obtaining information about life and death matters, and pervasive uncertainty. The tools of supply and demand analysis must be used with care and sometimes must be modified to conform to the realities of the health care market.

11. **Management** is necessary to make labor and capital productive and requires **converting economic principles into rules of behavior** that can be clearly communicated to employees, bosses, clients, and other partners. Management is not simple, because it is people, not things, that have to be managed, and because **decisions** must be made under **uncertainty**, based on **expectations**, without ever really knowing all the facts one would like to have.

12. **Efficiency** of the health care system depends not only on how effectively it is producing medical services and reducing costs, but also on its **dynamic** ability to generate new medical technology and on the performance of the system in meeting broader **social welfare** goals.

PROBLEMS

1. What is the difference between Mr. Axel's demand for physical therapy and his need for physical therapy?

2. What determines the value of a knee brace? How can an economist maintain that I am better off if I paid $7,000 for an operation that made my twisted knee worse rather than better?

3. Which are more elastic: dental visits or visits for the treatment of diabetes? Physician visits or hospital days? Psychiatry or orthopedics? Why?

4. If the price of office visits increases from $20 to $22 and the number of visits per family per year declines from 12 to 10, what is the price elasticity of demand?

5. If most college students are poor, why do they spend so much on discretionary goods, such as CDs? Are the ones who go on to medical school richer or poorer than the ones who take jobs right after graduation?

6. In the year 2005, in Anytown, suppose that one person is willing to pay $1,000 for relief from hay fever; another two are willing to pay $350; about five more are willing to pay $50; one is willing to pay $40; one is willing to pay $35; one each is willing to pay $34, $32, $30, and $28; about a dozen are willing to pay $10; four are willing to pay $5; and half of the rest of the town (another 75 people) are willing to pay $1.

   a. Draw the demand curve for hay fever relief in Anytown.

   b. What is the potential total benefit from relief of hay fever if it is provided to everyone who asks? To everyone willing to pay $35 or more?

   c. If the price of hay fever medication is $20, what is the quantity demanded? What is the quantity demanded if the price is $50? $5?

7. Suppose Betty's demand for physician visits is Quantity = 10 − (0.2 × Price).

   a. Draw Betty's demand curve.

   b. What is the quantity demanded at a price of $10 per visit? $25?

   c. At what price will she buy four visits? Eight visits?

   d. If the government agrees to pay half of her health care bills, what would her quantity demanded be at a price of $10 per visit? $25? Draw the new, subsidized demand curve.

   e. What is the elasticity between a price of $5 and $6 per visit? Around a price of $30? Around a quantity demanded of eight visits?

   f. Calculate the elasticity of the new, half-subsidized demand at a price of $30 per visit and compare it with the elasticity you obtained from the original demand curve. What is the new elasticity around eight visits?

8. Is chemotherapy a substitute for or a complement to cancer surgery?

9. Provide your own example of a diamonds–water paradox in medicine, in which the clearly more valuable service is provided at a much lower price.

10. In what units is Prozac purchased? What are the units in which psychotherapy is purchased?

11. If the price of a postoperative follow-up visit is reduced from $40 to $30, the number of patients returning for follow-up increases from 18 to 25.

a. What is the marginal revenue (MR)?

b. What is the price elasticity?

c. What would your estimate of MR and price elasticity be if the quantity demanded moved from 18 to 20 (instead of 25)?

12. Dr. Old requires that all services be paid for at time of treatment, in cash. If he decides to allow patients to pay with credit cards, will this increase or decrease demand? Will it increase or decrease price elasticity?

13. Which is more price elastic: the demand for Cesarean sections or the demand for vaginal deliveries? Why?

14. Ask four people what they have paid for (a) a drug, (b) minor care (office visit, physical therapy session), and (c) major care (hospitalization, surgical procedure). Find out how price sensitive they think they were for each. Do they think that everyone else receiving similar care paid the same amount as they did?

15. Our Lady of Dollars Hospital needs to increase total revenue to build a new chapel. The hospital wants to keep the total number of patients in each service area (emergency room, obstetrics ward, operating room, laboratory, cardiac ward) the same. How can the hospital use price discrimination to achieve this objective?

16. Give an example that shows how the health care system is willing to give up some current efficiency in the production of medical services to (a) increase dynamic efficiency by providing money for research and (b) increase social welfare.

17. Explain how current proposals to increase insurance for mental health services would affect the market for psychiatrists. Discuss short-term and long-term effects, equilibrium, and disequilibrium. Illustrate with supply and demand graphs.

18. If people are healthier, will their demand for medical care increase or decrease? (Be careful, this is a tricky question. Consider some analogies: If people become more coordinated, will their demand for athletic equipment rise or fall? If they become more knowledgeable, what happens to their demand for books?)

ENDNOTES

1. Barron H. Lerner, *Breast Cancer Wars* (New York: Oxford University Press, 2001); R. Rettig et al., *False Hope: Bone Marrow Transplantation for Breast Cancer* (Oxford, UK: Oxford University Press, 2007).
2. Although, it is, of course, opposite in sign due to the law of downward sloping demand—as price goes up, quantity goes down.
3. Video rentals cost the same whether you get them in the morning (when demand is low) or in the evening, because the customer can hold on to the disc and play it when they want to. However, video stores can still practice a form of "time price discrimination." My local store allows you to return a video "late" (until noon the next day) without penalty, since almost no one wants to watch videos in the early hours.
4. This perfect correspondence holds only under many simplifying assumptions. Supply curves may deviate from marginal costs, may be flat or upward sloping as well as downward sloping, and so on. These are complexities that must be faced, but are beyond the scope of this textbook. Too much attention to technical details relying on unreal assumptions (constant technology, perfect information, no charity) tends to obfuscate rather than clarify the workings of medical markets for most readers. A useful overview of some of the issues is provided in *The Economics of Health Reconsidered* by Thomas Rice, which is listed among the suggestions for further reading.
5. John Eisenberg, *Doctor's Decisions and the Cost of Medical Care* (Ann Arbor, Mich.: Health Administration Press, 1986).
6. Robert Fogel, *The Escape from Hunger and Premature Death, 1700–2100: Europe, America and the Third World* (New York: Cambridge University Press, 2004). See also the variety of sources cited in Chapter 16.
7. Joseph Schumpeter, *History of Economic Analysis* (New York: Oxford University Press, 1954).

CHAPTER 3

COST-BENEFIT AND COST-EFFECTIVENESS ANALYSIS

QUESTIONS

1. Is the effort expended to save one more life a total, average, or marginal cost?
2. How much is too much to spend to save someone's life? Is one life worth more than another?
3. Is it more beneficial to screen high-risk or low-risk people for disease?
4. Can the statistical probability of death among teenagers be compared to mortality among the retired elderly?
5. Is there necessarily a trade-off between health and money?
6. Which are better measures of the value of care: patient choices or professional judgments?
7. Why do decisions based on the average benefit from treatment lead to too much medical care?

Every choice involves a trade-off, giving up something to get something else (see Section 1.3). **Cost-benefit analysis** (**CBA**) replicates on paper the balancing of pros and cons, of advantages and disadvantages, that occurs implicitly in the marketplace.[1] CBA is also used for public decision making to protect the interests of children, homeless people, people with mental illness, people with substance abuse problems, and other disenfranchised individuals, as well as people of future generations who are not adequately represented in the marketplace. Moreover, many health care decisions are sufficiently complicated and threatening that the individual, even though otherwise competent, may have to depend on the judgment of physicians and other professionals to identify alternative treatments and determine the relative value of medical outcomes, rather than depending on his or her own informed choices. When decisions must be made involving third-party financing or multiparty public issues, an explicit decision-making process such as CBA replaces the independent market decisions of consumers. **Cost-effectiveness analysis** (**CEA**) is a truncated form of CBA, fully analyzing the cost side but not translating the benefits (lives saved, illnesses prevented, a patient's additional days of activity, extent of a patient's sight restored) into dollars. CEA is used in decision making to determine which alternatives are cheaper. A study evaluating whether hypertension screening, nutrition counseling, medication, or cardiac bypass surgery would provide the most additional years of life expectancy for each dollar spent is a cost-effectiveness study. A study evaluating whether cardiac bypass surgery adds a sufficient number of years to life expectancy to justify the amount spent on care is a cost-benefit study.

3.1   COST-BENEFIT ANALYSIS IS ABOUT MAKING CHOICES

"It is best to think of the cost-benefit approach as a way of organizing thought rather than as a substitute for it."

— *Michael Drummond*[2]

Every decision—whether in the market, the public sector, or the family—involves a form of CBA. Usually the consideration of costs and benefits is informal and internal; therefore, we are not conscious of it. All we can observe is the behavior that results from this internal weighing of costs and benefits. A study by Orley Ashenfelter and Michael Greenstone addressed the increase in traffic fatalities caused by the decision to raise speed limits on major interstate highways from 55 mph to 65 mph.[3] Raising speed limits allows cars to go faster and can reasonably be expected to cause more traffic fatalities. This study showed that higher speed limits led to slightly faster travel, about +2 mph (many people routinely exceed posted speed limits), saving approximately 45 million hours of travel time each year. However, faster travel led to more deaths—approximately 360 additional fatalities per year. Doing some simple calculations translates these findings into a cost of 125,000 hours per life. Valuing time at a wage rate $12.80 per hour yields an estimate of the value of time gained per life lost of $1.6 million. Differences in assumptions or in the estimation procedure can lead to a higher or lower value (the range here was $940,000 to $10 million). The point of the study is that the lives lost were not the result of a mistake or bad luck—they were a choice. We, the public, decided that it is worthwhile to have more people die on the road to save travel time for the rest. While economic analysis reveals the implied dollar value of this legislative choice, it is people's behavior, not economic analysis, that puts a value on human life.

An Everyday Example: Knee Injury

Life, and the health care system in particular, confronts us with difficult choices every day. Is it worth taking three hours, and possibly paying $80, to go to the emergency room (ER) so that a doctor can examine the throbbing knee you injured playing soccer? Since pain makes it difficult to think, it can be helpful to make a list of the pros and cons, such as the one in Table 3.1.

TABLE 3.1   Cost-Benefit Analysis (CBA) of Knee Injury (first step)

Pros (go to ER)	Cons (don't go to ER)
It might stop the pain.	It will cost $50, $100, or more.
It could prevent long-term injury.	It will take at least two, maybe four, hours.
I will feel stupid if something was wrong and I did not go.	Even if the injury is serious, surgery could make it worse.
I can't get any work done anyway while I sit here worrying.	My friends on the team will think I am not tough.

If you believe that the benefits of going to the ER outweigh the costs, you will go to the ER. Even if you do not write down the pros and cons, a similar sort of balancing takes place inside your head. CBA is the explicit and formal presentation of that mental balance sheet. Economics does not provide answers or make it easier to take bitter medicine, but it does clarify *how to ask the questions* to make decisions more rational and more consistent. First, you must *enumerate* the benefits and costs. Then, you must *quantify* each benefit and cost as accurately as possible, given what is known about the situation. For example, it is impossible to tell exactly how much time it will take in the ER, but you think a range of two to four hours is likely. You must then place a value on each benefit and cost. A balance sheet can be added up only if every line is expressed in the same terms, usually dollars. It does not make much sense to compare a benefit of $50 with a cost of ¥910 (yen), and there is no rule for determining how many hours of pain are worth avoiding a permanent limp; however, it is very clear that a cost of $500 is less than a benefit of $1,000.

This hypothetical knee injury can be used to illustrate CBA. The direct dollar cost of the ER visit is expected to be about $80, and you expect to wait for three hours. Since you could have been at a job where you were making $7 per hour, we can add $21 for the *opportunity cost* of the waiting time. (We will later consider the fact that surgery could make you worse instead of better.) Feeling that you are not as tough as other members of the team seems silly, but it is worth something. How much? Suppose that you were willing to pay $40 for crutches you really did not need, just to keep your friends from making fun of you. This $40 is your willingness to pay (WTP) to avoid a "wimp" label. Adding all the items, your estimated comprehensive total cost for going to the ER is $80 (charges) + $21 (time) + $40 (WTP fear) = $141 (see Table 3.2).

It is reasonable to assume that if your knee does not get better, you will eventually seek treatment, even if you don't go to the ER immediately. Let's suppose that before you injured your knee, you already had an appointment to go to the sports medicine clinic a week from Thursday. Therefore, the relevant costs and benefits are for treatment today versus treatment ten days from now, rather than for treatment versus no treatment. *Only count items that change as a result of your decision—the marginal benefits and costs.* The potential that an ER visit will stop the pain is counted on the list of pros and cons as a benefit. The labeling of pros and cons is somewhat arbitrary, and it is equally correct to say that the potential for continued pain is a cost of not going to the ER. A reduction in cost is the same as a benefit, since both are expressed in dollar terms. It is this equivalence that makes it possible to create a balance sheet for decision making. If benefits and costs are not expressed in the same terms (dollars) with opposite signs (+ or −), one cannot say which is greater.

What is it worth to stop the pain? Suppose that instead of going to the ER, you call the clinic and ask that someone phone in a prescription to the pharmacy. How much would you be **willing to pay** (**WTP**) to get the prescription rather than endure the pain? It is difficult to study, and may be impossible to work, when you are in pain. It is also difficult to sleep or even enjoy watching television. You might be willing to pay as much as $150 for relief from pain for the next ten days. This WTP is the correct measure of the value of benefit received. WTP is the mirror image of opportunity cost, the "highest-valued opportunity forgone." Different people put different values on what it is worth to endure pain. Furthermore, your estimate of its worth to you will be imprecise, because you don't frequently make deals trading money for pain. However, let's assume that if the pills cost $200, you would not buy them. That refusal would demonstrate that the value of pain relief is less than $200 for you. The value is somewhere between the lower ($0) and upper ($200) bounds. Is pain relief worth $40, $50, or $150? There is no way to tell unless we observe your entire demand curve.

There is an overstatement of benefits here, since the pills are virtually certain to relieve pain, whereas the visit to the ER may not. Clearly a chance of reduced pain is worth less than

TABLE 3.2	Knee Injury as an Example of Cost-Benefit Analysis

Scenario: I injured my knee playing soccer this afternoon. I called and got an appointment to go to orthopedics/sports medicine clinic in ten days, next Thursday. However, it has now begun to hurt a lot and I wonder if I should go to the emergency room (ER) right away.

CONS (don't go)

Visit to ER will cost $50, $100, or more.	Average = $80
(direct personal cost, ignores cost to insurance)	
I will have to wait for at least 2, maybe 4 hours.	3 hours × $7 = $21
(opportunity cost)	
My buddies on the team will think I am a wimp.	Willingness to pay = $40
(willing to pay $40 for crutches just to look good)	
Even if the injury is serious, surgery could make it worse.	Sunk cost = $0
(The issue is treatment today vs. Thursday, rather than	
treatment vs. no treatment, so only incremental costs count.)	
	Total cost $141

PROS (go to ER now)

Might stop the pain.	$150 × 1/3 = $50
(pills stop pain with certainty,	
going to ER just a 1-in-3 chance)	
Could prevent long-term injury.	$50,000 × 1/200 × .71 = $178
(WTP knee surgery $50,000, 1/200 chance,	
discount 7 years @ 5 percent)	
Will feel stupid if something was wrong and I did not go.	Willingness to pay = $20
("worried well" WTP for regular office visit)	
I can't get any work done anyway while I sit here	
worrying about it.	6 hours × $7 = $42
(time has same $ value for benefits and costs)	
	Total benefits $290

Observed behavior just gives us a lower bound that benefits exceed costs (>$141). Another observation, that I did not go when the wait was five hours and ER charges were $250, could provide an upper bound as well (<$325).

the certainty of reduced pain, but how much less? An approximate **adjustment for risk** can be made by calculating the **expected value**. Assume that we have made enough observations to know that the average person would be willing to pay $150 for relief of knee pain. If we think there is a one-in-three chance that going to the ER now will stop the pain, the expected benefit of this one-third chance of pain reduction is one-third of the $150 I would be willing to pay for certain pain reduction (i.e., $50).

The most important benefit of prompt treatment is probably a reduction in the risk of permanent injury. People are willing to pay thousands of dollars and undergo multiple operations to try to fix their knees. Although your personal valuation is the only one that is truly relevant, the values established by other people may provide a useful guide, since you have not had hundreds of opportunities to figure out how much an injury is worth. Let's say your estimate of the loss imposed by a bad knee is $50,000. This is a lot of money, but the possibility that going to the doctor this week rather than next week will make a difference is slight, maybe 0.5 percent (1 in 200). Thus, the expected value of prompt versus delayed treatment is one two-hundredths of $50,000, or $250. Furthermore, it is likely that if the knee does cause you a problem, it will be some years in the future. Although that is still bad, it is not as bad as being harmed today. To take into account the fact that the problem will not occur for a while, we should **time discount** the $250, using the methods provided in Section 3.6. This reduces the expected marginal benefit of prompt treatment to $178.

The fear of looking stupid for failing to seek treatment for a problem that could have been cured if treated promptly is common. Indeed, some studies have estimated that more than 70 percent of all initial visits to the doctor are made by the "worried well," people who have some vague symptom and just need evaluation and reassurance rather than treatment.[4] A modest lower bound for the value of worry reduction might be the price of a brief diagnostic office visit, or $20. What about the loss of work time due to pain and worry? These hours should be valued the same as the waiting time in the ER, or $7 an hour (the assumed hourly wage). If you think that a prompt visit will help you avoid six hours of wasted time between now and the appointment next Thursday, the prompt visit is worth 6 × $7, or $42. The sum total of all the benefits is $50 (pain) + $178 (prevention) + $20 (worry) + $42 (time) = $290.

You go to the ER. You may not realize it, but you have done a CBA—even if you never thought about the injury in these quantitative terms. Your action (going to the ER) reveals that your subjective estimate of total benefits ($290) outweighs your subjective estimate of total costs ($141). You don't find yourself being wheeled into the ER saying "I'm happy because I've got a projected consumer surplus of $149 ($290 − $141) from coming here." You just do it, or you don't. An economist considers your choice the true indicator of your personal and largely unconscious CBA. Your preferences would be revealed in more detail if we could observe you in another situation in which you chose not to go to the ER. Suppose you arrived at the ER and found that the wait would be five hours instead of three and that the clinic charge was $250 instead of $80, and you chose to leave without waiting to be seen. This would provide an analyst of your behavior with a second set of costs ($325), which in this case exceeded benefits and set an upper bound on estimated total benefits.

Stepwise Choices: Yes or No? How Much?

The initial decision, whether or not to do something, is decided by looking to see whether total benefits are likely to be greater than total costs. Given that you should seek medical care, the secondary decision then becomes "how much?" Suppose that going to a physical therapist two times per week helps to strengthen your knee, making it less painful to walk and run, seems well worth the time and money involved. If two times a week helps enough that you feel that paying the $50 ($25 for each visit) and using three hours (45 minutes for each therapy, 45 minutes to get there and back each time) is worthwhile, the question then becomes: would you be better off going three times a week? Perhaps going just once a week would be better? It is possible to make this secondary decision regarding "how much" by examining every possible course of action and evaluating which one gave the greatest net gains (Total Benefits − Total Costs). However, it is often easier to approach this decision incrementally, by asking whether doing a bit more increases benefits more than it increases costs. Going three times per week may make your knee significantly better, more than enough to outweigh the incremental "**marginal cost**" of $25 and 1.5 hours. Marginal cost is defined as the cost (all costs, not just the money paid out) of one additional unit.

Suppose you try going four times per week, and you think maybe it feels better, but not much different. In that case the marginal benefit (the incremental benefit of four visits compared to three visits) is small, less than the $25 and 1.5 hour marginal cost. Then consider going just once per week. You can save some time and money, but now you find that your knee does not seem to be healing properly, and frequently hurts after walking. We can summarize the decision process as follows: try increasing the visits a little, and if the additional (marginal) benefit is worth more than the additional (marginal) cost, keep going more and more as long as the marginal benefits exceed the marginal cost; stop at the point where marginal benefit = marginal cost. Conversely, when the increased visits result in the marginal cost being more than the marginal benefit, then you should reduce the quantity of medical care. Keep reducing as long as the marginal costs saved are greater than the marginal benefits given up; stop when marginal cost = marginal benefit.

Decision Rule:

Marginal Benefit > Marginal Cost	*Try doing more*
Marginal Benefit < Marginal Cost	*Try doing less*
Marginal Benefit = Marginal Cost	*Stop—this is the best one can do*

Notice how the additional benefits of therapy (usually) decline as more and more visits are used. This is an example of the principle of declining marginal productivity—and of the first law of demand (see Chapter 2). The first visit each week is much more valuable than the second, and once a person is going twice per week, they get little benefit from a third. A fourth visit is worth almost nothing to the person—not even worth the time it takes to get to the clinic. Therefore it is incorrect to ask what is "the" value of a physical therapy visit, since it depends on how many the person is already receiving. Only rarely would we try to decide whether we should get "some" or "no" medical care—and that would be when the condition to be treated is considered not very serious. Most medical decisions are marginal: should the patient get more medical care or less? The new pills or the old ones? It is important to recognize that *total*, *average*, and *marginal* costs convey different types of information for these decisions.

Calculating Marginal and Average Costs

Marginal and average cost per unit are accounting interpolations. The underlying quantity is "Total Cost." Usually, there is some cost just to have an organization, even if it is not producing goods and services. For any specific level of service, adding up all the bills (input costs plus fixed/sunk costs) provides an estimate of total cost for that level of production. If the quantity is increased (decreased), then Total Costs will increase (decrease). **The *difference* in Total Costs (divided by the number of additional units) is an estimate of *marginal* cost** at that level of production. The **Total Cost divided by the total number of units is an estimate of average cost**. (More thorough discussion of marginal, average, and total costs are found in most economics and accounting textbooks.) Estimation is considerably more rough and uncertain for any actual medical organization, such as a hospital, where most inputs are used in a wide variety of services and there is no single satisfactory measure of "quantity" (Days of care? Admissions? Surgeries performed? Number of lab tests? Should the ICU be counted the same as the outpatient radiology? See Chapter 8 for more discussion).

In Table 3.3, it can be seen that when the clinic has produced a quantity of 99 visits, the Total Cost is $2,000. With 100 visits, the Total Cost rises to $2,017, so the marginal cost of that visit is ($2,017 − $2,000)/(100 − 99) = $17. The average cost per visit of 100 visits is $2,017 ÷ 100 = $20.17 per visit. Similar calculations provide the marginal and average costs for the 101st and 102nd visits. Above that, the table provides larger leaps. To calculate the marginal cost per visit between 102 and 110 visits, the difference in cost must be divided by the 8-unit difference in units, and between 110 and 120 visits, the difference in total cost must be divided by the 10-unit difference in total units. Average cost is always calculated by the total cost divided by total quantity. Note, however, that this is only a calculation—an estimate based on total costs. There is no separate and definitive cost of the 105th visit, since it depends on sunk costs, how many units were already produced, production of other services

TABLE 3.3	Calculating Marginal and Average Costs Per Unit		
Units	**Total Cost**	**Marginal Cost**	**Average Cost**
Number	*Sum of All Fixed and Variable*	*Difference in Cost/ Difference in Units*	*Total Cost/ Total Units*
99	$2,000		
100	2,017	$17.00	$20.17
101	2,034	17.00	20.14
102	2,052	18.00	20.12
110	2,200	18.50	20.00
120	2,390	19.00	19.92
130	2,600	21.00	20.00
140	2,900	30.00	20.71

in the building, and other factors. "Costs per unit" are guidelines for making decisions based on accounting data, not elements of absolute truth.

Defining Marginal: What Is the Decision?

The term "marginal," much favored by economists, means "the change in *xxxx*." The decision being made defines the margin. The change in *how much* treatment a patient receives is called the intensity margin. In the example above, intensity is measured by the number of physical therapy visits per week. It could be the number of lab tests, the number of pills taken in a week, or the number of milligrams of the drug in each pill, or whether the treatment was given by a family doctor, a specialist, a hospital, or the intensive care unit of a medical center. All represent increases where greater **intensity** of treatment costs more. The decision of *how many* patients to treat is often called the **severity** or risk margin, and is usually stated in terms of the qualifications for treatment: for example those with blood pressure >200, between 160 and 199, between 140 and 159, between 120 and 139, or anything over 100. The looser the criteria, the more patients treated and the greater the costs. In an accident, the risk margin might be (a) all patients with open fractures and unconscious, (b) any fractures, (c) anyone bruised or hurt. For a screening program it could be (a) infants, (b) children, (c) mothers, (d) everyone else. The important point to recognize is that some patients will benefit more than others.

Intensity Margin Example: How Much Treatment?   Most diseases can be treated in different ways, but often the newest or most powerful treatment costs more than a commonly used treatment that is effective most of the time. Suppose that a patient is admitted with cancer, and without treatment there is only a 30 percent chance that the patient will be alive one year later. With the standard drug A (generic) treatment, average one-year survival increases to 62 percent. Somewhat better results, 65 percent, are sometimes achieved with drug B, but it is still under patent and thus costs significantly more for a year's treatment: $5,500 instead of $400. There is a brand new drug C, just out, and a preliminary trial indicates that it might provide 67 percent one-year survival. The company claims, correctly, that survival is doubled, and justifies a premium price of $80,000.

Using drug A provides a gain of 32 percent (from 30 percent to 62 percent), whereas for drug B and C the gain (compared to no treatment) is 35 percent and 37 percent, respectively. The cost per year of life saved using drug A is $400 ÷ 32 percent = $1,250, an amount that

TABLE 3.4	Marginal Analysis: What Quality/Intensity of Treatment?		
	Survival Rate	Cost	Cost per Year of Life Saved
No treatment	30%	$ 0	
Drug A	62%	400	$ 1,250
Drug B	65%	5,500	15,714
Drug C	67%	80,000	216,216
Compare B to A	3%	5,100	170,000
Compare C to A	5%	79,600	1,592,000
Compare C to B	2%	74,500	3,725,000

no one would question is worthwhile.[5] For drug B and drug C the cost per year of life saved is similarly calculated and is $15,714 and $216,216, respectively. The cost of drug C is high, but most people would agree that spending $200,000 or more to save a life is still worthwhile.

This initial analysis does not reflect the actual decision facing the doctor, which is whether to use drug C, drug B, or drug A; giving no treatment is not really an option, and thus is not a valid basis for comparison. The doctor should compare drug C with the alternatives, as shown in the lower section of Table 3.4. Compared to drug B, the expensive drug C provides only a 2 percent gain in survival (from 65 percent to 67 percent) at an additional cost of $74,500 (from $5,500 to $80,000), so each additional year of life saved has an estimated cost of $74,500 ÷ 0.02 = $3,725,000. To obtain such a small gain for so much expenditure might make many people hesitate, and suggest that it might be worthwhile to use the extra $3 million for additional primary care or vaccinations, and stick with the less expensive drug B or even drug A.

The benefits of drug C depend on what it is compared to. When compared to nothing at all, the cost ($80,000) seems high but not exorbitant relative to the gain (an increase in survival from 30 percent to 67 percent). By applying the concept of *opportunity cost*, the economic analyst makes a more valid comparison to the best available alternative, drug B, and sees that the cost (an additional $74,500) is very large relative to the small potential gain (increasing survival from 65 percent to 67 percent). Comparing drug C to nothing gives the analyst average cost ($216,216 per year of life saved). The appropriate comparison is marginal (incremental), taking account of opportunity cost by comparing drug C to the best available alternative, and shows an added cost of $3,725,000 per year of life added.

An intriguing study of the effect of more intense treatment on patient outcomes was conducted by Mark McClellan, Barbara McNeil, and Joseph Newhouse of Harvard (McClellan, a physician and Ph.D. economist, subsequently became head of the FDA and then head of the Medicare/Medicaid Programs).[6] They examined what happened to Medicare patients who had an acute myocardial infarction (MI). This is a useful group to study because virtually all of them get admitted to the hospital and receive some treatment, and thus have records that can be tabulated. The study separated the patients into two groups: those who lived close to hospitals with cardiac catheterization facilities and those that lived more than 2.5 miles from such hospitals. Examination of more than 200,000 medical records showed that patients living closer to hospitals with catheterization facilities were six times more likely to be admitted to hospitals with such facilities, were twice as likely to get catheterized within seven days, and about 50 percent more likely to get a coronary artery bypass graft (CABG) or percutaneous transluminal coronary artery angioplasty (PCTA) within 90 days. These results are not surprising: those closest to hospitals with facilities for advanced invasive procedures are more likely to be admitted there, and to receive such procedures, even if their medical conditions are no different from those of patients living farther away. There was a significant initial benefit from getting more intense care: only 7.5 percent of the patients living close to an advanced hospital died within one day, compared to 8.9 percent of those living farther away. Other than avoiding mortality in the first 24 hours, the use of more procedures of the patients living closer to advanced hospitals did not seem to provide much benefit, and the long-term mortality of the two groups was essentially the same. One speculation is that rapid advanced treatment temporarily saved a few lives, but most of these patients did not fare any better than others receiving less treatment, and a substantial fraction of the 1.4 percent of patients whose lives were prolonged past 24 hours were in fact still very seriously ill, sufficiently so that more than half of them died within two years. Taxpayers funding Medicare have to ask: was it worth millions of dollars to provide extra treatments to perhaps save less than 1 percent of elderly heart attack patients, or should some of those funds have been spent on prevention efforts?

Severity Margin Example: Which Patients to Treat? How Many?   Is every patient the same? Obviously not. How should an economic evaluation account for the differences in patients? Any given therapy is likely to benefit some patients quite a lot. Other patients may obtain only moderate benefit, and some very little. Usually it is the people who are most severely ill who stand to benefit most. Consider cardiac surgery and heart transplants. It could be life saving for someone whose heart is very weak and about to give out. Severe angina can be a symptom of serious disease. Patients with mild angina are usually less ill. Sometimes three or four heart vessels are occluded, but those with only one-vessel occlusion do not stand to benefit as much. Malfunctions of the heart valves can cause death, but many minor valve malfunctions that do not seriously threaten one's health can be heard through a stethoscope. Much of the work of medicine is diagnostic, trying to determine who will benefit, and how much, from a particular therapy. Imagine patients going into a hospital to receive surgery that restored their hearts to perfect health, or a transplanted heart that was totally healthy. The greatest benefit would accrue to those most seriously ill, the next largest benefit to those who are seriously ill but not quite as bad off, then those who are moderately ill, then to those with mild illness, and so forth. Hypothetically, let us classify patients by degree of illness/likelihood of benefit into groups called Stage V, Stage IV, Stage III, Stage II, and Stage I disease, and also those who seem to have symptoms but on further examination are found not to have any heart disease as Stage 0. Typically, there are a few patients who are very seriously ill and stand to benefit quite a lot, and a rather large number of patients with minor illness who stand to benefit only slightly. Table 3.5 presents the data for our hypothetical example illustrating changes in the criteria used to determine which patients receive treatment.

The "gain" is assumed to be additional years of life obtained from having a healthier heart. The most seriously ill patients (Stage V) gain a lot: 30 extra years of life. Seriously ill patients (Stage IV) gain 10 years, while ill patients (Stage III) gain half that much. Moderately ill patients (Stage II) gain just 2 years of life, and slightly ill patients (Stage I) gain 1 year.

TABLE 3.5   Marginal Analysis: Severity (Which Patients to Treat? How Many?)

	Stage V	Stage IV	Stage III	Stage II	Stage I	Stage 0	Cumulative Total
Gain (each person)	30	10	5	2	1	0	274
Number of Patients Coming to the Clinic	4	6	10	12	20	48	100

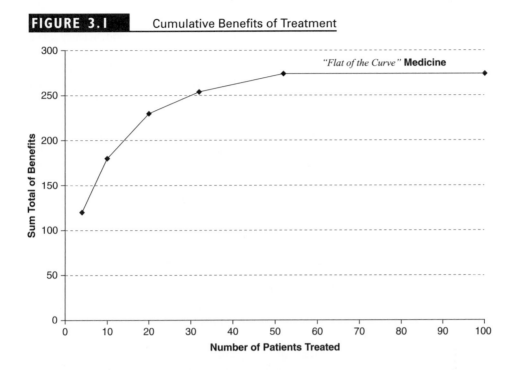

FIGURE 3.1   Cumulative Benefits of Treatment

Diagnostic exams show that almost half, 48 percent, have no defects that would benefit from surgery (Stage 0). If the 4 patients with most severe illness were treated, the total gains would be 120 additional years of life (gain of 30 years each times 4). If all 100 patients were treated, the total gains would be 274 years of life, or an average of 2.74 each. Most clinics would be very happy if they could increase the lifespan of the average patient by more than 2 years—but note how much more effective the clinic would be if it did not treat the 48 people whose diagnostic workup showed no defects: the average gain for the remaining 52 patients would be 274 ÷ 52 = 5.3 years of life gained per person. The more the therapy is concentrated on those who benefit most, the greater the gains for each surgery performed. The marginal analysis shows that more than half of the total gains are obtained just by treating the two sickest groups of patients, Stage IV and Stage V.

Assuming that the clinic does what most doctors would want to do, and treat first those patients who are sickest and stand to benefit most, then the total benefits obtained by treating more and more patients are displayed graphically in Figure 3.1. Since there are no additional benefits after 52 patients are treated, the total benefits line flattens out. This is what many analysts call "flat of the curve medicine": extending a useful therapy to so many patients (including those that do not need it very much or at all) that there are no additional benefits. Note that the average benefit is still large, because those few patients who really benefited a lot bring the average up even though the many patients with little or no benefit add little or nothing.

Opportunity Cost: Looking at Alternatives

> "Growing old is a pretty lousy thing to have happen to you, until you consider the alternative."
>
> — *George Burns* (and lots of others who were not comedians)

Costs and benefits are not intrinsic or absolute values; they are comparative values. Once a patient is diagnosed with pancreatic cancer or human immunodeficiency virus (HIV) infection, all of the alternatives are pretty bad, but four years of life might be a lot better than two years of life, and the ability to play tennis a lot better than continuous nausea. On the other hand, all of the alternatives facing a student graduating with a master's degree in medical information systems may look good, yet living in San Francisco might be more appealing than living in San Antonio, and the possibility of moving up into corporate systems management within a national health care chain might be more appealing than remaining the director of records in a small community hospital. To make a decision, the relevant question is not how good or how bad the situation is, but rather: What are the options? The appropriate measure of economic cost is **opportunity cost**, determined by the highest-valued alternative forgone when a decision is made. Thus, in choosing a $45,000 job in San Francisco, the graduating student who gives up a $50,000 job in San Antonio is "paying" an opportunity cost of $5,000. The cost of not taking an experimental drug is the forgone chance of living an extra two years or feeling better.

It is important to consider opportunity cost in relation to "the next best" option. Supporters of a medical treatment or program sometimes compare it with an alternative that is obviously bad, which makes it possible to overstate costs and benefits (e.g., "Do you want to go to the dentist today, or would you rather have all your teeth fall out?" or "The proposed health insurance program can save the country from socialized medicine.") Most of us are able to detect such bias in the presentation of arguments, but we may miss more subtle distortions. Often a decision is presented as all or nothing, when the real alternatives are between different levels of action. The choices are not limited to flossing your teeth every day or never; they include flossing occasionally, every other day, or after each meal.

Expected Value

The general principle is to make a decision in which benefits (B) are greater than costs (C), or B > C. Suppose, however, that benefits or costs are uncertain. Five hundred grams of Xloxidine might cure you or leave you in the same condition. Surgery may cause you to miss one or five weeks of work. A choice must be made, based on the best possible information or the best guess, long before the outcome of treatment is revealed. The estimate of what is likely to happen is called the **expected value**, a core concept of risk analysis. If the analysis concerns many people, in which case the law of large numbers applies, the expected value is just the average.[7] For a single person facing an event that either will or will not happen, the expected value is the value of that event (benefit or cost) multiplied by the fraction of the time that the event will occur:

Expected Value of Z = (Probability that Z will occur) × (Value of Z)

A patient receiving chemotherapy with a 70 percent chance of death may live, while a patient receiving surgery with a 20 percent chance of death may not. Yet the decision must be made in advance and should maximize expected welfare in the face of this uncertainty. Of course, after the fact, the patient's family may wish that they had done something differently. To say that the optimal choice sometimes turns out worse is simply to recognize that life is full of risks. CBA is based on the best available estimate of probability. It may be a guess or, preferably, an extrapolation from well-designed studies reported in scientific journals to which the analyst refers. "I don't know," or "I need more information," are not valid responses, since a decision is going to be made regardless of how much is known. The job of the analyst is to get the best estimate and indicate the sources of information and the range of variability. A clear discussion of the alternatives in specific terms is required. Under this useful shorthand formula, an option is chosen if

$$(\text{Probability of Gain}) \times (\text{Benefit}) > (\text{Probability of Loss}) \times (\text{Cost})$$

In this formula, attention is focused separately on the uncertainty and the relative values that interact in the decision-making process. Judgmental advice, such as "it is better to get the operation and risk dying than not get the operation and remain impaired" jumbles probabilities and values together, hiding information and making communication more difficult. Such commingled statements do not make the patient think about how much it is worth to live impaired compared with dying, or to consider specifically the percentage probability of partial recovery or death. An explicit recognition of benefits, costs, and risks provides a better ground for shared decision making between physician and patient.

For situations involving many people and events with more than one outcome, the expected value is a weighted average of all possibilities. The calculation must be summed (Σ) across all categories of people and all possible outcomes to arrive at the expected value for the group as a whole:

$$\text{Expected Value} = \frac{\sum (\text{number of people for whom } \mathbf{Z}_i \text{ occurs}) \times (\text{Value of } \mathbf{Z}_i)}{\text{Total number of people}}$$

3.2 MAXIMIZATION: FINDING THE OPTIMUM

Economists use a powerful analytical rule to simplify decision making: **the decision between alternatives depends only on factors that change**. Therefore it is not necessary to examine the full range of possibilities but only to look at doing a little more or a little less (i.e., to consider changes at the margin) to determine whether a decision is optimal. If the marginal benefits of a therapy are greater than the marginal costs, more should be done. If marginal costs are greater than marginal benefits, less should be done.

If two alternatives share a common feature, that feature will not play a major role in determining which alternative to choose. For example, consider how many days a woman should remain in the hospital after delivering a baby. One proposal might be discharge from hospital after 24 hours ($10,000 for the delivery and $1,000 for one day in the hospital) and another proposal could be discharge after 48 hours ($10,000 for delivery and $2,000 for two days in the hospital). Both alternatives include the cost of delivery (and one day in the hospital), so their difference will cancel out the factor(s) that are the same. The extra cost of the 48 hour proposal is $1,000 ($12,000 − $11,000). The insight from economics is that it is the "extra" or "marginal" amounts that matter. Thus, the extra cost should be compared with the extra benefits.

More medical care usually makes people healthier. Physicians, rightly, concentrate on benefits as opposed to costs and often try to do as much as possible. However, people who use more resources to obtain medical care have fewer resources available for food, entertainment, housing, and other goods they want. Economics is concerned with trade-offs. What is the appropriate balance between medical care and other goods? How many doctors, nurses, and hospitals should there be? Economists insist that both costs and benefits be considered in making a decision. Economists also approach the decision differently from most physicians, asking not what is right or wrong, but whether a little more or a little less would make things better or worse. An economist will use marginal analysis to **optimize**, moving toward a maximum net benefit in small steps. To apply principles of maximization and use mathematics to estimate values, economists must abstract from other elements, ignoring some of the complexity of medical conditions and framing the issues in terms of dollars. Prices, costs, taxes, bids, contracts, and so on are the language used by economists to communicate human desires and limitations. The task of CBA is to make that language clear and applicable to the situation at hand, and to present the essential facts and trade-offs in a way that is easily understood by physicians, the public, and politicians.

Declining Marginal Benefits

The **marginal benefit** is the value to consumers of one more unit of service. Willingness to pay for additional care declines as more and more is provided; therefore, the marginal benefit curve slopes downward. It looks like the demand curve; in fact, the marginal benefit curve and the demand curve are the same. To see why, remember that the demand curve is a schedule showing what quantity a consumer will buy at different prices. As long as marginal benefit exceeds the price, consumers will continue to buy. The quantity at which they have had enough and stop buying is the quantity at which the marginal benefit has fallen to the point where it is just equal to price. The quantity bought at price $P is the same as the quantity at which marginal benefit is $P; the marginal benefit (stated in dollars) of one more unit for a consumer who already has quantity Q is the same as the price they are willing to pay for one more unit.

Even though society benefits from having more medical care, the additional increment of benefit from each additional hospital day or doctor visit tends to become smaller and smaller as more services are provided. There are two reasons for declining marginal benefits. As more treatments are provided, they are given to less and less severely ill people, who are less likely to benefit. In ERs and Army field hospitals, the process of giving treatment first to those who are most likely to be helped is known as triage. Although it does not use mathematics or geometry, triage operates on the same principles as economic maximization—and both field triage and economic optimization suggest that efficiency is gained by treating the patient most likely to benefit first.

The other cause of declining marginal benefits is that for any single person, the benefit from having additional units of medical service tends to decline as more and more services are used, just as benefit from consuming additional pizzas or sodas or pretzels per day tends to decline as the second, third, and fourth are consumed. In Figure 3.2 (top), the fact that more medical care will improve health is shown by the rise in the total benefit curve. The fact that marginal benefits become smaller as more and more services are used shows up as a lower rate of increase, reducing the slope to make it flatter.

Optimization: Maximum Net Benefits

Costs are the other side of the decision. Every additional unit of treatment adds to total costs. After start-up, the marginal cost of producing another unit of medical treatment is usually constant or rising as the total number of treatments increases. Each additional hospital bed tends to cost as much as or more than the last one, and each additional nurse who is hired expects to get paid as much as or more than the last one hired. At some point, the additional costs of extra treatments will outweigh the additional benefits. An optimum is where the net gain (benefits − costs) is largest. This can be found diagrammatically by plotting both benefits and costs on the horizontal axis and choosing the point where the distance between them is greatest (Figure 3.2, top), equivalently by plotting net gains on the horizontal axis and choosing the quantity of care where it peaks (Figure 3.2, middle), or finally by plotting the marginal benefit and marginal cost curves and choosing the point where they cross (Figure 3.2, bottom).

| FIGURE 3.2 | Total, Net, and Marginal Benefits and Costs |

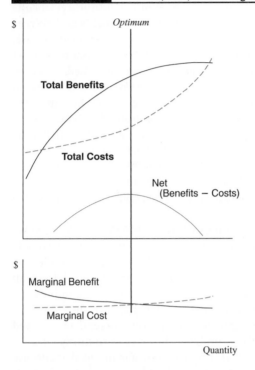

A geometric property in Figure 3.2 is frequently used by economists to determine the point at which a maximum is reached: at the peak of the net gains curve it is flat (horizontal); therefore, its slope is 0 (Figure 3.2, middle). The total benefit and total cost curves (Figure 3.2, top) have a corresponding property: at the point where net gains are maximized, their slopes are equal; therefore, the difference in the slopes is 0. More generally, since "net gains" are defined as (benefits − costs), $slope_{net\ gains} = slope_{benefits} − slope_{costs}$, and at the maximum, $slope_{net\ gains} = 0$. These principles of maximization common to geometry and calculus can be stated in everyday terms. As any curve or function approaches a peak, the incremental increases become smaller and smaller. The maximum occurs at the turning point, where the curve goes from rising (positive) to falling (negative). To the left, marginal gains are positive, and to the right, marginal gains are negative. Here, as the optimum is reached, the marginal gains from adding a bit more or a bit less are 0. To determine the maximum distance between two curves, the focus is on the incremental or marginal change of one curve relative to another. If the additional (marginal) benefit from providing one more treatment is larger than the additional (marginal) cost, providing more treatments will make society better off (Figure 3.2, bottom). If the additional benefit from providing one more treatment is smaller than the additional cost, providing more treatments will make society worse off. At the optimum, the additional benefit will just offset the marginal cost; therefore, there is no change in net gains (marginal gain = 0).

Maximum net gains at   Marginal Benefit = Marginal Cost   *so that*   MB − MC = 0

Why Marginals Are "the Max," and Averages Are Misleading

Although we can use geometry or calculus to determine the average cost and average benefit (the slope of a line from the origin to the total benefit curve or total cost curve, respectively), these common accounting measures are not especially useful for determining optimization. The largest average gain usually occurs to the right of the point at which marginal costs have long exceeded marginal benefits. **A society that uses average benefits and average costs to make medical decisions usually ends up providing far too much medical care.** To see why, look back at Table 3.5 and Figure 3.1. The average benefit from treating all 100 patients coming to the clinic is 2.74 years of life gained per person treated. However, focusing treatment on the more seriously ill patients and refraining from treating those who are not very sick (Stages 0 and I) allows the clinic to obtain more than 80 percent of the benefits by treating just 20 percent of the patients—and for this group the average gain is more than 10 life-years per person. Treating patients who are not very sick is "flat of the curve medicine," wasting good therapy by applying it to a mass of patients who do not stand to benefit very much. It is not that surgery X or drug Y is not worthwhile, it is that because it is so valuable for a few well chosen patients, its use is extended to all kinds of patients who think they might benefit but in fact do not benefit very much (although sometimes the providers benefit a lot from increased sales).[8]

Reviewing economic evaluations of medical care, such as the 1975 classic, "What Do We Gain from the Sixth Stool Guaiac?" discussed at length in earlier editions of this textbook, reveals several important elements of CBA.[9] First, the marginal cost is often considerably different from the average cost. Second, the direct cost (screening) may be much less than the indirect costs of dealing with unintended side effects (e.g., from the barium enema test to rule out cancer among those with false positive results). Together, these observations suggest the following *rule for making medicine cost-effective:* **target diagnosis and treatment to persons at highest risk.** This basic principle, however, is routinely violated. Our desire to do as much as possible for as many people as possible means that effective screening programs are extended to everyone—including healthy young people with almost no risk of disease—making the marginal cost per case very high. At least some of the rapid increase in medical care costs can be attributed to this general failure to distinguish average costs from marginal costs, when marginal costs are most relevant to the question of how much medical care should be provided. Thousands of lives are saved by modern medicine each year, and more than 90 percent of those lives could still be saved even if half the medical care system were eliminated, as long as we continued to screen and treat those at highest risk.[10]

3.3   MEASURING BENEFITS

For most medical programs, the three major types of benefits are as follows:

- Health
- Productivity
- Reductions in future medical costs

Health

Better health is the most direct and important gain from medical care. Yet it is often difficult to determine how much change in health status actually results from medical care and how much results from waiting for things to heal, random variation, nutrition, and other factors. If a cancer patient lives eight months, is that six months longer than the patient would have had without treatment, or four months fewer, since chemotherapy is so toxic?[11]

Such obstacles to valid measurement of the effects of treatment usually limit CBA to studies of large groups of patients in which statistics can be used to estimate average effects. After the effect of therapy is measured (comparing one treatment to an alternative), the problem of placing a dollar value on the improvement in health must be faced. If faster treatment can give a heart-attack victim four more months of life, is that worth $1,000? $100,000? $1,000,000? Or perhaps $19.95? Most people would agree that gaining an extra year of life is worth more than $1,000 and less than $1,000,000. However, deciding exactly where within that range the appropriate value lies is crucial in such determinations as whether it is worth spending $50 million to upgrade the 911 emergency telephone system in order to treat people quicker. Some innovative techniques for measuring the value of life are explored in Section 3.5, but it is important to recognize now how difficult and ambiguous the measurement process is. Most health care provides more subtle gains (e.g., physical therapy improves mobility, medication lessens the pain from a headache), which are even harder to measure in dollar terms.

A significant fraction of all visits to the doctor, perhaps as many as half, do not make a difference in health status. Either the symptoms that led people to seek care were not caused by anything serious, or the condition was such that medical care could not change the course of the disease. These visits provide care, reassurance, and social support, but not cure. The benefits of caring are often left uncounted because they are small relative to the gains from a dramatic cure. Also, much the same benefit can often be obtained regardless of the type or scientific validity of the treatment (e.g., a naturopath may provide sympathy as well as or better than a trained neurologist). When one considers how many more people obtain the benefits of caring from medical professionals than obtain large health gains from cures, the cumulative importance of subjective personal assessments look quite large.

Productivity

The earliest economists were not so much interested in the value of health itself as in how much a healthier workforce could contribute to the economy. In 1662, Sir William Petty proposed a plan to improve the treatment of the plague in England, and wrote an analysis showing that the additional costs would be more than covered by the additional taxes obtained from having more people at work.[12] When modern economists turned their attention to evaluating health programs in the 1950s and 1960s, the difficulty of directly measuring and valuing health improvements led them to consider increases in earnings due to greater life expectancy and reduced sick days as proxy measures. Such gains can be measured with precision, are objectively verifiable, and are easy to obtain from existing labor statistics. These advantages made earnings the primary measure of benefits in CBA for the next twenty years, but now they are considered inadequate. Are women's lives worth less than men's because women's earnings are lower on average? Are elderly people worthless once they stop working? Contributions to society through the labor market are a clear benefit of health care, but by themselves form an incomplete and biased measure.

Reductions in Future Medical Costs

Many diseases are less costly to treat if care is given early and if treatment is done correctly the first time. Vaccination now can prevent hospitalization in the future. Better infection control allows patients to be discharged from the hospital sooner. Yet good medical care is not always, or even usually, cheaper. The least expensive way to treat heart attacks is never to attempt resuscitation. A transplant may mean ten more years of life, but it will certainly mean hundreds of thousands of dollars in additional care. Reductions in cost, while not insignificant, can hardly constitute the primary justification for medical care.

3.4 MEASURING COSTS

Following are the primary types of medical costs:

- Medical care and administration
- Follow-up and treatment
- Time and pain of patient and family
- Provider time and inconvenience

Medical Care and Administration: Charges versus Costs

Unlike prices for other goods, most medical prices are overstated to cover related expenses for education, research, community outreach, and care for patients who cannot pay. Health economists use three methods to determine the direct costs of medical care: adjusted charges, cost accounting, and extrapolation from comparable services.[13] **Adjusted charges** for U.S. hospital care are usually estimated by multiplying billed charges by the Medicare cost-to-charge ratio (see Section 8.2). The actual cost of hospital services is, on average, only about 60 percent of billed charges. The cost of some services, such as laboratory work and drugs, may be as little as 15 percent of charges, whereas for ER and obstetric services, actual costs may be as much as 125 percent of billed charges. Per unit costs are always estimates and are subject to interpretation, since they depend on numerous assumptions regarding overhead allocation, counting, and the averaging of quality and quantity. **Cost accounting** for CBA uses the same principles as job costing in other industries. Resources (e.g., nursing hours, technician time, space, supplies) are estimated from direct observation, and their costs are estimated using prevailing wages, prices, and so on. An overhead charge is then applied for administration, utilities, and other central services. Specialized job costing studies for the most expensive elements of care are often combined with the more readily available adjusted charges for other services. **Extrapolation from comparable services** is used when charges are not available and cost accounting is too time-consuming. For example, the cost of keeping patients in the hospital when they need only custodial care could be extrapolated from the cost of a day in a nursing home. Likewise, the cost of services provided by salaried physicians in a public health clinic may be extrapolated from adjusted charges for similar services in nearby communities.

Follow-up and Treatment

Whereas direct costs are almost always counted, most medical care creates **secondary treatment costs**, which are not always counted. In the colon cancer example, the largest cost is not the screening test itself, but the additional laboratory work done on those who never had the disease but whose initial test results were positive (i.e., false positives). Similarly, the surgical cost of a knee operation for a seventy-year old widower may be much less than the cost of postoperative admission to a nursing home for weeks of recovery because he cannot climb the stairs of his apartment. With surgery, it is usually necessary to include as a cost the possibility of serious complications and death, which are worse than the condition being treated. The point is that most medical care (and other human attempts to do good) involves many secondary or unintended effects that must be included to ensure that the cost accounting is comprehensive.

Time and Pain of Patient and Family

The time patients lose and the pain they suffer often outweigh direct medical costs. It is common to value patient time at the average wage rate for all employed workers, as was done for the traffic fatality (55 mph versus 65 mph) study discussed in Section 3.1.[14] Using different rates for men, women, children, elderly people, and minorities usually contributes little to the analysis and may incorporate institutionalized discrimination. However, such differentials may explain many individual differences in behavior because they are very real to the person choosing whether to obtain care. Pain, suffering, anxiety, and death are most appropriately valued according to a person's willingness to pay. An analyst may not consider a particular patient's point of view and his or her specific pain and time costs, but these factors could explain why many beneficial treatments are not sought. For example, programs that offer free flu shots do not result in 100 percent of the population at risk getting an immunization, and offer little benefit to people whose time is worth a lot. Providing more advertising about the free flu shot program may not increase the uptake if time costs and pain are the main deterrents to getting immunized.

Provider Time and Inconvenience

The supply-side reason for not undertaking many medical activities is that providers are not compensated for their time and inconvenience. For example, although there is a tremendous need for organ donations, the physicians who must obtain the families' consent are often the ER doctors, neurosurgeons, and internists present at death who find it burdensome to speak with the families to try and get them to agree to donate their loved ones' organs. Taking time to explain the issues, dealing with emotional distress, and facing frequent refusals are costs for which they obtain no direct benefits. Such "hassle costs" are a disincentive that greatly reduces the number of organs made available for transplant. Similarly, the requirements that every hospital admission or referral to a specialist be documented imposes a hassle cost on the primary physician, and leads predictably to a lower number of hospital days and specialist referrals. This reduction in services may make it look as if managed care plans ration the number of services to reduce costs and make profits. However, it is important to remember that the services forgone are those that the patient's physician was unwilling to write a letter or make a phone call to support and, therefore, are unlikely to have been considered critically important.

3.5 EVIDENCE-BASED MEDICINE

Cost-benefit analysis will provide a definite answer only in clear-cut cases. Often, to arrive at an assessment many assumptions must be made, judgment must be used, and measurements replaced with estimates. Why take on such an exercise if precision is so hard to come by? The primary reason for engaging in CBA is not to find the exact ratio of benefits to cost, or a measure of cost per life saved down to the penny (or dollar, or even thousand), but to begin the process by asking the real questions: What is the evidence that this treatment actually works? What are the consequences, in pain, in risks, and in resources diverted from other patients? Evidence-based medicine is a development of the scientific attitude toward medical practice that says "prove it" rather than "we do it this way because we always treat that kind of patient this way."[15] The need for evidence, rather than tradition, is apparent in the discussion of radical mastectomy to treat breast cancer in Chapter 2, endnote 1. A similar process of reassessment may be under way for the use of lung volume reduction surgery for lung cancer. After initial favorable reports and a large increase in the number of surgeries (despite the high operative mortality), a randomized clinical trial reported its results in 2003: no improvements in survival for those receiving lung volume reduction. Some of the many therapies that have faded from use after evidence finally accumulated that they were not worthwhile include X-ray screening of healthy juveniles and adults for lung cancer, antibiotics for viral infections, extended bed rest for cardiac patients, massive vitamin C doses (for a variety of ailments), gastric freezing for stomach ulcers, and on and on.

Why do so many useless or low-benefit treatments continue to be used in practice? One reason is that we want to do something. No one wants to leave a patient in pain without trying to help. Perhaps even more important are logical failures due to "regression to the mean," "opportunity costs," and "selective reporting." These all can make a useless treatment look as if it is helping, or even like a miracle cure. Most acute illnesses get better with or without treatment. When a patient feels bad and a new treatment is tried, and the patient then improves (regression to the mean), that improvement is often attributed to drug X even though it would have occurred anyway. Placebos are the most important opportunity cost ignored. People who get treated (or think they are being treated—maybe they just get sugar water) almost always report feeling better, and actually do heal faster. It has even been discovered that bitter-tasting liquids make better placebos than sugar water. Tests have also been done to test the placebo effect of surgery using fake operations, which showed significant positive results. Probably the most important logical failure is due to selective memory: patients and doctors remember and report successes more than failures. It is like playing twenty games and then remembering to tell only about the four that you won. Selective reporting often leads to a dramatic overstatement of benefits, which is why we read so many newspaper articles about medical breakthroughs that are "coming soon" that seem to just disappear because they did not work out. Conversely, have you ever seen headlines that another promising drug or surgery just didn't seem to be much of an improvement? Only a well-controlled randomized study that reports all results, the good and the bad, and compares the new treatment to the baseline benefits from placebos while guarding against mistakes from regression to the mean, can provide a valid measure of real therapeutic benefits.

3.6   THE VALUE OF LIFE

> "A man who knows the price of everything and the value of nothing."
> — *Oscar Wilde's definition of a cynic*

Isn't health priceless? Some patients and physicians protest that it is impossible to measure the priceless benefits of medical care with the crude yardstick of money. Regardless of whether people think it is right or proper, their actions place a dollar value on human life when they make a decision to provide or deny treatment. If an 87-year-old patient in heart failure is transferred from a nursing home to a cardiac care unit for ten days, the physician affirms through this action that the potential gain in lifespan is worth more than the $15,000 cost of the hospital admission. Immediately discharging this patient with instructions to give him four aspirin every six hours affirms the physician's belief that it is not. Our actions place a dollar value on life even if we do not choose to recognize this fact. We live in a world of scarce resources and must make decisions within these limitations. We place a value on (and a limit on the value of) health whether we wish to or not, with money as a generalized expression of this value.[16] Perhaps the most important role of economists in the CBA of health care is pointing out this reality.

Valuing human life places special but unavoidable demands on economists. For activities that are traded in the market, such as medical care, work time, drugs, and transportation, valuation may be complicated by risk and discounting, or blurred by overhead allocation and wage differentials. Nevertheless, the process of connecting resources and program effects to specific dollar amounts is understandable and familiar. Considerations of life and death or pain and suffering are not so clear. Since there is no explicit market for postoperative pain and mortality, a way must be found to reflect the value that people place on these events. By choosing to buy a car that is cheaper but less safe, a person is making an implicit trade between money and the risk of dying. That trade-off is also made when buying smoke detectors, choosing to accept a more dangerous job assignment for higher pay, refusing to fill a prescription because it costs too much, and flying to the Mayo Clinic to get the best possible treatment for a rare disease. People buy and sell health all the time, but they do not do so in an organized market like the New York Stock Exchange. **Economists do not put a value on life or illness; they measure the value that consumers put on life and illness as shown by their behavior.**

One attempt to provide an explicit dollar value for life is described by Michael Jones-Lee.[17] It was observed that people would run across a highway (at a small but noticeable risk of dying) rather than spend the time going around to a pedestrian overpass. Through observations and questionnaires, it was established that people were willing to accept a risk of 0.000002 of death to save seven minutes (0.117 hours) of walking. Valuing their time by an average wage rate of $20, the value of life as can be extrapolated as follows:

Value of Life: Jones-Lee Approach

$$\text{Value of Life} = \frac{(\text{Value of Time}) \times (\text{Hours used})}{(\text{Rick of death per hour saved})} = \frac{\$20 \times 0.117}{0.000002} = \$1,170,000$$

A more sophisticated approach is to consider the value of life as the additional wages required to get someone to take a more dangerous job. A statistical regression[18] of the association between wages and risk showed that for each 0.0001 increase in risk of death, there was an additional $240 in annual salary; therefore, the estimated value of life measured by the method used in this study was $240 \div 0.0001 = $2.4 million. Other studies using similar methods have estimated values of life from $800,000 to $6 million.[19] One problem with occupational risk estimates is selection bias: the people who are less risk-averse or mistakenly underestimate the true risk are the ones most likely to apply for the more dangerous jobs. A study that captures the behavior of the more safety-conscious individuals was conducted by Rachel Dardis, a researcher who measured the number of people purchasing smoke detectors as a function of price.[20] From these data she constructed a demand curve (Figure 3.3). In 1974, the price of a smoke detector was $52, and only 1.8 million were sold (adjusted for inflation, $52 in 1974 is worth $198 in 2010, with an annualized operating cost per household of $27 in 2010 dollars). By 1979, the price had declined to $12, and 10 million were sold (which is $31, inflation adjusted, and yields an annualized cost of $4 a year). Each smoke detector was estimated to result in a 0.000036 reduction in the risk of death and a 0.000023 reduction in the risk of injury. Using these probabilities, Dardis estimated that those who purchased smoke detectors when they first came on the market at $198 made decisions

| FIGURE 3.3 | Value of Life: Smoke Detector Study |

Changes in the number of smoke detectors purchased as prices fell from $150 in 1974 to $24 in 1979 are interpreted as a derived demand for life saving, implying a "value of like" demand that exceeds $2,000,000 for early purchasers, and $305,000 for late purchasers.

Source: Rachel Dardis, *American Economic Review* 70 (1980): 1077–1082.

consistent with a value of life of $2 million; those who waited until prices dropped to $30 implied a lower value of life—less than $400,000. This smoke detector study brings home the relevance of the first law of demand: even for life itself, people will buy less as the price increases.

We must all die sometime; therefore, no medical treatment can truly save a life forever. A problem with efforts to estimate the value of life is that the rhetoric itself reinforces denial, making it seem as if the purpose of medical care is to save lives. The real task of medicine is to reduce suffering and anxiety while extending the expected length of life by a few years. Glorified language can thwart clear thought and practical action. It may provide a convenient way to avoid admitting in public that the life of an eight-year-old child is valued more than the life of an eighty-year-old grandparent. Such avoidance does not make the difference in valuation any less true. Economists use the decisions made by state legislatures, families, and patients to show that they value the length and quality of life, which can be changed by medical care, rather than the fact of mortality, which cannot.

3.7 QUALITY-ADJUSTED LIFE YEARS (QALYs)

The extra dollar cost of providing one additional year of life expectancy has become a standard method for evaluating many health programs. Yet a year spent sick and in pain is worth less than a year lived in perfect health, free of symptoms. It is important to account for both quality and length of life when assessing the outcomes of new medical treatments. A significant risk of surgical mortality may be worth accepting to treat a disease and alleviate pain—but how much risk? Researchers use econometrics, surveys, and professional judgments to estimate the value of a year spent in different states of disability.[21] Such **quality-adjusted life years** (**QALYs**) rate quality of life between 0.0 (death) and 1.0 (good health). In the survey results presented in Table 3.6, respondents indicated that living for three months confined to a hospital for tuberculosis treatment was worth only 1.8 months (0.60 × 3 months) of regular time spent at home in good health.[22] The value of living in the hospital declines further when it is not temporary but permanent. Living ten more years confined in a hospital being treated for a contagious disease was considered to be worth only 1.6 years of normal life. Although such conditions were not included in this survey, people consider

TABLE 3.6	Quality of Life Adjustment Factors	
Duration	**Health State**	**Adjustment**
	Reference State: Perfect Health	**1.00**
3 months	Home confinement, tuberculosis	.68
3 months	Home confinement, contagious disease	.65
3 months	Hospital dialysis	.62
3 months	Hospital confinement, tuberculosis	.60
3 months	Hospital confinement, contagious disease	.56
3 months	Depression	.44
3 months	Home dialysis	.65
8 years	Mastectomy for injury	.63
8 years	Kidney transplant	.58
8 years	Hospital dialysis	.56
8 years	Mastectomy for breast cancer	.48
8 years	Hospital confinement, contagious disease	.33
Life	Home dialysis	.40
Life	Hospital dialysis	.32
Life	Hospital confinement, contagious disease	.16
	Reference State: Dead	**.00**

Source: D. L. Sackett and G. W. Torrance, "The Utility of Different Health States as Perceived by the General Public," *Journal of Chronic Diseases* 31 no. 11 (1978): 697–704.

some illnesses to be worse than death; therefore, each additional year lived in such misery could be counted as having negative value.

Discounting Over Time

The value of a dollar obtained fifteen years from now is worth less than a dollar today. The value of potential increases in life expectancy fifteen years from now is worth less than the same increase in the probability of living today. The *present value* of an additional year of life obtained fifteen years from now is calculated by discounting over time, just like the present value of a dollar obtained fifteen years from now is calculated. If the rate of discount (interest rate) is 5 percent, the present value of receiving a dollar next year is $1 \div (1.05) = \$0.952$, and the present value of receiving a dollar in fifteen years is $1 \div (1.05)^{15} = \$0.479$. Analogously, the 5 percent discounted value of an additional year of life fifteen years from now is about half the current value (see further discussion of discounting and present value in Chapter 12).

QALY League Tables

The costs of medical care can be compared with benefits by calculating the cost per adjusted year of life gained. On the benefit side, each additional life year is discounted for risk (expected value), time, and quality of life. On the cost side, adjustments are made for any differences between charges and actual costs, expected reductions in days lost from work, and reductions in the cost of medical care for related conditions. Consider the hypothetical example in Table 3.7. The patient can expect to live three years with medications alone but will live five years, with a better quality of life, if the surgery is successful. However, the surgery is effective only 40 percent of the time, it costs $30,000, and there is a 3 percent chance of immediate death due to surgical mortality. The estimated cost per QALY gained

TABLE 3.7	Hypothetical QALY Calculation Example					
	Year 1	Year 2	Year 3	Year 4	Year 5	Total
Time discounting factor	1.00	.95	.91	.86	.82	
Baseline						
Quality of life	.60	.50	.40	*(Dead)*	*(Dead)*	
Discounted value	.60	.48	.36	.00	.00	1.44
Quality adjusted life expectancy without surgery, 1.44 years						
Successful surgery						
Quality of life	.90	.80	.70	.60	.50	
Discounted value	.90	.76	.63	.52	.41	3.23
Quality adjusted life expectancy without surgery, 3.23 years						
Net gain in QALYs			1.79	*(3.23 – 1.44 discounted years)*		
Probability			40%			
Expected value			.72			
Less surgical mortality			−.04	*(3% of baseline 1.44 years)*		
Expected net QALY gain			.68			
Cost of surgery			$30,000			
Cost per QALY gained			$44,000	*($30,000 ÷ .68)*		

is $44,000. Similar estimates have been made for a number of medical interventions so that relative costs can be calculated and presented in QALY league tables, such as Table 3.8.[23] From these results, it can be seen that it costs more than 7 times as much ($14,000 versus $1,900) to increase QALYs by one year with a heart transplant as it does with a pacemaker implant. Trying to extend and improve life by using coronary artery bypass grafting to treat minor two-vessel disease with mild angina is still more expensive, $35,000 per QALY gained. QALY rankings can be used to assess which medical treatments should be expanded and which should be cut back to optimize system efficiency. When the state of Oregon decided in 1993 to enroll more poor residents in its Medicaid program, funding those extra people

TABLE 3.8	QALY "League Table"
Treatment	**Present Value of Extra Cost per QALY**
Physician advice for smoking cessation	$450
Pacemaker implantation for heart block	1,900
Hip replacement	2,000
CABG for severe angina LMD	2,800
Control of total serum cholesterol	4,600
CABG for severe angina 2VD	6,200
Kidney transplant	8,200
Breast cancer screening	9,500
Heart transplant	14,000
CABG for mild angina 2VD	35,000
Hospital hemodialysis	38,000

CABG, coronary artery bypass graft; LMD, left main disease; 2VD, two vessel disease.

Source: A. Williams, "Economics of Coronary Artery Bypass Grafting," *British Medical Journal*, 291 (1995): 326–329.

by eliminating coverage of medical services deemed to be of lowest benefit, legislators used a decision-making process analogous to the construction of a QALY league table.

3.8   PERSPECTIVES: PATIENT, PAYER, GOVERNMENT, PROVIDER, SOCIETY

How much has to be paid for treatment, and how much the treatment is worth, depends on whose perspective the cost-benefit analyst is taking. From the individual's point of view, treatment that makes an infectious disease less communicable is of no direct benefit, and medical costs may be relatively unimportant because he or she has insurance. From a group perspective, reducing communicability to neighbors is a major benefit of treatment, and hospital charges are important because total insurance premiums for the group as a whole will rise. The broadest perspective is that of society as a whole, including future generations.

Many of the conflicts over health policy arise from the difference in perspectives of different groups. For gay men, research and prevention of AIDS may be the most important health issue of our time, whereas finding drugs to assist in stroke rehabilitation is not.[24] For women over 65 with hypertension, these priorities may be reversed. An economist hired by Medicare to do a CBA on whether a new type of surgery should be covered must ask, "Am I to consider primarily the effects on the Medicare budget, or should I also include benefits to hospitals, doctors, and state legislatures?" The treatment of taxes and transfers is crucial in this regard. If new Medicare regulations cost Medicare $100 but reduce state Medicaid expenditures by $40, is that reduction to be counted? From the state's perspective, it is a windfall gain of $40. From the perspective of the U.S. budget and the Medicare administrator, it is a cost of $100. From a social perspective, the shifting of costs from state to federal budgets is irrelevant, and the cost is the net amount, $60. Consider also the effect of taxes. If a 10 percent tax on health care raises the price of a visit to the doctor from $20 to $22, the extra $2 is a relevant cost to the patient or the insurance plan but not to society. If there were no "health taxes," that $2 would have to be obtained elsewhere by raising other taxes or by reducing government spending, perhaps on roads or defense.

Distribution: Whose Costs and Whose Benefits?

In the real world, people may think that they should consider benefits to society as a whole, but they act according to a more immediate calculus of benefits and costs to themselves as individuals and to the groups (teenagers, steelworkers, residents of Lancaster, Hispanics, senior citizens) to which they belong. A major barrier to actually implementing a project is raised by the following question: What about the losers? Laser surgery for cancer may help thousands of people who would not have survived with the chemotherapy previously used, but it will kill some people who would have lived. Development of a new home health system means that the hospital down the street will find even more of its beds empty and will have to lay off some employees. It is almost impossible to make a major change that hurts no one. Unfortunately, it is also almost impossible for a politician to vote for a project that clearly hurts some identifiable person. Programs are more likely to pass when the costs are diffused over a large number of people and thus are difficult to identify. For example, a requirement for more extensive testing of drugs or better disposal of toxic waste leads to a general rise in the cost of medicine. Even though in total it amounts to millions of dollars, it takes only a few pennies per prescription and thus is ignored. Conversely, imposing a loss of a few thousand dollars on a single individual or firm is sufficient to get them to file a lawsuit to stop the program. The relative power of the group that must bear most of the costs often determines the political feasibility of any change.

CBA Is a Limited Perspective

Although CBA is a powerful tool for policy analysis, it can be quite limited. It is difficult to do a useful economic analysis unless the medical facts are well known. How many people have the disease, what is the cure rate from therapy, and what levels of disability are likely to result? These clinical questions must be answered before any assessment of costs and benefits is attempted. The strength of CBA as a tool lies in its ability to interpret medical issues as choices in a market. Yet to do so, it must force health and human caring into such a rigid economic model that it tends to overemphasize efficiency and may entirely fail to recognize the most important ethical and social values that underlie medical practice. Medicine as a profession rests on the dignity and sanctity of life, a philosophy and practice that resists overt commercialization.

CBA and Public Policy Decision Making

Cost-benefit analysis is a way of looking at past behavior, at decisions actually made, so that future decisions can become more clear, rational, and consistent. A decision being made by a single person was used in the knee injury example. In practice, CBAs are almost never done for a single case since it takes too long, costs too much, and depends on statistical assumptions that are more valid for large groups. When a single person is involved, that person knows his or her personal costs and willingness to pay better than any analyst. Formal analyses are apt to be most useful under the following circumstances:

- Large amounts of resources (millions or billions of dollars) are involved.
- Responsibility for decisions is fragmented (government agencies, large corporations).
- The goals and objectives of different groups are at odds or unclear.
- Alternative courses of action are radically different.
- The technology and risks underlying each alternative are well understood.
- A long time frame is involved (e.g., strategy versus management).

Econometrics, balance sheets, surveys, decision trees, and other tools of the economics trade are usually applied to large projects and long-standing problems. For example, is screening blood donors for HIV and hepatitis worthwhile? How often should they be screened, and with what tests? Is inpatient alcohol treatment better than outpatient and, if so, is it enough to justify the increase in costs? The treatment of millions of people costing billions of dollars over many years is involved in these issues, each of which has been given full formal CBA. The test of what is important ultimately lies in the judgment of those who are most affected by the decision. Health CBA almost always counts two things, death and money, because they are routinely recorded. A good analysis is able to capture other factors that are significant and yet keep the presentation simple enough that the costs and benefits of alternative courses of action are clearly seen.

SUGGESTIONS FOR FURTHER READING

David M. Cutler and Mark McClellan, "Is Technological Change in Medicine Worth It?" *Health Affairs* 20, no. 5 (September 2001): 11–29.
A. S. Detsky, "A Clinician's Guide to Cost-Effectiveness Analysis," *Annals of Internal Medicine* 113, no. 2 (July 15, 1990): 147–154.

Michael F. Drummond, Mark J. Sculpher, George W. Torrance, Bernie J. O'Brien, and Greg L. Stoddart, *Methods for the Economic Evaluation of Health Programmes* (Oxford, U.K.: Oxford University Press, 2005).

J. M. Eisenberg, "Clinical Economics: A Guide to the Economic Analysis of Clinical Practices," *Journal of the American Medical Association* 262 (1989): 2879–2886.

Victor Fuchs, *Who Shall Live?* (New York: Basic Books, 1974).

Mark McClellan, Barbara McNeil, and Joseph Newhouse, "Does More Intensive Treatment of Acute Myocardial Infarction in the Elderly Reduce Mortality?" *Journal of the American Medical Association* 272, no. 11 (1994): 859–866.

Martin I. Meltzer, "Introduction to Health Economics for Physicians," *The Lancet* 358 (September 22, 2001): 993–998. Available free from www.theLancet.com.

B. J. O'Brien, D. Helyland, W. S. Richardson, M. Levine, and M. F. Drummond, "Users Guides to the Medical Literature XIII: How to Use an Article on Economic Analysis of Clinical Practice (B)—What Are the Results and Will They Help Me in Caring for My Patients," *Journal of the American Medical Association* 227 (1997): 1802–1806.

M. A. Testa and D. C. Simonson, "Assessment of Quality of Life Outcomes," *New England Journal of Medicine* 334 (1996): 835–840.

SUMMARY

1. **Every act is a judgment about value**. When people act, they show by that act that they think the gains are worth more than the costs. Economists look at decisions that patients and physicians have made in the past to estimate the value they place on health outcomes.

2. **Cost-benefit analysis (CBA)** does not make decisions. It is a **framework** that can be used to make the decision-making process more rational, more consistent, and more clearly communicated. The cost-benefit analyst organizes the facts provided by clinicians and the public's values to present data in a way that is useful for making policy decisions. Although some form of cost-benefit trade-off occurs in virtually all decisions made by consumers, a formal CBA is used only for large-scale government or corporate projects with a long time frame and many parties involved in the decision-making process.

3. **Cost-effectiveness analysis (CEA)** compares the cost of two different methods of reaching the same goal (immunizing 100 children, preventing 10 cases of flu, adding one extra year of life) but does not attempt to measure the benefits in dollars.

4. The appropriate measure of costs is the **opportunity cost** (i.e., what is given up). The appropriate measure of benefits is **willingness to pay (WTP)**, what the patient or society is willing to give up to attain an improvement in health.

5. In choosing between alternatives, it is the change in benefits (**marginal benefits**) and the change in costs (**marginal costs**) that matter, not the average value.

6. **Marginalism** is the process of trying out small adjustments and moving always in the direction of adjustments that make things better until no further improvements are possible. With marginalism, we do not need to know whether a decision is good or bad, only whether it makes things better or worse. If a manager keeps choosing in a way that makes things better, eventually the organization will reach the best possible decision (i.e., its **optimum**). Economists have found that to evaluate an organization they need not look at everything, but rather need only to examine the organization's **behavior at the margin** to determine whether it can do better.

7. The primary **benefits** to be accounted for in health care projects are as follows:

    a. Health (extend life or reduce morbidity and pain)

> **b.** Productivity (decrease time lost from work)
>
> **c.** Reductions in future medical costs

8. Following are the major categories of **costs** to be accounted for:

> **a.** Medical care and administration
>
> **b.** Follow-up and treatment damages (side effects)
>
> **c.** Time and pain of patient and family
>
> **d.** Provider time and inconvenience

9. Since marginal benefits are usually declining and lower than the average benefits as health programs increase in size, it is important to **target treatment toward those most in need**. Many useful medical technologies become wasteful when they are expanded to include low-risk individuals.

10. Benefits are rarely certain. The **expected value** of a medical treatment is the product of the likelihood of success multiplied by the magnitude of the health gain that will occur if treatment is successful. A useful shorthand for dealing with risk is to examine whether:

$$\textit{Probability of Gain} \times \text{Benefit} > \textit{Probability of Loss} \times \text{Cost}$$

11. Years of life must be discounted if the quality of life is reduced. Questionnaires are used to estimate how many years of life a person with a disability would be willing to give up to gain one additional year of life without the disability or to reduce the risk of death. In this way, **comparisons can be made between treatment alternatives in terms of quality-adjusted life years** or **QALYs**. Since an additional year of life expectancy in the distant future is worth less than an increase in health now, it is also necessary to use an interest rate to discount benefits over time.

12. Comparing medical therapies in standardized units, such as cost per QALY gained, can help decision makers determine which programs should be expanded and which should be cut back, and thus lead to better public policy.

PROBLEMS

1. {*expected value*}

    (**A**) Successful rehabilitation of a shoulder injury obviates the need for reconstructive surgery costing $6,000. However, rehabilitation is successful only 70 percent of the time. What is the expected value of rehabilitation?

    (**B**) Treatment for endocarditis is risky. The patient will either (a) die in the hospital, (b) partially recover, or (c) fully recover. With full recovery, the patient can expect to live for another 20 years, but only 25 percent of patients fully recover. With partial recovery, the patient can expect to live 10 more years. However, 20 percent of patients die in the hospital. Assuming that patients usually live just one year without treatment, what is the expected value of the treatment expressed as additional years of life?

2. {*marginal cost*}

    (**A**) A course of chemotherapy costs $8,000. If given to patient A, it will increase life expectancy by two months; for patient B, by six months; for patient C, by one month; for patient D, by five months; and for patient E, by four months. If all five patients are treated, what is the average cost per year of life gained? If only one patient can be treated, which one should it be? If only two patients are treated, which ones should they be? What is the marginal cost per additional year of life for the patient most likely to benefit? What is the marginal cost per additional year of life for the patient least likely to benefit? Draw the total and marginal benefit curves (label the Y axis "Years of life gained" and the X axis "Number of patients treated"). If all five patients are treated, what is the average cost per year of life gained? The marginal cost? If patients are treated in alphabetical order, which one determines the marginal cost per year of life gained: patient A, patient E, or some other patient?

   (B) {*demand curve*} Assuming that each additional year of life is worth $60,000, draw the demand curve for chemotherapy. Draw the supply curve. What is the relationship between the demand curve and the total and marginal benefit curves you drew in part A of this question?

3.   {*marginal cost, quality dimension*} Those who suffer from allergies can take medicine to relieve their suffering. Without treatment, they will have 118 bad days per year. Generic drug G costs $76 for an annual prescription, whereas Brand name drug B costs $680. With drug G, most people suffer only 42 days of allergy symptoms, whereas drug B seems a bit better, usually reducing symptomatic days to just 38. What is the average cost per day of symptom relief with drug G? With drug B? What is the marginal cost per additional day of relief if a patient is switched from drug G to drug B?

4.   {*direct versus indirect costs*} A school district determines that less than 70 percent of first-grade students have completed all recommended immunizations. A task force suggests two ways to reach the goal of 95 percent immunization: (1) hire 20 visiting nurses to do outreach in the community or (2) pass a law mandating that children will not be allowed to attend school unless they bring documentation showing evidence of complete immunization. How is the distribution of costs and benefits different under the two plans? Which plan is more cost-effective?

5.   {*need versus demand, opportunity cost*} Many experts recommend that people get at least 30 minutes of vigorous exercise three to five times a week; however, is actual participation in exercise less than the amount (a) needed or (b) demanded? Why do most college students get more exercise in summer than in winter? Does need, demand, or a difference in the opportunity cost of time account for the fact that most actors get more exercise than most accountants?

6.   The World Health Organization (WHO) is considering sending in a team of experts to deal with an outbreak of schistosomiasis in a distant country. Sending a larger team will allow WHO to prevent more fatalities, and they estimate the following effectiveness:

Number of Team Members	Number of Deaths
0 (i.e., no action)	1,200
5	500
10	200
15	100
20	60
25	40
30	30
35	25
40	22
45	20
50	20

(**A**) It costs $5,000 for each team member sent. Calculate the *total, average,* and *marginal* cost of life saving through this effort and display it on a graph. If saving a life is valued at $100,000, what is the optimal number of people WHO should send to combat the epidemic? If saving a life is valued at $10,000, what is the optimal number? What team size gives the most "bang for the buck" (i.e., the largest number of lives saved per dollar spent)?

(**B**) Each person sent must be taken away from a disease-fighting team at work elsewhere in the world. What is the appropriate opportunity cost measure of sending people to fight the new epidemic: the transportation cost of $5,000 or the reduction of life-saving efforts from the job they are pulled away from?

7.   {*willingness to pay*} What determines the value of a cure for acne? For ALS (amyloid lateral sclerosis, or Lou Gehrig's disease)? For Alzheimer's disease? Which discovery is worth more to a pharmaceutical firm that is able to patent a cure?

8.   {*QALYs*} Patient BN is a 36-year-old female with a type of organ failure that reduces her quality of life to half of what it would be in good health. Without treatment she can expect to live only two years. With a successful transplant, BN can expect to live four years and have a quality of life that is near (80 percent) what she would enjoy in good health. However, the transplant costs $100,000, plus $10,000 each year for drugs and follow-up care, and carries a 15 percent risk of rejection resulting in immediate death. What is the cost per additional year of life gained (without discounting for time or quality of life)? What is the cost per discounted QALY gained (assuming a 5 percent time discount rate)?

9.   {*interest rates and future value*} As a health economist for the U.S. Centers for Disease Control and Prevention, you have been asked to analyze a number of programs targeting different diseases and recommend which should receive priority, given that budgets are limited. As part of your analysis, you will have to determine what interest rate is appropriate for discounting future costs and benefits. You are going to be visited by an economist from AARP, formerly the American Association of Retired Persons, and another economist from the Children's Defense Fund. Which group will lobby harder for a lower discount rate? Why?

10.   Should a new, expensive ($250,000+ per year) cancer drug be covered by insurance or not? Who might argue for covering the drug? Who might argue against coverage? What effect would the usefulness of this drug have? What effect would the quantity of patients who potentially would use this drug have? What role could the economic analysis play?

ENDNOTES

1.   This chapter has benefited from extensive review and revisions by Jeffrey Hoch of the Centre for Research on Inner City Health at St. Michael's Hospital and the University of Toronto.

2.   Michael Drummond, *Principles of Economic Appraisal in Health Care* (Cambridge: Oxford University Press, 1981), p. 17. Several sources and texts are listed at the end of this chapter as suggestions for further reading. Good current examples of cost-benefit analyses and reviews of the literature can be found in journals such as *Health Economics, American Journal of Public Health, Medical Decision Making, New England Journal of Medicine,* and *Journal of the American Medical Association.*

3.   Orley Ashenfelter and Michael Greenstone, "Using Mandated Speed Limits to Measure the Value of a Statistical Life," *National Bureau of Economic Research Working Paper w9094,* August 2002 (http://www.nber.org/papers/w9094).

4.   S. R. Garfield et al., "Evaluation of an Ambulatory Medical Care Delivery System," *New England Journal of Medicine* 294, no. 8 (1976): 426–431; P. J. Wagner and J. E. Hendrich, "Physician Views on Frequent Medical

Use: Patient Beliefs and Demographic and Diagnostic Correlates," *Journal of Family Practice* 36, no. 4 (1993): 417–422.

5. The usual threshold for the value of adding one year of life is now usually considered to be somewhere in the range of $100,000 to $250,000, and certainly not less than $50,000.

6. The "law of large numbers" says that the observed average will be close to the "true" mean if the number of observations is large enough.

7. Mark McClellan, Barbara McNeil, and Joseph Newhouse, "Does More Intensive Treatment of Acute Myocardial Infarction in the Elderly Reduce Mortality?" *Journal of the American Medical Association* 272, no. 11 (1994): 859–866.

8. Victor Fuchs, *Who Shall Live? Health, Economics and Social Choice* (New York: Basic Books, 1974); Bengt Jonsson, "Economics of Drug Treatment; For Which Patients Is It Cost-Effective to Lower Cholesterol?" *The Lancet* 358 (2001): 1251–1256. Analogous "flat of the curve" purchases might be Sunday hikers who buy specialized and expensive boots and equipment needed mostly for climbing the Himalayas, a student buying a top-end computer just to send and receive email, or an investment banker buying a Ferrari to drive to a local restaurant. It is not that the special equipment is not valuable–just that the special features provide little extra benefit for most people.

9. Duncan Neuhauser and Ann Lewicki, "What Do We Gain from the Sixth Stool Guaiac?" *New England Journal of Medicine* 293 (1975): 226–228.

10. David Cutler, Angus Deaton, and Adriana Lleras-Muney, "The Determinants of Mortality," *Journal of Economic Perspectives* 20, no. 3 (2006): 97–120; Jonathan Skinner and Douglas Staiger, "Technology Diffusion and Productivity Growth in Health Care." NBER working paper #14865, April 2009.

11. Michael Ibrahim, "Rules of Evidence," in *Epidemiology and Health Policy* (Rockville, Md.: Aspen Press, 1985), 39–49.

12. Sir William Petty, *The Economic Writings of Sir William Petty*, ed. Charles Henry Hull, [1662–1687] reprint (New York: AM Kelley, 1963), 108. This anthology includes *A Treatise of Taxes and Contributions* (1662), *Political Arithmetik* (1676), and other writings. Petty's plan primarily involved the forced closure of houses where the plague appeared, with resettlement of the families at government expense at farms forty miles outside of London for three months. Arguably the first real economist, Petty was no stranger to self-interest or pride. He asked that 2 percent of the net increase in tax revenues from his plague treatment plan be given to him as a reward from the King for his brilliant idea. He did not fully specify how those gains would be figured. Had he done so, health economists today might be much more effective, competing for millions of dollars in health benefits royalties.

13. Thomas E. Getzen, "Medical Care Price Indexes: Theory, Construction and Empirical Analysis of the U.S. Series 1927–1990," *Advances in Health Economics* 13 (Greenwich, Conn.: JAI Press, 1992): 83–128.

14. See the discussion in the Suggested Readings by Drummond et al. and others.

15. A. C. Gelijns et al., "Evidence, Politics and Technological Change," *Health Affairs* 24, no. 1 (2005): 29–40; Mark A. Hlatky, Gillian D. Sanders, and Douglas Owens, "Evidence-Based Medicine and Policy: The Case of the Implantable Cardioverter Defibrillator," *Health Affairs* 24, no. 1 (2005): 42–51; Scott D. Ramsey and Sean D. Sullivan, "Evidence, Economics and Emphysema: Medicare's Long Journey with Lung Volume Reduction Surgery," *Health Affairs* 24, no. 1 (2005): 55–66; David M. Eddy, "Evidence-Based Medicine: A Unified Approach" *Health Affairs* 24, no. 1 (2005): 9–17.

16. A decision maker's preferences are said to be "lexicographic" when everything depends on one factor, with other factors allowed to affect choice only when they are equal to the primary factor. For example, a parent might say to a physician, "Do whatever you can to minimize my child's chance of dying. Given that, if one treatment is less painful, or costs less, you can do that one." This decision is lexicographic since one factor, the probability of the child's survival, dominates all others. In such a case, there are no trade-offs and hence no necessity to make an economic analysis such as a CBA. Computers sort alphabetical lists lexicographically: by the first letter, then by the second, and so on. People often claim that one thing is important above all others (survival, honor, religious purity) even though most behavior indicates that trade-offs are made. Even saints respond to pain, and parents are not acting nobly if they do everything to try to save one child and in the process harm their other children and their own lives. Arguing that medical decisions should only be based on costs when there is no chance that doing so will affect quality or risk lives is the same as saying that money does not matter in the real world.

17. Michael W. Jones-Lee, *The Economics of Safety and Physical Risk* (Oxford: Blackwell, 1989), p. 67, based on data and extrapolations from S. J. Melinek, "A Method of Evaluating Life for Economic Purposes," *Accident Analysis and Prevention* 6 (1974): 103–114.

18. *Regression Analysis* is covered in virtually all standard statistics textbooks. There is also a short description provided in S. Folland, A. Goodman, and M. Stano, *The Economics of Health and Health Care* (Upper Saddle River, N.J.: Prentice Hall, 2001), 59–67.

19. M. Moore and W. Kip Viscusi, "Quality Adjusted Value of Life," *Economic Inquiry* 26 (1988): 369–388.

20. Rachel Dardis, "The Value of a Life: New Evidence from the Marketplace," *American Economic Review* 70 (December 1980): 1077–1082.

21. M. E. Backhouse, R. J. Backhouse, and S. A. Edley, "Economic Evaluation Bibliography," *Health Economics* 1 (Supplement) (1992): 1–236; John Hutton and Alan Maynard, "A NICE Challenge for Health Economics," *Health Economics* 9, no. 2 (2000): 89–94.

22. D. L. Sackett and D. W. Torrance, "The Utility of Different Health States as Perceived by the General Public," *Journal of Chronic Diseases* 31, no. 11 (1978): 697–704.

23. Alan Williams, "Economics of Coronary Artery Bypass Grafting," *British Medical Journal*, 291 (1985): 326–329; Julia Fox-Rushby, Anne Mills, and Damian Walker, "Setting Health Priorities: The Development of Cost-Effectiveness League Tables," *Bulletin of the World Health Organization* 79, no. 7 (July 2001): 679–680; Tammy O. Tengs et al., "Five Hundred Life-Saving Interventions and Their Cost-Effectiveness," *Risk Analysis* 15, no. 3 (1995): 369–390.

24. T. R. Fanning et al., "The Epidemiology of AIDS in the New York and California Medicaid Programs," *Journal of Acquired Immune Deficiency Syndromes* 4 (1991): 1025–1035.

CHAPTER 4

HEALTH INSURANCE: FINANCING MEDICAL CARE

QUESTIONS

1. Who pays for losses: insurance companies or the people who buy insurance?
2. What is an "actuarially fair" premium?
3. Does pooling of funds reduce losses or reduce variance?
4. Do insurance companies take risks, or do they just put a price on risks?
5. Who takes care of people when they need medical care they cannot afford?
6. Is a favor from a friend similar to a loan from a bank?
7. Are people who think they will become sick more likely to obtain insurance?
8. Are people with insurance more likely to sustain a financial loss?
9. Does employer-provider health insurance make people work more hours or less?
10. Does insurance increase or decrease the demand for medical care?

Breaking an arm, catching pneumonia, having a heart attack—there are a dizzying array of risks that could disrupt your life. We hope none of these bad things will happen, but if they do, most of us can rely on insurance to cover some of our financial losses. From an individual perspective, insurance generates net benefits by allowing trade between two possible states of the world: a little money in the usual state (when a person is healthy) is given up to get a lot of money in the unusual and more difficult state (when a person is sick). From society's point of view, insurance is a method of pooling risk so that one person's loss is shared across many people rather than being borne by that person alone. If all people contribute, the pool of collected funds will be sufficient to compensate the unlucky few. All participants gain peace of mind, knowing that they can obtain necessary medical care with limited financial risk. Chapters 4 and 5 examine the operations, history, and theory of health insurance. To grasp how insurance works, it is necessary to understand that it is a means both for individual maximization of utility and for social promotion of group values such as respect for life, care of people with disabilities, equal opportunity, and political unity.

4.1   METHODS FOR COVERING RISKS

What would you do if you broke your arm? Who would take care of you? How would you eat and pay your rent while you were out of work? Who would pay for the doctor and hospital care? There are several ways this loss could be covered.

Savings

The first economic consequence of a loss is to use savings to pay for current expenses. *Savings* can be thought of as a trade between time periods. People do not save to pile up money. They save so that they can consume more in the future, either because they plan to do so (e.g., for retirement or a vacation) or to protect themselves against the unexpected (e.g., accident, illness). Savings provide a buffer against random losses, smoothing out consumption over time so that you can still eat if you are not working, still pay the rent if you incur a $600 doctor bill immediately after your vacation, and still pay tuition bills if you need expensive prescription drugs to get you through your final exams. The ability to smooth out the amount of consumption over time improves utility. The difference between a planned variation (a vacation trip) and a risk (a broken leg) is the element of uncertainty. Saving is limited as a risk management tool because it allows individuals only to trade with themselves at different time periods; it does not spread a catastrophic loss over a large group of people so that it can be borne more easily. Although people can plan a vacation or retirement within their budgets, they may face an extraordinary loss (e.g., spinal injury, cranial fracture) that is far too expensive to be handled by their own resources.

Family and Friends

Young people who have not had a chance to accumulate their own savings must depend on their families' financial resources to carry them during an illness. Although family assistance may be freely and generously given, it creates an obligation to pay your family back when you are well, to be grateful, and to help other family members in the future when they need it. Thus, the family engages in a form of exchange among people as well as among time periods.[1] Your current loss is covered by someone else's current savings, which gives you an obligation to cover someone else's loss in the future. Whereas individual savings allow one person to trade among his or her own time periods to optimize consumption, families trade over time and people; therefore, they can absorb the shock of a loss without a disastrous decline in living standards more effectively than an individual alone.

  Favors that friends do for each other occur so frequently and unconsciously that it seems strange to look at them as trades. When I carry books for someone whose leg is in a cast or take notes for a classmate who has the flu, I am simply being nice and not looking to receive anything in return. Yet ultimately, families and friendship are based on a sense of mutual obligation and reciprocity. If someone consistently fails to help me, eventually I will stop being helpful to him or her. Furthermore, I might let others know how inconsiderate and selfish that person is so that they won't waste their time assisting him or her. It is by such means that the informal rules of exchange among friends and families are enforced. Helping out might not be legally binding, but it is socially binding.

Charity

The obligation to help extends beyond friends and family to people we have never, and may never, meet and who can do nothing for us in return. We still care about people even if we don't know them. Mutual caring makes people a society rather than just a random collection of individuals.[2] The first hospitals were caring institutions, substitute homes for people who did not have a home and for people who were ill or had a disability but whose families were too poor to take care of them.[3] Charity as a means of social exchange predates formal insurance contracts by thousands of years and has been far more important as a way to pay medical bills for most of that time. Yet charity is limited in scope and the extent to which most people feel responsible for someone else's misfortune has declined as formal market institutions have arisen to provide coverage for risks.

Private Market Insurance Contracts

Bad things happen. We cannot always do anything about them. When we can do something, it often costs a great deal of money. Suppose that I am one of one hundred middle-aged executives sent by XXumma Corp. to Eastern Europe for a year. We can assume that several of us will get sick during the year. Suppose we knew that one of us was going to have a heart attack. An operation could help, a coronary artery bypass graft (usually known by its initials CABG and pronounced like "cabbage"), but this operation, with all its attendant aftercare, costs about $50,000. The person who has the heart attack will suffer financially as well as physically. A way of making a bad situation a little better is for us to form a club. Each person puts in $500 and the unlucky one who has a heart attack gets the operation paid for. This is known as **risk pooling**, and it is the essential feature of all insurance.

Although no one can predict who will be the unlucky one, for large numbers of people, the **risk**—the variance and expected value of all losses averaged over all people—is quite predictable. From the individual perspective, insurance is a trade between two possible states of the universe: one in which the person has a heart attack and one in which he or she does not. Money is shifted from the state in which individuals have more (when they are healthy) to the state in which they have less (when they are sick), similar to the way saving shifts money from good periods to pay for the bad periods. From a societal point of view, insurance is a collection of trades between people. Money is shifted from people who have plenty of money (those who are healthy) to people who suffer losses (those who are sick).

Insurance pools losses; it does not get rid of the losses or even reduce them. The group members must pay for all losses (plus some administrative fees or "load") with the **premiums** they pay. Insurance companies do not like to take risks. They like to sell insurance to large groups of people with predictable (average) losses. This way the insurer's revenues and expenses, and therefore its profits, are very stable and predictable from year to year. Insurance companies specialize in pricing risks, not in taking risks. They try to predict exactly how large premiums need to be to cover all the predicted losses. This specialty, known as actuarial science, uses information on previous losses to make accurate predictions of the amount of money required to pay for future benefits. For this example, the probability (one in one hundred) and size ($50,000) of the loss is well known, so it is simple to determine the **actuarially fair premium**, $1/100 \times \$50,000 = \$500$. An actuarially fair premium is the same as the *expected value of a loss* discussed in Chapter 3 with regard to cost-benefit analysis.

Insurance must be priced above the actuarially fair premium to cover the expenses of administering the insurance plan, to provide a cushion for contingencies, and to provide profit to the owners who put up their expertise and capital. The difference between the actual premium and the actuarially fair premium is known as the **loading factor**. It may be as small as 5 percent or 10 percent for group policies covering large businesses and may exceed 100 percent for individual policies.

Traditional insurance plans simply paid for all (or a defined part) of the medical bills a person incurred. Such **indemnity** plans have become rare. People want insurance companies to bargain for lower prices with hospitals and physicians, to evaluate whether new variations on an old drug are really worth twice as much, and to process all paperwork. **Managed care** plans provide a package of services at a cost lower than people could obtain if they tried to do it all on their own (see Chapter 5).

Social Insurance

Market contracts are mutually beneficial to people who purchase insurance and to the companies that act as financial intermediaries. However, they do nothing for people who cannot afford to buy insurance or for people excluded from purchasing insurance (e.g., people with disabilities). Market contracts do not pay for medical research or education programs to promote healthy lifestyles, nor do they provide outreach to teenage mothers or people with mental illness. In short, they do nothing to strengthen the social contract that binds the people of a nation together in support of each other. The informal obligations of citizens to society expressed in charitable giving are extended and formalized in social insurance programs such as Medicare and Social Security in the United States, the National Health Service in the United Kingdom, universal Medicare in Canada, and the health care systems of most countries.[4] Contributions to social insurance are not voluntary but mandatory through the tax system. Who will pay and who will receive are determined by concerns common to all and the political process rather than through individual choices made in the marketplace.

WHY DO POLICE OFFICERS AND FIREFIGHTERS HAVE SUCH COMPREHENSIVE INSURANCE?

Medical coverage for those who put their lives on the line for the good of the community remains comprehensive even though many employers and government agencies are cutting back on benefits. There is a symbolic importance to this insurance that goes beyond financial considerations. If the community is not willing to do everything possible to protect the health of these public servants, why should these servants continue to risk it all to save lives? Similar considerations lie behind the willingness of an Army troop to go to great lengths to recover a wounded or dead comrade when such efforts don't seem to be worthwhile from a cost-benefit perspective and also have led to the creation of a $20 billion system to care for disabled veterans.

As explained in Chapter 1, the U.S. health care system is a blend of private and public financing. Medicare, a social insurance program that covers medical bills for most elderly people in the United States, is larger than the many private for-profit companies combined. Even when insurance is privately paid and managed by profit-making firms, government regulations mandate who is covered, what services are offered, and how prices are set. Therefore, even private insurance is forced into some conformity with social insurance principles.

Strengths and Weaknesses of Different Forms of Risk Spreading

Individual savings are quite limited as a form of risk management since the resources of only one person are used. There is no way that a person born with a genetic defect can save money to cover that risk. Most young people cannot save the $20,000 or so required to treat a broken leg, and a serious illness would exceed the financial capabilities of all but the wealthiest individuals. Trades involving more than one person are needed for coverage. Taking money from family and friends spreads the risk more widely, but this larger group

TABLE 4.1	Types of Risk Protection	
Method	**Reduces Effects of Loss By**	**Depends On**
Savings	Shifting consumption between periods	How much I personally have now
Family, Friends, Charity	Sharing between people	How much people care about me
Insurance Contract	Trading between possible states of the world through financial markets	Ability to price risk

may have difficulty telling whether you really need assistance. In addition, if family and friends do contribute toward your medical bills, they may also want to give you lots of unwelcome advice and intrude in your personal affairs. Charity brings in an even broader group, but the sick individual has less incentive to minimize waste, since he or she is spending other people's money. Charity also tends to be unreliable and even more meddlesome. The extent of resources available is limited by how much people care, and charity alone could never fund a modern medical system.

Markets create impersonal contracts to pay for services. They can draw on financial resources from around the world. Your insurance may be handled by a company in the Netherlands that neither knows nor cares about you as a person, but fully meets your needs as long as the doctor bills get paid on time. Yet markets are driven by profits, not love, and each participant must pay his or her own way. Nothing will be done for a child with a genetic defect unless a parent has a policy that includes dependents. A lawyer's interpretation of a contract replaces family concerns as the factor determining which kind of medical care will be provided. The movement from individual to group to market financing reveals a trade-off: the individual is most sensitive to his or her own needs, but has the smallest span for risk pooling (savings, trade over time periods). The market is global in reach, but impersonal and willing to help only when there is a profit to be made (see Table 4.1).

Social insurance combines the humanitarian thrust of charity with the financial strengths of the market, but it provides only a compromise, not a reconciliation. Social insurance can be comprehensive only if contributions are made compulsory through taxes. As the financing base is broadened to include more people, social insurance grows ever more divorced from personal empathy and becomes just one more government service provided through the political process. As taxpayers, we are willing to provide some medical care for everyone, but not necessarily the best quality in the best rooms of the most modern hospitals. In addition, some taxpayers may be downright hostile about spending millions of dollars on patients who, for example, spent their money on entertainment rather than medical care or who have worsened their own illnesses through substance abuse or unhealthy lifestyles. Social insurance requires that society reach a consensus on who deserves what and how medical care should be delivered. Such a consensus currently exists in the United States only for the elderly under Medicare, and even that can fall apart, as it did in 1989 when revisions to cover pharmaceuticals and catastrophic expenses were passed, implemented, and then repealed by Congress after a revolt by older taxpayers.[5]

4.2 INSURANCE: THIRD-PARTY PAYMENT

As medical care became more expensive, the potential cost of illness went from burdensome to overwhelming. In 1929, $200 was an unusually large medical bill. In today's high-tech intensive care units (ICUs), hospital costs of $100,000 or more are common, with extra payments needed to cover surgery, anesthesia, laboratory tests, and drugs. Few individuals can afford to pay the high cost of advanced modern treatment for serious illness, but few are willing to forgo treatment if they become seriously ill. Insurance makes it possible for most people to obtain care when they need it without going bankrupt. Regular withholding of premiums and taxes spreads the financial risk across many people and makes catastrophic expenses bearable.

Why Third-Party Payment?

Insurance would not be necessary if everyone's medical expenses were near the average. Instead, there is a great deal of variation—much more than there is for food, housing, clothing, transportation, and other major expenses. Most people are healthy during any given year, so that over half of them have minimal costs (less than $600) for medical care (see Table 4.2 and Figure 4.1).[6] However, each person in the top 1 percent had medical expenses above $175,000, and the average for the top 10 percent of the population, which includes most people that needed hospitalization during the year, was over $50,000. Most people will find that their actual costs for the year will be much lower than the premiums for any reasonable health insurance policy, and 90 percent will be well below average (i.e.,

TABLE 4.2		The Concentration of Personal Health Expenditures			
		Top		Upper-Middle	Bottom
	All	**1%**	**Next 9%**	**40%**	**50%**
Persons (millions)	310	3	28	124	155
Health $ (millions)	$2,624,400	$582,617	$1,112,746	$845,057	$83,981
Per person	$ 8,459	$187,809	$ 39,855	$ 6,810	$ 541

FIGURE 4.1   Distribution of Individual Medical Care Expenditures

Note: The 1 percent of individuals with highest cost consume over 20 percent of total services, and the top 5 percent consume about 50 percent.

less than $8,459). Yet who can afford the risk that they will be among the one in ten that requires significant medical care and end up paying $50,000 or more?

Although each of us would prefer to pay nothing, most of us can afford to pay for at least some of the cost of the care we expect to receive if we get sick. Even if we are healthy, it is reasonable to be asked to contribute something toward the expenses of those who are not— but how much? A $175,000 bill could be staggeringly difficult to pay. We might not even think that we can afford $8,459, which is the average annual cost of medical care per person. However, whether we wish to pay that much or not, an average of $8,459 per person must be extracted through taxes, bills paid by individuals, insurance premiums paid by employers (who must therefore reduce wages), or some other means, such as charitable giving, to keep the system running. These funds are needed to keep hospitals open; pay doctors, nurses, custodians, and clerks; keep research laboratories researching; and so forth.

Most of us are not aware of the financial burden we bear for health care provided to ourselves and others. For most workers, employers pay about $2 an hour (8 percent of total wage and benefit compensation) for health benefits, reducing the amount that can be paid out as wages.[7] Even if an employer does not provide health insurance, something is deducted each week as taxes, which is often labeled "H.I." or "FICA:M." This is hospital insurance, not for the employee, but for the elderly and people with disabilities on Medicare. Every time we buy a candy bar or a gallon of gasoline, we pay state taxes that fund Medicaid for indigent people. On the other hand, senior citizens might complain bitterly about the cost of drugs and hospitals and nursing homes, with little awareness of how much subsidy they are receiving. Even if senior citizens pay thousands of dollars out of pocket, more than 90 percent of hospital bills, half of nursing home bills, and almost one-third of the costs of their drugs are being borne by other people, mostly younger working people.

Variability

The chance that an insured group will have extraordinarily high or low losses declines sharply as the number of people in the group increases. Figure 4.2 shows how risk declines with the size of the risk-bearing pool. It assumes that each person in the group has a one in one hundred chance of sustaining a $50,000 loss. The expected loss ($500 per person) is the same regardless of the number of people insured. With just 10 people insured, it is virtually impossible for the loss to be equal to the expected loss of $500. With 100 people in the risk pool, it is possible (37 percent of the time, assuming a standard normal probability

---

FIGURE 4.2   Variability Declines as the Size of the Risk-Sharing
Pool Increases

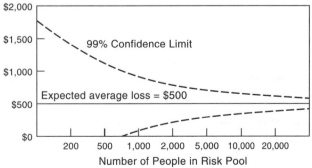

distribution) that one of them will get sick, thereby making the loss equal to the expected value of $500. Just as often (37 percent of the time), however, no one will get sick and losses will be 0. About 18 percent of the time two people in the group will get sick, making the average loss $1,000, and 8 percent of the time three or more people in the group will become ill. With 1,000 people in the group, it is unlikely (0.005 percent) that no one will have an illness. Most (99 percent) of the time the average loss will be between $100 and $900 per person. These are known as 99 percent confidence intervals, which are represented in Figure 4.2 by the dashed lines that start far from the mean and gradually move closer as the number of people in the group increases. With 10,000 people in the risk-pooling group, the chances of no one getting sick are vanishingly small, as are the chances that the average loss will exceed $1,000. The group will experience losses between $370 and $630 per person 99 percent of the time. An insurance company is quite confident doing business with a group this large. On the other hand, a company with fewer than 25 insureds has a sizable chance of losses that are more than double the expected value (about 22 percent of the time).

Third-Party Transactions

Insurance modifies the nature of economic exchange by redirecting the flow of money. It changes who negotiates prices, who bears responsibility for mistakes, and who has the right to profit from directing business to one hospital instead of another. The standard market model with one group (consumers) determining demand and a different group (firms) determining supply is left behind when we enter the medical world with patients (who receive care but do not directly pay for it), insurance companies (who neither supply nor consume, but pool risk and profit from handling funds), and providers (who are reimbursed by a *third party*, insurance, on behalf of a group of patients rather than being paid directly—see Figure 4.3).

What does each of the three parties in an insurance contracting network gain? *Patients* gain by pooling risks to eliminate financial uncertainty and to make expensive treatments affordable. *Insurance companies* benefit from profits. Even when the underwriting gains (the difference between premiums paid in and benefits paid out plus administrative costs) are negative, an apparent loss, companies may still make money because they will hold the premiums for 6 to 24 months before paying out benefits. At 8 percent, the interest on $1 million dollars in premiums for two years is $(1.08) \times (1.08) \times (\$1,000,000) -$ $(\$1,000,000) = \$166,400$, which is not a bad profit for a firm that some reports might claim made no money because benefit payouts exceeded premium revenues. In addition, insurance

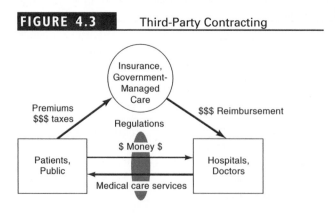

FIGURE 4.3   Third-Party Contracting

companies usually get higher returns on investments than individuals because insurers are so large, with better opportunities and specialized investment staffs. Insurance companies are regulated and taxed as large financial investment institutions, with underwriting gains and losses treated as secondary. This does not mean that underwriting and risk selection are not important, only that expected investment returns are already built into the price of the premium.

Providers gain from an increase in demand and regularity of payment. When patients are covered by insurance, they are more apt to come in for care and less likely to argue about price. Traditionally, patients have expected doctors and hospitals to be more lenient than landlords and bankers about late payment, and many medical bills went unpaid or were paid only in part. Falling demand and irregular payment during the Great Depression in the 1930s forced many hospitals to close due to bankruptcy and led to the start-up of the largest private insurance plan in the world (Blue Cross) as a method of insuring patients so that provider revenues could continue.[8] Like all great ideas, insurance had to benefit all parties so that all parties would enthusiastically cooperate.

Benefits from Exchange

Patients	*Insurers*	*Providers*
risk pooling	profits	increased demand

Who Pays? How Much?

There is a popular misconception that when insurance pays for something, it is free. Unfortunately, while we may not realize who pays because third-party transactions are indirect, every dollar spent on medical care is paid by you, by me, or by someone just like us. Insurance companies and the government never really "pay" for anything. For the most part, individuals pay for medical care by paying higher taxes and/or taking home lower wages. Even the tax advantage for employee benefits does not mean that we are able to get something for nothing. (There are no free lunches!) The government still has to pay its bills. If fewer dollars are collected through wage taxes, more dollars must be collected through gasoline taxes, property taxes, income taxes, Social Security taxes, or other taxes to make up the difference. When a hospital provides "free" care to someone as charity, it must raise charges to those who are insured (and the few who cover their bills out of their own pockets) to pay for it. Insurance does not reduce the cost of medical care; rather it redistributes costs so that different people end up paying.

Under third-party payment systems, the connection between what the first party (the patient) pays and what the second party (the provider) receives is indirect at best. The "charges billed" for a visit to the emergency room often bear little resemblance to what you have to pay or what the hospital receives. In health economics, one must give up the familiar realm of simple two-party transactions in which "bought" and "sold" happen at the same price. This chapter discusses how much the patient (or his or her family) pays, not how much the doctor or hospital actually receives, which is usually quite different (see Chapters 6 and 8). As pointed out in Chapter 1 (Table 4.1 and Figure 1.4), the total of all money paid by patients and families (as out-of-pocket charges, premiums, and taxes combined) will automatically match the total money received by all providers (e.g., hospitals, physicians, drug companies, nursing homes). However, for any particular subgroup or set of transactions, this equivalence is unlikely. Insurance breaks the linkage between what the patient pays and the amount the provider is paid.

People pay premiums to be insured, but then do not pay directly for the medical care they use. Health insurance is similar to having a credit card that allows you to buy whatever you need, but for which payment is set at $100 per month regardless of the number of purchases you make. As you might expect, since one does not have to pay any extra for more purchases, the amount spent tends to rise uncontrollably (see Figure 9.6 for one illustration). That is why most **indemnity insurance plans** providing unlimited reimbursements in return for a fixed premium have disappeared from the market. Most people are now covered by **managed care** plans (see Section 5.5) in which they allow the insurer to exercise some control over the number and type of services covered in return for more affordable premiums. Managed care plans use their control over purchasing to negotiate lower prices from hospitals, doctors, and drug companies. In a sense, managed care represents the evolution of the insurer from a passive financial intermediary to an active purchasing agent.

How Are Benefits Determined?

Insurance is a legal contract that is specific regarding how much will be paid, to which providers, and under what conditions; the evidence of loss required; and who will arbitrate disputes. Health insurance isn't based on sickness at all, but rather on incurring an expense for medical treatment. Most people will never see the complete contract drawn up by their employer and the insurance company; they will only see informational pamphlets, hear descriptions during new employee orientation, and so on. All such benefit descriptions, even in an advertisement or brochure written in Spanish or another language, are legally binding contracts. If a policy states that it covers eye examinations, it covers eye examinations. If a policy states that it will pay $16 for filling a tooth cavity, it will pay $16. In some sense, every set of documents constitutes a slightly different insurance plan. The insurance plan must pay any amount that a court decides a reasonable person reading such descriptions would expect the insurance plan to pay. Furthermore any benefits routinely paid in previous years and not explicitly revoked become a precedent, even if those benefits are not mentioned in the contract. The use of fine print to leave the insured burdened with thousands of dollars of unexpected bills is simply not allowed and in fact would be self-defeating for an insurance company. Over time, premiums will be adjusted upward to cover whatever medical costs are incurred.

4.3 RISK AVERSION

Would people be willing to pay even a 10 percent load (mark-up) just to get their premium money back as benefit payments? To the extent that people can easily fund routine losses through personal savings, they won't be willing to pay the mark-up, which is why most routine losses are not insured. Only large and potentially catastrophic losses are worth paying extra to insure against.

Suppose the premiums required in the earlier heart attack example were not the actuarially fair $500, but $750, or $1,000, or even $1,500? This is still better than having to sell your house, being in debt for 20 years, or—perhaps worse—not being able to have an operation that could save your life if catastrophe strikes. To an economist, the fact that people are willing to pay more than the expected value of the loss for insurance is evidence that they think they are better off with insurance than without it. The desire to replace an uncertain loss with a steady and certain premium payment is known as **risk aversion**. Some people feel very strongly about risk and will go to great lengths to avoid it. Most people choose not to take financial chances unless they have to or are well paid for doing so

---

ARE YOU RISK AVERSE?

Here's an easy test. Imagine your boss offering to flip a coin to determine whether to double your monthly paycheck or take it away. If the prospect of losing your paycheck is much more unpleasant than the chance of doubling it, you, like most people, are risk averse and a good candidate for insurance.

(e.g., risky investments provide a higher rate of interest than safe government bonds). Others are willing to take some chances. To some extent this is a matter of taste, similar to how spicy you like your food. Your aversion to risk also depends to some extent on how much income you have—going from $2 million a year to $50,000 is not nearly as scary as going from $200,000 to $5,000, which would provide you with less than $100 a week to spend on food, rent (forget it—you're living at your parent's place again or homeless), and travel (mostly by bus).

With insurance, people can obtain medical care they otherwise could not afford. What if a $350,000 liver transplant could extend your life expectancy by 10 years? If you value your life at $100,000 per year (see Section 3.6), the benefit-to-cost ratio of treatment is 3 to 1 and clearly worthwhile. Yet you, like most people, do not have $350,000 in cash to spend and cannot get a bank loan for that amount, without collateral, just to possibly extend life. Insurance expands the choice set of patients facing serious illness and gives us all peace of mind. Economist John Nyman estimates that this **access to treatment** (affordability) gain is more valuable than pure risk sharing in ordinary financial insurance by an order of magnitude.[9] When it comes to life and death, being able to get help is extremely important.

Given that most people are risk averse, why aren't all risks insured? Life is full of risk. I buy an airplane ticket for a spring vacation even though I could die before I ever get to use it. My bicycle might be stolen. Some people study for a profession, such as accounting or computer science, only to find that job market conditions have changed by the time they graduate. As you take the exam for this course, at least some of the result (I hope not all) will be random (e.g., which questions were asked during class, when television commercial breaks occurred during your study time). Only a few risks in life are insured. Why? For one reason, it is costly to write up and specify insurance contracts, pay claims, and so on. Most small losses will, on average, balance out over time and thus can be handled by savings. In addition, several structural incentive problems occur with insurance such as adverse selection and moral hazard, discussed later in this chapter, that reduce its value.

In most property and casualty insurance, the losses that are insured are large, infrequent, and random (unpredictable). Many medical expenses meet these criteria, but not all do. For example, most doctor visits for colds and the flu are small, frequent, and fairly predictable. Although the magnitude of the financial losses incurred might explain why some medical expenses are insured, it does not explain why insurance coverage is so extensive in health care, covering many minor and routine services as well as catastrophic events. Three special factors must be recognized in considering the market for health insurance. One is the belief that everyone has a right to medical care. Another is the effectiveness of medical providers in promoting insurance because it provides benefits to them, not the least of which is removing the doctor–patient relationship from the world of commercial trade and haggling over price. Third, and perhaps most important, is the near impossibility of patients acting as informed consumers and smart shoppers. Trying to determine what medical care to get, whether treatment A is really worth $1,500 more than treatment B, or whether having an operation now will save money in the long run, is too difficult. We turn to intermediaries, to doctors and insurance plans, to make many of these decisions for us.

The fact that we are not insured against all risks raises an interesting question: If people are so risk averse, why do they gamble (by playing the lottery or at casinos)? It is clear why people may gamble on an investment in stock or land. They are compensated by getting (on average) higher returns than they can obtain with less risky investments. However, in the casino form of gambling, you don't get paid for taking risks; you have to pay for the privilege of taking on risk. The truth is, people gamble this way mostly for fun. It is something exciting to do, like going to a sports event. Sometimes people gamble because they do not understand that the odds are against them—that if they keep playing long enough they are bound to lose. Then there are a few people who gamble because it is their job, and like casinos, they almost always win when we put our money on the table. Don't envy the professional gambler too much, though. For this person, gambling is work rather than a diversion, and the hardest thing is finding willing customers—which is also the case for insurance salespeople.

4.4 ADVERSE SELECTION

Risk pooling works well because everyone in the group is at risk and therefore has an interest in making sure that solid insurance benefits are provided. Consider the heart attack example again, and suppose that instead of the risk being purely random, you knew that you were the one who would end up in the hospital. In this case, you would make sure that you got insurance and might even be willing to pay an astronomical premium to get it. However, if you were certain that you were not going to be the one ending up in the hospital, you would not try very hard to be part of the insurance group and might not be willing to pay $500 or even $50. Whenever the group of people actually insured is not average, but disproportionately composed of those at higher risk, then adverse selection has occurred.

If higher risks result from something the insurance company can observe in advance and that both the insured and the company acknowledge, varying premiums by risk category causes no difficulties. For example, pricing by age is common, such as charging $300 per month for people 35 and younger, $500 for people 35 to 50, $650 for people 51 to 60, and $900 for people 61 and older. Adverse selection creates difficulties when some risk factors are known to the insured, but not to the insurance company (e.g., my chest hurts every time I go walking, I enjoy fried foods and recreational drugs, my brother and sister recently died from heart attacks). Difficulties arise even when the risks are well known but it is considered "unfair" to charge for them (e.g., women employees paying less than men, doubling the premiums for people age 61 and older, charging unmarried men more because of the perceived higher risk of HIV/AIDS). If an employer subsidizes an optional health plan for its workers, the ones most likely to buy insurance are those at high risk. This is called **adverse selection** and means that the average losses in the insured group will be larger than the expected value for the employees as a whole. If young, healthy workers do not participate, premiums have to increase. At the extreme, the plan may be left with only those who were ill to begin with and who knew that they would collect benefits, which is not considered insurance at all because there is no risk pooling. For this reason, insurance companies usually require that all or at least a majority of the employees in an organization be insured.

A more subtle form of adverse selection occurs when a company offers two kinds of plans, a basic plan and a more comprehensive option for which employees pay extra. Who will choose the comprehensive plan? Some people will choose it because they are very risk averse and therefore willing to pay extra for the more comprehensive benefits. This causes no difficulty for the insurance plan since the actuarial risk (expected loss) of such people is about average. The difficulty arises because there will also be a disproportionate number of high-risk individuals (e.g., those who are older or overweight) who buy the comprehensive plan. As more and more high-risk people sign up for the comprehensive plan, their medical expenses will exceed the expected value, and even the "high" premium will not be sufficient to pay the bills. Thus, the extra premium for comprehensive insurance must be raised still higher. As the premium goes up, fewer and fewer low-risk people are willing to pay for the better coverage. Eventually, only the chronically ill who are certain to sustain a big loss will sign up for the comprehensive plan. As the difference in premiums between the basic and high-option plan becomes greater, fewer and fewer people at low risk are left in the high-option pool. The principle of risk sharing is defeated by the progressive separation of risks between the groups. This death spiral ends with the termination of the high-option plan (see the box "Adverse Selection at Harvard").

The more differences there are in expected costs of illnesses and the more inside information people have about their own health, the greater the potential for adverse selection (see the box "Do People Choose to Die?"). The elderly are particularly problematic because many of their medical expenses are for chronic illnesses that are well known to them and not random. Insurers' major method for reducing adverse selection, insisting that all employees

---

ADVERSE SELECTION AT HARVARD: GETTING PUSHED OUT OF THE PPO

In 1994, Harvard University faced a substantial deficit in the employee benefits budgets. For years, Harvard had offered both HMO and PPO health insurance plans, with the more expensive PPO plans being more generously subsidized by the university. In order to reduce cost, Harvard in 1995 implemented a new program in which it contributed the same dollar amount regardless of which plan the employee chose (although the amount contributed is larger for low-income employees). Although employee contributions went up for all plans, they went up more for the relatively generous PPO Flex plan (see Table 4.3). In response, enrollment in this high-option plan began to fall. David Cutler and Sarah Reber examined the characteristics of those employees who switched out of the high-priced plan.[10] As theory predicts, those who switched were more likely to be healthy; they were younger on average and had spent less on medical care in prior years than those who elected to pay more and stay in the high-option plan. Hence it is not surprising that the high-option PPO Flex lost money in 1995. To compensate, PPO premiums were raised an additional 16 percent for 1996, which pushed even more young healthy employees into the HMO plans, and the PPO lost even more money. In 1997, the pattern was clear and the high-option plan was discontinued, completing an adverse selection death spiral in only three years.

TABLE 4.3 — Changes in Employee Premiums and Enrollment at Harvard

		Employee Pays		Enrollment			
	Premium	Old	New	1994	1995	1996	1997
Individual							
PPO Flex	$2,773	$555	$1,152	16%	13%	8%	Discontinued
HMO	1,980	277	421	84%	87%	92%	100%
Family							
PPO Flex	$6,238	$1,248	$2,208	22%	18%	11%	Discontinued
HMO	5,395	776	1,191	78%	82%	89%	100%

Source: David M. Cutler and Sarah J. Rebler, "Paying for Health Insurance: The Trade-off Between Competition and Adverse Selection," *Quarterly Journal of Economics* 113 (May 1998):433–466.

DO PEOPLE CHOOSE TO DIE?

Actuaries have found that people who buy life insurance are more likely than average to die prematurely.[11] The reasons have less to do with the drama depicted in Arthur Miller's *Death of a Salesman* (since suicide invalidates many policies) than with mundane adverse selection. For example, people who know that their parents died young or that their heart palpitates, or who worry about their lack of physical activity since they turned fifty, are more apt to buy life insurance when it is offered. Conversely, those who buy annuities (policies that pay insureds a certain amount per year as long as they live) show positive selection and are less likely than average to die prematurely. Questionnaire respondents who reply "yes" when asked, "Do you expect to live a long time?" do, in fact, enjoy longer lives than those who respond "no," even after adjusting for the effects of age, blood pressure, cigarette smoking, and all other measurable health risks. This indicates that individuals do have private knowledge that they can use to select coverage that is most favorable to them but costly to the insurer.

---

in a company be included in a group plan, is not available for the elderly since most of them are retired. The ultimate solution for adverse selection is to include everyone in a social insurance system, similar to what the United States did for the elderly by creating Medicare.

4.5 MORAL HAZARD

A person with medical insurance is more likely to go to the doctor because of a sore throat than someone who is not insured. If sent to the hospital, an insured person is more likely to pick a nicer and more expensive facility than an uninsured person. These changes in behavior cause the expenditures of people with insurance to be greater than what an actuary would have predicted from observing the records of people without insurance, and this increase in loss is known as **moral hazard**. One form of these behavioral changes can be illustrated using ordinary demand curve analysis (see Figure 4.4). The demand for physician visits by people without insurance is shown in line D. With insurance picking up 80 percent of the

FIGURE 4.4   Moral Hazard

"Moral hazard" increase in
consumption due to insurance

costs, the net "price" (P_i) that a patient has to pay personally is just 20 percent of the actual price; therefore, consumption will increase to Q_i. This increase in visits resulting from being insured is attributable to moral hazard.

Insurance obviously makes patients less aware of and sensitive to the price of care, but is it likely that people will use services having little or no health benefit just because they are free? For heart surgery, no. Pain and the loss of time are sufficient to keep most people from undertaking surgery just for the fun of it. What about routine office visits? Many of them are for minor symptoms that will go away without treatment. Insurance makes people much more likely to seek treatment for minor symptoms and thus to increase the overall cost of insurance. Even some surgical procedures are of limited value and are likely to be undertaken only if insurance pays. Suppose 76-year-old Uncle Al has a liver infection. It is probable that he will die from the infection no matter what we do, but there is a chance that he could live several more months or even years with a liver transplant—at a cost of $100,000 for the surgery and $5,000 per month after that for drugs and after care. If Uncle Al or the family had to pay directly out of their own pockets, they would probably decide that it was not worth paying so much for such an expensive operation that is unlikely to be successful. However, if insurance is picking up the tab, or if Medicare is passing the cost on to all other taxpayers, Uncle Al and the family might go ahead and try for an improbable cure.

Figure 4.5 shows that the extent of expenditure increase due to moral hazard increases with the price elasticity of the demand curve. For services that are not very price sensitive (D_1), the fact that people are insured will not cause them to purchase many more services; therefore, there will not be much of a distortion in consumer behavior due to insurance. On the other hand, for services that are very price elastic (D_2), the fact that people are insured can cause a very large increase in the quantity they consume (which insurance will pay for), thereby making moral hazard a large problem. This theoretical result provides us with a hypothesis about which services will be covered by insurance. Since moral hazard reduces gains from risk pooling, types of medical care for which there is considerable moral hazard (services with high price elasticity) will be less likely to be covered by insurance than services for which there is very little moral hazard (those with low price elasticity). A number of studies have shown that this is the case.[12] Services such as hospital care and surgery with lower price elasticity of demand are more likely to be insured than services such as nursing home care, physical therapy, mental health care, dentistry, and drugs, which have a higher price elasticity of demand. Exchange must make all parties better off, and when problems

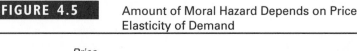

FIGURE 4.5   Amount of Moral Hazard Depends on Price Elasticity of Demand

such as moral hazard reduce the value of transacting, there will be less pooling of risks through the insurance market.

Welfare Losses Due to Moral Hazard

The extra services people consume just because they are covered by insurance result in some economic waste. If it costs $20 to produce an X-ray, but the X-ray is only worth $5 to the patient, there is a net loss of value of $15. This loss of value is often called the **welfare triangle** because the area of the triangle between the price that the insurance company must pay and the demand curve yields a good measure of the size of the loss (see Figure 4.6). If insurance pays 80 percent of the bill, the number of X-rays consumed rises from five to nine. The cost of each X-ray stays the same, $20. The sixth X-ray is worth only $16, for a loss of $4; the seventh is worth $12, for a loss of $8; the eighth is worth $8, for a loss of $12; and the ninth is worth $4, for a loss of $16. The total amount paid for the four extra X-rays is $80, and the **welfare loss** is about half that, $40.[13]

Who loses? All members of the insured group lose because their premiums must be higher to cover this excess use of services. In fact, even the person getting the extra service probably would prefer a tighter contract that provided only worthwhile services at a lower premium. This is why so much work is done using contract exclusions, fee limits, second opinions, and so on to make sure that reimbursement is provided only for necessary services. There is a demand for the "hassle" of making patients and physicians justify their use of services because it reduces premiums. Evidence of this demand is that consumers choose policies that include restrictive contractual language rather than policies that pay for everything without question but cost more. This does not mean that it is pleasant when you are sick to go through all sorts of bureaucratic hoops to get a claim paid; it does mean that the effort is justified in terms of reduced premiums—or else you would choose a different plan. Insurance companies will give customers whatever they want, including aggravation, to make a profit.

Welfare losses due to moral hazard are to some extent unavoidable. They are part of the cost of insurance, the way that an unwanted orange peel is part of the cost of an orange. On net, people are better off with the insurance (including moral hazard) than without it. If people are buying insurance, the gains from trade due to risk pooling must be exceeding the

FIGURE 4.6   Welfare Loss due to Moral Hazard

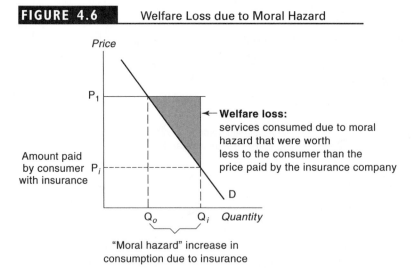

welfare losses from moral hazard. If the losses were larger than the gains, people would not buy. However, when the purchase of insurance is subsidized by the government, this may no longer be the case. The extra insurance bought due to tax subsidization creates additional excess utilization of services that are not highly valued by consumers (see Section 4.6).[14]

There is a systemwide welfare loss caused by insurance that is more difficult to see. Insurance tends to increase demand and make patients less price sensitive, which increases prices overall. Whether or not one person becomes insured will have little effect on the price of X-rays. Yet if everyone who now has insurance had it taken away, demand would fall and the price of X-rays would surely decline. People who are uninsured are worse off because other people are insured, because those other people's insurance raises the price that uninsured people have to pay in order to obtain care.[15] It is even possible that we all would be better off if we were all uninsured, even though each one of us individually is better off with insurance. This paradoxical (and quite unlikely) result would only occur if the gains from risk pooling were smaller than the increase in prices resulting from universal insurance.[16] However, the systematic distortion of prices resulting from insurance raising overall demand may create a larger welfare loss than the moral hazard welfare triangle attributable to tax subsidy. Such systemwide effects are difficult to gauge, because looking at individual behavior may not tell us what is happening to the system as a whole. One way to measure systemwide effects is to compare different health care systems in different countries that use different types of insurance to see how well each one works and what they cost, but this ambitious effort is left for later (see Chapter 17).

4.6 TAX BENEFITS

There is a less visible and more diffuse fourth party in most third-party insurance transactions—the government. Many governments take on the social obligation to provide medical care directly, as is done by the National Health Service in the United Kingdom and by the Swedish health system. Some countries have chosen to build on employee health insurance plans to create universal coverage for all citizens, such as the German Krankenkassen or the Japanese employment societies. The United States is somewhat unique in that insurance is encouraged but not universally required. The U.S. government, through Medicare, directly provides insurance for all people 65 and older and through Medicaid for many people who are classified as being indigent or disabled. The U.S. government also provides tax incentives for many others to be insured through the private sector. The primary tax incentive is that health benefits are nontaxable compensation for employees but still allowed as deductible expenses for the employer. The following example shows how this tax incentive works.

Employee Pays for Medical Care		**Employer Pays for Insurance**
$1,000	Company labor cost	$1,000
None	Insurance premium	($200)
$1,000	Gross paycheck	$800
($350)	Taxes (at 35 percent)	($280)
$650	Net paycheck	$520
($200)	Medical bills	None
$450	**Available for spending**	**$520**

The employer spends the same for labor either way and does not care whether insurance premiums are taken out of a paycheck or paid later from the employee's bank account. With insurance taken out, the employees' gross income is less and therefore the amount of taxes paid is less. The employee with the larger paycheck, after paying for medical care with after-tax dollars, has less money left for spending than the employee whose health insurance premiums paid for the same amount of medical care on a pre-tax basis. As long as the administrative load is less than the tax rate, it is cheaper to buy medical care pre-tax using employer-paid insurance than for the employee to pay the bills directly. This tax break for employer-paid health insurance is a substantial (more than $250 billion per year) and important part of the voluntary system of health care that Americans have come to depend on.[17] Without the tax incentive, most working people would not have health insurance as an employee benefit.

4.7   EFFECTS OF HEALTH INSURANCE ON LABOR MARKETS

One of the reasons that people take a job is to obtain health insurance. It is a benefit to them, but it is a cost to the employer. However, it is a fixed cost per person: the premiums do not go up if an employee works 48 hours rather than 40 or go down if only 30 hours are worked. Thus it is cheaper to hire 10 employees and have them work 20 percent harder than to hire 12 employees and pay for two additional insurance premiums (unless the wage rate has to go up for overtime). As the cost of health care rises, the employer has a greater and greater incentive to get each employee to work harder for more hours so as to avoid hiring more people.[18] Another way for a company to avoid the rising cost of health insurance is to replace full-time employees with part-timers who do not receive benefits. The costs of providing health insurance benefits is similarly reduced by using independent contractors, long-term "temps," and adjunct instructors rather than regular faculty.

Looking at the supply and demand curves for labor, it is evident that increasing the benefits cost per person should reduce not only the quantity of regular labor, but also its price. The total compensation (wage + benefits) rises, reducing quantity (number hired) and price (wage rates) (Figure 4.7). This result is confirmed by several studies showing that most, but not all, of an increase in health care premiums shows up as a decrease in take-home pay.[19]

Employers can also reduce their health insurance costs by having healthier employees. Whereas it is very difficult to get people to change their behavior by enough to significantly

FIGURE 4.7   Effect of Increased Benefits Cost on Price (Wages) and Quantity of Labor

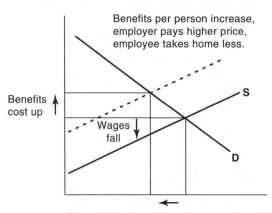

reduce the rate of costly illnesses, it is fairly easy to just not hire unhealthy employees—which is why nondiscrimination laws and policies make it illegal to refuse to hire someone because they are old, overweight, have HIV, or could get pregnant. It is also why certain benefits are mandated and legally required. Rather than not hiring women, a restaurant could just refuse to pay for births or gynecology. Although selecting only people who are healthy and inexpensive to cover might help the employer, it would make things worse not only for the people who are discriminated against, but also for the government, hospitals, and all the rest of us that end up paying and caring for all the sick people who cannot get employer provided health insurance.

Employees as well as employers respond to incentives. People who have health insurance through a spouse or family member are more likely to take time off, to switch jobs, or retire.[20] A poor single mother whose children are covered by Medicaid is not going to take a minimum-wage job that will cause her to lose her benefits. Studies have shown that potential loss of insurance benefits is a significant reason that people continue working when they would rather retire, and also stick with the same employer even when they would rather look for another job and switch.[21]

4.8   HISTORY OF HEALTH INSURANCE

In some sense, risk pooling has always existed—people have always taken care of each other during times of need. Financial contracts for pooling risk did not become important until the Industrial Revolution, when economies moved from the medieval manor system, where most people worked the land, to a wage-based economy centered in cities and towns. Freemen who left the medieval estates and gathered in town to practice skilled trades, such as printers and goldsmiths, often became quite wealthy, but were potentially subject to catastrophic losses if they become ill. Although gaining freedom, they had given up the protection and security that went with being part of an estate. If they became sick, they might have become destitute. The guilds were organized to further their interests collectively and became natural vehicles for sharing risks. Initially this took the form of soliciting donations from all other guild members—"passing the hat" when someone became ill or died. Then more formal institutions evolved that accumulated funds over time. A "subscription" would be regularly collected that could be used to pay benefits. In this early form of insurance, there was no distinction made between the loss of wages due to illness and the costs of medical care (or burial). Insurance was simply a way to provide money in time of need. The guild members knew each other well, and therefore the definition of loss was made by a consensus of the leadership, not by the existence of a doctor's bill.[22]

Early industrialists also recognized the need to provide wages and medical care for workers when they were sick. It is unlikely that funds were set aside for this purpose. Rather, sickness funds were drawn out of daily business receipts. Most such benefits were informal, provided at the discretion of the business owner, and not part of the official employment contract. In this sense, early industrial benefits were quite similar to the paternalistic obligations owed to the serfs by the manorial lords who owned the land they worked on, except that as factories and wages replaced farms and tenant shares, the benefits were money payments rather than direct care. By the nineteenth century, some industries that were particularly dangerous and remote (mining, timber) had developed contracts with a "company doctor" so that there was always regular medical care available. In other industries, it was the workers who organized to provide sickness benefits. As unions became an important means for furthering the interests of workers, they found that they needed some way to keep the membership involved (and paying dues) throughout the year and not just when a strike was threatened. Medical coverage became the preferred union benefit. It was always needed, made the workers and their families grateful, and attracted newcomers. In those days care could be provided at relatively low cost through clinics or "dispensaries" staffed by young doctors hired by the union to practice several nights a week. Company and union clinics, mutual benefit societies, and other forms of prepayment had become common by 1850, but still provided medical care financing to only a small fraction of the population, probably less than one-twentieth. As wages rose above the subsistence level and workers became more assertive, it became evident that insurance would have to be extended to cover more of the population.

The first national health insurance program was implemented in Germany in 1883. Bismarck, the chancellor who had unified the German Lander (provinces) into a nation, saw that his political successes were threatened by the popularity of socialist causes among workers. By putting together a social security system with medical insurance and retirement benefits for industrial workers, he preempted one of the main goals of the socialist movement and was able to maintain popular support.[23] National health plans were established in England in 1911, Sweden in 1914, and France in 1930. At first, only salaried workers in the major manufacturing plants were covered, usually with a lesser degree of coverage for dependents. Other workers, such as agricultural and retail workers, day laborers, shopkeepers, and the self-employed, had to take care of themselves. Over the next 50 years, coverage was successively broadened. By 1980, almost every developed country had health insurance coverage for all citizens, either through a national health service (United Kingdom) or a universal insurance plan (Canada) or by coordinating all employer-based plans and providing government insurance for the rest of the population (Germany, Japan).[24] Evolution of health insurance in the United States was much different, and a large segment of the population still lacks health insurance today.

The United States depended on voluntary private initiatives to develop health insurance, with much less reliance on government. There was a recognition that the population needed protection against losses due to illness, and in 1929 the independent Committee of the Costs of Medical Care began a fact-finding study, eventually producing a 28-volume report that was very influential in shaping the growth of voluntary insurance in the United States.[25] In this same year, Baylor Hospital proposed to the local teachers' association that it would provide all the care needed to anyone who would pay a premium of $0.50 a month. The plan proved to be very popular, and similar plans were started by other hospitals nearby. One problem with a "hospital prepayment" plan was that a patient whose doctor worked in a different hospital, or who needed a special type of care elsewhere, got no benefits. The solution was to combine all the separate plans under the sponsorship of the state hospital association so that one plan covered all hospitals; thus, Blue Cross was born. It grew rapidly, from 3,000 members in 1930, to more than 10,000 in 1932, and to more than 1,000,000 by 1936. In 2009, 102 million people were insured through 39 Blue Cross/Blue Shield plans, but many of these had changed during the last 10 years from local nonprofit community organizations to large multistate for-profit corporations.[26]

The imposition of wage and price controls during World War II provided an indirect, but powerful, boost to voluntary insurance. Employers were not allowed to raise wages, but they could provide additional benefits.[27] With wartime production booming and many laborers drafted into the military, most companies desperately needed to attract more workers. In less than 20 years, health insurance went from being an occasional perk that covered just 5 percent of the population to a routine benefit that was expected to be part of any good job and covered more than 50 percent of the population. Even with favorable tax treatments and active encouragement, voluntary insurance could not be extended to cover two of the groups who needed it most: the elderly and the poor. The poor were simply not able to afford health insurance. Furthermore, while policy makers and hospital administrators might think that paying premiums to prepare for future medical expenses was one of the most important things a family could do with its money, many of the poor did not. Since there was always some form of care available, usually in city clinics and hospitals, the poor often chose to spend what little discretionary money they had on better housing, better food, or some entertainment, rather than insurance premiums.

The difficulties of the elderly in obtaining insurance were largely attributable to adverse selection and the discounting of consumption over time.[28] While younger people were formed into risk-pooling groups on the basis of employment, many older people were not attached to an employer. There was no natural grouping by which risks could be shared, and there were no tax advantages to insurance premiums paid out of savings or retirement benefits rather than wages. Differences in the expected costs of medical care between individuals are much greater for older people, making it more difficult to constitute risk-sharing pools. Whereas many of the illnesses that strike younger people are essentially random events of low probability, many medical expenses of the elderly are for chronic conditions. There is no reason for a healthy 72-year-old to want to be in a group paying the same premium as someone with cancer or arthritis who is likely to have high medical expenses for many years. Elderly people often know much more about the potential cost of their health conditions than any insurance company can, thus creating adverse selection problems when allowed to purchase insurance individually. These difficulties are exacerbated by the need to save early in one's career to pay for medical expenses that come after retirement. There must be a mechanism for transferring dollars from consumption at early ages toward old age. The Social Security Acts of 1965, which established the **Medicare** (Title XVI) program for the elderly and **Medicaid** (Title XVII) for the indigent, brought fundamental changes in the U.S. health care system and made government a major partner in financing medical care.[29] Adverse selection was no longer a problem for the elderly, because everyone age 65 or older was insured. Poverty no longer excluded the indigent from health insurance, because the government made these benefits available at no cost.[30]

After a century of development, health care financing in the United States is still in flux, with a mixed public and private system in which government accounts for 48 percent of total funds (59 percent once tax subsidies are included), private insurance accounts for 34 percent (including Blue Cross/Blue Shield, self-funded employer plans, commercial insurance companies, and HMOs), charitable contributions and various programs account for 7 percent, and the remaining 11 percent is paid directly by patients and family members out of pocket. A sizable fraction of those out-of-pocket costs are for deductibles and coinsurance and thus, in one sense, could be considered part of the third-party insurance payments.

Among this variety of health insurance organizations, government (Medicare in particular) is now the dominant payer. During the 1950s, Blue Cross set the tone and structure for insurance coverage and Medicare copied the Blue Cross reimbursement system. Since then, the balance of power has changed dramatically. Blue Cross has fragmented, reducing what was once a pervasive community voluntary organization to a set of franchisees linked by a trademark, with the largest (California, New York) transformed into independent, and essentially faceless, for-profit insurance companies with no specific ideology or geographic ties. Conversely, Medicare has become so large that no hospital and few doctors can afford to be without a Medicare contract. Every provider is thus compelled to use the complex and highly regulated Medicare cost and activity reporting scheme. Other insurers find it easier to adapt the Medicare payment system than to develop their own, making the influence of Medicare even greater than its percentage share of the market.

4.9 FINANCING HEALTH CARE: INSURANCE AS A FUNDING MECHANISM

From the point of view of the patient, the problem is how to find enough money to pay for needed medical care or to get someone else (insurance, government) to pay. From the perspective of the government or the medical care system as a whole, the problem is how to extract enough money from the economy to cover all of the expensive personnel and new technology, regardless of who pays. From the point of view of insurance companies and medical corporations, the issue is how to make the most profit. Most market goods and services are paid for as a result of the individual decisions of many people and firms, without outside intervention, but all modern economies use taxes and insurance—prepaid funding— in order to pay for medical care (see Chapters 16 and 17). From a system perspective, it simply is not possible to get enough money from individual payments to finance a modern medical system. Very few patients, no matter how much they need chemotherapy and organ transplants, are going to be able to pay $150,000 at their moment of need. Unlike the similarly expensive purchase of a house, they are not going to start saving up in their twenties in order to make a down payment or take out a mortgage—and, if they did take out a mortgage, who would pay it off if they died? The public expects expensive and technologically sophisticated medicine to be available, but they cannot pay for it without some comprehensive financing mechanism.

The most common form of financing in most countries is a dedicated wage tax, as is used in the United States to fund Medicare. Some countries pay for most medical care out of general taxes (such as in the UK, Italy, Sweden, and Taiwan), some rely primarily on wage taxes (such as Germany and Japan), while some use a substantial proportion of private insurance and voluntary employer payments (such as Australia and the United States). Reliance on patients' personal payments to fund medical care is limited to relatively undeveloped economies, and none that has a modern and technologically sophisticated medical system.

Entitlements: Open or Closed Financing?

Most markets have "open" funding—consumers can spend as much as they want on food, on clothes, on cars, on books, and so forth. Limits are imposed only by the constraint that income puts on spending. In order to buy more books, one has to give up some food (or something else) or work more to earn extra money. When consumers are not paying directly, as in tax-supported government programs, limits on spending are usually set in advance through a fixed budget, and financing can be said to be "closed." The National Health Service (NHS) in the United Kingdom is a notable example of closed or "global" budgeting. [31] Parts of the U.S. health care system have had closed-end budgets (e.g., immunization programs, city health clinics, Department of Veterans Affairs hospitals, state mental hospitals). Yet traditionally, the United States has relied on a mixture that is both open and closed, termed "**entitlement** funding."

In Medicare, Medicaid, and most employer-based health insurance plans, patients are entitled to a specified set of services that the payer has to cover, regardless of the amount and types of services used or the prices charged. Historically, insurance companies did not care much about the size of the bill, since they were merely third-party intermediaries, raising premiums to match the rise in the cost of services. Patients had little incentive to moderate utilization, since services were being paid for with "other peoples' money" (i.e., taxes, insurance, employers' reserves). Hospitals, physicians, and other providers had even

TABLE 4.4 Comparison of Open-Ended and Closed-End Health Care Financing

Open-Ended Entitlement Funding

Patients	Providers	Insurance	Short-Run Problems	Long-Run Problems
Demand care	Produce services	Pays bills *(all risks are here and purely financial)*	Variability in costs	Costs escalate uncontrollably

Closed-End Budget Funding

Government	Providers	Patients	Short-Run Problems	Long-Run Problems
Allocates budget *(no financial risk—political unrest)*	Produce services *(consumer complaints)*	Receive care *(quality/quantity risk)*	Government blamed for everything	Stagnant, unresponsive system since customers carry no $$

less incentive to hold the line on costs, since larger total insurance reimbursements implied larger total payments to providers. The end result was that costs soared out of control. Eventually employers, Medicare, and Medicaid were all forced to make changes to reduce expenditures. In Medicare and Medicaid, the freedom of doctors and hospitals to charge what they wanted was replaced by controlled administrative prices under the prospective payment "Resource Based Relative Value System" (RBRVS) (see Chapter 6) and "Diagnostically Related Group" (DRG) system (see Chapter 8). Employers started to control health insurance costs by using managed care contracts (Chapter 5).

Both open and closed financing are subject to problems that are inherent in the structure of the financing contract (Table 4.4). In open-ended systems, if there are excess demands, either the insurance pool runs a deficit or individuals must reduce other consumption to pay medical bills. If excess demands are placed on closed systems with a fixed budget, no more money is spent, but troubles arise due to poor service, long waiting lists, and other frictional costs that lead to patient dissatisfaction. Mixing open and closed funding through entitlement financing reduces some problems but creates others. An entitlement system without a fixed budget lacks any strong set of cost controls. Yet at the same time it still requires open-ended government subsidy either directly, as in Medicare and Medicaid, or indirectly, as in the tax-exemption of employer-based health insurance. The various contractual innovations mentioned in the previous paragraph can all be viewed as attempts to combine open and closed funding in such a way as to simultaneously control costs and maintain patient satisfaction.

SUGGESTIONS FOR FURTHER READING

AHIP (America's Health Insurance Plans), www.AHIP.org

David M. Cutler and Sarah J. Reber, "Paying for Health Insurance: The Trade-Off Between Competition and Adverse Selection," *Quarterly Journal of Economics* 113 (May 1998): 433–466.

Employee Benefit Research Institute, www.ebri.org

Paul Gertler and Jonathan Gruber, "Insuring Consumption Against Illness," NBER working paper w6035, May 1997, available at http://nber.org/papers/w603

Institute of Medicine, *Employment and Health Benefits: A Connection at Risk* (Washington, D.C: National Academy Press, 1993).

John Nyman, *Health Insurance* (Palo Alto, Calif.: Stanford University Press, 2002).
Mark V. Pauly, "Taxation, Health Insurance, and Market Failure in the Medical Economy," *Journal of Economic Literature* 24, no. 2 (June 1986): 629–675.

SUMMARY

1. From an individual perspective, **insurance is a form of trade** between time periods or between different possible states (healthy or sick) in the future. From a societal perspective, insurance is a method of **pooling risks** so that the burden of financial loss is distributed over many people. An individual's **savings** can spread the cost of illness over time. **Family, friends, and charity** spread risk across people. **Private insurance contracts** spread risk through organized markets. **Social insurance** uses taxation to spread risk over all citizens.

2. Due to the **uncertain and uneven distribution of medical care costs**, with 70 percent of total dollars being spent on behalf of the 10 percent of people who become most ill during a year, most health care payments flow through **third-party insurance** intermediaries that pool and transfer funds, which differs from the direct exchange of money for services between two parties (consumers and providers) common to most markets.

3. An **actuarially fair premium** is equal to the **expected value** of a loss, the dollar amount multiplied by the probability of occurrence. The "law of large numbers" means that higher losses for some will be offset by lower losses for others; therefore, for a large group the overall loss usually will be close to the expected value. If each person contributes an average amount, the pooled funds will be enough to pay for all the individual losses.

4. **Insurance companies do not pay for losses**—people do. The entire cost of medical care, including the costs of administration and use of financial capital, is paid through premiums, taxes, or patient coinsurance (e.g., deductibles, copayments) collected for each service rendered. Therefore, only large, random, infrequent losses are worth insuring. Insurance covering small, regular losses raises costs while providing few benefits from risk reduction.

5. People prefer having an income that is certain rather than the same average income subject to random fluctuations. Because of **risk aversion**, consumers are willing to pay more than the expected value of a loss to obtain insurance coverage. From the supply side, the excess of premiums received over benefits paid is called the load or **underwriting gains** of the insurance company.

6. People who know that they are likely to sustain a loss are more likely to purchase insurance, resulting in **adverse selection**, a change in the composition of the insured group. This difficulty in the grouping of people for insurance is to be distinguished from an increase in the average loss due to a change in the behavior of individuals.

7. **Moral hazard** occurs whenever having insurance leads individuals to increase the amount spent or to increase the risk of loss. In health economics, moral hazard most commonly refers to the increase in utilization of medical services that result from being insured. The **welfare loss due to insurance** occurs because people who do not have to pay the bills tend to consume some care that is worth less to them than what it costs to provide. The gains from risk reduction must be worth more than these welfare losses or people would choose to go without insurance. However, the subsidy provided by exempting employer-provided health insurance benefits from taxes encourages extra

insurance coverage. There also may be a general rise in the price of medical care because insurance increases the demand for services. This clearly causes a loss of welfare to those who are uninsured and, by increasing overall costs, creates a systemwide distortion that reduces economic efficiency.

8. The premiums for health insurance count as an expense to employers and are not counted as income to employees, thus generating **tax benefits** when medical expenses are paid through insurance rather than by patients directly out of pocket. Employer **tax subsidy**, wartime restriction on wages increases that favored benefits, and the ability of companies to avoid adverse selection through risk pools covering all employees are major reasons for the rise of employer-based health insurance.

9. Historically, the development of voluntary insurance plans in the United States was led by groups of hospitals and doctors who were interested in **assuring payment to providers** as well as in protecting patients from losses.

10. The **escalation in costs** due to **open-ended entitlement financing** through indemnity insurance that paid bills without imposing restrictions on use has been the primary force driving the development of more extensive contractual solutions through managed care.

PROBLEMS

1. {*cost sharing*} Find four people who have been treated for illness in the past three years. Ask them the following questions.

   a. How much did you pay for insurance?
   b. How much did the insurance really cost (i.e., what you paid plus what the employer or government paid)?
   c. How much did you pay in medical bills?
   d. How much did the medical care really cost (i.e., what you paid plus what the insurance company or government paid)?

2. {*actuarially fair premium*} A company with 617 employees had the following experience this year:

	Cost (each)
14 hospitalizations	$5,600
37 physical therapy sessions	$340
9 births	$1,800
4.1 physician visits per employee	$55
2.4 prescriptions filled per employee	$21

   Assuming that the cost of medical care rises 7 percent over the next year, what would the actuarially fair premium per employee be for the next year?

3. {*size of risk pool*} Use the information in Figure 4.2 pertaining to a loss of $50,000 that occurs randomly with a probability of one in one hundred. If the insurance company charges $750 per person per year, what is the load above the actuarially fair premium? If 100 people are in the group, will the insurance company show an underwriting profit? Will the insurance company ever break even? How likely is it that the plan will show a loss next year? With 50 people in the group, is it more or less likely that the plan will show a loss? What about with 500 people? How large does the group

have to be before the insurance company can be 99 percent sure that it will show an underwriting gain for the year?

4. {*savings, social insurance*} Explain which mechanism (savings, charity and contributions from friends, private insurance, or social insurance) you believe would cover losses resulting from each of the following conditions:

> seasonal hay fever
>
> congenital birth defects
>
> schizophrenia
>
> Alzheimer's disease
>
> preventive dental cleaning
>
> posttraumatic jaw reconstruction
>
> cigarette-induced chronic pulmonary obstruction

5. {*load, gains from trade*} Give three good reasons why someone might choose to pay $1,150 for health insurance when the actuarially fair premium was only $900.

6. {*adverse selection*} In each of the following pairs, which situation (a) or (b) would pose the largest problems regarding adverse selection?

> **i. (a)** A policy covering accidents for all children attending YMCA camps
>
> **(b)** A policy covering accidents for college students traveling abroad

> **ii. (a)** Inclusion of HIV/AIDS treatment in the standard benefit package offered to teachers
>
> **(b)** An optional rider providing HIV/AIDS coverage for an additional premium

> **iii. (a)** Basic medical services insurance package offered to students entering college
>
> **(b)** Basic medical services package offered to professors seeking early retirement

> **iv. (a)** Optional mental health coverage offered to employees of ABC Inc.
>
> **(b)** Optional mental health coverage offered to children of ABC Inc. employees

7. {*moral hazard*} Explain which types of insurance coverage (a) or (b) within each pair would most likely cause more problems resulting from moral hazard.

> **i. (a)** Indemnity payments of $10,000 for each eye or limb lost
>
> **(b)** Indemnity payments of $50 for each day spent in a nursing home

> **ii. (a)** Treatment in an emergency room
>
> **(b)** Treatment in an intensive care unit

> **iii. (a)** Arthroscopic surgery for knee injuries
>
> **(b)** Amputation for foot injuries

> **iv. (a)** Family counseling
>
> **(b)** Electroconvulsive therapy

v. (a)   Decongestants

(b)   Antibiotics

8.   {*moral hazard*} The following table gives the demand curve for doctor visits for Ralph, who doesn't have health insurance. Assume that Ralph responds only to the amount he must pay out of pocket when deciding how much care to use. By filling in the blank lines, calculate Ralph's new demand curve if he obtained insurance coverage that paid 80 percent of the bill. If the charges are $100 (i.e., Ralph pays $20 out of pocket), how many of the additional services Ralph uses are worth less (to him) than what they cost? How many are worth less to him than what he pays?

Price per visit	Number of visits	Out-of-pocket cost with insurance	Number of visits with insurance
$0	20	—	—
$20	18	—	—
$50	15	—	—
$100	10	—	—
$150	5	—	—

9.   {*welfare loss*} Bill's new insurance policy contains a prescription plan that provides all drugs through a local pharmacy with a $2 copayment. Under the old insurance, Bill had to pay for his own medication and purchased nine inhalers at $16 apiece to help control his asthma. With the new plan, Bill purchased 15 inhalers, keeping some as spares in his glove compartment and desk, since he only had to pay a $2 copayment for each one. How much are the six additional inhalers worth to Bill? How much do they cost him? How much do they cost the insurance company? Is Bill better or worse off under the new plan? Who would be worse off?

10.   {*incidence*} When medical care is reimbursed through employer-provided insurance, whose welfare is ultimately affected when the cost of medical care rises: the owners of the firm that pays the premiums (employer), the government whose revenues are reduced because insurance benefits are not taxable as wages, or the public in their roles as workers, consumers, and taxpayers? Is there any difference between short-term and long-term effects?

11.   {*ownership*} Why was it more common for railroads and timber companies to provide health insurance in the early 1900s than for textile mills or accounting firms?

12.   {*ownership*} Who controlled Blue Cross when it was formed? Did this form of insurance generate profits for its owners?

ENDNOTES

1. Gary Becker, *A Treatise on the Family* (Cambridge, Mass.: Harvard University Press, 1981); Robert H. Frank, *Passions Within Reason: The Strategic Role of the Emotions* (New York: Norton, 1988).
2. Edward O. Wilson, *On Human Nature* (Cambridge, Mass.: Harvard University Press, 1976); Jerome H. Barkow, Leda Cosmides, John Tooby, eds., *The Adapted Mind: Evolutionary Psychology and the Generation of Culture* (New York: Oxford University Press, 1992).
3. Rosemary Stevens, *In Sickness and In Wealth: American Hospitals in the Twentieth Century* (New York: Basic Books, 1989); John D. Thompson, *The Hospital: A Social and Architectural History* (New Haven, Conn.: Yale University Press, 1975).
4. William A. Glaser, *Health Insurance in Practice: International Variations in Financing, Benefits, and Problems* (San Francisco: Jossey-Bass, 1991).

5. William Aaronson, Jacqueline Zinn, and Michael Rosko, "Medicare Catastrophic Health Insurance," *Journal of Health Politics, Policy and Law* (1993).

6. Stephen Cohen and William Yu, "The Concentration and Persistence in the Level of Health Expenditures over Time: Estimates for the U.S. Population 2005–2006. Statistical Brief #236, February 2009, AHRQ, www.MEPS.ahrq.gov; *Health Care Financing Review, Medicare and Medicaid Statistical Supplement, 1995*, p. 35; Marc L. Berk and Alan Monheit, "The Concentration of Health Expenditures, Revisited" *Health Affairs*, 20, no.2 (March 2001): 9–18. The distribution of costs across individuals can be measured only for personal health care costs that are billed to individuals, not overhead items such as public health, construction, insurance administration, etc. Such overhead items make up about 10 percent of national health expenditures, and hence the "all persons" average in Table 4.2 is only 90 percent as large as the per capita average for all national health expenditures reported elsewhere. In truth, many costs have overhead components and are difficult to unambiguously assign to a single person, although they are clearly concentrated on the most ill and not evenly distributed. Some economists would argue that costs are even more concentrated than Table 4.2 indicates, because hospitals and physicians typically overcharge the least complex patients to subsidize the most difficult and complex cases (see the discussion of "cost shifting" in Chapter 8).

7. Bureau of Labor Statistics, U.S. Dept. of Labor, "Employer Cost for Employee Compensation," March 14, 2006, http://www.bls.gov/ncs/ect/home.htm.

8. C. Rufus Rorem, "Sickness Insurance in the United States," *Bulletin of the American Hospital Association* (June 1932); Odin W. Anderson, *Health Services as a Growth Enterprise in the United States since 1875*, 2nd ed. (Ann Arbor, Mich.: Health Administration Press, 1990).

9. John A. Nyman, *The Theory of Demand for Health Insurance* (Stanford University Press, 2002) and "The value of health insurance: the access motive," *Journal of Health Economics* 18 (1999): 141–152.

10. David M. Cutler and Sarah J. Reber, "Paying for Health Insurance: The Trade-Off Between Competition and Adverse Selection," *Quarterly Journal of Economics* 113 (May 1998): 433–466.

11. Lewis C. Workman, "Life Annuities," in *Mathematical Foundations of Life Insurance* (Atlanta, Ga.: Life Office Management Association, 1982), 155–195.

12. Kevin F. O'Grady, Willard G. Manning, Joseph P. Newhouse, and Robert H. Brook, "The Impact of Cost Sharing on Emergency Department Use," *New England Journal of Medicine* 313 (1985): 484–490; Mark V. Pauly, "Taxation, Health Insurance and Market Failure in the Medical Economy," *Journal of Economic Literature* 24, no. 2 (June 1986): 629–675.

13. The size of the welfare triangle is $(P_{original} - P_{insured}) \times (Q_{insured} - Q_{original}) \div 2$, which for this example would be $(\$20 - \$4) \times (9 - 5) \div 2 = \$32$. This is slightly less than in the numerical example because with discrete units (i.e., one, two, . . . eight, nine X-rays, with no fractions) the demand curve is not a continuous straight line but a step function, and so the area between the original $20 line and the demand curve is somewhat larger. In most cases, economists use the continuous formula, since with many consumers buying many units of service, the individual bumps are less important and the demand curve approximates a continuous line.

14. Martin S. Feldstein, "The Welfare Loss of Excess Health Insurance," *Journal of Political Economy* 81, no. 2 (1973): 251–280.

15. Gina Kolata, "Medical fees are often higher for patients without insurance," *New York Times*, April 1, 2001(http://www.nytimes.com). However, it is *sometimes* the case that the profits that hospitals make from insured patients are used to provide charity services to the uninsured (see discussion of cost-shifting in Chapter 8). Whether or not an uninsured person is made better or worse off depends upon whether or not they receive services for free, or with sufficient subsidy that the price to them is less than the market price would be without insurance.

16. Adam Wagstaff and Magnus Lindelow, "Can insurance increase financial risk? The curious case of health insurance in China," *Journal of Health Economics* 27 (2008): 990–1005.

17. J. Sheils and R. Haught, "The Cost of Tax Exempt Health Benefits in 2004," *Health Affairs* 23 (February 2004): w106–w112; T. M. Selden and B. M. Gray, "Tax Subsidies for Employment-Related Health Insurance: Estimates for 2006," *Health Affairs* 25, no. 6 (2006): 1568–1579.

18. David Cutler and Bridgette Madrian, "Labor Market Responses to Rising Health Insurance Costs: Evidence on Hours Worked." *RAND Journal of Economics* 29, no. 3 (1998): 509–530.

19. Kate Baicker and Amitabh Chandra, "The Labor Market Effects of Rising Health Insurance Premiums," NBER working paper #11160 (2005); Jonathan Gruber and Alan Krueger, "The Incidence of Mandated Employer-Provided Insurance: Evidence from Worker's Compensation Insurance," in David Bradford, ed., *Tax Policy and the Economy, Volume 5*: 111–143 (Cambridge Mass.: MIT Press, 1991).

20. Thomas Buchmueller and Robert Valetta, "The Effect of Health Insurance on Married Female Labor Supply," *Journal of Human Resources* 34, no. 1 (1999): 42–70.

21. David M. Blau and Donna Gilleskie, "Retiree Health Insurance and Labor Force Behavior of Older Men in the 1990s," *Review of Economics and Statistics* 83, no. 1 (2001): 64–80; Jeannette Rogowski and Lynn Karoly,

"Health Insurance and Retirement Behavior: Evidence for the Health and Retirement Survey," *Journal of Health Economics* 19, no. 4 (2000): 529–539; Philip Cooper and Alan Monheit, "Does Employment-Related Health Insurance Inhibit Job Mobility?" *Inquiry* 30, no. 4 (1993): 400–416.

22. R. Munts, *Bargaining for Health: Labor Unions, Health Insurance and Medical Care* (Madison: University of Wisconsin Press, 1967); David T. Beito, *From Mutual Aid to the Welfare State: Fraternal Societies and Social Services 1890–1967* (Chapel Hill: UNC Press, 2000).

23. Peter A. Kohler and Hans F. Zacher, eds., *The Evolution of Social Insurance 1881–1991: Studies of Germany, France, Great Britain, Austria and Switzerland* (New York: St. Martin's Press, 1982).

24. William A. Glaser, *Health Insurance in Practice: International Variations in Financing, Benefits, and Problems* (San Francisco: Jossey-Bass, 1991).

25. Committee on the Costs of Medical Care, *Medical Care for the American People* (Chicago: University of Chicago Press, 1932).

26. Robert Cunningham III and Robert M. Cunningham Jr., *The Blues: A History of the Blue Cross and Blue Shield System* (DeKalb: Northern Illinois University Press, 1997); Laura B. Benko, "The Blues Rise Again," *Modern Healthcare* (September 9, 2002): 14–15.

27. Institute of Medicine, *Employment and Health Benefits: A Connection at Risk* (Washington, D.C.: National Academy Press, 1993), p. 70; Melissa A. Thomasson, "The Importance of Group Coverage: How Tax Policy Shaped U.S. Health Insurance," NBER working paper (February 2000): 7543 (www.nber.org/papers/w7543).

28. Herman M. Somers and Anne R. Somers, *Medicare and the Hospitals: Issues and Prospects* (Washington, D.C.: The Brookings Institution, 1967).

29. W.J. Cohen, "Reflections on the Enactment of Medicare and Medicaid," HCFR (supplement): 3–16; Theodore Marmor, *The Politics of Medicare* (Chicago: Aldine, 1973).

30. Note, however, that many people you might consider "poor" are not eligible for Medicaid, a major reason that there are still 40 million uninsured. Typically the "working poor" have income above the poverty line but lack employer-provided insurance. Single persons without children usually do not qualify, even if their incomes are very low (hence the acronym TANF, Temporary Assistance to Needy *Families*).

31. Alan Maynard and Karen Bloor, "Introducing a Market to the United Kingdom's National Health Service," *New England Journal of Medicine* 334, no.9 (1996): 604–608.

CHAPTER 5

INSURANCE CONTRACTS AND MANAGED CARE

QUESTIONS

1. Who is the largest health insurer?
2. Which is better: individual insurance plans, employer-provided insurance, or government insurance?
3. How is a state mandate to cover alcoholism treatment similar to a tax?
4. Why are so many Americans uninsured?
5. Who pays when the cost of medical care rises: employers, employees, government, or insurance companies?
6. How much profit can an HMO make? At whose expense?
7. What is the underwriting cycle? A retention ratio? A self-insured ASO? ERISA?
8. Do Managed Care and Health Savings Accounts (HSAs) reduce the cost of health insurance or just shift it around?
9. Who are the winners and losers in managed care? Do cost reductions mean that some doctors must earn lower incomes? Who are the winners and losers from HSAs?
10. Does a physician "gatekeeper" or "medical home" work for or against the patient?

5.1 TYPES OF INSURANCE PLANS

Of the 310 million people in the United States, most have some form of private health insurance, usually through an employer. Government programs, mostly Medicare and Medicaid, cover 28 percent of the population. Note that government is the largest payer in dollar terms because it covers more of the most expensive patients (disabled, chronically ill, elderly). Nine percent of the population, 27 million people, purchase private health insurance individually. That leaves about 46 million people, or 15 percent of the population, uninsured (see Table 5.1).[1]

TABLE 5.1	Health Insurance Coverage of the U.S. Population	
	Non-Elderly	**Elderly**
Total persons	272 million	38 million
With insurance	82.8%	99.2%
Employment	32.1	34.1
Employee (dependent)	30.0	***
Other private insurance	6.8	25.9
Military	2.9	7.1
Medicare	2.7	93.2
Medicaid	13.9	8.9
Uninsured	17.2	1.9

Source: U.S. Census Bureau, Current Population Survey and EBRI

Note: Percentages add to more than 100% because many persons have multiple coverage.

Medicare

Medicare is arguably the most important insurance plan in the United States even though it covers only 13 percent of the population because it sets a national standard, providing procedural definitions and payment levels used as references by hospitals, doctors, and private insurance companies in all 50 states to determine reimbursement. Created by Congress in 1965 to provide insurance for people over age 65 and some people with disabilities, Medicare covered everyone in these categories and thereby overcame the adverse selection issues that made it so difficult for them as individuals to purchase private health insurance. A substantial portion of the money for Medicare comes from a tax of 2.9 percent on all wages, half paid by the employer and half paid by the employee, with the remainder coming from general tax revenues and premiums. Medicare financing thus redistributes resources from high-income wage earners to relatively needy elderly and disabled people with disproportionately large medical expenses (see Chapter 14).

Medicare is split into two parts, Part A (hospital) and Part B (physician and outpatient services), plus a new Part D (drugs). Although the specifics of coverage can be complex, clear and detailed descriptions of benefits are readily available at www.medicare.gov. Part A coverage is provided on application to people age 65 or older and to those entitled to specified programs, such as Social Security and programs for people with end-stage renal disease. To obtain Part B coverage, beneficiaries must pay a premium ($96.40 per month in 2009 or more if personal income is above $85,000), which is supposed to cover a quarter of the actuarial cost but usually falls short because of the reluctance of politicians to offend groups that lobby for the elderly. Since Part B coverage is so heavily subsidized and Part A beneficiaries are usually enrolled unless they explicitly choose to opt out, almost all Medicare insureds (98 percent) have both Parts A and B. In addition, 88 percent of those with Medicare have supplemental "Medigap" insurance or HMOs that cover copayments, deductibles, drugs, and some other expenses (Table 5.2).[2] Part D coverage is more complicated, since the elderly may be covered by a qualified employee retirement plan or may enroll individually.

Employer-Based Group Health Insurance

Four factors explain why more than half of the U.S. population is covered by employer group health insurance:

- Covering a large group under a single contract reduces transaction costs.
- Group coverage mitigates adverse selection.

TABLE 5.2 The Twelve Standard Medicare Supplement Plans

Basic Benefits must be included in all plans, and cover Part A coinsurance plus hospitalization for 365 days after Medicare benefits end; Part B coinsurance (generally 20% of Medicare-approved expenses) and copayments, and the first 3 pints of blood each year. Note that many people choose to purchase a comprehensive HMO benefit under the MEDICARE+CHOICE plan rather than Medigap insurance—you do not need both.

A	B	C	D	E	F*	G	H	I	J*
Basic benefits	Basic benefits	Basic benefits	Basic benefits	Basic benefits	Basic benefits	Basic benefits	Basic benefits	Basic benefits	Basic benefits
		Skilled nursing coinsurance	Skilled nursing coinsurance	Skilled nursing coinsurance	Skilled nursing coinsurance	Skilled nursing coinsurance	Skilled nursing coinsurance	Skilled nursing coinsurance	Skilled nursing coinsurance
	Medicare Part A deductible	Medicare Part A deductible	Medicare Part A deductible	Medicare Part A deductible	Medicare Part A deductible	Medicare Part A deductible	Medicare Part A deductible	Medicare Part A deductible	Medicare Part A deductible
		Medicare Part B deductible			Medicare Part B deductible				Medicare Part B deductible
					Medicare Part B excess charge (100%)	Medicare Part B excess charge (80%)		Medicare Part B excess charge (100%)	Medicare Part B excess charge (100%)
		Foreign travel emergency	Foreign travel emergency	Foreign travel emergency	Foreign travel emergency	Foreign travel emergency	Foreign travel emergency	Foreign travel emergency	Foreign travel emergency
			At-home recovery			At-home recovery		At-home recovery	At-home recovery
							Basic drug benefit ($1,250 Limit)	Basic drug benefit ($1,250 Limit)	Extended drug benefit ($3,000 Limit)
				Preventive care					Preventive care

*Plans F and J also have a high deductible option. Plans K and L offer lower premiums with higher out-of-pocket costs subject to an annual limit.

Source: 2002 Guide to Health Insurance for People with Medicare, CMS Publication No. 02110, www.medicare.gov.

TABLE 5.3	Annual Premiums for Employee Health Insurance Coverage, 2008				
	HMO	**PPO**	**POS**	**HD (HSA)**	**Average**
Single					
Total premium	$ 4,754	$ 4,802	$ 4,647	$ 3,922	$ 4,704
Employee pays	$ 705	$ 731	$ 865	$ 468	$ 721
Family					
Total premium	$13,122	$12,937	$12,330	$10,121	$12,680
Employee pays	$ 3,380	$ 3,344	$ 3,730	$ 2,813	$ 3,354
% of all insured employees	20%	58%	12%	8%	100%

Source: Kaiser/HRET Employer Health Benefits Survey, http://www.kff.org

- Employer payment yields a tax benefit.
- Many of the most expensive patients are heavily subsidized or excluded.

An employee usually obtains insurance by choosing one of the options offered, deciding whether to include children and other dependents, and contributing a small amount toward the total premium (see Table 5.3). Almost all large employers provide health insurance benefits, but less than one-third of small employers (those with fewer than 10 employees) do so and often make the employee pay a large part of the premium, so that fewer people choose to participate (Figure 5.1).[3] The largest employee groups are usually self-insured (i.e., the employer bears the risk although it may use an insurance company to administer benefits). Even though employer-provided health insurance covers 60 percent of the population, it pays for only one-third of total medical bills due to copayments and deductibles and because many of the expensive cases (elderly, disabled, nursing home residents) are covered by Medicare, Medicaid, and other government programs.

FIGURE 5.1 Percentage of Workers Insured by Size of Firm

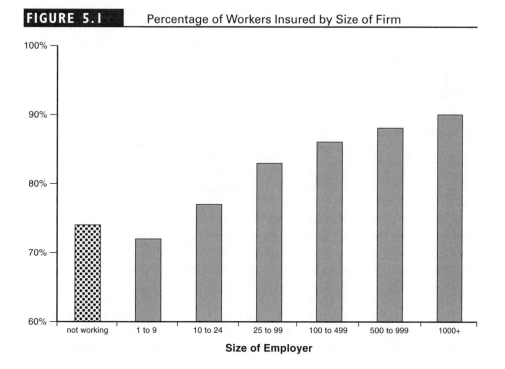

Size of Employer

Self-Paid Private Insurance

Nine percent of the population, mostly people who are self-employed or who work for small companies that do not provide employee benefits, purchase private health insurance individually. Individuals acting on their own behalf lack group purchasing power and often pay significantly higher premiums even for reduced levels of coverage.

Medicaid

People who are poor cannot pay for insurance and many of them (14 percent of the population) are covered under the government **Medicaid** program, which also provides supplemental coverage for a substantial number of elderly people, including a majority of those living in nursing homes. Medicaid is funded jointly by the states and the federal government. The federal government may pay as much as 80 percent of the total program cost for low-income states, but only half for wealthier states. Program design (which differs from state to state), beneficiary enrollment, and other factors, as well as per capita income, can affect both the total cost and the financing split. Medicaid benefits vary widely from state to state, covering from 12 to 32 percent of average medical costs. Although Medicaid was designed to cover mothers with low incomes and their children, it has become the dominant funding mechanism for nursing homes. This has occurred primarily because Medicare has very limited nursing home coverage; therefore, as the elderly incur expenses during long nursing home stays, they become poor enough to qualify for Medicaid and switch to government funding.

Other Government Programs and Charity

Charity paid for about $80 billion (3%) of health care in 2007. Workers' compensation, automobile accident insurance, and similar programs paid more than $25 billion. The Department of Veterans Affairs received $35 billion in funding, with a somewhat smaller amount being paid for dependents through the Department of Defense. Programs sponsored by the Maternal and Child Health Bureau, Substance Abuse and Mental Health Services Administration, Bureau of Indian Affairs, and a variety of other programs accounted for another $40 billion in health care. The government also provides a special tax break for families with very high medical costs (more than 7.5% of adjusted income).

The Uninsured

Despite the wide variety of health insurance plans, 46 million Americans, about 16 percent of the population, have no health insurance.[4] Uninsured individuals needing care must try to pay with their own limited resources, find a special government program, depend on charity, or simply present themselves at a hospital or clinic and ask to be treated free of charge. The percentage of the population without coverage depends significantly on the efforts of local and state governments. States choosing expansive Medicaid programs and broad outreach to the working poor can reduce the number of uninsured individuals substantially. Wisconsin, Minnesota, Hawaii, and Massachusetts insure all but 8 percent of their citizens, whereas Texas leaves 24 percent of its population without insurance.

   Although some uninsured individuals pay large sums out of pocket when they get sick, a much greater number stay healthy and pocket the cash or, having no resources, depend on charity when they are ill. That is why the problem of so many uninsured individuals is so intractable. For many of the uninsured, not having insurance is a rational economic decision. Three-fourths of the uninsured are under age 35, and people this young tend to be healthy, to be enrolled in college, or to earn low wages. For them, paying $500 a month or even $50 a month for health insurance may not make sense.[5] People over age 35 who are working in low-paying jobs often need the money to eat and pay rent more than they need it to provide protection from uncertain medical bills that may never materialize. There are also a small number of people who are chronically ill and would not pass even a cursory medical exam, and hence can be insured only if they take a job in a large firm that provides group coverage.

WHAT DO PEOPLE BUY WHEN THEY DON'T BUY HEALTH INSURANCE?

Most of the time, being uninsured is a matter of choice. It may not be a sensible choice or may be the result of a choice no one would want to face (buy the children food or buy health insurance), but it is a choice nonetheless. Knowing what people buy when they do not buy health insurance provides insight into their choice.

A study by Helen Levy and Thomas DeLeire from the University of Chicago indicates that what people buy with the money they save from not purchasing health insurance depends significantly on whether they are poor or relatively well-off.[6] According to the study, for people in the bottom quartile of the income distribution, the money they did not spend on health insurance went mostly toward food, rent, and other necessities. For people in the upper income quartile, the spending pattern was quite different— the largest type of spending increase was for transportation, specifically, for expensive used cars (Jaguar or Ferrari anyone?). The study indicates that programs trying to help people who are truly needy may inadvertently subsidize people who are uninsured simply because they want to spend on other things.

State Children's Health Insurance Program

The State Children's Health Insurance Program (SCHIP) was enacted by Congress in 1997 as Title XXI of the Social Security Act to provide $40 billion to increase coverage for the 10 million children under the age of 18 who were uninsured. However, the program works through state governments and some have used available funding for other purposes, leading to great unevenness in implementation. Almost 5 million children eligible for SCHIP or Medicaid have not been enrolled. Less than 5 percent of children in Rhode Island, Connecticut, and Pennsylvania are uninsured, and almost 20 percent of children in Texas and New Mexico are left uninsured.[7] The fact that so many children are still uninsured reflects the choices made by the public and their elected representatives. In this regard, it is probably worth mentioning that children do not vote, and that the parents of poor children are much less likely to vote than the senior citizens who qualify for Medicare.

5.2   HSAs, MEDICAL SAVINGS ACCOUNTS, AND HIGH-DEDUCTIBLE "CONSUMER-DRIVEN HEALTH PLANS"

Insurance provides protection against the cost of medical care. Inevitably, this protection makes people less sensitive to costs; that is, they are more willing to use extra services and less concerned about finding the best price for the services they use. Great interest has been expressed in making patients more direct participants in the financing of their own medical care through "consumer directed health plans." The details of the plans are still under development, and the various plans differ considerably, but certain core elements are common to most of them:[8]

- Patients pay most small and medium medical expenses on their own.
- There is a high deductible (>$1,000) for major illness and high cost care.
- The defined contribution by employer or government is limited to a fixed dollar amount.

Health savings accounts (**HSAs**) are the newest and currently most important form of consumer-driven health plans. Although authorized by the Medicare Modernization Act of 2003, which established Part D coverage for prescription drugs, HSAs have really been in operation only since 2005 because the rules and regulations for implementation are complex and took many months to work out. In essence, an HSA is a tax-favored savings account coupled with a high-deductible health plan. Patients must pay all of their expenses below the deductible (at least $1,000 for singles and $2,000 for families, rising with inflation after 2005) either out of pocket or from the HSA savings account. Any money left in the savings account can be carried forward to the next year, and any earnings on the savings are exempt from federal taxes. The savings account can be funded by either the person or the employer (in an amount less than or equal to the deductible), and such contributions are exempt from federal income taxes for both the employee and the company.

Health reimbursement accounts (**HRAs**), established by a series of U.S. Internal Revenue Service Rulings in 2002, are similar to HSAs but differ in that they are funded solely by the employer and can be offered with any type of health insurance plan (not only high-deductible plans), and any savings in the HRA account stays with the company if the employee changes jobs. **Medical savings accounts** (**MSAs**), an earlier type, linked a tax-advantaged savings account to a high-deductible health insurance plan and was limited primarily to self-employed persons. The argument for creating MSAs was that self-employed persons should be able to get the tax benefits available to people receiving insurance through their employer. Somewhat related are the **pre-tax spending accounts** where money is regularly deducted and deposited in accounts to be used for medical or dependent care and avoids income taxes. Pre-tax spending accounts have become very common, but they suffer from the disadvantage that any money not spent by the end of the year is taken away rather than rolling over from year to year or earning interest.

Defined Contribution Health Plans

The rising cost of health care has created major problems for American industry. General Motors has been called "A health-insurance plan for retired auto-workers with a side business that tries to make and sell enough cars to pay the premiums." Rising health care costs have contributed to bankruptcies in all sorts of manufacturing, as well as airlines and some service industries. Employers have begun to get out of the business of providing pensions by replacing them with defined-contribution 401(k) retirement plans, and many would like to get out from under the responsibility of paying for ever higher health care costs by making a fixed payment (defined contribution) of perhaps $500 or $750 per month. In this way, the responsibility for rising costs would be shifted to the employees, who "own" their own health plan, just as they own a 401k. This shifting of responsibility is clearly counted as a strength by employers, but may be considered a weakness by employees, who could see much more of future wage increases used to pay rising premiums or out-of-pocket medical expenses.

High-Deductible Insurance

A great advantage of a high deductible is that the majority of people who have few illnesses and only modest medical expenses will never have to use their insurance at all during the year. Ninety percent of the population has medical expenses below $5,000 per year (see Table 4.2) and most of them could be building a nice mutual fund account growing tax-free to add to their retirement. HSAs, MSAs, and other "consumer-driven" plans based on high-deductible ("catastrophic") insurance have become more popular with employers as a way of cutting costs while continuing to offer coverage to employees, but they still attract less than 10 percent of the market—and disproportionately the younger, healthier, and wealthier employees and dependents who are less difficult to cover.[9]

SAMPLE DEFINED CONTRIBUTION HSA PLAN

Employer: Contributes $100 (pre-tax) per month and provides catastrophic major medical insurance that pays 90 percent of all expenses above $5,000 in a calendar year.
Employee: Pays all bills, first using money in his or her HSA, and when that is gone, uses own money for the rest up to $5,000 and 10 percent of all bills in excess of $5,000. Any savings left over earns interest and may be used for retirement.

Although most of the people signing up for insurance have medical costs below a $5,000 limit, most of the costs are attributable to those few patients who get really sick and do have catastrophically high costs. If the high-deductible plan provides full coverage above a limit, then patients (and hospitals) have no reason to control costs; thus expensive organ transplants and brain surgeries may get used more frequently and priced even higher. Conversely, using coinsurance to make patients more cost-sensitive in this range might seem cruel and not work well in practice—the employee with a disability trying to come up with 20 percent of a $450,000 liver transplant bill is not going to be happy and will find many newspaper reporters sympathetic to his complaints that this kind of insurance is not fair. Furthermore, the person with a transplant or any serious chronic illness will have high expenses not only in the current year but next year and the year after as well. That person will never accumulate a surplus in his or her HSA savings account or a cushion to cover even minor bills, since the fixed employer contribution will start to run out in January or February.

"Ownership" of one's own health insurance plan in effect removes the pooling across persons, leaving only pooling over time (see Section 4.1). Whereas insurance usually equalizes premiums and cross-subsidizes, HSAs make the old and the sick pay more to achieve the same level of coverage, and a defined contribution means that a larger percentage is taken from the income of the poor than the wealthy (or more realistically that poor people buy cheaper health insurance plans and do without some care, just as they buy less clothes, smaller houses, cheaper food, and less travel).

Do patients really want to make financial choices and try to save money when they are seeking medical care? A benefit of insurance is that one no longer has to worry about the money, just get the doctor to do their best. The problems of information asymmetry (Section 6.4) in medical care are such that it is not obvious that most patients can make good choices about which treatments are worth spending a few dollars more for.[10] Accumulating information and making choices is costly, and almost no one seems to like keeping track of hundreds of medical bills and trying to get them submitted to an insurance company for reimbursement, or arguing over what is and is not covered, or how much, or who should be penalized if the doctor or the bill is in error.

5.3 A RANGE OF RISK BEARING: FIXED PREMIUMS, ADMINISTERED SERVICES ONLY, AND SELF-INSURANCE

An employer can purchase insurance at a fixed price and bear no risk, or it can pool its own funds, handle all claims, and self-insure while bearing all risks. In between these two options there are a range of contracts that split the risk and claims-processing burden: experience rated, retention ratio, minimum premium, and administered services only (ASO) plans (Table 5.4). Negotiating price is a major problem in contracting for insurance. **Experience rating**, by allowing the price to rise or fall to match the dollar amount of claims submitted by employees during the previous year (experience), avoids costly and contentious haggling. A **retention ratio agreement** makes a similar adjustment, but in the current year. The employer and insurer estimate losses, and if claims turn out to be smaller than expected, the insurer returns most of the difference, retaining only a percentage (the retention ratio) for administrative expenses and profit.

Two things make it difficult for an employer to act as its own insurance company: catastrophic losses and claims processing. To some extent these difficulties can be ameliorated through contractual arrangements. Economies of scale in risk-bearing can be obtained contractually through **reinsurance**, which is a type of major medical coverage for employers, a policy for the group as a whole that covers 90 percent of the cost of any individual above a specified amount (perhaps $50,000) or an aggregate loss of the group as a whole that is above the expected value (perhaps above $5 million). Of course, reinsurance is quite costly; therefore, coverage is usually purchased for extraordinary losses only. Claims processing is apt to create administrative difficulties, because a company is usually better at its own line of business than at the business of managing and paying insurance benefits. Economies of scale in claims processing can be obtained contractually through **administered services only (ASO)** contracts in which an insurance company processes the bills, pays the claims, and settles disputes for a set fee per year or per claim, but all funds for paying benefits come directly from the employer.

Under "normal" circumstances the costs of experience-rated, retention ratio, ASO, and self-insurance contracts should converge toward the same amount; however, circumstances are rarely normal. When a firm accepts bids for an experience-rated plan, it is not uncommon

TABLE 5.4	Range of Insurance Contracts			
Insurer Bears Risk, Processes Claims ←				→ **Employer Bears Risk, Processes Own Claims**
Fixed Premiums	**Experience Related**	**Retention Ratio**	**ASO**	**Self-Insurance**
Pay pre-set amount for coverage	Premiums changed each year to reflect last year's actual claims	If losses are less than expected, insurer gives back part of premium	Administrative services only, insurance company pays claims using the firm's own funds	Firm pays claims, acts as their own insurance company

for an insurance company to try to "buy the business" by setting the premiums very low in the first year. Then it will use the bad experience during that year to force a high premium in the following year. The employer who got such a good deal is now stuck and must accept a substantial premium increase or incur the costs of going out to bid again, often finding that with such a record of underwriting losses, few insurers want to bid. Also, a group with higher-than-expected losses may find that their insurer starts to give poor service and gets very nasty about paying claims (and thus is able to hold onto premium dollars longer). On the other hand, employee groups often try to take advantage of insurance companies by dropping them after a bad year (thus allowing no time to make up the extraordinary losses through experience rating) or repeatedly going into the market to search for low bids. The more flexible retention ratio agreement is like a partnership. The insurance company and the employee group get together in a long-term arrangement in which initial pricing is not so important. Year-to-year conflicts are avoided. However, the downside of this more integrated contract is that if things do go wrong, it is much worse for both parties.

The Underwriting Cycle

In the long run, the increases in premiums match the increases in underlying health care costs. However, in any given year the rate of increase could be higher or lower. Economists have observed that most insurance markets (e.g., property and casualty, malpractice, health) tend to have a cycle of overcharging and undercharging that lasts about 7 to 10 years.[11] At the peak of the cycle, premiums are high relative to costs, profits are fat, and competitors are attracted to start the cycle. As more insurance companies enter the market, premiums are driven downward. In the trough of the cycle, rates are low as insurance companies compete vigorously to gain market share. The lack of profitability eventually takes a toll, some insurance companies exit the market, and rates increase. Eventually, rising prices and good profits start the cycle over again. Figure 5.2 shows how premiums and costs have risen and fallen over the last decade. At the beginning of the 1990s, hefty double-digit premium increases built profitability. The rise of managed care and the overhanging threat of government intervention kept medical costs very low in the middle of the decade—but

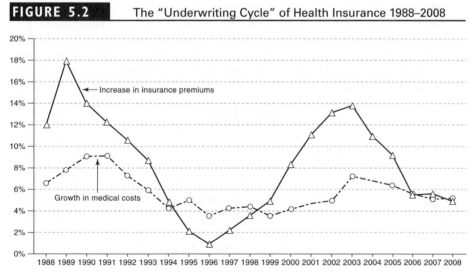

FIGURE 5.2   The "Underwriting Cycle" of Health Insurance 1988–2008

Source: Kaiser/HRET survey of employer health benefits and U.S. National Health Accounts.

insurers trying to get a larger piece of the market drove premiums down below costs. The combination of low premiums and rising costs crushed profits, pushing several HMOs and insurance companies to the edge of insolvency. The years 2001–2003 were catch-up time, with insurers once again trying to build reserves. After that, premiums started to fall. It is expected that premiums will continue to moderate but still exceed the rate of inflation and the growth in wages.

ERISA, Taxes, and Mandated Benefits

The employee benefits offered by a company are determined largely by competitive conditions in the labor market as the company tries to hire new workers or directly through negotiations with the unions that represent the workers. Companies view benefits as a way to retain workers, and workers view benefits as a way to protect themselves against losses. The interests of both companies and workers are represented in the final outcome.

Sometimes a broader public interest is imposed in the form of **mandated benefits**, regulations promulgated by the government stating that specific benefits (e.g., substance abuse treatment, AZT treatment for HIV infection) must be provided. If such benefits are a good thing, why don't they arise naturally in the course of competitive contracting? Consider the case of substance abuse benefits. Without such benefits, insurance will pay for treatment of liver damage, but not for treatment of the excessive drinking that caused it. From a social perspective, it is much more efficient to treat the underlying cause (alcoholism) than to treat just the symptom (liver damage). However, a company is not interested in the productivity of society as a whole, but in the productivity of its workforce. A quite reasonable profit-maximizing response to alcoholism is to fire the employee and push him or her out onto the streets, where the burden is borne by the rest of society. Adverse selection can also play a role. A company with especially generous benefits for HIV/AIDS treatment will find its premiums going higher and higher as more chronically ill people try to get jobs there. Eventually, if adverse selection is severe enough, only people with a very high risk of HIV/AIDS would be willing to accept the low wages paid by this company in order to get the benefits.

Mental illness poses similar problems of adverse selection because the benefits are highly concentrated, with most of the dollars spent on just a few people, who, with their families, are much more aware of the risks than the insurance company. In a competitive market, insurance contracts reflect the interests of companies and most employees but not society as a whole. If such benefits are not mandatory, only a few companies will offer them.

Insurance is primarily regulated by the states. Some states, such as Arizona, impose very few mandates, while Massachusetts has more than thirty. Employers operating in multiple states need uniform national laws because it is difficult to maintain many different sets of benefit plans and give more or less to an employee depending on place of residence. Under the **Employee Retirement and Income Security Act of 1974 (ERISA)** and later amendments, self-insured firms are regulated under national ERISA rules and thus are exempt from state mandates. Because only large firms are able to self-insure, the attempt to increase coverage through mandates may have the paradoxical effect of reducing the number of people insured, as small firms opt to provide no health insurance at all.

State taxes provide another incentive to self-insure. Most states impose a premium tax of 1 percent to 2 percent that can be avoided through self-insurance or ASO contracts. Minimum premium plans in which the employer pays the first $X million (usually about 90 percent of estimated losses) and the insurer pays the rest exist primarily to avoid state taxes, since they are no different from fixed-premium full insurance with regard to risk or claims processing. Several innovative state health care financing plans have been challenged under ERISA. For example, New Jersey funded a special program for the uninsured through a 30 percent surcharge on all hospital bills. After large companies won ERISA exemption, only small employers and individuals were left paying the surcharge; therefore, the state was forced to dismantle its program.[12]

If mandated benefits are a good idea, why don't the states just pay for them? The answer is that they would have to raise taxes to do so. A mandated benefit, although it operates like a tax on firms, is counted as a regular cost of business to the firm. It does not appear on the government's budget and thus is not recognized by many voters. Although the public ultimately will lose more in forgone wages than in taxes avoided, this fact is not obvious to voters when they go to the polls. For this reason, any national insurance plan enacted in the United States is likely to be based on employer contributions. People who would never vote to increase taxes to fund national health insurance will calmly vote to have government insist that every employer provide benefits—and so our government will rationally follow the path of least resistance.

Insurance, by channeling funds through different organizations and contractual arrangements, has a tendency to obscure the actual costs of medical care. Pretending that a mandated insurance benefit will somehow make these services cost less than if they were funded through a tax increase has misled some people, while companies have misled the public by claiming to have paid a "fair share" for their own workers but never dealing with the issue of how health care for people who are homeless, have a mental illness, or have HIV/AIDS will be paid for. A health care system that helps only the healthy is cost-effective in one sense and worthless in another. Perhaps the worst aspect of the complex system of health insurance that has arisen in the United States is this obfuscation of reality that allows interested parties to avoid responsibility and never face up to the hard decisions on how to pay for health care. It is, therefore, worthwhile to examine how this complex system came to be and why some organizations and contracts have dominated in the United States while different forms of insurance developed in other countries.

5.4 MANAGED CARE PLANS

Why *Managed* Care?

The primary impetus behind managed care has been the rise in health care costs, and in particular, the rise in the cost of employee health benefits. Traditional corporate health insurance for employees, Medicare, and Medicaid were open-ended **entitlement** systems. Patients had no reason to worry about costs. Hospitals, doctors, and insurers, being recipients of funds, actually benefited from increased spending. From 1970 to 1980, health care expenditures by businesses rose from 3.1 percent of employee compensation to 4.9 percent. Then costs grew even more rapidly, and by 1990 these expenditures reached 7.1 percent of employee compensation.[13] The value of health benefits, equal to 36 percent of after-tax profits in 1970 and 43 percent in 1980, actually exceeded (108 percent) total corporate profits in 1990 and are almost certain to continue to exceed total profits in 2009. Indemnity insurance premiums for Blue Cross and Blue Shield coverage rose as much as 30 percent a year in many markets during the early 1980s.

In the face of these large increases, prudence and survival demanded that something be done to reduce the cost of health care to businesses. The problems of businesses had actually been made worse by government cost-containment efforts in the 1980s because reductions in Medicaid and Medicare rates forced hospitals to shift costs by charging more to insured patients (see Section 8.4 for a discussion of cost-shifting). Businesses became increasingly willing to turn to an outside contractor that could stabilize benefit costs, even if it meant having to accept some constraints and employee complaints. Health Maintenance Organization (HMO) contracts and membership exploded, rising from 3 million in 1970 to 9 million in 1980, 36 million in 1990, and 77 million in 2005, with employer group contracts accounting for 90 percent of total membership.[14]

In a system characterized by a lack of financial restraints, it is not surprising that the United States was spending far more on health care than any other country in the world (Chapter 17); the surprise was how little health the nation was able to buy with all the extra money spent. Despite years of insistence by politicians and physicians that the United States had the best medical care in the world, there is scant evidence that the additional expenditures led to improvements in longevity, infant mortality, morbidity, or days lost from work relative to other countries spending less than half as much per person.[15] What has become apparent is that the real inflation-adjusted hourly wages of workers have stagnated, and even declined, while the cost per hour of employer-provided health benefits has soared, and that the federal government has been burdened by billions of dollars in deficits attributable to the soaring cost of Medicare benefits. The nation has searched for an organizational structure that would add the missing elements of planning, coordination, and control to the health care system to improve efficiency and limit total expenditures.

Management: The Distinctive Feature of Managed Care

The fundamental difference between traditional medical practice under fee-for-service (FFS) indemnity insurance and managed care is that **a manager** intervenes to monitor and control the transaction between doctor and patient (Figure 5.3).[16] An outside party, such as the plan medical director, a trained utilization review nurse, or a software program, identifies care that is potentially at variance with accepted clinical practice. This may be done through a statistical profile of each physician's practice, assessment of laboratory testing, a review of individual cases, or a combination of techniques. The manager examines the process of care and controls the flow of funds, facilitating payments in some circumstances and holding back in others. Since the **managed care organization** (**MCO**) takes financial responsibility for medical care, it has an incentive to provide care efficiently. To remain viable, the MCO must compete on the basis of both quality and cost. A delicate balance must be maintained between expenditure control, administrative process, and medical uncertainty.

The most loosely organized MCOs are referred to as **preferred provider organizations** (**PPOs**) or **point-of-service plans** (**POSs**). The insuring MCO negotiates contracts with a

---

FIGURE 5.3   Flow of Funds with Managed Care

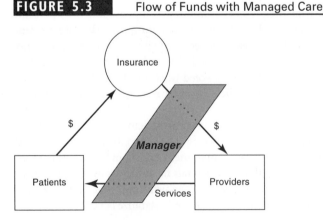

set of doctors and hospitals (the network) to obtain care at a discount. Patients receiving care within the network pay only a small copayment. Patients may obtain care outside the network, but may have to pay substantially more or receive a referral from their regular doctor stating that such specialty care is medically necessary. In a **health maintenance organization** (**HMO**), referrals are necessary for most specialty care, the insurance only pays for care within the network, and the networks are usually more limited than under POS or PPO plans. A **closed-panel HMO** is an organization that provides all care in-house using its own doctors and hospitals. The largest closed-panel HMO is Kaiser Permanente, which has more than 8 million members, mostly in the western United States.

Contractual Reforms to Reduce Costs

Indemnity insurance is a contract to pay for care. The premium must be sufficient to pay for all medical care provided and administrative overhead:

$$\text{Total Premiums} = \Sigma(\text{Price} \times \text{Quantity}) + \text{Overhead (load)}$$

Total costs can be reduced only by reducing one or more of these three elements. Since a managed care organization adds management, overhead increases. This leaves price and quantity. Of these two, *prices are the easiest to cut*. Most of the early successes of managed care plans came from the ability to cut the amounts paid to doctors and hospitals. Sometimes these prices were reduced because of excess supply; sometimes because the MCO became a big buyer and could exercise market power; sometimes the mere threat of taking patients away, or sending more, was sufficient to obtain discounts; and sometimes it was just because no buyer had ever before haggled aggressively in a system that had grown fat and soft. It is worth remembering that during the reign of the indemnity insurance plans, no one, not even the insurance company, stood to gain very much from hard bargaining—so all parties avoided it (to the insurance company, higher medical costs meant larger premiums; to employers, cost of benefits were offset by declines in wages, not profits; to employees, the gains from reducing costs were seen as too distant, or barely perceived—even though ultimately it was the employees who paid the cost).

Cutting prices does not change the amount of actual resources used (physician hours, X-ray machines, hospital beds). It simply means that one group (buyers) is paying less, and thus another group (sellers) receives less. In economic terms, it is a pure transfer. Presumably buyers are happy to pay less, but sellers are not happy to receive less. Indeed, faced with an onslaught of discounts, hospitals and physicians finally revolted, creating a "backlash" that blamed managed care for all sorts of evil in the service of greed. Thus, while price cuts are the most readily used method to reduce costs, and the source of most savings that MCOs have achieved,[17] there are clear limitations to such a strategy.

The second method for reducing costs, cutting the quantity of medical services, has proven to be much more difficult. Despite the rhetoric of "restrictive" managed care plans, the reality is that the total volume of services is rarely reduced by enough to make a substantial difference in total spending. To reduce quantity of services, both the patient and the physician must agree. The initial idea was that medical services that do not have much of an impact on health could be removed without conflict ("cutting out the fat"). Yet whether a service is medically useful or not has little to do with its effect on physician income—both vital and merely marginal services bring in the same fee. Thus, physicians are harmed (by reduced incomes) even if patients are not. Furthermore, although it is relatively easy to discover services that are relatively unimportant ("the need for this service results from a rare side effect"), it is almost impossible to say that such services would never be helpful, that they would not be important in one in a hundred (or one in a million) cases.

What did happen was that the use of services was bent to follow the contract more closely. For example, since many contracts with hospitals specified a set payment per day, the number of days a patient could stay in the hospital was reduced. However, patients still needed the same amount of surgery, after care, drugs, and so on, so the intensity of services was increased—more hours of nursing care and more procedures performed each day. The net result of fewer days and more inputs per day was that the total cost of hospital care was not reduced. As long as more nurses are hired, more drugs are used, and more tests are performed, total expenses cannot fall even though the number of patient days is falling. Over time, the reduction in ALOS (average length of stay = number of days per patient admission) was more than offset by an increase in the cost per day (see Chapters 8 and 9).

The third method for reducing cost was to **substitute cheaper forms of care**—prescribe generic rather than brand-name drugs, have patients see a nurse practitioner rather than a doctor, treat patients with medicine rather than surgery, perform hip replacement rather than long-term nursing home care, and so on. The idea was that a manager could identify an alternate form of care that was just as (or almost as) effective but significantly less expensive. Substitution has been practiced effectively for pharmaceuticals (see the box in Section 5.5), but has been less successful for other categories of medical care. Even in pharmaceuticals, the savings from use of cheaper generic substitutes has been more than offset by the rise in the total number of prescriptions and increased use of expensive new compounds, so total drug costs per patient have continued to rise.

A Fourth Way: Reforming the Organization to Reduce Cost

The rigid equation of Cost = (Price × Quantity + Overhead) holds as long as one considers managed care only as a contractual modification that leaves the underlying organization of medical practice the same. An alternative, more radical, reform is to change the organizational structure. Instead of having an insurance company/MCO that pays bills and a separate set of hospitals and physicians that provide care, a single unified organization could integrate both functions. Kaiser, Group Health Cooperative, and others had begun using closed-panel group practice (CPGP) to do so in the 1940s. In a CPGP, the physicians work on salary for the organization, the hospitals are owned by the organization, and the drugs are purchased by the organization. A **single entity combines all the complex functions of providing and paying for medical care**.

Since a CPGP offers a package rather than a set of parts, there are no meaningful prices and quantities, no distinction between insurance overhead and clinical management. It is like getting a package trip to Cancun rather than paying separately for airfare, hotels, meals, excursions, taxis, and a travel agent's fee. This "**fourth way**" of reducing costs was, in fact, the original form of managed care, and the term "HMO" originally applied only to such comprehensive CPGP health plans (since they could presumably save money by maintaining health rather than treating illnesses) (Table 5.5). The challenge for an integrated CPGP HMO

TABLE 5.5	How Managed Care Can Reduce Total Costs

Contractual: Reduce Total P × Q by:

1. Reducing prices
2. Reducing quantities
3. Substituting cheaper types
4. **Organizational**: integrate insurance and production in a comprehensive closed-panel group practice (full service package in a single organization; no prices or quantities as such).

is to keep premiums low and satisfaction high—the itemized prices and quantities fade out of existence and relevance.

Changing organizational structure offers great potential for savings but is hard to bring about, and most CPGPs have rather timidly tried to stay close to "regular" medical practice (see the discussion of the Kaiser health plan in Chapter 10). The potential for organizational change to reconfigure consumption can perhaps most easily be grasped through a familiar example—music. For 200 years, people have listened to string quartets performing Brahms compositions. To perform a 20-minute piece, it takes four musicians playing 20 minutes each (and practicing for years) to bring music to the audience. Whether it is 1710 or 2010, it still takes four musicians and 20 minutes. There is little room to cut price (musicians have never been all that well paid), and playing the entire prelude in 15 minutes is not a satisfactory way to achieve efficiency. However, focusing on the needs of the consumers rather than the producers reveals a new way, and a new organization—a recording company. The performance can be played around the world (OK, so it is not quite as good as being there) for a per person cost that is a fraction of the four musicians' hourly wages. Indeed, once the music is digitized and placed on a compact disc, a person can listen to it at home, in the car, or at a picnic dinner on the beach rather inexpensively. If the revolution in musical consumption seems exceedingly far-fetched as an analogy, consider the health effects of small pox vaccination, sanitation, heart pacemakers, and the Internet on the practice of medicine between 1910 and 2010.

Medical Loss Ratios

Almost 77 million people, 21 percent percent of those with private insurance, were in either contractual or organizational HMOs in 2005, a 500 percent increase in just twenty years.[18] Eighteen million Medicaid enrollees were in HMOs, as were 7 million Medicare enrollees. Except for Medicare, the old-style indemnity insurance that paid bills automatically without managerial intervention now accounts for less than 5 percent of private insurance. There has been consolidation in the industry, with the number of operating HMOs dropping to 465 in 2005. By far the largest are the CPGP Kaiser health plans with 8.4 million enrollees. Yet the 55 CPGP/staff model HMOs are outnumbered by the 410 contractual independent practice association (IPA)/network HMOs, which account for 78 percent of total enrollment.

Most contractual HMOs take 15 to 20 percent of the premiums they receive for administration, marketing, and profit,[19] with the bulk of the funds used to pay medical expenses (see Table 5.6). This fraction is known as the "medical loss ratio." The largest expense category is physician services. Although hospitals are the largest expenditure item in the National Health Expenditure accounts, HMOs' tight controls over hospitals and coverage of a generally younger and healthier population means that less than a third of HMO premiums are used to pay for inpatient hospital services. Some of the HMOs' other expenses are reinsurance (to keep the plan solvent and ensure that patients' bills are paid even if the plan

TABLE 5.6	HMO Expenses as a Percent of Premiums
Physician and outpatient	41% ⎤
Inpatient	31% ⎥
Outside referrals	7% ⎬ "Medical loss ratio" = 82%
Emergency	3% ⎦
Administrative	13%
Profit	5%

should have a catastrophic loss), taxes, emergency out-of-area services, and certain highly specialized treatments that must be paid for on a FFS basis to noncontracted providers. Over time, the HMO business has become much more price competitive. Administrative expenses and profit margins have been cut as plans become more efficient; therefore, the percentage of total dollars going to treatment (the medical loss ratio) has risen. In earlier years, wide variations of ± 25 percent were not uncommon. With more experience and better information, competitive standards have been set so that most HMOs offer a similar price (perhaps ± 10 percent) for most benefit packages (see Table 5.6).

5.5 THE RANGE OF MANAGED CARE PLANS

The variety and possible configurations of managed care are too diverse for any single definition. It is better to think in terms of a range from unmanaged to tightly managed as illustrated in Figure 5.4. At the looser end, under FFS medicine with indemnity insurance, the health plan takes all the financial risk but exercises no medical management. Whatever hospitalization, surgery, or drugs any physician decides to order are paid for by the insurance company without question. There is no haggling over prices. Any difference between premiums and expenses becomes a gain or loss to the insurance company but has no effect on the hospital or physician. The only "control" comes from making the patient pay for some deductibles, coinsurance, or excess over the plan maximums. At the other end is the closed CPGP HMO, in which a single organization combines the functions of medical provider and insurance company. It enrolls members; builds hospitals; employs physicians, nurses, and therapists on salary; purchases drugs, beds, cardiac pacemakers, and so on; and controls all finances. Any difference between premiums and expenses is a gain or loss to be shared with the physician group.[20] In between these two ends are a range of contracts that link medicine and insurance but stop short of combining them into a single organization. For example, Independence Blue Cross has a set of relatively unrestricted contracts ("personal choice") and a more restrictive set ("Keystone HMO"). Both are administered out of the same office and cover most of the same doctors and hospitals, but the HMO plans require prior authorization by the primary care doctor for many services and more frequently limit the choice of specialty care providers.

Provider Networks

The differences between POS, HMOs, PPOs, and other managed care structures usually do not matter much to the average consumer, but are significant in the contracting and business relations between the insurers and providers. Under pure indemnity insurance, the contract is solely between the patient and the insurance company. Upon evidence of loss (a bill), the insurance company sends a check to the patient, who is responsible for all relationships with the providers. A managed care organization arises when the insurance company begins to make contracts with physicians and hospitals, forming a network of providers. A **preferred provider organization** (**PPO**) limits the patient's choice of physicians and hospitals by paying in full (or a larger percentage) only for care received from approved providers within

FIGURE 5.4   Range of Managed Care Plans

Indemnity FFS	UR	PPO	Open HMO	Closed HMO

No management controls ← → *Tight management controls*

TABLE 5.7	Hypothetical PPO Payment	
	Within Network	**Outside Provider**
Hospital	100%	80%
Physician	90%	75%
Therapist	90%	50%
Pharmacies	No copay	$10 copay
Drugs		
In formulary	Covered	50%
Not in formulary	Not covered	Not covered

the network. Patients can choose to see a physician outside the plan or to stay in a hospital that is not part of the preferred group if they are willing to pay a larger portion of the bill (see Table 5.7).

A PPO is a contractual intermediary—a corporate entity created by a group of doctors, an entrepreneur, a hospital chain, a union, an employer coalition, or the insurer.[21] It will have procedures to certify providers (check license validity, meet standards, produce reports and statistics) and set specifications for reimbursement (per diems, discounted fees, other), some of which may depend on restrictions ("we get all of your heart surgery") or volume discounts. Contracts may be open or exclusive—a physician may belong to one or many PPOs, an MCO may have one PPO or many, a PPO may contract with one hospital or many, a PPO may contract with one MCO or many. The overlapping contracts and gaps can make the relationships and flow of funds rather complex. Usually, the term "HMO" is applied to a plan offering care through a single, fairly limited network. A hybrid HMO-**POS** (**point of service**) allows patients to obtain care cheaply within the HMO network but also to opt-out "at the point of service" and see any other provider by paying extra. The differences between a PPO, HMO, and an HMO/POS can be subtle, so much so that patients may not even know exactly what type of plan they are covered by unless they examine the contract closely. Many large insurers such as Blue Cross now offer **triple-option** plans, in which the enrollee can chose the HMO, the PPO, or indemnity insurance, with the premium increasing in steps as the controls over utilization become weaker.

Gatekeeping

Two restrictions tend to mark the transition from partially managed PPO and POS plans to HMOs: (1) mandatory authorization for hospitalization, and (2) primary physicians who act as gatekeepers. Mandatory authorization means that the physician must get on the phone to the health plan and explain why the patient needs hospitalization and document the severity of illness to obtain approval before admitting the patient. Under a **gatekeeper** system, patients must receive all their primary care from a single physician, and any specialist referrals, surgery, prescriptions, and hospitalizations must be approved in advance by the gatekeeper primary physician. In this way, the plan is able to delegate responsibility for cost control and appropriateness to the **primary care** physician (PCP).

Capitation

Gatekeeper physicians are commonly paid a **capitation** rate, a fixed amount **per member per month** (**PMPM**) (currently about $20–$40) for each person enrolled with them.[22] They must provide all primary care for each person and act as a manager by coordinating

MANAGING PHARMACY COSTS: CARVE-OUTS AND TRIPLE-TIER BENEFITS

In the past, Medicare and most employer indemnity insurance plans did not pay for the cost of pharmaceuticals taken by patients outside the hospital. Outpatient drugs were fairly inexpensive, billing information was hard to obtain, and therefore benefits were limited. As the cost of pharmaceuticals rose and information systems expanded, it became easier and more valuable to provide prescription coverage. It is now common for employer plans to have a pharmaceutical component, and Medicare has added drug coverage as "Part D." Yet dispensing prescriptions is sufficiently different from other types of medical services that most insurance companies subcontract with specialized firms called pharmacy benefit managers (PBMs). Thus, it is actually the PBM (not Blue Cross or Aetna) that processes the claims and pays the pharmacy. Drugs have become a carve-out benefit because the PBMs can do the job better, at lower cost.

How do PBMs manage care to save costs? First, they obtain **rebates** (payments for volume) and **price discounts**. PBMs are large, handling millions of prescriptions a year, and can use their market power at both ends: manufacturing (pharmaceutical companies) and retail (pharmacy chains). Second, they can use **substitution**. A recent study showed that mandatory generic substitution (MGS) reduced average costs by 8 percent.[23] In such a contract, the insurance only pays for the generic version of a drug if the Food and Drug Administration (FDA) has deemed it equivalent to the more expensive brand-name version, regardless of how the prescription is written. While 8 percent may not seem like a lot, it is larger than the profit margins in most retail businesses.

More sophisticated contracts divide drugs into tiers to provide incentives for patients to actively cooperate in **reducing the use** of expense drugs. In the three-tier plan shown here, the most favored tier 1 drugs have only a $2 copayment. These are generic versions of expensive brand-name drugs or brands for which the PBM has negotiated a large discount or rebate. Tier 2, with $10 copayments, is made up of drugs on an approved list (formulary): drugs with no generic equivalent, drugs with small discounts, and the like. Tier 3, in which patients face a hefty $30 copayment, is reserved for the expensive brand-name drugs that have a generic equivalent in tier 1, drugs of limited usefulness, drugs that are frequently prescribed for off-label (i.e., not approved by the FDA) purposes, or expensive drugs whose benefits seem relatively minor (Viagra, Cox-2 inhibitor, and low-dose antihistamines might fall into this tier).

Triple-Tier Drug Benefit Plan

Category	Patient Copayment	Types of Drugs
Tier 1	$2	Generics, sole source
Tier 2	$10	Approved formulary
Tier 3	$30	Off-patent brands, lifestyle

Tiered pharmacy benefit plans were relatively rare a decade ago but are now found in 85 percent of large employee health insurance plans.[24] They have been shown to reduce total costs by increasing rates of generic substitution and by (slightly) reducing the number of prescriptions filled. What may be even more important to employers, though, is that they provide a relatively simple way of shifting more of the cost to the employee (all those copayments add up). Indeed, dissatisfaction with large and repeated copayments make the integrated CPGP HMO solution, in which the HMO has an in-house pharmacy and uses salaried pharmacists to distribute drugs, look more attractive—and is one reason for the sudden influx of veterans who have other insurance plans moving into the Department of Veterans Affairs (VA) health system.

and approving all other services. Capitation is sometimes used for hospitalization, for laboratory services, and even for certain types of specialty care (heart transplants, oncology, mental health, and substance abuse treatment). These are often referred to as "carve-outs" or "subcapitation." Paying for the number of people enrolled rather than the number of services rendered changes the economic incentives from "doing more" (FFS) to "doing less" (capitation). With fixed payments per member made in advance, profits are greater when fewer services are used.

What, then, keeps the HMO from doing less and less until it maximizes profits by providing no services at all? Quite simply, the need to attract new members and keep the old ones. Competition and the potential loss of enrollment makes HMOs strive to maintain quality and patient satisfaction. In FFS, profits increase as more is done. What keeps a surgeon from performing an unnecessary operation in order to make more money? Control over excessive surgery under FFS is largely a matter of professional ethics and disapproval by peers, since there is no external reporting and no manager who intervenes to question the appropriateness of treatment.

Withholds

All HMOs must use FFS payment for some types of care, especially for specialty services in which use by enrollees is rare and unpredictable. **Withholds** are a way of incorporating part of the cost-control incentive of capitation into FFS payment. An HMO specialty referral withhold plan might work as follows: Each specialist receives 80 percent of the agreed amount at the time the patient is treated. The other 20 percent goes into the withhold pool. The HMO projects a total dollar expenditure for specialty referral services for the year. If the total of referral bills from all specialists is at or below that amount at the end of the year, the withhold pool is distributed in accordance with the amounts billed. In this case, the specialist receives 100 percent of the amount billed but has to wait until the end of the year to receive the last 20 percent. However, if the total billings are more than 20 percent above the projected total, the HMO keeps the withhold pool to help pay for the unanticipated extra volume. In this way, part of the risk of overutilization is shared with the specialists. If the total bills are more than 100 percent of the projected total but less than 120 percent, the specialists and the HMO split the withhold pool at the end of the year.

Utilization Review

Some of the other management interventions used to control cost and utilization include the following:

- **Second opinion**—A second doctor must review the record and concur with the initial doctor's recommendation before surgery is performed.
- **Pre-certification**—Approval must be obtained in advance from the insurance company before elective surgery is performed.
- **Pre-admission testing**—A requirement that many tests be performed in advance on an outpatient basis so that the patient spends fewer days in the hospital.
- **Concurrent review**—Regular evaluations are made by a case control nurse to authorize a continued stay in the hospital or additional procedures.
- **Database profiling**—Graphs and charts indicating the number of services used per 1,000 patients by each doctor or hospital are maintained to identify abnormally high or low patterns of utilization.
- **Intensive case management**—A nurse in the insurance company follows and manages any case expected to cost more than $10,000.

- **Generic substitution**—A prescription for a brand-name drug is filled with a cheaper generic version if the two are deemed equivalent by the FDA.

- **Discharge planning**—A social worker meets with the patient and family early to facilitate rapid transfer back home or to a nursing home.

- **Retrospective review**—An evaluation is conducted after the patient is discharged from the hospital to deny payment for any medically unnecessary services.

- **Audits**—An insurance company representative ensures that all services billed for were actually performed.

5.6 MANAGED COMPETITION AND THE FEHBP

The Federal Employees Health Benefits Plan (FEHBP) has operated successfully for more than forty years with a rather unique structure that provides for consumer choice and price competition between plans. Within each area many companies make bids (i.e., advertise a premium per month) to provide standard coverage plus additional optional benefits. Although employees can choose among any of the qualified plans, the FEHBP pays only up to the cost of the lowest bid. The employee must personally pay the extra amount (if any) by which the plan chosen exceeds the premium for the low-cost plan. In this way the individual bears the full marginal cost of extra benefits, amenities, and inefficiencies.

Based on the experience of the FEHBP, economist Alain Enthoven published a provocative proposal for a Consumer Choice Health Plan in the *New England Journal of Medicine* in 1978, envisioning a future in which managed care was the norm and FFS was the secondary alternative.[25] His proposal was based on a recognition that consumers, confronted with thousands of possible illnesses, millions of possible prices, and indemnity coverage that was (a) difficult to understand and (b) comprehensive enough to make the effort of comparing costs not worthwhile, actually made decisions that were very remote from the market in which suppliers operated. Consumers looked for plans with low copayments, or coverage of eyeglasses and orthodontics, or benefit maximums set at reassuringly astronomical amounts—factors that had nothing to do with the average total cost of most medical care or the rising premiums that employers had to pay each year, which were reducing profits and wages. In contrast, "consumer choice" as presented by Enthoven was based on making a choice between two or three competing plans, each with a price that was known in advance and for which the consumer would have to pay the full difference between the low-cost plan and the high-cost plan if he or she preferred to obtain greater choice, more coverage, or higher quality.

Although by 2009 it was evident that managed care had indeed pushed indemnity FFS into a small corner, few of the specifics of the Enthoven proposal came to pass. No universal guarantee of basic care for all Americans has been made, employer tax subsidies still favor more expensive plans, and most HMOs do not compete on the basis of care (since they have overlapping lists of hospitals and physicians) but rather on minor contractual stipulations regarding copayments, dental benefits, referral procedures, and extent of coinsurance. It will be interesting to see what the next decade will bring (see Chapter 18).

5.7 INCENTIVES—TO PATIENTS, TO PAYERS, AND TO PROVIDERS

Which type of insurance plan encourages patients to use a more expensive, higher quality hospital? Which type of plan encourages longer stays? The insurance contract not only provides coverage for risks and access to high cost specialty services, it also structures the incentives. Being reimbursed a fixed number of dollars per hospital day gives patients an incentive to (a) find a hospital that is priced near that amount but not below and (b) stay as long as they want since each additional day is covered. It may also make patients try to bargain with the hospital to accept the amount of reimbursement provided as payment in full. If the per day maximum applies only to hospital charges, both the hospital and the patient may have an incentive to get laboratory fees, drugs, physical therapy, and other care billed separately by an outside firm.

HMO and PPO contracts use reduced deductibles and copayments to provide incentives for patients to use only hospitals for which the HMO or PPO has negotiated volume discounts—and it is the promise of additional volume that makes hospitals offer discounts. Most drug reimbursement is now of the "triple-tier" form: a low per prescription fee for generic drugs, a moderate per prescription fee or percentage for drugs on an approved list (formulary), and a higher per prescription fee or percentage for "off-list" drugs (see the box on "triple-tier" pharmacy plans in Section 5.5). Indeed, often it requires a physician to write a letter (a significant disincentive) for the patient to get any reimbursement at all if the prescribed drug is not on the list. By structuring incentives this way, insurance contracts can reduce or increase the use of certain services, steer patients to approved providers, and affect the sort of price negotiations that take place.

Insurance, like many other business arrangements, tends to serve the interests of those who write the contracts. Thus, the original Blue Cross plans, developed by hospital associations, were beneficial to hospitals; the generous reimbursement with no patient charges and community rating kept hospital beds full and revenues flowing. The entry of commercial insurers depended on their ability to offer a lower-priced product using copayments and deductibles to reduce premiums and reduce services (not something in the interest of hospitals, which wanted more business, not less). If these contractual stipulations caused some "positive selection"—discouraging sick people from purchasing commercial insurance and making them stick with Blue Cross—this was fine with the commercial insurers and the companies that purchased coverage for their employees from them, who had no desire to cover more "high-cost" people. Of course, the hospitals worried because they still had to care for the high-cost people and the uninsured regardless of how much they could get paid.

In the long run, contracts must meet the needs of all parties, but it can take a long time to get there. Also, it is possible to structure contracts so that the interests of some smaller groups lacking influence are ignored. For example, a corporation may be willing to eliminate coverage for alcoholism since it could just fire those employees rather than rehabilitate them, or it may be willing to put an annual maximum on the number of days of hospital treatment to discourage people with HIV/AIDS from taking a job there.

Universal national health insurance coverage would put everyone under the same contract so that no one could be excluded. However, with everyone insured under the same plan, no one has incentives to shop around for better prices, no ability to pick and choose which coverage is or is not worthwhile, and no chance to go somewhere else if the service provided by the insurer is unsatisfactory. Insurance contracts in the real world represent a balancing of incentives and interests, a balance that is changing all the time.

SUGGESTIONS FOR FURTHER READING

David M. Cutler, Mark McClellan, and Joseph P. Newhouse, "How does managed care do it?" *RAND Journal of Economics* 31, no. 3 (Autumn 2000): 526–548.

Employee Benefit Research Institute, *Employment Based Health Benefits, 2008* (serial publication) (www.ebri.org); and Paul Frontsin "Sources of Health Insurance and Characteristics of the Uninsured," EBRI Issue Brief #321, November 2008.

Alain Enthoven, *Theory and Practice of Managed Competition in Health Care Finance* (Amsterdam: North-Holland, 1988).

Kaiser Family Foundation and HRET *Employer Health Benefits, 2008* Annual Survey, (www.kff.org).

Peter R. Kongstvedt, *Essentials of Managed Care*, 4th edition (Gaithersburg, Md.: Aspen, 2003).

Managed Care Digest (annual), (www.managedcaredigest.com).

Diane Rowland, "Medicaid at Forty," *Health Care Financing Review* 27, no. 2 (Winter 2006): 63–78; http://www.cms.hhs.gov/HealthCareFinancingReview/.

SUMMARY

1. Paying medical bills with **insurance makes health care a third-party transaction**. All three parties—patients, providers, and insurers—must benefit from the transaction. However, **separating the flow of funds from the flow of services obscures the real cost** of medical care. Health care is paid for by people (as patients, taxpayers, or employees giving up some wages to get health benefits), not by corporations.

2. The **government is the single largest insurer**, paying for 48 percent of all medical care. **Medicare**, which pays for the medical care of the elderly, is the largest and most influential government program, although the state/federal **Medicaid** program dominates long-term care reimbursement. Tax advantages have fostered the growth of health insurance as an employee benefit. Private health insurance covers 60 percent of the population but pays only 34 percent of the total bills. About 12 percent is paid for out of pocket by patients or their families.

3. About 46 million Americans, **16 percent of the population, are uninsured**. For many of them it is a rational decision to go without insurance based on their youth, good health, and/or low current earning power. For some, going without insurance is the result of a chronic disease, bad luck, or the size of the company they work for.

4. Insurance comes in a range of contractual forms, from pure insurance with fixed premiums, to various forms of risk sharing, to administered services only, to self-insurance plans in which the employer bears all the risk. Obtaining **tax benefits and exemption from state-mandated** coverage under ERISA has been a major reason for companies to self-insure.

5. **Managed care** is a diverse set of contractual and management methods used to arrange the financing and delivery of medical services. Its distinctive feature is that *a manager* intervenes to monitor and control the transaction between doctor and patient. Traditional insurance provides value through risk pooling so that medical expenses can be covered by an actuarially fair premium equal to the expected average loss. Managed care adds value by systematically **reducing the average** loss through utilization review, negotiating discounts, preauthorization, formularies, case management, statistical profiling, and other process controls.

6. **Escalation in costs** under open-ended entitlement financing from Medicare, Medicaid, and employer-provided health insurance has been the primary force driving the development of managed care. HMOs **reduce costs** by saving money on both the demand and the supply side. They obtain **discounts** by contracting in volume with physicians and hospitals, **substitute** less expensive services (e.g., home care instead of hospital stays), and **control utilization** through the approval process. HMOs may use one-third to two-thirds fewer inpatient hospital days per thousand people than traditional fee-for-service insurance, although they often use more ambulatory services.

7. A **pharmacy formulary** limiting payment to those drugs listed, a **preferred provider network** that makes patients pay extra for using hospitals and physicians not on the list, **capitation**, primary care **gatekeepers**, and **utilization review** are some of the ways that managed care firms control costs. However, simple **price cuts** obtained through hard bargaining appear to be the major source of savings. Managed care has made many doctors bitter, since these savings reduce the income and professional autonomy of physicians.

8. Managed care attempts to create a much greater degree of **vertical and horizontal integration** in a medical system that has resisted organizational change. Changes in telecommunications and **information technology** make it possible for management to practice utilization review and monitor quality of care. Managed care has been shown to **reduce costs**, but it is probably not the answer to all of America's health care problems. Some HMOs have made money by **risk selection**, accepting mostly healthier patients. Other HMOs may find it hard to maintain **quality of care** once the easy savings from discounting and substitution have been taken, and thus may be tempted to reduce services in precisely those areas where patients, hampered by information asymmetry, depend most on professionals for monitoring quality.

9. Insurance **contracts create incentives** for patients, providers, and insurance companies to behave in ways that affects the market. Almost any contract will favor some interests and harm others.

PROBLEMS

1. {*gains from trade*} Who benefits from a three-party transaction?

2. {*accounting, incidence*} How can a patient benefit if the premiums paid are more than the cost of the medical care received? How can an insurance company benefit if the medical care it provides costs more than the premiums paid in?

3. {*marginal incentives*} Explain how one insurance contract can provide incentives to:

    a. Choose a more or less expensive hospital.

    b. Spend more or less days in the hospital.

    c. Choose a more or less expensive surgeon.

    d. Use more or less drugs.

    e. Use more or less expensive drugs.

4. {*uninsured*} The law now gives a worker who becomes unemployed the right to buy continuing health insurance coverage after leaving the company. Why might it be rational for a factory worker who loses his or her job to give up this legal right to purchase coverage and become uninsured, even knowing that he or she is at risk for high medical expenditures?

5. {*mandated benefits*} Prior to 1970, maternity was usually treated differently from other medical expenses, either excluded entirely from coverage or subject to a flat lump-sum cash (indemnity) benefit. Why? During the 1970s, 23 states mandated that treatment related to pregnancy be covered the same as any other type of treatment, and in 1978, such coverage became uniform throughout the United States. Would mandated maternity benefits make working in a salaried position more or less attractive to women? Would it make women of childbearing age more or less attractive as employees? Would it increase or decrease the number of births performed by

Cesarean section? Who do you think bore the expense of implementing this mandate? (For a discussion of these issues see "The Incidence of Mandated Maternity Benefits," by Jonathan Gruber, *American Economic Review* 84, no. 3 (April 1994): 622–641.

6. {*adverse selection*} Which government insurance program is more affected by adverse selection: Medicare or Medicaid?

7. {*incentives*} Which surgeons are more subject to financial incentives when deciding between alternative courses of therapy: FFS physicians who own their own practices or salaried physicians working for an HMO?

8. {*industrial organization*} If an HMO reduces the patient's marginal cost of surgery, hospitalization, chemotherapy, and other expensive items to zero, how can it provide incentives for reduced utilization?

9. {*industrial organization*} Is an HMO able to obtain the biggest discounts where it has a large market share or where it has a smaller market share?

10. {*transaction costs*} Since managed care firms must hire managers to review all hospitalizations and surgeries, isn't managed care necessarily more expensive than unmanaged FFS care due to this extra administrative cost?

11. {*incidence*} If ABC corporation shifts from an indemnity plan to an HMO plan that lowers its cost of employee benefits by 35 percent over three years, who benefits? Who loses?

12. {*selection bias*} If a company offers both an HMO and an indemnity plan, which employees will choose which? (Assume the company pays 80% of the premiums and the employee 20%).

13. {*selection*} Would an HMO entering the Medicare market expect to experience favorable or adverse selection? Would the magnitude of the selection bias be larger or smaller for an HMO entering the commercial employee benefit market? The Medicaid market?

14. {*costs*} What are the three main ways HMOs act to reduce the cost of care? What is the fourth way?

15. {*dynamics*} Will a contract that lowers the amount an HMO pays providers be more important with regard to the HMO's short-run or long-run profitability? The providers' short-run or long-run profitability? Why?

16. {*information*} In what ways can an HMO use information to increase profits? As information technology has become more efficient and cheaper to use, have health care firms invested more or less in computers?

17. {*distribution*} Why do "star" surgeons rarely work for HMOs, even the largest and wealthiest ones?

18. {*physician behavior*} What is the purpose of a withhold fund? Do HMOs have substitutes for financial incentives in controlling physician behavior? What factors make these substitutes more or less effective?

19. {*dynamics*} What technological change has been most important in fostering the growth of managed care?

20. {*selection*} Is a person who is chronically ill and has a long-term relationship with a physician more likely to choose an HMO, PPO, or indemnity plan? How will this affect HMO capitation rates?

21. {*incentives*} What incentives does a capitated physician have to keep his patients happy? What incentive does an FFS physician have? If Mr. Jones is a cranky old man who smokes and drinks so much that his liver and other organs are going downhill, which payment system provides more incentive to keep Mr. Jones satisfied? Which provides the most incentive to render extra care? Which provides the most incentive to make sure that the level of care is optimized?

22. {*marginal cost*} Ralph says he pays $960 per month for his employer's HMO plan. Since the employer also offers a PPO and POS plan from another insurance company, why doesn't Ralph switch plans?

23. {*marginal cost*} Suppose a family physician has HMO patients who are capitated for primary care, HMO patients who are capitated using a withhold for hospital care, and FFS patients. For which patients is the marginal cost to the physician of doing additional laboratory services highest? For which patients is the marginal cost to the physician of admitting them to the hospital the highest?

24. {*incidence*} Which groups tend to win by a general move toward capitated managed care? Which groups tend to lose?

ENDNOTES

1. Estimates of coverage from EBRI and the Kaiser Family Foundation 2008 annual publications, based primarily on the U.S. Census Bureau "Current Population Survey."
2. Mary A. Laschober et al., "Trends in Medicare Supplemental Insurance and Prescription Drug Coverage, 1996–1999," *Health Affairs* 21, no. 2 (April 2002): 11.
3. Kaiser and HRET, *Employer Health Benefits, 2008 Annual Survey*.
4. C. DeNavas-Walt, B. D. Proctor, and C. H. Lee, "Income, Poverty and Health Insurance Coverage in the United States, 2004." <http://www.census.gov/prod/2005pubs/p60-229.pdf> and Kaiser Family Foundation, "The Uninsured and Their Access to Health Care" Publication 1420-07, November 4, 2005, <www.kff.org>.
5. The 19–24 age group is more than twice as likely to be uninsured as other age groups (35% versus 15%). J. P. Vistnes and S. H. Zuvekas, *Health Insurance Status of the Civilian Noninstitutionalized Population, 1997* (Rockville, Md.: Agency for Health Care Policy and Research, July 1999). MEPS Research Findings #8, AHCPR Pub. No.99-0030.
6. Helen Levy and Thomas DeLeire, "What Do People Buy When They Don't Buy Health Insurance?" Harris Graduate School of Public Policy Studies, University of Chicago, working paper, June 26, 2002 (www.jcpr.org/wpfiles/levy deleire.pdf).
7. Lisa Dubay, Ian Hill, and Genevieve Kenney, "Five Things Everyone Should Know About SCHIP," Series A, No.A-55, The Urban Institute, October 2002. (www.urban.org/url.cfm?ID=3105707); Elizabeth Thompson Beckley, "Missing the SCHIP," *Modern Physician* (September 2002): 10; also see www.insurekidsnow.gov.
8. Gary Claxton et al., "What High-Deductible Plans Look Like: Findings From a National Survey of Employers, 2005." *Health Affairs* Web exclusive W5 (September 14, 2005): 434–441; Debbie Welle-Powell, "HSAs—Friends or Foes?" *Healthcare Financial Management* (March 2006): 76–79.
9. Colleen M. Barry et al. "Who Chooses a Consumer-Directed Health Plan?" *Health Affairs* 27, no. 6 (December 2008): 1671–1679.
10. Jeffrey Liebman and Richard Zeckhauser, "Simple Humans, Complex Insurance, Subtle Subsidies," NBER working paper #14330, September 2008; Nicole Maestas, Mathias Schroeder, and Dana Goldman, "Price Variation in Markets with Homogenous Goods: The Case of Medigap," NBER #14679, January 2009.
11. Joy M. Grossman and Paul B. Ginsburg, "As The Health Insurance Underwriting Cycle Turns" Health *Affairs* 23, no. 6 (2004): 91–102; Alice Rosenblatt, "The Underwriting Cycle: the Rule of Six," Health *Affairs* 23, no. 6 (2004): 103–106.
12. Howard S. Berliner and Sonia Delgada, "From DRGs to Deregulation: New Jersey Takes the Road Less Traveled," *Journal of American Health Policy* 3 (July/August 1993): 4448.
13. The U.S. Bureau of Labor Statistics Employee Compensation measures have varied over the years, and the various issues of the *BLS Handbook of Methods* should be examined to understand the vagaries of comparison (www.bls.gov). Bradley R. Braden and Stephanie L. Hyland, "Cost of Employee Compensation in Public and Private Sectors," *Monthly Labor Review* 116, no. 5 (May 1993): 14–21.

14. *2005 HMO-PPO/Medicare-Medicaid Digest*, Aventis Pharmaceuticals, (www.managedcaredigest.com). This is a standard compilation of HMO statistics that has been published for a number of years under various titles and corporate sponsors.

15. The United States ranked 26th in male life expectancy among 191 nations in 2000 (28th for females), a bit behind most other developed countries. The risk of dying between ages 15 and 59, a perhaps more significant measure, was even worse (36th for males, 38th for females). Overall, the World Health Organization ranked performance of the U.S. health system 37th, *World Health Report 2000* (www.who.int/whr). See also Victor Fuchs, "The Best Health Care System in the World?" *Journal of the American Medical Association* 268, no. 7 (1992): 916–917; Jack Hadley, *More Medical Care, Better Health?* (Washington, D.C.: The Urban Institute Press, 1982); OECD, *OECD Health Data: Comparative Analysis of Health Systems* (Paris: Organization for Economic Cooperation and Development, 2002).

16. Neelam K. Sekhri, "Managed Care: the U.S. Experience," *Bulletin of the World Health Organization* 78, no. 6 (2000): 830–844 (www.who.org or www.who.int); C. Liu, R. Frank, and T. McGuire, "Demand Response of Mental Health Services to Cost Sharing under Managed Care," *The Journal of Mental Health Policy and Economics* 11 (2008): 113–125.

17. David M. Cutler, Mark McClellan, and Joseph P. Newhouse, "How Does Managed Care Do It?" *RAND Journal of Economics* 31, no. 3 (Autumn 2000): 526–548; Daniel Alman, Richard Zeckhauser, and David M. Cutler, "Enrollee Mix, Treatment Intensity and Cost in Competing Indemnity and HMO Plans, NBER working paper no. 7832, August 2000 (www.nber.org); Ann Barry Flood et al., "How do HMOs achieve savings?" *Health Services Research* 33, no. 1 (April 1998): 79–99.

18. *Managed Care Digest 2005*, www.managedcaredigest.com; Robert H. Miller and Harold Luft, "Managed Care Plans: Characteristics, Growth and Premium Performance," *Annual Review of Public Health* 15 (1994): 437–59.

19. *Managed Care Digest: HMO-PPO Digest 1995* (Kansas City, Mo.: Hoechst Marion Roussel, 1995). In an integrated CPGP HMO, administrative and medical expenses all occur within the same organization and cannot meaningfully be separated. In reports, Kaiser or Group Health often say their administrative expenses are very low, 2 percent or so, but this low figure comes from counting only the central office staff, and not all the clerks, secretaries, medical directors, information specialists, etc., who are at work in the clinics.

20. In principle, an integrated closed HMO could be run as a for-profit corporation benefiting stockholders, a division of a voluntary hospital chain, or a consumer co-op with all profits used to increase community benefits. In practice, the residual ownership interest has de facto resided primarily with the senior physician group, even when they are technically employees of the HMO.

21. The term "PPO" is commonly used to refer to two things: an insurance plan and a corporate entity. The two are distinct. Your "PPO" insurance may actually have contracts with a dozen PPO organizations. Conversely, a single PPO organization with 50 physicians may have contracts with more than one insurance company (and at different prices).

22. Marsha Gold et al., "A National Survey of the Arrangements Managed-Care Plans Make With Physicians," *New England Journal of Medicine* 333 (1995): 1678–1683; Gerard Anderson et al., "Setting Payment Rates for Capitated Systems: A Comparison of Various Alternatives," *Inquiry* 27, no. 3 (1990): 225–233.

23. Geoffrey F. Joyce, Jose J. Escarce, Matthew D. Solomon, and Dana Goldman, "Employer Drug Benefit Plans and Spending on Prescription Drugs," *Journal of the American Medical Association* 288, no. 14 (October 9, 2002): 1733–1739. See also the comment on the article by Donald M. Steinwachs, "Pharmacy Benefit Plans and Prescription Drug Spending," on pages 1773–1774.

24. Kaiser Family Foundation and HRET, Employee Health Benefits, 2002 Annual Survey, Chart #12 "Percentage of Covered Workers Facing Different Cost Sharing Formulas for Prescription Drugs: 2000, 2001, 2002," (www.kff.org/content/2002/20020905a).

25. Alain Enthoven, "Consumer Choice Health Plan," *New England Journal of Medicine* 298 (1978): 650–658, 709–720; *Theory and Practice of Managed Competition in Health Care Finance* (Amsterdam: North-Holland, 1988), and "Management of Competition in the FEHPB," *Health Affairs* 8, no. 3 (1989): 33–50.

CHAPTER **6**

PHYSICIANS

QUESTIONS

1. How are physicians paid?
2. Which types of physicians earn the highest incomes?
3. How much does it cost to practice medicine?
4. Are rising malpractice insurance premiums a major cause of higher doctor bills?
5. Is medical care "sold" like other goods and services? Why does a doctor serve as the patient's "agent," making choices about which hospital and what medicine to use?
6. Why are licensure restrictions more strongly enforced for some types of medical care than for others?
7. Is the American Medical Association (AMA) a professional society serving science or a union serving the economic interests of its members? Is it both?
8. Which is more competitive: the market for health insurance or the market for medical care?

At the center of medical practice stands the physician. Physicians direct the flow of patients by controlling admissions, referrals, regulations, insurance reimbursements, and prescriptions. A very powerful and special bond exists between doctor and patient. This relationship is based on medical science—and ethics and emotions—as well as economics.[1] Even when a transaction does not directly involve a physician financially, the physician still plays a dominant role. In the preceding chapters we discussed health care from the perspective of the patient. Now we switch to the perspective of the provider—not the payer, but the payee. For the physician, medical expenditures are not *costs*; they are *revenues*.

6.1 FINANCING PHYSICIAN SERVICES: REVENUES

Whereas most of the labor force is employed and paid a salary by a large organization, most physicians are independent entrepreneurs or partners running what are, in effect, small businesses.[2] The income of physicians in solo or group private practices mostly comes from **fee-for-service** payments, a specified amount paid for each visit or procedure, although an increasing amount is coming from complex, negotiated third-party contracts. In the 1930s, physicians were essentially free to charge whatever they decided was appropriate but often collected much less than what they charged. Today, 89 percent of physician revenues come

TABLE 6.1	Types of Physician Payment

Charges: The amount appearing on the bill, without insurance.

Fee-for-Service: A specified payment for each unit of service provided.

Fee Schedule: A set "menu" of prices for each service agreed upon in advance.

UCR: A method for denying bills that are out of line with the "usual, customary and reasonable charges made by this and other physicians for the same service last year."

RVS: A schedule based on objective standards showing relative value points for each service compared to a common unit (i.e., regular office visit). Deciding a dollar value per point converts it into a fee schedule.

RBRVS: The relative value schedule set by Medicare for physician fees.

Capitation: A set payment per person per month regardless of the number of services used.

Salary: A paycheck from an employer.

from third-party payments,[3] and most fees are subject to some form of external review or control (see Table 6.1).

It is important to distinguish between what the physician **charges** (i.e., the amount that appears on the bill) and the actual payments made by the insurance company, which may be considerably less. One of the initial steps in the evolution of physician payment in the United States was the development of **usual, customary, and reasonable (UCR)** fee schedules. The Blue Shield plans, which then provided the largest portion of physician insurance and operated with the support of local medical societies, collected information on what each physician charged for each service in a local area during the previous year. When a physician submitted a bill, it was checked to determine whether it was above his or her median charge for the same service the previous year (usual), above the 75th percentile of charges by all doctors in the area (customary), or justifiably higher because of a patient's complicating secondary illness or another acceptable reason (reasonable). When Medicare was implemented in 1966, it adopted the Blue Shield UCR method of paying physicians.

An effort to reduce payments, particularly for certain services, led insurers to promulgate **fee schedules**. A fee schedule is like a menu that specifies how much the insurance company will pay physicians for particular services. Fee schedules can be proposed by the sellers (physicians) to try to keep prices up or by the buyers (Medicare, insurance companies) to try to keep prices down. A major difficulty with fee schedules is the amazingly large number of services that must be priced. It is easy to come up with a reasonable price for a coronary bypass operation or services associated with a normal birth, but what about for oblique lateral pelvic X-rays, measurement of bilirubin or potassium levels, management of schizophrenia, and a host of other medical services?

To bring order to fee schedules, organizations have devised **relative value scales**, which give each service a point value. A common service (e.g., standard office visit, hernia repair surgery) is usually given a weight of 1 point, and all other services are given point values relative to that standard unit of service (e.g., 5 points, 0.2 point). After the physician and insurance company agree on the value per point, payment for each service is determined (e.g., if value per point is $20, a physician providing a 3.5-point service is paid $3.5 \times \$20 = \$70$). In 1992, the Medicare resource-based **relative value scale (RBRVS)** was implemented. A team of health economists and health services researchers, led by William Hsiao of Harvard University, studied the resources used in providing physician care to estimate a point value for each service based on (1) physician time, (2) intensity of effort, (3) practice costs, and (4) costs of advanced specialty training.[4] The Centers for Medicare and Medicaid Services (CMS) of the U.S. Department of Health and Human Services, which administers the Medicare program, set the dollars per point for 2003 at $34.59, with adjustments for geographic variation in practice costs and for malpractice insurance (see the RBRVS fee schedule box).

The Medicare physician reimbursement system provides a kind of "public good" (see Chapter 15) for other insurance programs; that is, a universally understood and practiced standard fee schedule they can adopt or easily modify by changing the dollar conversion factor or separating certain categories. Medicaid, Blue Cross, and commercial insurance contracts that cover the 87 percent of the population under age 65 often base their payments on a modified form of the Medicare RBRVS or use Medicare payment levels as a benchmark.

RBRVS FEE SCHEDULE

Medicare relies on a resource-based relative value scale (RBRVS) to determine the fees it will pay physicians to treat its beneficiaries. A fee is calculated by multiplying a service's relative value units (RVUs) by a conversion factor, adjusting for geographic cost variations. Medicare also uses the RBRVS to pay for certain services furnished by allied health professionals (e.g., physician assistants, nurse practitioners, certified registered nurse anesthetists, and physical therapists).

Relative Value Scale

An RBRVS is a list of physician services with RVUs assigned to each service. The units indicate a service's cost relative to that of the typical physician service, which has a relative value of 1.0 units. A service with 1.559 units is therefore 55.9 percent more costly to provide than the typical service, whereas a service with 0.693 units is 30.7 percent less costly to provide than the typical service.

A service's total RVUs are spread over the following three major components:

- Physician Work (pw)—The time spent, effort exerted, and skills used by the physician to furnish the service. This component includes preservice, intraservice, and postservice work related to the physician's encounter with the patient.

- Practice Expenses (pe)—The wages, salaries, and fringe benefits the physician provides office staff and money spent on other office expenses, such as rent and supplies. Many physician services have two practice expense RVUs—facility practice expense units and nonfacility practice expense units, the latter almost always higher than the former. This site-of-service differential recognizes that the physician does not absorb the full cost of services provided in a facility setting. Part of the cost is paid by the facility and, therefore, is included in the amount the facility is reimbursed.

- Malpractice Insurance (mi)—Separated from other practice expenses, largely because it varies significantly among specialties and across states and fluctuates markedly with oscillations in malpractice awards. Recently, malpractice expense has significantly increased.

Physician work accounts for approximately 55 percent of total RVUs, followed by 42 percent for practice expenses and 3 percent for malpractice insurance.

Level 1 of the CMS Common Procedure Coding System is used to identify the physician services a patient receives. Level 1—Current Procedural Terminology, fourth edition (CPT-4)—is the most widely used coding system for office visits, consultations, surgery, imaging, and other physician services. Approximately 7,500 CPT codes are paid under the

(Continued)

RBRVS FEE SCHEDULE (CONTINUED)

RBRVS fee schedule. Certain physician services may be performed by nurse practitioners, nurse midwives, or other midlevel or nonphysician practitioners. These practitioners may practice independently or under a physician's supervision, depending on state law. The same CPT code is used to document a service, regardless of who performs it.

Table 6.2 shows Medicare's RVUs for calendar year (CY) 2003 for selected physician services, which range from under 1.0 to nearly 29. The table shows the following:

- The RVUs for a new patient's office visit exceed those for an established patient's office visit; the units for both types of visits vary directly with the level of care.

- The RVUs for major surgical procedures (e.g., CPT 69501) include the cost of services and items that are bundled with the procedure, such as the surgeon's initial consultation, preoperative visits, treatment for complications after surgery, and postoperative visits to the surgeon for 10 to 90 days after surgery.

- Diagnostic and therapeutic radiology services have a professional and technical component. The professional component represents the portion of the service associated with the interpretation of the test. The technical component is the portion associated with the performance of the test. Often, a physician is paid for the professional component while the hospital where the service is furnished is paid for the technical component.

The RVUs are adjusted for geographic variations in wage rates and other prices that physicians pay for the resources used to produce patient care. The adjustment is based on geographic practice cost indexes (GPCIs) for physician work, practice expenses, and malpractice insurance. As of January 1, 2003, there were about 90 Medicare payment areas nationally, including statewide areas and metropolitan statistical areas. GPCIs vary noticeably across payment areas.

TABLE 6.2   Proposed Relative Value Units for Ten Physician Services, CY 2003

HCPCS/CPT Code	Description	Physician Work	Practice Expense Facility	Practice Expense Nonfacility	Malpractice Insurance	Total Units Facility	Total Units Nonfacility
99202	Office or other outpatient visit, new patient, level 2	0.88	0.32	0.77	0.05	1.25	1.70
99204	Office or other outpatient visit, new patient, level 4	2.00	0.72	1.49	0.10	2.82	3.59
99212	Office or other outpatient visit, established patient, level 2	0.45	0.16	0.52	0.02	0.63	0.99
99214	Office or other outpatient visit, established patient, level 4	1.10	0.40	1.03	0.04	1.54	2.17
99283	Emergency department services, level 3	1.24	0.32	NA	0.08	1.64	NA
30400	Reconstruction of nose	9.83	8.81	NA	0.80	19.44	NA
35501	Artery bypass graft	19.19	7.43	NA	2.33	28.95	NA
42800	Biopsy of throat	1.39	2.62	3.09	0.10	4.11	4.58
69501	Mastoidectomy	9.07	8.07	NA	0.65	17.79	NA
70336	Magnetic image, jaw joint	1.48	NA	11.67	0.56	NA	13.71
	Professional component	1.48	0.51	0.51	0.07	2.06	2.06
	Technical component	0.00	NA	11.16	0.49	NA	11.65

NA = not applicable.
Nonfacility = outside of hospital.

Source: Federal Register, "Medicare Program," vol. 67 (December 31, 2002), Appendix B.

(Continued)

RBRVS FEE SCHEDULE (CONTINUED)

Conversion Factor

The dollar value of an RVU is called the conversion factor (CF). This factor ($34.59 for CY 2003 for all physician services except anesthesia) is multiplied by the RVUs to calculate the fee for a given service. At times, Medicare's conversion factor serves as a floor for private health plans and ceiling for state Medicaid programs. Given the following assumptions for CPT 99283, CF = $34.59, RVU_{pw} = 1.24 (RVUs for *physician work*), RVU_{pe} = 0.32 (RVUs for *practice expenses*), RVU_{mi} = 0.08 (RVUs for *malpractice insurance*), $GPCI_{pw}$ = 1.032 (GPCI for *physician work*), $GPCI_{pe}$ = 1.109 (GPCI for *practice expenses*), and $GPCI_{mi}$ = 1.215 (GPCI for *malpractice insurance*), the fee would be $59.90.

$$\text{Fee} = \text{CF} \times [(RVU_{pw} \times GPCI_{pw}) + (RVU_{pe} \times GPCI_{pe}) + (RVU_{mi} \times GPCI_{mi})]$$
$$\$59.90 = \$34.59 \times [(1.24 \times 1.032) + (0.32 \times 1.109) + (0.08 \times 1.215)]$$

If the annual Medicare Part B deductible has been met, Medicare would pay 80 percent of the lower of the calculated fee or the amount the physician actually charged for the service (see Section 5.1). The patient would be responsible for paying the balance plus any extra amount that Medicare allows a nonparticipating physician to charge.

Fee Updates

In general, the conversion factor is updated annually for changes in the costs physicians incur to provide patient care. Medicare's update factor equals the compound rate of change in the following items:

- Medicare Economic Index—Measures the weighted rate of change in the cost of physician and nonphysician labor, supplies, and other resources used to produce patient care. The calculation includes a downward adjustment for productivity growth.

- Performance Adjustment—Made when actual and allowed Medicare expenditures for physician services differ. The allowed amount is a target designed to slow spending growth. Spending above the target is deducted from future fee increases; spending below the target is added to future fee increases.

- Other Factors—May cause Medicare spending to increase or decrease. Examples include an expansion of the physician services that Medicare covers or new statutory or regulatory requirements that affect practice costs (e.g., the Health Insurance Portability and Accountability Act [HIPAA].

Note: This box on RBRVS was prepared by health finance consultant and lecturer Paul L. Grimaldi, Ph.D. © 2003. For additional discussion on this topic, see Paul L. Grimaldi, "Medicare Fees for Physician Services are Resource-Based," *Journal of Health Care Finance* (Spring 2002): 88–104.

Copays, Assignment, and Balance Billing

Medicare and other insurers' contracts not only state what they will pay the physician, but also often specify what the patient must pay. A **copayment** of $5 or $10 per visit is often required, both to reduce premiums and, by forcing the patient to bear some costs, to reduce the number of services utilized. Some plans may also have a **deductible**, which requires the patient to pay the first $100 or $500 out of pocket per year or per illness. **Coinsurance**, with patients paying 10 percent or 20 percent of the bill, is a common part of major medical benefits. The contracts are so complex that it is often difficult for either the patient or the physician to know exactly who is responsible for which part of the bill. Two forms of payment can be distinguished: individual reimbursement and assignment. Under **individual reimbursement**, the patient pays all the charges, sends copies of the bills to the insurer, and is reimbursed for the medical expenses that are covered. Under **assignment**, the physician sends the bill to the insurer. The patient is charged for the copayment and may be **balance billed** for the difference if the physician's charges exceed the maximum fee allowed by the insurance contract. Under the Medicare participation agreement, a physician who accepts assignment agrees not to balance bill for any charges over the Medicare payment. Patients like assignment because they do not have to handle paperwork and are not stuck with additional fees. Physicians like the fact that they are paid directly and more rapidly, but do not like being denied the right to charge as much as they believe their services are worth. Indeed, the prohibition of balance billing in Canada led to a national physician's strike when the rule was first imposed.

Under current U.S. Medicare rules, physicians are limited to an additional 15 percent above the Medicare fee for balance billing if they choose not to accept assignment and are penalized by receiving only 95 percent of the regular fee schedule for services. In effect, Medicare has ruled out balance billing by making it economically unattractive. Medicaid rules are often more stringent and have significantly lower payment rates, which is why many physicians choose not to participate in the Medicaid program. Some physicians choose not to participate in Medicare to avoid the payment limits imposed by the RBRVS system, but since 20 percent of all physician bills are paid for by Medicare, this is difficult to do unless their practice is mostly obstetrics, sports medicine, or another specialty in which they treat few elderly clients.

Physician Payment in Managed Care Plans

As insurance companies have tried to control their costs by exercising market power, the passive payment of bills has given way to a system of **negotiated fees**. For some common and easily specified services purchased in large volume (intra-ocular lens implants, psychiatric evaluations for drug abuse), the insurance company can often obtain a low fixed price set in advance in return for guaranteeing the physician a certain number of patients or procedures. When individual fees are not negotiated, it is common for managed care contracts to specify **discounted fees**, offering perhaps 75 percent of what the physician would ordinarily bill other patients. The complexities of per unit service pricing are bypassed completely under **capitation**, a fixed payment per person per month regardless of the number of services used (see Chapter 5). A **health maintenance organization (HMO)** using a capitation rate of $100 per month pays that amount to the physician for each of the HMO members enrolled with that physician whether the member visits the doctor's office once, twice, ten times, or not at all. **Independent practice association (IPA) HMOs** that contract with many physicians use capitation rates to pay physicians, but a staff HMO hires physicians to work exclusively in the HMO's facility and pays physicians a **salary**, with perhaps some bonus based on productivity or on the profitability of the HMO. With this arrangement, the physician, in effect, becomes an employee of a large medical care firm (even though legally the physician may still be considered an independent practitioner because of laws in many states prohibiting the corporate practice of medicine). Salaried physicians are also found in hospitals providing emergency room and inpatient care, in administrative posts, and in research and teaching organizations. About 40 percent of physicians are now salaried employees, and the number continues to grow as health care organizations become larger and more complex. Chapter 5 presents a more extensive discussion of managed care contracting.

Incentives: Why Differences in the Type of Payment Matter

How physicians are paid determines the incentives they face to work harder, raise prices, or admit patients to the hospital. Under fee-for-service insurance, a physician gets paid more for doing more. Under HMO capitation, the payment is the same regardless of the number of services provided; therefore, a physician may do less. Under a relative value scale, payment is based on the number of points; therefore, physicians may push to classify the service in a higher point category (the ensuing gradual rise in total points while the number of services provided remains constant is known as "code creep"). In an intriguing experiment, half the doctors in a pediatric clinic were randomly selected to be paid on a fee-for-service basis and half were selected to be paid a salary.[5] The fees were set so that the average doctor seeing the average number of patients would earn the same on either a fee-for-service or salary basis. In practice, the fee-for-service doctors saw more patients, recalled them for more visits, and generally exceeded the normal guidelines for the amount of services, whereas the doctors who were on salary saw fewer patients, had them return less frequently, and were in less conformity with standard guidelines. This randomized control trial demonstrates that economic predictions regarding the incentive effects of different types of payment are borne out in a practice setting.

Payment type may affect patients' access to physician care as well. The Medicaid program has come under severe budgetary constraints and thus tends to pay physicians less well than Blue Shield, HMOs, and commercial insurance. Although physicians are constrained by ethics and law to provide high-quality care to all who need it, economic theory predicts that government imposition of mandatory price controls leads to shortages. A group of experimenters called 300 physician offices and requested an appointment, identifying their type of insurance as Medicaid.[6] Almost half the physician offices said that they were not accepting new patients, and when the experimenters did get an appointment, the average wait was two weeks. The experimenters then called back, identifying themselves as having commercial insurance, and 78 percent of the doctor's offices gave them an appointment within two days. Physicians try hard to provide adequate care to the poor, but if the payment levels are consistently lower, the level of service will be lower.

A Progression: From Prices to Reimbursement Mechanisms

As the medical care system moved away from individual fee-for-service toward third-party insurance, the financial linkage between patients and physicians was attenuated and finally severed. Although there may be some "price" attached to each service under Medicare RBRVS, the price bears almost no resemblance to what that would mean in a normal market: the patient does not pay the price, nor does the price allow the supplier to match output to demand, because it is imposed externally by the government. In such an environment, equilibrating varied interests through individual decisions based on price is replaced by a collective political market. Who is paid and how much is determined in part by concerns about how the elderly will vote in the next presidential election, the effectiveness of insurance lobbies, or a need to find the least difficult way of balancing the budget. Tracking the flow of funds to and from physicians is further obscured by referring to all payments as *reimbursement*, even though insurance companies do not "reimburse" physician costs (physician time is the bulk of the expense) and payments are more accurately termed physician *fees* or *revenues* or *salary*.

6.2   PHYSICIAN INCOMES

Physicians are among the most highly trained and well-compensated workers in the United States. The median physician income is about $225,000 in 2010, five times the average worker's salary. Physician earnings grew more rapidly than average workers' earnings for most of the twentieth century. During the period 1982 to 2004, when average workers' earnings were almost flat (up only 3 percent in 22 years after adjustment for inflation), real physician earnings rose more than 25 percent. To a large extent, these high earnings were attributable to the quality of those who entered the profession (almost all were in the top quarter of their college graduating classes), the long years of post-college training required, the extra effort (most physicians worked about 50 percent more hours than the average salaried worker), and compensation for having to act as entrepreneurs and manage a medical business (self-employed physicians earned 50 percent more than those who chose to work on salary). However, even after adjusting for all these factors, there is still a premium obtained for becoming a physician. Perhaps even more important than higher incomes is the implied "floor"; physicians virtually never face unemployment, and many are able to accept "low-paid" positions (i.e., those that pay less than $100,000 per year) to follow their own interests in helping the poor, working with children, traveling to exotic locations, or studying interesting diseases.

Even during training in residency programs, physicians earn about $42,000 a year, which is about the same as the average worker, although certainly less than the opportunity cost of their time (see discussion of the costs of time and returns in Chapter 12). As with most workers, physicians' earnings grow rapidly early in their careers, rise to a peak around age 50, and decline thereafter (see Table 6.3).

There is a marked difference in earnings by specialty. Pediatricians and family practitioners are at the low end, with psychiatrists only slightly above. The high end is made up of the surgeons, cardiologists, and radiologists. Although numerous factors are involved, much of the difference in incomes among specialties is attributable to the reimbursement system: physicians get paid more for doing something (e.g., reading an X-ray, performing an operation) than for caring or thinking (e.g., listening to a patient's history, deciding which path of treatment to follow, helping the family of a dying person). The reimbursement system is driven by the "billable event." Although a colleague or a manager might be able to assess all the work a physician does on behalf of patients, the financial system is not able to do so. A physician always finds it easier to get paid for a procedure, since it is observable and has a standard billing code, than for a personal interaction or conceptual effort.

A desire to rebalance incomes across specialties and provide more payment for thinking and caring was a goal of the Medicare RBRVS system, but it was not very successful at doing so. Health insurance is designed to protect individuals against potentially large but infrequent losses while minimizing moral hazard from excess purchase of discretionary services. Although correct from a risk management perspective, in practice this means that fees for some specialties are almost fully covered (e.g., surgery, anesthesia), leading to increased demand and higher incomes, whereas other specialties are subject to copayments and deductibles that limit demand and incomes (e.g., pediatrics, psychiatry). The bottom line for the physician is that the income potential from choosing a particular specialty has more to do with how the services of that specialty are treated by insurance than with the work or training involved.

TABLE 6.3	Physician Characteristics and Incomes	
941,304	total number of U.S. physicians	
732,234	active in patient care	
98,688	residents in training programs	
243,457	International Medical Graduates	

Median Income		
$225,000	All Physicians	100%
175,000	Pediatrics	8%
182,500	General/family practice	10%
190,000	Internal medicine	17%
196,000	Psychiatry	5%
252,000	Emergency medicine	3%
264,000	Obstetrics/gynecology	5%
309,000	General surgery	4%
335,000	Dermatology	1%
361,000	Anesthesiology	4%
370,000	Plastic surgery	1%
393,000	Cardiology	2%
440,000	Orthopedic surgery	3%
444,000	Radiology	4%
193,000	Employee or contractor	42%
194,000	Self-employed solo	25%
300,000	Self-employed group	33%
250,000	2 physician partners	
272,000	3 physician group	
275,000	4 physician group	
312,000	5–25 physician group	
300,000	25+ physician group	
174,000	Under 35 years	15%
216,000	35–44	23%
248,000	45–54	24%
225,000	55–64	18%
187,000	65 or older	20%

Sources: AMA Physician Characteristics and Distribution in the U.S., 2009;
AMA Physician Socioeconomic Statistics, 2000–2002 and earlier years;
Medical Economics, compensation survey, 2008.

6.3 PHYSICIAN FINANCING: EXPENSES

Physician Practice Expenses

The expenses of maintaining a practice take up about half of all the funds flowing into physician offices. Physicians must pay for other medical professionals and assistants who help them take care of patients, as well as taxes, rent, utilities, supplies, malpractice insurance, and so on, as shown in Table 6.4. In addition to all these ongoing expenses, it usually takes at least $100,000 in start-up capital to equip even the most basic office, and an elaborate suite housing an active practice in specialties such as plastic surgery could cost several million dollars. One reason for physicians to work together in group practices is to obtain economies of scale from sharing office space, equipment, and information systems. Only a large group can afford to have assistants who specialize in support functions, such as laboratory technicians, billing and appointment clerks, physical therapists, and so on. Yet closer examination of the data reveals an apparently anomalous finding: even though it

TABLE 6.4		Physicians' Office Practice Income and Expenses		
$440,000	100%	Gross revenues		
			Private insurance	53%
			Medicare	24%
			Medicaid	12%
			Patients paid	11%
$225,000	51%	Net income		
$ 74,800	17%	Non-physician employee wages (4 FTE per physician)		
$ 13,200	3%	Employee physicians		
$ 52,800	12%	Office rent and expenses		
$ 17,600	4%	Medical supplies		
$ 22,000	5%	Malpractice liability insurance		
$ 8,800	2%	Equipment		
$ 25,800	6%	Other expenses		

Worked an average of 57 hours per week, seeing 105 patients, and giving 4 hours of charity/uncompensated care. The average charge for a patient visit was about $100 in 2006.

Source: AMA Physician Socioeconomic Statistics, 2000–2002, *Medical Economics* survey, 2006.

seems that a large group practice would use ancillary help and equipment more efficiently, such expenses take a greater percentage of total revenues for groups than for solo physicians who practice alone. To understand why a more efficient practice uses more, rather than less, nonphysician inputs, it is necessary to consider a basic result from the microeconomic analysis of firm production. To reduce per unit costs, firms must use more of the inputs whose output per dollar is higher and/or use less of the input whose output per dollar is lower (see Section 2.5).[7] At the optimum, the ratio of marginal productivity to input price is the same for all inputs.

$$\frac{\text{Marginal Productivity}_{\text{input A}}}{\text{Price}_{\text{input A}}} = \frac{\text{Marginal Productivity}_{\text{input B}}}{\text{Price}_{\text{input B}}} = \ldots$$

$$= \frac{\text{Marginal Productivity}_{\text{input Z}}}{\text{Price}_{\text{input Z}}}$$

Larger and more organized physician groups are able to make better use of nonphysician inputs, raising their marginal productivity. Therefore, groups use more of these inputs relative to physician time. Efficiency is not defined as having the lowest amount of overhead, or even the highest number of patient visits per physician hour, but rather the lowest cost (physician and nonphysician) per visit. This raises the following question: What "price" should be applied to physician time?

The Labor–Leisure Choice

A physician-entrepreneur has an income of revenues less expenses, which is called profit by the Internal Revenue Service (IRS). Most of the income is not economic profit but compensation for all the hours of work put in. How should this time be valued? What is its opportunity cost? For a young physician starting out with relatively few patients, it is common to take on a temporary part-time moonlighting job in a hospital emergency room or in a well-established senior practice with many patients for wages of $75 to $150 per hour. Since doctors give up those jobs as their practices become established, their time must be worth more than that, but what forgone opportunity defines this higher hourly rate? What a busy physician gives up is leisure: time to be with family, time to run and swim and watch television, and even time to sleep. The more lucrative each hour of practice and the more hours the physician puts in, the more each hour of forgone leisure is worth. Most doctors work very hard, averaging more than 50 hours per week. Furthermore, once they make $150,000 or $250,000 per year, a little time off may well be worth more to them than earning an extra $5,000 by working late. This is one reason the supply of physician time is not very elastic; even doubling or quadrupling physicians' income could not get them to double the number of hours worked. Indeed, it is even possible that for some physicians, supply is "backward bending"—higher income per hour may make them feel sufficiently rich that they work fewer rather than more hours.[8] If backward-bending supply seems difficult to understand, think about how much you would work if I paid you $100 per hour, $1,000 per hour, or $100,000 per hour. Eventually you would decide to work less and enjoy leisure more because additional money simply would not mean that much to you. One difficulty physicians have in making the labor–leisure choice is that their income often depends on putting in many hours per week early in their careers, when the rate of pay is low or even zero. This is similar to the problem facing most college students: getting into the best business or law school and making partner depends on excess hours put in now to obtain future income. To fully analyze the trade-off between labor and leisure, it is necessary to recognize that some work is done more for its value as investment in future earnings than for current earnings.

The Doctor's Workshop and Unpaid Hospital Inputs

Almost every doctor needs to use a hospital to provide patient care. Some specialties (anesthesiology, thoracic surgery, pathology) are practiced almost entirely inside hospitals. Yet physicians do not pay the hospital for the privilege of working there and usually are not employees of the hospital. In terms of an influential model proposed by Mark Pauly and Michael Redisch, the hospital functions as the "doctor's workshop" and is a source of unpaid inputs in production.[9] Since the efforts of hospital nurses, laboratory technicians, and record keeping professionals do not "cost" the physician anything, physicians tend to overuse them to supplant the use of similar inputs in their offices. It is easy to see how they might favor a system of nonprofit hospitals supported by the community and government subsidy because the value added to their practices by these hospitals far exceeds the hours physicians are expected to "give" to hospital educational and administrative functions.

The hospital-based specialties of radiology and pathology are a special case, with high incomes that clearly depend on hospital practice. Since physicians in these specialties spend virtually all their professional time within the hospital, have a regular flow of work, and do not meet individually with patients, it appears that they might most readily be paid on salary. Yet historically, radiologists have strongly opposed salaried practice, favoring fee-for-service arrangements, contracts in which they operate the diagnostic facility for a percentage of gross or pay rent to the hospital. Their opposition was sufficient to force Medicare to separate the professional fee for reviewing X-rays and specimens from the hospital charges for producing them. The primary issue is control—over professional activity and over money. If the pathologist runs the lab, he or she in effect "owns" the captive block of business constituted by the hospital's patients. However, if the hospital runs the lab, pathologists must compete on the basis of price (i.e., take a lower salary) and accept hospital direction over their working conditions. Consider the case of a 60-year-old pathologist who has been head of the lab for 20 years and is friendly with most of the surgeons on staff. If it is his lab, he can bring in a junior pathologist to do the day-to-day work and go into semi-retirement to play golf with the hospital administrator and his surgeon friends, living off the "rents" he collects as an owner of the practice. If it is the hospital's lab and he is on salary, the hospital can threaten to fire him and hire the junior pathologist to save money, unless the senior pathologist is willing to accept a pay cut and work harder. The issue of who "owns" the patient's business and can collect the additional income (rents) arising from control over volume and referrals arises repeatedly in our examination of the organization of medicine and is central to managed care (see Chapters 5 and 12).

Malpractice

One of the most contentious physician practice expenses is malpractice insurance. The rationale for allowing medical malpractice suits is that they improve incentives for safety by forcing doctors to behave more carefully when treating patients. Malpractice is not a good way of compensating patients for harm done to them, since it costs $1.20 in legal fees for every $1 a patient receives.[10] About one in twenty physicians will incur a malpractice claim in any given year, and two in five will be sued at least once during their careers. The premium for a physician's malpractice insurance averages about $22,000 (5 percent of gross revenues), but ranges from just $5,000 or less for family practitioners to $100,000 and more for orthopedic and neurosurgeons. Although malpractice premiums have risen rapidly in some years, virtually all the additional costs are quickly passed on to patients and their insurance companies in the form of higher fees, and one recent study showed that after adjustment for inflation over the last 30 years, premiums were actually level or lower in a majority of specialties.

Malpractice is a real problem, but the current malpractice system may not be the best solution. Studies have shown that a negligent iatrogenic injury (i.e., caused by the physician) occurs approximately once in every 100 hospital admissions. Only a tenth of those injured will file a claim, and less than half will gain compensation through the courts. At the same time, there will be a larger number of suits filed when there was no negligence, and some of these patients will win despite the lack of any physician error. The randomness of the legal process, as well as the fact that most physicians are almost fully insured for losses due to malpractice, limits the effectiveness of the system to change behavior. However, being sued is costly in terms of lost time and increased anxiety, and most physicians exercise extraordinary care in treating patients. After all, they became physicians because they wanted to care for patients, not because they wanted a job that was easy. Although some physicians have claimed that the fear of being sued has raised medical costs by forcing them to practice "defensive medicine," some studies have shown that higher levels of liability or a greater number of suits do not necessarily lead to much higher numbers of tests per patient, more admissions, or more prescriptions.[11] Since most suits are filed for a procedure that a doctor has done, rather than for something not done or for a diagnosis that was missed, the lack of excessive testing or other medical treatment attributable to malpractice is not surprising.

Does the malpractice system deter negligence by physicians? Only to a limited extent, and at considerable cost. Yet while the ability of malpractice suits to compensate patients for damages or to force doctors to practice better medicine has been roundly criticized with good reason, it has not been easy to find a solution that is clearly more efficient or acceptable to both doctors and patients.

6.4 THE TRANSACTION BETWEEN DOCTOR AND PATIENT

The bond of trust between doctor and patient is one of the strongest professional relationships in society. When patients show up at a doctor's office, they are apt to ask two questions: "What is wrong with me?" and "What should I do about it?" If told that they have a disease, most patients trust the doctor to perform the right diagnostic and therapeutic procedures, with little idea of what those might be or what the charges will add up to.[12] If a surgeon is called in, he or she is likely to be a complete stranger who asks for thousands of dollars to make an evaluation and incision. Patients who agree to surgery can only hope that in the long run it will do some good, since postoperative pain and mortality will make them worse off in the short run. Unlike a person shopping for a car, a suit, or a haircut, patients do not know what they need, what it should cost, and even, once paid for, how much good the treatment actually did. Instead of a clear specification of what is to be expected from both parties, the patient must trust the doctor to do what is right and to bill fairly for the necessary care (which will mostly be paid for by insurance).

Asymmetric Information

It is the superior ability of the physician to answer those two questions that tends to make the doctor–patient relationship so much different from an ordinary commercial transaction. Although the physician's information is not perfect, it is much better than that of the patient, and the physician is able to seek additional information required for treating an illness at much lower cost. This disparity is known as **information asymmetry**. When it is necessary to decide which test to perform, which drug to prescribe, and whether to perform surgery, all these choices can be made better and at lower cost by a physician. An exchange relationship in which one party makes choices on behalf of the other is known as **agency**.[13] Just as a purchasing agent buys supplies for a company and an actor's agent represents the actor in negotiations, a physician is the patient's agent in deciding which treatment is appropriate and which medical services to buy. The reason that agents act on behalf of another is that the agent's information and transaction costs are lower. It is cheaper for a physician to make medical choices on behalf of a patient than for the patient to go to medical school to make a decision.

Agency: Whose Choices?

When ordering food or renting a movie, personal tastes and preferences determine the best choice. Markets excel at matching myriads of consumers with thousands of products. Complex tradeoffs between price, quality, and individual desires are made with little difficulty or cost. Medicine is different. The best choice of treatment depends upon illness, not tastes and preferences. Value for money is achieved in the markets for food and movies by allowing consumers to choose among the many alternatives available in the marketplace. In medicine, most choices must be made by the doctor. The patient often would not even know what illness they have, much less the pros and cons of each treatment option, without expert advice. The patient cannot choose his or her own medicine, but must have a prescription written by the doctor. The choice among specialists and diagnostic facilities is called a referral because it is made by the doctor, not the patient.

Although many goods and services are transacted under conditions of less-than-perfect information, it is the magnitude of the disparity that sets medical care apart. For example, although I may not know what my mechanic is doing, I can readily observe whether my automobile is working better when it comes back from the shop. Poor-quality parts can be repaired or replaced. At most, I might ask for my money back. Bad surgery is not only difficult to detect, it also can be disabling or even fatal. Once you are dead, repairs, replacements, and even outrageously large malpractice settlements are irrelevant. To an extraordinary degree, the demand-side choices normally made by consumers are delegated to providers in medical markets.

6.5 UNCERTAINTY

In what is perhaps the most well-known and often-cited paper on health economics, Nobel laureate Kenneth Arrow stated: "The special economic problems of medical care can be explained as adaptations to the existence of uncertainty in the incidence of disease and in the efficacy of treatment."[14]

As discussed in Chapter 4, uncertainty "in the incidence of disease" refers to the random occurrence of illness—one never knows when one will get sick or how bad the illness will be. The problem of randomly occurring losses can be offset to some extent by pooling risks through insurance. The losses still occur and must be paid for, but the financial uncertainty is removed.

Uncertainty "in the efficacy of treatment" refers to the inability to know whether the chosen treatment will work. In theory, it might be possible to "insure" against such losses, but in the real world there are no meaningful guarantees for medical care. A cardiologist treating you for a heart attack does not guarantee that you will be able to run marathons again, nor does an oncologist guarantee that she can cure your cancer. The most either will promise is to provide you with everything modern medicine has to offer. Why can't they give a guarantee? First of all, because it is so difficult to tell how ill you were in the first place, it is often impossible to tell whether treatment has improved your health. Second, unlike a car or a house, there is no way to replace your body. Although almost any ordinary loss can be fixed with sufficient compensation, a monetary guarantee is an empty promise if you are dead.[15]

The distinction between the two types of uncertainty and the economic response to them is shown in Figure 6.1. Note that in each case, there is a transfer of responsibility away from the patient. Under insurance, the responsibility for payment is transferred to the insurance company, relieving all actual and potential patients of the uncertainty of financial losses due to illness. Under agency, the responsibility for making a decision on appropriate care is transferred from the patient to the physician. Agency creates gains because it substitutes professional control for costly patient monitoring of quality. It is much cheaper for an experienced and highly educated physician to determine which treatment is best than for a patient to try to do so.

6.6 LICENSURE: QUALITY OR PROFITS?

Licensure is a collective extension of the doctor–patient relationship of agency. Not only do individual patients trust their physicians to act as their personal agents, all of us together have collectively chosen to let the medical profession act as our public agent, deciding

FIGURE 6.1 Uncertainty in Medical Care

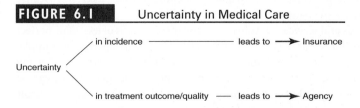

Uncertainty in the incidence of illness can be ameliorated by the use of insurance. Uncertainty in the outcome and quality of treatment can be ameliorated by exchange using an agency relationship; licensure and trust in physicians, nonprofit ownership, and government regulation.

who is qualified to practice medicine. Through the institution of **licensure**, the medical profession serves as a sort of quasi-governmental body making decisions of behalf of all consumers.[16] Consumers do not examine each doctor's credentials and legal records; they turn that responsibility over to licensure boards. It is cheaper for knowledgeable professionals to do this once for all consumers rather than having each patient individually try to determine whether the person listed as a "doctor" in the phone book is qualified to practice medicine. The government does not make laws regarding the practice of medicine, but uses laws to enforce the decisions made by voluntary and independent professional boards.

It is often debated in the media and among economists whether licensure serves the interests of patients (by improving the quality of care) or of physicians (by raising prices and incomes).[17] Such a debate, framed in terms of one side or the other, misses the point: any public policy in a democracy is in fact a form of trade that must serve the interests of both parties if the policy is to be upheld. By the fundamental theorem of exchange, both physicians and patients must be made better off by licensure.

How Does Licensure Increase Physician Profits?

Licensure radically changes the market structure. A flexible supply curve is replaced by a fixed supply—diagrammatically a vertical line, since quantity does not change as prices rise or fall (see Figure 6.2). To the extent that the supply of doctor services is reduced under licensure, prices are higher so that all doctors enjoy higher incomes (of course, this means that some people who wished to become doctors are not allowed to do so). These profits are maximized if the profession acts as a monopoly in determining how many doctors are allowed to practice. Supply can also be reduced by work rules that control total productivity. For example, it is common for dental practice regulations to determine how many assistants each dentist can supervise (and therefore the number of total patients who can be seen). Extending the physician's training period also serves to reduce the effective doctor supply, since each graduate has fewer remaining years of productivity.

Thinking of the demand for physician services as derived demand suggests two further possibilities for raising income: (1) increasing the price of substitutes such as chiropractors and nurses and (2) increasing demand for output. The effective price of many physician substitutes can be made prohibitively large by forbidding them to perform some acts (prescribing drugs, performing surgery, admitting a patient to the hospital). Less extreme, but also effective, are rules that limit health insurance to reimbursement for services performed

FIGURE 6.2   Demand and Supply with Licensure

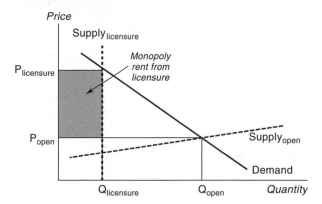

by or under the supervision of a physician. Even if a substitute provider is willing to provide services at a much lower price, it will still cost patients more because they will have to pay the entire bill out of pocket. Insurance has been the most important factor in increasing the overall demand for medical care. Physicians have played a major role in the spread of insurance and the creation of payment system rules (e.g., UCR fees, separate professional fees for radiologists and pathologists), which increase physicians' economic power. Hospital-based specialists such as radiologists and pathologists have fought the implementation of RBRVS and bulk-purchase managed care contracts that tend to give more control to payers and increase price competition among suppliers. Professional activities also directly increase demand both through new medical discoveries and by monitoring and controlling quality so that patients are more willing to visit any licensed practitioner.

Supply and Demand Response in Licensed versus Unlicensed Professions

To illustrate the differences in market dynamics between licensed and unlicensed labor supply, physicians are compared with health administrators in Figure 6.3. Health administrators often earn a master of health administration (M.H.A.) degree early in their careers, but many rise through the ranks without attending graduate school and others obtain master of business administration (M.B.A.) or master of science (M.S.) degrees in schools of business, medicine, public health, public policy, or human services.[18] The crucial point is that there is no central control over the number of people who can enter the profession, no licensure or specific educational requirement, and no legal restriction on practice by outsiders. Administrators usually start at modest salaries ranging from $40,000 to $80,000, like most people with an M.B.A. degree, and work their way up the organizational ranks. Although some administrators eventually earn large salaries, many tend to get stuck in the middle ranges and some are pushed out of the field entirely. Thus, administrator earnings are related to individual characteristics and experience and hence are rather variable. Physician earnings are in part monopoly "rents," increased profits shared by the profession as a whole, and

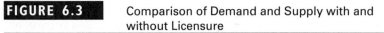

FIGURE 6.3   Comparison of Demand and Supply with and without Licensure

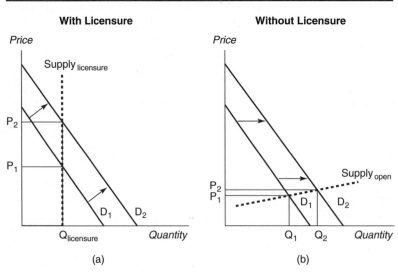

thus are not only higher but also more stable. Although both physicians and administrators see their earnings increase as they gain more experience, for physicians, the growth is more regular and virtually never interrupted by unemployment.

The comparative effects of an increase in demand are shown in Figure 6.3. For physicians, who are licensed, virtually all the increase in demand goes into higher incomes because there is no flexibility for supply to increase. For unlicensed administrators, higher wages attract more and better entrants so that part of the increase in demand goes into an increase in the quantity of labor supplied and only partly into an increase in incomes. Although increased demand leads to more applicants to medical schools, no new medical schools will be built because these numbers are controlled by the AMA, American Association of Medical Colleges (AAMC), and affiliated professional bodies. In contrast, increasing demand for health administrators has caused graduate programs to spring up around the country as universities compete to attract students.

How Does Licensure Improve Quality?

It is possible to improve quality by revoking the licenses of physicians whose medical practices are shown to be inferior, but such removals are rare.[19] The quality of physicians in practice depends much more on the initial selection of who is allowed to enter the profession, the training they receive, and efforts by practicing physicians to monitor one another and impose informal sanctions (ostracism from professional groups, denial of hospital privileges, refusal to refer new patients or share business opportunities).[20] *The ability of sanctions and selection to improve quality would be greatly reduced if there were no monopoly profits.* Because licensure restrictions guarantee successful applicants a career with high income and prestige, many outstanding students seek admission to medical school. After becoming doctors, they work very hard not to lose that title. The money and power that come with being a physician, a form of monopoly profits, are too attractive to give up. If a doctor could earn more money and satisfaction working in a bank, an insurance company, or another career, why worry about losing a medical license? The opportunity cost of losing a license is so significant that the threat of losing a license is enough to make it rarely necessary for the profession to actually revoke a license and terminate a physician's right to practice.

The value of a license depends on the prestige of the medical profession as a whole; therefore, each doctor has an incentive to maintain the professional franchise by selecting only the best candidates to enter the profession and by continuing to make sure that all doctors are as good as they can be at caring for patients so that demand remains high.[21] Choosing only the best candidates for admission to medical school means that the graduates will be superior regardless of how much they learn during medical school. Prestige and income play a large part in attracting outstanding students. The incentive for a student to train long and hard is also related to the expectation of high income in the future. After graduation, the threat of losing these extraordinary returns provides an incentive to maintain competency and support licensing boards. The existence of monopoly profits serves as a monetary performance bond that can be lost, a kind of collective collateral put up by the profession to ensure good service on the part of all its members.

Observing that some specific restrictions on medical practice have no direct bearing on quality has led some economists to question whether licensure boards are committed to protecting the public interest or the private economic interests of their members. Application of the fundamental theorem of exchange indicates that there is no conflict between the two objectives and that they may reinforce each other. A particular restriction on medical practice may not directly improve quality, but removing it could cause quality to deteriorate by reducing the monopoly profits that provide incentives for the profession to police itself.

A better test of whether licensure improves quality is to look at how the strength of licensure restrictions varies by type of medical practice—where and when the "licensure contract" is most apt to be approved by both patients and physicians.

A Test of the Quality Hypothesis: Strong versus Weak Licensure

The timing of licensure legislation suggests that until the level of a doctor's training can significantly affect quality and the probable outcome of treatment, effective professional licensure is unlikely to occur or will be very weakly enforced. Before 1900, licensure was clearly desired by physicians to improve their economic status, as demonstrated by their vociferous support of such laws in state legislatures. Yet licensure laws could not get popular political support until medical science advanced to the point at which knowledge made a real difference.[22] The strength of licensure was related not only to the increased effectiveness of new treatments, but also to the increased danger posed by the use of surgery and powerful drugs.

Some types of medical care, such as cardiac surgery, are inherently dangerous and demand great skill. Bad heart surgeons may have a mortality rate five times higher than good heart surgeons.[23] Given the great impact of measurable physician-quality indicators (training, medical practice records, opinions of peers), we would expect licensure restrictions to be very strong for heart surgery (see Table 6.5). That is indeed the case. Although legally one need only be licensed as a physician in order to perform heart surgery, in practice doctors are virtually prohibited from doing so unless they have completed a residency, completed a fellowship in the specialty, and been given special hospital privileges after a review by peers who have observed them acting as assistants on a number of operations. These additional mandatory checks make it evident that heart surgery has strong licensure restrictions. Conversely, there are other types of medical care that are much less dangerous and demanding, such as surgery to remove corns from the foot. Although such surgery can be practiced with greater or lesser skill, it is not likely to cost a life. One does not need a residency or hospital medical staff review to remove corns, and indeed corns are often removed by podiatrists, who are not licensed doctors of medicine (M.D.s), although they are usually licensed doctors of podiatric medicine (D.P.M.s). The lack of special medical staff restrictions and the existence of alternative professional certification show that care of the foot has weak licensure. Refractions to prescribe eyeglasses are similarly performed by competing professions (M.D. opthalmologists and O.D. optometrists) under weak licensure. Mental health is a specialty with a wide array of professionals—psychiatrists (M.D.s), psychologists (Psy.D. doctors of psychology or Ph.D. doctors of philosophy), family therapists and counselors (C.A.C., M.S.W., A.A.M.F.T., and other designations), and even psychics (palm readers, speakers for past lives, aura visionaries)—and such weak licensure that virtually anyone can offer to help you with your problems. There are substantial risks to life in mental illness, and more people die from substance abuse and depression than from many other conditions, but the professional does not always have substantial advantage over the client in choosing

TABLE 6.5	Weak versus Strong Licensure
Weak ⟵────── **Licensure** ──────⟶	**Strong**
Consumers can choose	Only trained professionals choose well
Low risk	High risk
Uncertainty small	Information asymmetry high
Examples: podiatry, eyeglasses	*Examples: neurosurgery, organ transplants*

therapies and therapists, because personality match is so important. It is hard to gain insight from a psychologist you despise, or who despises you, but a cardiac surgeon can be totally lacking in human interpersonal skills and still perform a good operation.

As the extent and value of the information asymmetry between patients and professionals increases, licensure becomes stronger. For heart surgery, technical quality is paramount and well evaluated by professional standards. Medical licensure is supplemented by hospital privilege reviews, insurance restrictions, and other forceful measures. However, for types of care in which the information differential is small, licensure is weak. For a broken heart, an M.D. psychiatrist may be no more effective than a sympathetic psychic whom the patient trusts and, for counseling, there are multiple forms of licensure, all rather weakly enforced.

SUGGESTIONS FOR FURTHER READING

American Medical Association, *Socioeconomic Characteristics of Medical Practice*, published annually until 2004 (www.ama-assn.org).

Kenneth Arrow, "Uncertainty and the Welfare Economics of Medical Care," *American Economic Review* 53, no.3 (1963): 941–973.

Atul Gawande, *Complications: A Surgeon's Notes on an Imperfect Science* (New York: Holt & Co., 2002).

Paul L. Grimaldi, "Medicare's Physician Fees Are Resource Based," *Journal of Health Care Finance*, (Spring 2002): 88–104.

Institute of Medicine, *To Err Is Human*, (National Academy Press, April 2000), (www.nap.edu/books/0309068371/html); and *Crossing the Quality Chasm* (July 2001), (www.nap.edu/books/0309072808 html).

George D. Lundberg, *Severed Trust: Why American Medicine Hasn't Been Fixed* (New York: Basic Books, 2001).

Michael Millenson, *Demanding Medical Excellence: Doctors and Accountability in the Information Age* (Chicago: University of Chicago Press, 2000).

SUMMARY

1. **The relationship between doctor and patient stands at the center of the medical care system**. Although payments to physicians constitute only 21 percent of total health care expenditures, the special characteristics of this exchange influence the organization and financing of all other parts of the system.

2. Over time, physician payment has changed from fee-for-service prices similar to prices of most other economic goods and services to complex reimbursement plans based on administrative formulas and negotiation. Increasingly, physicians are involved with managed care plans that pay a **capitation** rate (physicians receive a certain amount per member per month) or **discounted fee schedules** based on **relative value scales**.

3. Most physicians are owners or partners in small businesses rather than employees. They work long hours but do not face much business risk. On average, **self-employed physicians earn** about $251,000, while those who work as employees and are somewhat younger earn $190,000. Physicians who practiced in cognitive and caring specialties (family practice, psychiatry, pediatrics, internal medicine) earned less than those who practiced in procedure-oriented specialties (surgery, obstetrics/gynecology, radiology).

4. The average office medical practice hired **four allied health workers per physician** and had overall expenses equal to 51 percent of gross patient revenues. Although malpractice insurance is the expense category most frequently complained about, **malpractice takes only 3 to 7 percent of gross** revenues for most physician practices.

5. **Uncertainty** creates or exacerbates most of the information problems in medical care. Whereas financial uncertainty due to the random occurrence of illness can be reduced by insurance, uncertainty about the quality of care and outcome of treatment cannot; thus, collective agency mechanisms such as licensure and strong ethical traditions for physicians have been established.

6. **Information asymmetry** arises from the difference between the physician's and the patient's knowledge of medical treatments. Because of this disparity in the cost of knowledge, patients must trust physicians to act as their agents and make decisions on their behalf. In most economic exchanges, the point at which goods and services are transacted is the point at which information cost differentials are lowest. Since a low-cost valuation of well-defined goods is not possible in medicine, a trust relationship of agency has been established to ameliorate this potential market failure.

7. **Licensure** is a collective extension of the doctor–patient relationship of agency. It helps solve the problems caused by uncertainty and information asymmetry. **Licensure increases profits by restricting supply**, thus changing the traditional supply and demand curve analysis. The supply curve is fixed, or vertical, and increases in demand do not result in an increase in quantity but in increased profits for suppliers known by economists as "rents." Licensure **increases quality by** (a) ensuring that only the best students are selected to enter medical school; (b) mandating that students have three years of medical school, four years of residency, and periodical refresher courses thereafter; and (c) having physicians monitor each other. All these depend on having some excess profits or monopoly rents to serve as an incentive. Licensure is intended both to increase profits and to increase quality. Like any law, it **must satisfy both parties** (physicians and the public/patients) to be a self-enforcing political exchange. The importance of quality concerns is evidenced by comparing the types of care for which licensure is strong (cardiac surgery, chemotherapy) with those for which it is weak (removing corns, prescribing eyeglasses, counseling).

PROBLEMS

1. {*incentives*} Which type of payment gives a physician the most incentive to do the following:

    a. Spend more time with each patient? Spend less?
    b. Provide more laboratory services to each patient? Provide less?
    c. Modify the listing of diagnoses to increase revenues? Be objective?
    d. Reduce hospital utilization? Increase hospital utilization?
    e. Ask patients to return frequently? Try to handle problems once and for all?

2. {*compensation*} Do you believe that radiologists prefer to be compensated in a fee-for-service manner, by relative value scale, on salary, or as part of a capitated rate? Why? Why might practitioners of different specialties prefer different forms of payment?

3. {*organization*} Which organization provides the largest amount of payment to physicians in the United States? How does this organization choose to make these payments? Has the form of payment changed over time? Why?

4. {*earnings differentials*} What are some of the reasons that most pediatricians earn less than most neurosurgeons?

5. {*age earnings profile*} Generally, most physicians' incomes increase as they get older. Is the rate of earnings increase greater for some specialties than others? Why? Do you expect that male and female physicians have the same age-earnings profile? Why or why not?

6. {*earnings differentials*} Would you expect that physicians who earn significantly more than their peers have office practice costs that are above or below average? Are they more or less likely to hire other physicians?

7. {*valuation*} How are the values determined in setting up a relative value scale?

8. {*malpractice*} What are the objectives of the current medical malpractice system in the United States? How well does it work in achieving these objectives?

9. {*uncertainty*} If uncertainty regarding the occurrence of losses can be dealt with through insurance markets, why can't uncertainty regarding the outcome or quality of medical care be similarly priced and transferred?

10. {*agency*} What is an agent? How does employing an agent reduce the costs of making a transaction? Does employing an agent create any problems that would not occur if the consumer acted alone?

11. {*licensure*} Does licensure raise the quality of medical care, or does it raise the profitability of medical practice?

12. {*information asymmetry*} How do agency and information asymmetry lead to licensure? Are there more or less gains from trade as the degree of information asymmetry increases?

13. {*information asymmetry*} What does it mean to say that licensure is weak or strong? Why does the strength of licensure vary?

ENDNOTES

1. Atul Gawande, "Piecework: Medicine's Money Problem," *The New Yorker*, April 4, 2005, pp. 44–53; Eliot Freidson, *Profession of Medicine* (New York: Dodd, Mead, 1970); Victor R. Fuchs, *Who Shall Live? Health, Economics and Social Choice* (New York: Basic Books, 1983).

2. Most of the information here is from surveys done by the American Medical Association and reported in *Socioeconomic Characteristics of Medical Practice*, an annual/biennial monograph. A good sense of the entrepreneurial flavor of medical practice can be obtained by perusing several issues of *Medical Economics*, the "*Business Week*" of physicians.

3. U.S. National Health Accounts (www.cms.gov/statistics/nhe), see discussion and references in Chapter 1.

4. W. C. Hsiao, P. Braun, D. Dunn, and E. R. Becker, "Resource-Based Relative Values: An Overview," *Journal of the American Medical Association* 260, no. 16 (1988): 2347–2353; William C. Hsiao et al., "Results and Impacts of the Resource-Based Relative Value Scale," *Medical Care* 30, no. 11 Supplement (1992): NS61–79.

5. G. B. Hickson, W. A. Altmeier, and J. M. Perris, "Physician Reimbursement by Salary or Fee-For-Service: Effect on Physician Practice Behavior in a Randomized Prospective Study," *Pediatrics* 80 (1987): 344–350; Rose Anne Devlin and Sisira Sarrna, "Do Physician Remuneration Schemes Matter?" *Journal of Health Economics* 27 (2008): 1168–1181.

6. Medicaid Access Study Group, "Access of Medicaid Recipients to Outpatient Care," *New England Journal of Medicine* 330 (May 19, 1994): 1426–1430.

7. Uwe Reinhardt, "A Production Function for Physician Services," *Review of Economics and Statistics* 54, no. 1 (1972): 55–66.

8. Frank A. Sloan, "Physician Supply Behavior in the Short Run," *Industrial and Labor Relations Review* 28 (July 1975): 549–569.

9. Mark V. Pauly and Michael Redisch, "The Not-for-Profit Hospital as a Physician Cooperative," *American Economic Review* 63, no. 1 (1973): 87–99.

10. Patricia Danzon, "Liability for Medical Malpractice," *Journal of Economic Perspectives* 5, no. 3 (1991): 51–69; and A. J. Culyer and J. P. Newhouse, eds., *Handbook of Health Economics* (Amsterdam: Elsevier, 2000),

1339–1404; Marc A. Rodwin, Hak J. Chang, and Jeffrey Claussen, "Malpractice Premiums and Physicians' Income Perceptions of a Crisis Conflict with Empirical Evidence," *Health Affairs* 25, no. 3 (2005): 750–758; Marc A. Rodwin et al., "Malpractice Premiums in Massachusetts, a High-Risk State: 1975–2005," *Health Affairs* 27, no. 3 (2008): 835–844.

11. Peter A. Glassman, John E. Rolph, Laura P. Petersen, Melissa A. Bradley, and Richard L. Kravitz, "Physician's Personal Malpractice Experiences Are Not Related to Defensive Clinical Practices," *Journal of Health Politics, Policy and Law* 21, no. 2 (1996): 219–241.

12. This special economic character of the "trust" relationship with doctors has long been noted, and is discussed in Adam Smith's seminal 1776 treatise, *The Wealth of Nations*.

13. Michael C. Jensen and William H. Meckling, "Agency Costs in the Firm" and "Theory of the Firm: Managerial Behavior, Agency Costs and Ownership Structure," *Journal of Financial Economics* 3 (1976): 305–360. The extensive economic analysis of agency has focused primarily on the manager of a firm who makes decisions on behalf of shareholders. Many of these models are applicable, but since medical outcomes are not as readily measured as the profits of a firm, and since death has even more moral overtones than bankruptcy, the doctor–patient bond has important aspects above and beyond those that characterize the relationships of owner-to-shareholder or supervisor-to-employee. See the books by Gawande and Millenson in Suggestions for Further Reading; and Mark V. Pauly, "Taxation, Health Insurance, and Market Failure in the Medical Economy," *Journal of Economic Literature* 24, no. 2 (1986): 629–675; Robert L. Kane and Matthew Maciejewski, "The Relationship of Patient Satisfaction with Care and Clinical Outcomes," *Medical Care* 35, no. 7 (1997): 714– 730.

14. Kenneth J. Arrow, "Uncertainty and the Welfare Economics of Medical Care," *American Economic Review* 53, no. 3 (1963): 941–973.

15. To give a guarantee means to provide a contract stipulating what you will receive if something goes wrong (replace the item, money back, etc.). What would a "medical guarantee" look like? The broken transmission of a car can be repaired for $700, making money a fully satisfactory replacement. There is no such replacement for health or the pain of disease. Even if we could agree on a monetary amount, it would be different for every illness, different for every person, and different even if it was the same person and illness at a later time of life. There is no way to write a satisfactory contract in advance, hence the need for a substitute form of commercial relationship.

16. Richard Shryock, *Medical Licensing in America, 1650–1965* (Baltimore: Johns Hopkins University Press, 1967).

17. Elton Rayack, *Professional Power and American Medicine: The Economics of the American Medical Association* (Cleveland, Ohio: World Publishing, 1967).

18. U.S. Bureau of Labor Statistics, *Occupational Outlook, BLS Bulletin 2450* (Washington, D.C.: U.S. Government Printing Office, April 1994).

19. Formal licensure actions against physicians are rather infrequent, and usually for misconduct (drug abuse, fraud, sexual advances) rather than poor quality of care, which has led some observers to conclude that the institution of licensure was never intended to improve quality. However, note that revoking of a driver's license is similarly rare. The quality of daily driving is measured by a 15-minute test when a person is first licensed, but not thereafter, and revocation of drivers' licenses reflects a similar pattern of egregious personal flaws rather than the traits associated with quality (vision, eye–hand coordination, etc.)

20. Eliot Freidson, *Professional Dominance: The Social Structure of Medical Care* (New York: Atherton, 1970); *and Professional Powers: A Study in the Institutionalization of Formal Knowledge* (Chicago: University of Chicago Press, 1986).

21. Unfortunately, the desire to maintain the value of physician licensure also provides an incentive to cover up cases of poor quality. Admitting that some licensed physicians were actually bad doctors would reduce demand, and thus diminish the value of all licenses. Therefore, sometimes physicians will act to protect their own by hiding evidence of malpractice or other failures even when they strongly disapprove and could get rid of the offender.

22. John Duffy, *From Humors to Medical Science: A History of American Medicine* (Urbana: University of Illinois Press, 1993).

23. *A Consumer Guide to Coronary Artery Bypass Graft Surgery*, Vol. IV, 1993 Data. PHC4 (Harrisburg, Pa.: Pennsylvania Health Care Cost Containment Council, 1995).

CHAPTER 7

MEDICAL EDUCATION, ORGANIZATION, AND BUSINESS PRACTICES

QUESTIONS

1. Who controls the supply of physicians: the government or the American Medical Association (AMA)?
2. Are doctors more or less productive than they were twenty years ago?
3. Why do patients in Boston undergo more surgeries than patients in San Francisco?
4. Why are there more foreign doctors practicing in the United States than U.S. doctors practicing overseas if the needs are much greater there?
5. Can medical groups advertise to attract more patients and increase market power? Are bigger practices more efficient?
6. Is price discrimination legal? Why are some patients charged more for the same service? Why and how are doctors giving discounts on fees?
7. Do physicians trade patients? Are payments between doctors for referrals legal, ethical, or efficient?
8. Are chiropractors a substitute for physicians, or are they a complement?
9. Who sets the standards of practice to guide clinical decisions?

7.1 MEDICAL EDUCATION

A select and hard-working group of 17,000 students will graduate with doctor of medicine (M.D.) degrees from one of 127 U.S. medical schools this year.[1] For most of them it will be the middle of an arduous process that has taken over most of their lives since high school, and it will forever change the way they view the world and how the world views them. Many first thought about becoming doctors in elementary school, but some decided after pursuing other careers. All had to take premed courses in chemistry, biology, and so on and did rather well on average—almost half of them had an A average as undergraduates (grade point average (GPA) of 3.6 or higher). Getting into medical school was serious business that took substantial effort, and many applied to ten or more schools. Much of the selection, however, was self-selection. Weaker students generally chose not to apply. Less than half of the applicants to medical school were rejected. Of those who were admitted, 98 percent chose to enroll, and of those 95 percent will graduate, almost all of whom will then enter a hospital-based residency training program lasting three years or more before becoming generalist family practitioners or specialists in one of the other 22 recognized areas of medical practice eligible for board certification.

Although much has been made of the cost of medical education, most of that cost is borne indirectly by the government and the health insurance system. Just 4 percent of medical school costs are covered by tuition payments from students, whereas 46 percent comes from patient fees, 30 percent from research, and 20 percent from government appropriations and gifts.[2] Although tuition might run as high as $40,000 per year and most medical students (83 percent) are left with debts from student loans when they graduate, the amount of those loans (which average about $110,000) is not very large in relation to the income a physician can expect—less than 1 percent of lifetime earnings.[3] Far more onerous than the monetary obligations are the years of toil spent in learning the practice of medicine.

7.2   THE ORIGINS OF LICENSURE AND LINKAGE TO MEDICAL EDUCATION

At the time of the American Revolution, there were about 3,500 established medical practitioners in what was to become the United States, but only 400 had received any formal training and fewer than 200 held degrees. The ability to read and quote some Latin and an apprenticeship were considered sufficient qualifications for hanging out a shingle and calling oneself a doctor. As late as 1830, the University of Virginia provided all its students with instruction in medicine. Yet before 1900, there was little scientific basis for the way most doctors practiced medicine, and indeed the treatments prescribed were about as likely to harm health as to improve it. Since there was really no benefit from seeing a trained professional, there was no support for restricting the practice of medicine through licensure. Although state medical associations repeatedly pushed for licensure and were sometimes temporarily successful, the lack of public benefit doomed such efforts. In New Jersey, licensure laws were passed and then repealed at least 16 times between 1800 and 1900.[4] In other states, licensure laws were on the books but did not mean much because they were not enforced.

Two major technological breakthroughs radically changed the nature of medicine: anesthesiology (pain killing) and antisepsis (germ killing). Although surgery had been practiced since the dawn of humankind, the lack of anesthesia meant that most operations could last only a few minutes, and even then many patients went into shock and died. The other problem was postsurgical infection, which claimed almost as many lives as the injuries that were treated. Very few of the hundreds of thousands of soldiers who died during the Civil War were actually killed in battle; most died in hospitals days or weeks later. Today, most of those wounded soldiers could easily have been saved. Anesthesia and antiseptics changed surgery from a last resort for the desperate patient who would otherwise die, into a routine procedure used in the treatment of many diseases. The fact that twentieth-century surgery was more effective also paradoxically increased the risks. Patients who never before would have considered letting themselves be cut open went under the knife willingly.

Anesthesia, antiseptics, and a host of other scientific breakthroughs changed the promise, and the politics, of medicine. There was no longer any question that doctors must be educated and examined before they were allowed to practice. The Flexner Report of 1910 to the Carnegie Commission, which was supported by the AMA, called for the closure of all medical schools that did not require an undergraduate college degree for admission and provide laboratory training in biology and chemistry, clinical internships, and full-time faculty members. These standards, first viewed as utopian, were implemented with increasing force over the next three decades.

Legal control over physicians resides with state licensure boards, yet supply is actually determined by control over the number of students allowed to enter medical school (and the number of foreign medical graduates allowed to come to the U.S. for training, who often stay to practice). Unlike law school, in which there are many students who fail to graduate, or who graduate and fail the bar exam, or who pass the bar exam and cannot find a job, almost all medical students graduate and practice medicine. There are exams in school and afterward, but almost everyone passes, and the limitation of numbers is sufficient to ensure that everyone who wants to can find a position practicing medicine. By the end of the depression, the old laissez-faire system of unregulated physician practice with open entry had been entirely replaced by a modern system of medical licensure, with control over supply resting in the hands of the medical schools (which, in turn, were largely controlled by the joint AMA and Association of American Medical Colleges (AAMC) Committee on Medical Education).

A major practical difficulty in implementing licensure was how to handle all the existing physicians then in practice who had not received such an education. Although many were poorly trained and lacked ability, others were good physicians who had the respect of their communities and their colleagues. In order to allow these experienced doctors to continue to practice while upgrading standards for new entrants to the profession, they were "**grandfathered**" in. That is, a doctor could become licensed either by graduating from an acceptable medical school or by being an accepted member of the county medical society. Over time, the more highly qualified new graduates would replace the older cohort of nonuniversity physicians. Analyzed in terms of property rights, the existing physicians owned the rights to vote on standards. It would not be in their self-interest to vote for higher standards that would put them out of a job, yet a higher quality standard would increase demand and benefit all physicians. The grandfather clause allowed them to reap the rewards from licensure reform and in a sense became a form of payment for their property—control over the future of the profession. As usual, all parties, including the incumbents, must be made better off for a successful political exchange to occur.

AMA Controls over Physician Supply, 1930–1965

With reform curtailing new entrants and forcing unqualified older practitioners out of business, physician supply declined steadily from its 1900 level of 1.73 M.D.s per 1,000 population to 1.33 M.D.s per 1,000 population in 1930 (Figure 7.1). The supply of physicians held constant at this level for the next 35 years. Yet improvements in medicine greatly increased public demand, as did the rise in personal income over these four decades. With supply constant and demand increasing, earnings of physicians rose, as depicted in Figure 6.3. Concern was voiced that not enough physicians were available and that a shortage had arisen.[5]

There are several ways this shortage could have been rectified. The steep price rise that did occur held quantity demanded in check and made physicians happy, but did little for the public. Supply could have been expanded by increasing the productivity of physicians, changing the organization of medical practice, and using more ancillary health workers; some illnesses could have been treated by physician substitutes such as doctors of osteopathy (D.O.s) or chiropractors; or physicians could have been imported from overseas. These alternatives would have undercut organized medicine's control over physician supply and

FIGURE 7.1   Physician Supply per 1,000 Population

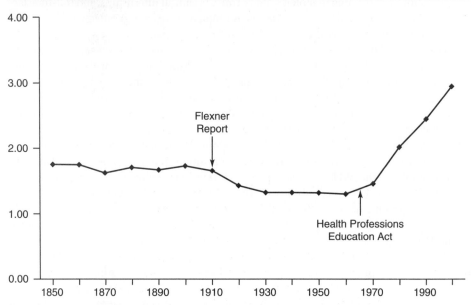

Source: U.S. Historical Statistics of the United States (New York, NY: Cambridge University Press, 2000 and prior census publications.)

incomes, and were strongly resisted by the AMA. Productivity improvements and lower prices were most strongly identified with prepaid group practices such as the Kaiser Health Plan in California and the Group Health Association in Washington D.C. (see Chapters 5 and 12). Concerted opposition by local medical societies led to the expulsion of group practice doctors and an obstinate denial of hospital privileges to physicians who were clearly qualified by education and experience.[6] In 1941, the Washington, D.C., Medical Society and the AMA were indicted, found guilty, and fined by the U.S. Department of Justice for having conspired to monopolize trade in physician services. This is but one of many in a string of cases across the country that left group practices bruised and hampered, but alive. Relations slowly improved, but opposition to prepaid group practice did not end until the 1970s.

The response of organized medicine to substitute providers took two forms: co-opting the competition and all-out war. D.O.s emphasized spinal manipulation in addition to standard medical practices and formed a separate type of care in 1900 with their own D.O. hospitals, but carried out many of the same Flexnerian educational reforms in those transitional years. Over time, M.D. and D.O. cooperation increased through sharing of hospital privileges, enrollment in each other's residency programs, and formation of joint political and social groups.[7] D.O.s were tolerated by the AMA and ultimately brought into the fold as slightly less polished M.D.s. Today, the differences between an M.D. and a D.O. degree are almost nonexistent, except that D.O.s are more likely to be general practitioners and do not control any of the high-prestige medical schools. In many states a single licensure board covers both types of physicians, and in California the M.D. and D.O. societies merged in 1961, although separate boards were later reestablished. Until about 1990, the number of D.O.s relative to M.D.s remained roughly constant at around 5 percent, and hence osteopathy had become more a partner to the AMA in controlling supply rather than a competitive threat.

Chiropractors, who often rely exclusively on spinal manipulation to treat disease and still train some practitioners in for-profit schools, have been severely and relentlessly attacked by the AMA.[8] Licensure acts explicitly exclude chiropractors from the practice of medicine, and this opposition has not changed even though the AMA has not been able to ban chiropractic practice, or indeed to prevent some of its own members from referring patients to chiropractors. Although some of the AMA opposition to chiropractic care is based on the lack of scientific foundation for manipulative treatments, much of it is motivated by economic concerns.

Breaking the Contract: The Great Medical Student Expansion of 1970–1980

Under the control of the AMA and the medical schools, enough new M.D.s and D.O.s were being produced to keep pace with the growth in the U.S. population (about 1 percent a year), but not with the increase in demand due to improved technology or higher disposable incomes. As the benefits of modern medicine became more evident, access to care was increasingly seen as a necessity in the rising American standard of living, one that workers had already paid for through their health insurance premiums. The constraints on supply caused longer waits for an appointment, less time for a patient to talk with an increasingly rushed physician, fewer old-style general practitioners willing to make house calls, and other deteriorations in service. The public was unhappy, and the politicians, who now provided most of the financing for medical schools, were willing to do something to redress the imbalance.

In essence, frustration with the inaction of the AMA led the government to unilaterally disrupt the old system. Congress passed the Health Professions Educational Assistance Act of 1963, forcing medical schools to admit more students and allowing more foreign physicians to immigrate to the United States. In response to the act and subsequent amendments, physician supply rose steadily to 1.61 physicians per 1,000 population in 1970, 2.02 in 1980, 2.44 in 1990, and 2.94 in 2000—more than twice the level of supply that prevailed from 1930 through 1965 (see Figure 7.1 and Figure 7.2). The number of entering students

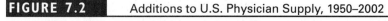

FIGURE 7.2 Additions to U.S. Physician Supply, 1950–2002

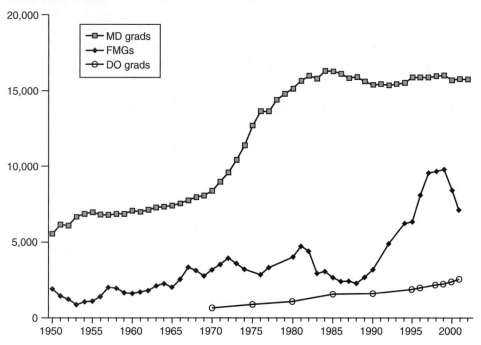

almost doubled in ten years, from 8,759 in 1965 to 15,351 in 1975. The government used two methods to bring about this increase.[9] First, it built more medical schools. Second, it offered additional funding on the condition that existing schools increase the number of students enrolled by at least 5 percent each year. By this time, federal and state funding accounted for 63 percent of medical school financing; hence, the schools were not in a good position to resist, even if they had wanted to. At the same time, changes in immigration rules were made to favor "shortage" occupations, including physicians. Foreign graduates made up just 6 percent of all physicians in practice in 1960, but by 1965 that fraction had doubled to 12 percent and further increased to 17 percent in 1970 and 20 percent in 1980.

Building Pressure: Fixed Domestic Graduation Rates 1980–2008

As the number of residents in training grew rapidly during the 1970s, it began to seem as though there were already plenty of physicians. The AMA complained loudly about a potential surplus, commissioning several studies to show that the United States was training an excess of physicians and that foreign graduates were no longer needed. These arguments were successful in helping the profession reestablish control over supply, and by 1980 the tide of public opinion had turned. The 1981 Report of the Graduate Medical Education National Advisory Committee, widely known as the GMENAC Report, projected a growing surplus, raising the possibility that in the future some physicians would face unemployment.[10] The flow of foreign graduates had already been severely restricted by changes in immigration law included in the Health Professions Educational Assistance Act of 1976. Moves were now made to reduce the rate of growth in the number of U.S. physicians. No more new schools were to be built. Class sizes were fixed at the current level.

The number of first-year M.D. students peaked at 17,268 in 1981 and was held below that number until 2005, then rose to 18,287 in 2007. There has recently been a growing recognition that instead of a surplus, a future shortage of physicians may occur.[11] Since the number of U.S. medical graduates has not kept pace with the growth in U.S. population, much less the growth in technology and incomes that raised effective demand, all the expansion in supply over the last 20 years has had to come from three other sources: (1) the delayed effect of the 1965–1975 "physician boom," (2) increased immigration of non-U.S. physicians, and (3) increased production of non-M.D. physicians.

7.3 ADJUSTING PHYSICIAN SUPPLY

The Flow of New Entrants and the Stock of Physicians

Although the number of students entering medical school jumped by 50 percent between 1968 and 1973, this had no immediate effect on physician supply because these extra students were still in school for four years. Even then, the sudden increase in the number of new M.D.s caused only a gradual rise in the supply of physicians. To see why, it is necessary to trace the life cycle of work, distinguishing the stock of physicians (the number available at any point in time) from the flow of entrants and retirees into and out of the labor force. Suppose that the average physician began practice at age 33 and retired at age 66. If the same number of physicians started work each year and retired after 33 years, 1/33, or 3 percent, of all the physicians in practice would leave each year and another 3 percent would join. The number of physicians in practice (the physician stock) would stay the same from year to year in

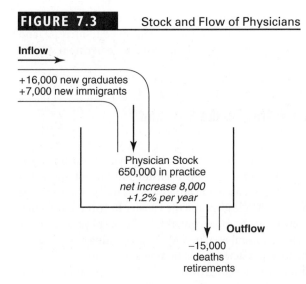

FIGURE 7.3   Stock and Flow of Physicians

this steady state. What would happen if the nation decided to double the physician supply by doubling the number of new graduates each year? In 33 years there would be twice as many, or 100 percent more, practicing physicians, but in the first year there would only be 3 percent more. The number of new additions would be twice as much as before, or 2 × 3% = 6% of the total, and the retirements would be the same, 3 percent, so that net growth would be 3 percent in the first year, 6 percent after two years, 9 percent after three years, and so on. The actual response would be even slower, because there is a lag of eight years from the time new students are admitted until they complete their residencies and become practicing physicians. The full effects of the 1965–1975 "doctor boom" (and subsequent bust) will not be fully realized until this cohort of new physicians has moved through the professional ranks and completed their work lives, some time between the years 2000 and 2025 (see Figure 7.3).

Immigration of International Medical Graduates

The number of foreign medical graduates practicing in the United States doubled in just three years, from 15,154 in 1960 to 30,925 in 1963, with 15,000 more arriving in the next four years. By 1980 there were 97,726 international medical graduates (IMGs) practicing in the United States, 20 percent of the total physician supply. Despite continued restrictions on immigration, the number of IMGs doubled from 1980 to 2000 and now constitute 26 percent of practicing physicians.[12] Although the number of IMGs entering U.S. residency training programs has leveled off at around 6,000 per year since 1995, the effects of the entry bulge from 1988–1995 will continue to expand this component of physician supply for decades to come.

Growth in Non-M.D. Physicians

Although smaller in number, the growth in non-M.D. physicians (primarily D.O.s) has been even more dramatic. In 1970, some 12,600 D.O.s constituted just 4 percent of the total physician supply. Whereas the number of M.D. graduates was essentially held constant at

17,000 from 1980 to 2000, the number of D.O. graduates jumped from 1,059 to 2,304.[13] The number of schools of osteopathy rose from 14 to 19, class size continued to increase, and D.O.s constituted an ever larger fraction of the U.S. medical graduates entering residency programs.

Balancing Supply and Incomes: Tracing the Past and Projecting the Future

The development of scientific medicine created the need for a new type of doctor in the twentieth century, and the history of physician supply and licensure must be interpreted in that context. To raise the quality of the individuals in the profession (as well as their prestige and incomes), the reforms envisioned by AMA leaders and the Flexner Report required that most of the inadequately trained practitioners be forced out, thus reducing physician supply from 1900–1930. From then until 1965, the number of new M.D.s graduating each year was held steady at about 4 percent of the total physician stock, numbers just sufficient to offset the 3 percent who retired each year and a 1 percent growth in the U.S. population, so that the physician-to-population ratio remained constant at about 133 per 10,000.

For a professional thinking technically in terms of medical "need" (a specific, fixed number of physicians required to treat a given number of illnesses), a constant physician-to-population ratio was sufficient to meet demand. From an economic perspective emphasizing responsiveness to prices and incomes, it is clear how inadequate both the concept and the numbers used by the medical profession were. Changing expectations, new technology, and a rising standard of living meant that demand was increasing, and the 1 percent growth in physicians set to match the 1 percent increase in population was not enough to forestall market stress, public dissatisfaction, and growing perceptions of a shortage.

What evidence does the market provide about whether too many or too few physicians were trained or allowed to immigrate? Pent-up demand kept physician incomes from falling during the 1970s as supply rose. Although real earnings dipped in 1985, and again during 1989–1990, physicians have done much better than the average American worker over the last 15 years. Groups that had to make an extra effort to enter the profession (IMGs, D.O.s) clearly found it worthwhile to do so, and pushed for access in record numbers. Such effort and expansion in auxiliary sources indicates that demand was growing faster than regular domestic supply. However, fewer college students were applying to medical schools. About 2 percent of those admitted to medical school did not attend. Although this fraction refusing the opportunity of a medical education was still quite small, it was fourfold above the rate between 1975 and 1985, when just 0.5 percent of those offered a place in medical school turned it down. Although projecting the future is always to some extent speculative, it is possible to give a reasonable assessment of the economic situation and prospects of physicians from these trends.[14] Becoming a doctor still offers above-average rates of return on postcollege education (see Chapter 12). However, the very high earnings growth that physicians enjoyed during the 1960s and 1970s was a temporary historical aberration, brought about by rapid growth in demand due to new technology in the context of fixed supply. In the future, doctors will have high, but not such extraordinarily high, earnings. Although they still will do much better than most graduates from other fields, new physicians will face more competition as they enter the market, and thus will be more likely to become employees holding salaried jobs and to hold on to such positions for longer during their careers. The few who become truly wealthy will be those who have worked their way up the ladder in large health care organizations or who have taken substantial risks as entrepreneurs.

7.4   GROUP PRACTICE: HOW ORGANIZATION AND TECHNOLOGY AFFECT TRANSACTIONS

Physicians who join together in groups have higher net earnings than those who practice alone: $194,000 for solo doctors compared with $250,000 for those in two-physician partnerships, $272,000 for those in three-physician groups, and $300,000 for those in larger groups (see Table 6.3). Physicians in group practices usually have better life styles: more interaction with colleagues, more support services, and fewer nights spent handling patient emergencies.[15] Economists must ascertain which factors lead to greater efficiency and hence higher incomes for group practice and, conversely, which factors limit the attractiveness of groups so that one-third of all physicians still choose to practice alone. There are fundamentally three ways that group practices serve to increase net income:

- Economies of scale raise the productivity of inputs, and hence lower costs.
- Added market power brings in greater revenues.
- Sharing spreads risk.

What does it mean to have **economies of scale** that make larger practices more efficient in the use of inputs? To a physician owner, it could mean either (a) that the cost of inputs required to produce a given amount of output has been reduced or (b) that the output in visits per hour of physician time has been increased. Analysis of group practice expenditures shows that some of both occurs.[16] Equipment and office space comes in discrete units and therefore is inefficiently used in small practices. An X-ray machine that can handle 10,000 patients may cost only 50 percent more than one that can handle 2,000, and even the smaller one is frequently idle for a doctor practicing alone. A large group can match equipment needs to the total patient volume of the group as a whole, and thereby achieve economies of scale. Similarly, each physician may need from one to four exam rooms at a time to maximize patient flow and from two to six assistants. A solo doctor will compromise by having an office with three exam rooms and four assistants, and thus sometimes the ancillary inputs will be overcrowded and limit productivity, while at other times they sit idle and waste money. A group can plan for an average, since it is unlikely that all the physicians will be busy or inactive at the same time, and thus achieve a better match. Office rent takes up 12 percent of the gross revenues of solo practices, 10 percent of two-physician partnerships, and only 7 percent of large group practices.

On the other hand, labor costs and full-time equivalent (FTE) employees per physician increase as practice size increases. A large group can allow for more specialization in the use of labor, so that a ten-physician group can have a laboratory technician, billing specialists, receptionist, intake nurse, exam room assistant, and so on, whereas a solo practice must make do with a general-purpose medical assistant or nurse. Increasing the productivity of an input can either decrease or increase its share of total expenditures depending on the elasticity of substitution with other inputs. (While increased productivity means that the same amount of output could be produced with less input, the fact that the input has become so much more productive may make the group shift to use more and more of it—computers are a good example.) Office space apparently cannot be substituted for physician time; thus, as it becomes more productive per square foot, it takes up a smaller fraction of total practice expenditures. Ancillary labor can be substituted for physician time, and as this labor becomes more productive, physicians use more employees rather than fewer. It is worth paying for more assistants to save the physicians' time because their net profit per hour of work increases.

Risk sharing across the members of the group also creates economies of scale. Just as random variation in the number of exam rooms required by each doctor can be averaged

COMPARATIVE ADVANTAGE AND PHYSICIAN ASSISTANTS

The principle that people and firms should produce the things at which they are *relatively* more efficient and use others to produce the things at which they are relatively less efficient is known as **comparative advantage**. There are gains from trade when relative costs differ, even if one party is better at everything. That is why investment bankers let someone else balance their checkbooks, great artists let helpers fill in the background scenery, great athletes let someone else play on punt returns, and even countries for which production of everything is inefficient export some goods to get the things they are most inefficient at producing. It makes sense to trade even when you can produce the item for less cost, if doing so frees up time and resources that can be used more valuably elsewhere. For example, suppose that a physician takes 15 minutes to do an intake examination and 5 minutes to do a follow-up. The physician assistant (PA) takes 40 minutes to do an intake examination and 30 minutes to do a follow-up. Even though the PA is less efficient at both tasks, the medical group will use the principal of comparative advantage and make the PAs do intakes, not follow-ups. Why? Because in eight hours a PA could do 12 intakes, freeing up three hours of physician time to do high-value surgery, while having the PA do 16 follow-ups would free up just 1 hour and 20 minutes of physician time. It is not the "cost" of using the PA to provide services that matters, it is the value of the additional services that the physician can provide. Trade should follow the course of comparative advantage, even though absolute productivity will determine rewards—the physician will earn more per hour than the PA.

It is worth noting how the principle of comparative advantage can work against some of the human traits we value in doctors. Both nurses and doctors can listen and show compassion, and spending more time yields better results. However, the physician can accomplish more high-tech diagnostic procedures per hour than the nurse and will tend to specialize in that direction, at the expense of listening. Even if we tell our doctors that we want them to spend more time with us and they are very good at listening, they are apt to hire assistants to do so because their comparative advantage lies in the application of medical technology.[17]

out in a large group, so can other revenues and expenses, so that the group can collectively enjoy a smoother and more certain income stream. Perhaps even more important, the emergency calls that interrupt the home life of every doctor are much less disruptive when combined and redistributed in a group. A solo practitioner must be "on call" every night or find someone else who is willing to cover. On Sunday, one emergency call could interrupt a football game, and there might be no more calls until a sleep-shattering call at 3 a.m. For a group, it is usual for each doctor to accept all the calls for a single day. The group doctor might handle seven emergencies on a Sunday but know that Friday night and Saturday are free, since any patients who need assistance will be handled by one of the partners. The burden of emergencies is not the time spent in caring for patients but the uneven spacing. This is the risk that is shared, and thus effectively reduced, in a group.

Since it is obviously so much more efficient for a doctor to handle ten patients in one night than one to three patients each night per week, why don't solo doctors contract with each other to do just that? For that matter, why can't independent physicians arrange to share office space or nurses? To some extent they do, and to that extent they start to become a group. As the contracts and sharing become more complete and cover more aspects of practice, the doctors who trade with each other become a single firm—that is, a group practice.

However, it is difficult to share. All the doctors must agree to standardize certain practices, coordinate efforts, pick a leader, accept the leader's ruling on disputes between them, and so on—in short, to be managed. It means being an employee or partner rather than the boss. Management is costly, and good physician managers, like all good managers, are rare and valuable commodities. Some studies of physician productivity overestimated economies of scale because they did not account for the time physicians must spend in management and how that management time increases as the size of the practice increases.[18] For some physicians, it is cheaper (and more fun) to put up with some inefficiencies and lack of specialized inputs to be their own bosses and not have to listen to, or give orders to, anyone else.

Contracting between many parties and managing larger operations create the costs that limit the attractiveness of group practice. Transaction costs are also the source of the economies of scale in marketing and revenue generation, which are often more important than production cost economies. Consider what happens when a successful older doctor combines his practice with that of a younger physician who is just starting out. The older physician has too many patients, and must turn some away or provide poor service. The young physician has too few patients, and must spend hours waiting for people to show up or moonlighting as an employee in a hospital emergency room. By combining their practices, the successful doctor is, in effect, selling some patients to the younger doctor in return for a part of the younger doctor's income. For such a transfer to occur, patients must be convinced that the junior doctor is as good as the senior one. The senior doctor guarantees the quality of the junior doctor by the act of forming a partnership. In effect, the senior doctor is saying, "I trust this doctor; so should you." Transfer is also facilitated by arranging for the junior partner to take a disproportionate share of night emergencies, the new patients who show up at the door for the first time, and those who do not want to wait weeks to see the senior partner. It is the patient's concerns about quality and trust that make the doctor–patient relationship special, and that makes it hard to obtain economies of scale by treating patients en masse. For a group to act as a collective, the guarantee of quality must extend to all the physicians in it. Just as all licensed physicians benefit from monitoring the quality of care provided by the profession and eliminating or reforming bad doctors, a medical group practice benefits from increased demand to the extent that it can closely monitor and control the quality of all its members.[19] The Mayo Clinic is a premier example of a medical group practice that acts as a "brand-name firm" and gains a marketing and revenue advantage from being perceived as a group with identifiable quality rather than just a random collection of individual physicians who happen to work in the same building.[20]

7.5   KICKBACKS, SELF-DEALING, AND SIDE PAYMENTS

> "... and if a doctor shall cheat his patient by overcharging for medicaments, then shall a finger of his left hand be cut off."
> — *Code of Hammurabi, 2300* B.C.

From the beginning, the AMA code of medical ethics has dealt with economic issues, rightfully noting that doctors must put the health of patients above profits if people are to trust them. The agency relationship is most threatened in day-to-day business by the practice of paying "referral fees" or **kickbacks**. The agent is supposed to be, and is, paid for acting in the principal's (the patient's) best interest. When doctors accept a fee for referring patients to one hospital rather than another, or for giving a surgical case to Dr. B instead of Dr. A, they may be tempted to go with the one who will pay them the most, not the one who will provide the best care. In ordinary business dealings, such a payment would be termed a bribe or a kickback. Corporate purchasing agents are sometimes caught accepting presents or kickbacks from suppliers in return for steering business their way. For suppliers to pay for business is not bad—they can give rebates or provide customer treats or price discounts. The problem is the distortion caused by directing a payment to the agent who is supposed to be making an objective choice, rather than the principal, who is supposed to get the benefits of any discounts. Before medicine became established as a profession, such practices were common. Surgeons in the large cities would advertise in rural newspapers their willingness to pay $100 or more for each case sent to them. Although such behavior seems unthinkable now, kickbacks keep cropping up. What was once the largest chain of psychiatric hospitals was investigated and convicted for paying physicians and social workers who sent in clients. The kickback scheme had become so well established that there was a standard going rate of $70 for each patient day.[21]

Why do kickbacks continue to occur if everyone knows that they are bad and they are condemned by all the official governing organizations? They continue because an agent's control over who gets the business is valuable property. To not make use of that value—that is, to act ethically and follow professional standards that put the interests of patients first—forces a doctor to put aside his or her own narrow self-interest. In the short run, it is easy to profit by betraying a trust to make a dollar. The violator hopes not to get caught. Even if an unethical physician does get caught, much of the punishment actually falls on other doctors because the profession as a whole gets blamed for a lack of standards and suffers from a reduced demand and falling prices for services. Trust and agency build professional value, and taking a kickback is one way for a member to steal part of that value, benefiting personally while harming others.

One of the major activities of physicians is prescribing drugs. If drug companies made payments to physicians, those dollars could distort the physicians' choices on behalf of their patients, perhaps by prescribing a drug that is less effective or one that is effective but three times as expensive as all the substitute drugs that would work just as well.[22] An even more difficult problem arises when the physician is not only prescribing the drug but also selling it. Knowing that the patient is in pain and trusts the physician, physicians could fatten their profit margins by overcharging for drugs. That such a problem is not new is evidenced by the quote from the code of Hammurabi at the beginning of this section. The potential for abuse is so high that physicians in this country have been legally prohibited from selling drugs or owning pharmacies since 1934. Even a pharmacy in a medical clinic must be run as a separate business to avoid conflicts of interest. In Japan, where no such law exists, the government sets price controls to keep physicians from overcharging, but that does not stop them from overprescribing. General-practice physicians in Japan get about a third of their net income from sales of pharmacy items, and their patients are prescribed twice as many drugs as similar patients in the United States.

In the quote from the code of Hammurabi, the prohibition is on overcharging for *medication*. Why isn't overcharging for service similarly condemned? The issue with kickbacks is not price, it is deceit. If Dr. Andrews says, "I am better than the others, and I want $20 more for each visit," that is her privilege. Patients can agree or go somewhere else. There is no fraud. To prescribe a drug and accept a $20 rebate from the manufacturer, or to send a surgical case to Dr. Jones knowing that he will send a case of wine in return, is fraud. The patient is unknowingly paying and has an agent whose decisions may be influenced by kickbacks rather than the patient's welfare. The patient going to Dr. Andrews, *and unaware that Dr. Andrews has any business arrangement with another doctor*, has a right to expect Dr. Andrews to choose objectively the surgeon who is best and to negotiate the lowest price.

As medicine has become more complex, with more transactions involved in each episode of patient care, it has become even more difficult to avoid conflicts of interest. Of particular concern in recent years have been incidences in which for-profit companies providing ancillary services (e.g., diagnostic radiology, home intravenous therapy) offer physicians "investments" in these businesses in return for sending patients.[23] So many such abuses took place that in 1976 federal anti-kickback laws were passed prohibiting any Medicare or Medicaid payment from companies to physicians based on the volume of patient referrals. The 1989 "Stark law" (named after its sponsor, U.S. Representative Fortney Stark of California) banned physicians from referring patients to clinical laboratories in which they have a financial interest. The 1993 "Stark II" law widened the ban to prohibit self-referrals to hospitals or radiology laboratories in which physicians are invested. The law also prohibits bonus plans within group practices based on the volume of laboratory referrals. Only a minority (less than 10 percent) of physicians invest in businesses that raise conflict of interest issues from self-referral, and only a few engage in profiteering at the expense of the government and patients.[24] Yet the actions of these few are so troubling to a public already dismayed over the high cost of health care that it is likely that further restrictions will be placed on independent diagnostic and therapeutic facilities owned by physicians.

7.6 PRICE DISCRIMINATION

One of the characteristics of the medical markets first noted by economists was that different patients pay different prices for the same service.[25] Some price differences are attributable to differences in cost or value (e.g., surgery by an experienced board-certified specialist versus a new resident still in training, midnight treatment in the emergency room versus a routine visit to the doctor's office). However, even after these factors are taken into account, there is still a sizable and systematic variation in charges. It is frequently noted that people who are well insured or have high incomes pay more, laboratory and other small ticket items are overpriced, and that services for which patients can "shop around" (e.g., eye exams, normal births, physical therapy) show less price variation than emergency medical care where immediate treatment is required.

A major reason for **price discrimination**, charging different prices for the same service to different types of patients or patients in different types of care, is that it increases total revenue. The change in revenue, marginal revenue, depends on price elasticity as well as price (see Section 2.3). More formally,

$$\text{Marginal Revenue} = \text{Price}(1 + 1/\text{Elasticity})$$

To maximize revenues when providing two different types of care, physicians should charge different prices even if their costs are the same for each service and should *charge a higher price where demand is least price sensitive* (i.e., where price elasticity, which is always negative, is smaller in magnitude). Conversely, where demand is very price sensitive, a reduction in price will bring in many more patients and increase revenues (see Figure 7.4). Pain, fear of dying, and wealth all serve to reduce price sensitivity. However, the most important factor making medical consumers less price sensitive is insurance (see Figure 7.5). Therefore, we would generally expect physicians to charge more for those services that are more fully covered by insurance, more life-threatening, more painful, and for which patients have the least ability to shop around. Some ancillary services (lab tests, X-rays, sonograms) are not very price sensitive even when insurance coverage is incomplete, because they are considered secondary and inevitable by-products, and thus rarely receive the kind of scrutiny given an operation or other major expense.[26]

FIGURE 7.4   Price Discrimination by Patient Type

FIGURE 7.5   Price Discrimination by Insurance Status

There is an important empirical discrepancy at odds with the revenue maximization model of physician price discrimination: the lower price is sometimes clearly below the cost of providing the service (sometimes care is even free) and, therefore, must decrease rather than increase physician income. Indeed, when queried about differential pricing, some physicians respond angrily to the suggestion that they are maximizing profits and assert that they act from a benevolent impulse, charging high prices to those who can afford to pay (or are well insured) so that they can take care of the destitute. Under closer examination, however, it becomes evident that there is a mixture of motivations that includes both charity and higher incomes in a blend that is not always clearly separable. Charging students less helps out a group that is usually poor and might not get care if they had to pay full price— and brings in more revenue for exactly the same reason. (Why do you think movie theaters and airlines give student discounts—is it a charitable impulse or a smart business practice to raise revenues because they know students have little discretionary money and wouldn't come to the theater or fly as often otherwise?) Price discrimination is pervasive in medicine and well accepted by patients, the government, and insurance companies. Yet if two people come into a shop and one is charged twice as much for oil, food, or rent, the person charged extra will complain or threaten to sue. The unusual willingness of people to accept or even praise price discrimination in medicine is one of the factors that has convinced economists that health care markets differ in significant ways from markets for most other goods and services.

7.7 PRACTICE VARIATIONS

The agency relationship arises because the patient trusts the physician to do what is right. What happens when the physician confronts a lack of information or when medical science provides no clear guidelines on what to do? The professional concept of "need," which assumes there is a right way to treat an illness and hence no necessity for examining trade-offs among costly alternatives, falters if the clinical pathway becomes ambiguous. The fact that some medical practices have been widely used with confidence, only to be later discarded as ineffective or harmful, fosters some doubts about the infallibility of medicine. In a 1934 study, the American Child Health Association chose 1,000 schoolchildren to be examined by physicians to determine whether or not they should have their tonsils removed.[27] Six hundred children had already had the procedure. The remaining 400 were examined, and the physicians recommended that 45 percent of them have a tonsillectomy. Then the 220 not recommended for surgery in the first round were examined by another group of physicians, who recommended that 46 percent of them have their tonsils out. A third exam by another set of physicians on the 118 who were left resulted in recommendations that 44 percent have their tonsils removed. After these three examinations, only 65 of the original 1,000 children were not recommended for a tonsillectomy! From this study, the experimenters concluded that the decision about whether a child needed a tonsillectomy was not primarily based on signs or symptoms or any objective evidence, but on a generally held opinion among the doctors consulted that they should give tonsillectomies to one-third to one-half of all the children they treated in that age range.

Today, tonsillectomy is a much less commonly performed procedure, in part because of these pioneering epidemiological experiments (epidemiology is the study of the distribution of diseases in populations, applying statistical methods to groups rather than studying individual patients). However, the insights regarding the range of uncertainty in common diagnoses were essentially ignored during the glory years of medicine after World War II, when it seemed that science could diagnose and cure every ailment. This optimistic conviction that medical advances would be continuous and consistently beneficial faded as the Vietnam War, an oil crisis, and rising environmental concerns led to a more cautious and critical assessment of technology. In what was then (in 1973) a little-noticed study, John Wennberg and colleagues found that the rates of many common types of surgery varied widely across counties in Vermont, with differences as large as six-fold, which were not explainable by differences in insurance, availability of hospitals, or illness rates.[28] For tonsillectomies, the rate varied from as few as 8 per 10,000 to as many as 60 per 10,000. In a subsequent study, Wennberg found that the people of Boston, Massachusetts, had more hospital beds, had more employees per bed, and paid 87 percent more on average for hospital care than the people of New Haven, Connecticut, yet in both cities the average health statistics were about the same and most people received high-quality medicine, with many patients treated in academic medical schools. Interestingly, Wennberg found that while the overall rate of surgery was higher in Boston, for certain conditions the rate of surgery was instead significantly higher in New Haven. Thus, it is not simply a question of more or less, but of a large degree of unexplainable variation (see Figure 7.6).

This phenomenon of **practice variation** or **small area variation** has been confirmed by a number of researchers. It suggests that there is a large element of ambiguity that can

FIGURE 7.6   Variation in Age-Adjusted Rates of Hospitalization for Different Diagnoses and Procedures. (Each dot represents one hospital market area.)

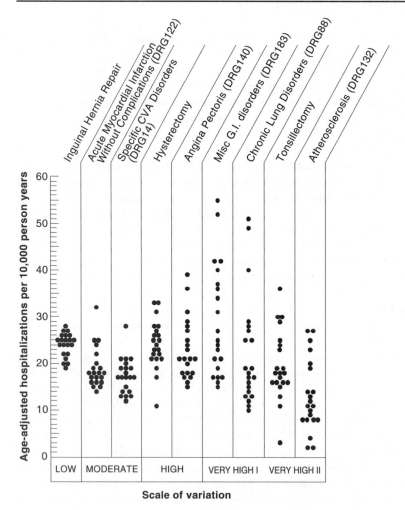

Source: J. Wennberg, K. McPherson, and P. Caper, *New England Journal of Medicine* 311 (1984): 298.

make widely different treatment choices constitute acceptable medical practice. Conditions in which indications are not so clear, or for which there are good alternative forms of treatment, show large variations (e.g., knee replacement, spinal surgery for back pain, tonsillectomy, treatment of psychoses). However, for conditions in which there are clear indications and a generally accepted treatment, the range of variation is much smaller (e.g., hernia repair, open-heart surgery, lung resection). Work is now under way to develop more formal **clinical pathways**, sets of instructions developed by medical professionals based on verified results of scientifically validated studies. These clinical pathways suggest how a particular illness should be managed, including which tests to perform, which medications to give, how long to wait for symptoms to improve before surgery, and so on. Many doctors denigrate such efforts as "cookbook medicine," while others recognize that clinical pathways, although not able to replace the physician's personal judgment, can help make treatment more efficient. What is important to recognize is that repeated demonstrations of wide variations in practice patterns have called into question the role of the individual doctor as final arbiter of right and wrong treatments. Impetus has been given to health policy promoting **evidence-based medicine**, which relies on the results of carefully constructed clinical studies with verifiable costs and outcomes of care, rather than accepting current practices as a standard or relying on the opinions expressed by professional associations.

UNCERTAINTY REGARDING HORMONE REPLACEMENT THERAPY

For many years, estrogen and progestin were routinely prescribed for postmenopausal women to replace hormones their bodies could no longer produce in quantity. Clinical judgment suggested that such hormone replacement therapy reduced the risks of heart disease, stroke, and osteoporosis that accompanied aging. Observational studies indicated that risk reductions on the order of 40 percent to 50 percent could be obtained, but there were no randomized studies that established the magnitude of effect with certainty.

The Women's Health Initiative was begun in 1991, and it eventually screened 373,092 women for participation. Of these, 16,608 were enrolled in clinical trials and randomized to receive either hormones or a placebo (inert pill). Participants were to be followed and repeatedly assessed medically for 8.5 years. However, the trial was stopped after only five years of observation because there were excess deaths and adverse events among the group receiving the hormones. The negative impact was small but conclusively demonstrated. Hormone replacement therapy did not help overall and on average probably harmed those who received it. No single physician, or group of physicians practicing together, would ever have been able to see these effects. Among 8,000 women over five years, there were approximately six excess heart attack fatalities and three excess stroke deaths— an annualized difference of only 0.01 percent. Only statistical methods and rigorously planned, carefully recorded observations of thousands of patients at many hospitals and clinics can distinguish effects such as these. In retrospect, the reliance placed on individual judgment and clinical experience resulted in many useless or harmful treatments.[29]

Small area variation is one form of **population medicine**, which uses groups rather than individual patients to define quality of care.[30] Although long used in public health (see Chapter 15), it is only with the spread of managed care contracting for large numbers of people that population medicine has become recognized as a valuable tool for assessing the quality of physician practice. As hospitals become integrated into health care systems to organize and better manage the care they provide to the community, decisions regarding treatment will be shaped more by analysis of statistics on large numbers of patients and less dependent on the experience of a single physician.[31]

NO MORE DR. WELBY

Marcus Welby, M.D. was one of the most popular shows on the ABC network from 1969 to 1976. Like the earlier Dr. Kildare (played by Joel McCrea in 1937 and Richard Chamberlain in the 1960s), the noble, warm, and caring physician played by Robert Young was everyone's ideal of what a doctor should be. However, like the wise dad Young played in *Father Knows Best*, the character of Marcus Welby was a Hollywood fiction that pleased audiences because it conformed to an ideal rather than to reality. When Robert Young died at the age of 91 in 1997, the era of happy TV families and kindly doctors who acted solely out of altruism had already passed.[32]

7.8 INSURANCE, PRICE COMPETITION, AND THE STRUCTURE OF MEDICAL MARKETS

The twinned effects of medical uncertainty, agency, and insurance, are combined in the health care system so that prices are almost uniquely *un*important for consumer behavior or well-being. Licensure and other monitoring procedures try to guarantee that any doctor available to serve you will provide excellent treatment using up-to-date technology, while insurance takes away the impact of cost and any incentive to spend time comparison shopping. Consider how unusual this market is. For cars, clothing, and housing, one expects that better quality will cost more and that only the wealthy will buy the superior brands. Not so for hospitals or surgery. It all costs the same more or less—a small copayment, a deductible, or nothing. In picking a movie or a pair of shoes, consumers assume that they will suffer the consequences of some inevitable bad and poorly informed choices on their part. Not in medical care. It is the doctor's fault, not mine, if the treatment does not fit or does not work properly. Nowhere else is price so irrelevant. Surgeons don't even list their fees, much less put up sale signs offering 40 percent off to increase business. If you buy expensive clothes, you will have to give up your expensive car, or your new apartment, or your tuition for graduate school. However, a person can get the best medical care in the world and walk out with their checkbook balance nearly unaffected.

For a patient seeking medical care, quality rather than price is paramount. Medical care must be purchased at the time it is needed, often under great stress. Serious illness may strike at any moment, without warning, or a person may go for years without visiting the doctor or the hospital. Medical services must be performed on the person. The outcome of treatment is uncertain and depends on quality of care, which patients are usually not sufficiently knowledgeable to judge. Even though quality is the most important characteristic, it is hard to measure and even more difficult to translate into dollars to enable the patient to rationally consider whether a highly regarded physician is really worth an extra-high fee. Indeed, in many cases, patients are not even sure exactly what is being done for them; therefore, they can hardly be sure that they're getting their money's worth. Furthermore, if a mistake has been made, no amount of money can readily compensate the patient for having been crippled or killed by poor quality. Experience in purchasing care for one illness may be of little help the next time you get sick, because you may have pneumonia instead of a broken leg.

Although prices do not play a major role in contracting for medical services, health *insurance* markets are very price competitive. Every year, people renew their insurance, and the choice can be planned and researched ahead of time. Insurance is not a direct personal service that must be performed in person; the check can be sent from anywhere. Insurance offers money, an absolutely standard and universal commodity, so that there is little quality variation (friendliness of service and amount of paperwork vary among insurance companies, but these are trivial compared with the variations among good and bad surgeons). If a mistake is made by the insurance company, its effects could be entirely erased by sending another check. Insurance is a regularly purchased routine product that is easy to buy in advance and for which small price differences are meaningful. This is not to say that consumers have no difficulty determining the value of their health insurance coverage and whether they got what they paid for, but that these problems are orders of magnitude less formidable than the problems faced in the purchase of medical care. Furthermore, the actual purchasing of insurance is carried out mostly by groups through brokers or full-time company benefits specialists, whereas consumers must go out and purchase medical care on their own.

WHY THE HEALTH INSURANCE MARKET IS MORE PRICE COMPETITIVE

Unlike medical care, which suffers many market failure problems from lack of consumer knowledge to variable incidence, the market for health insurance meets most of the conditions for purely competitive goods.

- Insurance is a homogeneous product. It provides dollars in reimbursement; thus, there is little "quality" variation.
- Insurance can be bought far in advance, when there is no time pressure or illness.
- Insurance can be bought far from home, in a national market.
- Purchasing is done by large and sophisticated buyers (corporate benefits offices, broker agents) who can afford to compare and examine the contracts being offered.

Although the health insurance market itself is very competitive, *the existence of insurance tends to make price competition more difficult to maintain in the medical care market*. Insurance breaks the linkage between buyer and seller, splitting payment "for" services by patients from payments "for" services to providers. The reimbursement provided by an insurer to a hospital may have almost no relation to the bill the patient receives, or to what the insurer would have reimbursed the patient if the bill were paid out of pocket. In third-party transactions, there is often no longer a single "price" in any meaningful sense, and the role of prices as information is seriously degraded. Prices can no longer communicate to suppliers what the value of services is to consumers, nor do they reflect the costs of inputs in production. By design, insurance removes the burden of medical costs from the patient. There is no longer any need to worry about whether it is worthwhile to go to the doctor or whether an extra visit is worth the additional cost. Insurance acts as a price subsidy by increasing demand and by removing the incentive to use less expensive substitutes. Once the insurance premiums are paid, everything costs the same. Price competition is replaced by quality competition since prices no longer matter.

Insurance tends to distort production behavior as well. Under many reimbursement systems, hospitals and doctors are paid according to the cost of care rather than according to the value of services (primarily because value is too difficult to measure). Hence, there is little incentive to work hard for increased efficiency. Some additional costs will be incurred for no reason other than the fact that the insurance will pay for them. With revenues coming from insurance rather than from patients, the connection between consumer service and profits is eroded. It may become easier to make money by providing what the insurance company thinks is important (detailed bills with lots of documentation) rather than providing what patients want or need.

Control over health care is exercised by control over the money that goes to doctors and hospitals. Thus, *insurance and reimbursement rules, rather than legislation, have become the dominant regulatory force in health care.* The government does not need to pass a law telling hospitals to do or not to do something. If reimbursement rules are shifted so that only hospitals that meet certain standards get paid, then hospitals will do what the flow of money directs them to do. It is not necessary to exhort doctors to provide examinations. If the money is made available through insurance, the services will appear in the marketplace.

7.9 CHOICES *BY* AND *FOR* PHYSICIANS

If medicine were totally different from all other goods and services so that the principles of rational choice did not apply, then there would be no reason to study the economics of health. If medicine were the same as every other market, then there would be little reason to separate out the field of health economics. Medical economics is different, but not entirely so. Physician choice of specialty, work hours, partners, prices, and many other aspects of practice are well described by economic models and show traditional responses to incentives. Patient's choices are not, mainly because so many of these choices are made collectively as "public choices" or regulations about licensure, labeling, or insurance (see Chapters 14 and 15), and most individual treatment choices about are delegated to the doctor who acts as the patient's agent. Even the choice of a personal physician does not appear to conform well to standard economic choices, being dominated by habit, informal recommendations of friends and family, and convenience, but only occasionally showing the conscious trade-offs between quantity, price, and quality that are typical of other markets.

Medicine is a vital service with broad public and professional interest. What that means in practice is that there is often a rhetorical cover blanketing the operation of self-interest by any party. Insurance companies, consumers, and providers all talk about the public interest while trying hard to maintain their own position or to get ahead. Physicians are skilled professionals who care for patients, and as professionals their incomes depend entirely on what can be earned from patients and insurance. Caring is a business, with revenues and expenses, not just a calling. The advice of economists is that following the path of dollars financing the system will often tell a student more about what is really going on than listening to the arguments presented in newspapers or on television, or by reviewing the most recent congressional testimony or transcripts from legal cases. Money talks, even to physicians and nonprofit hospitals. For those willing to listen, it speaks loudly and clearly about how the health care system works.

SUGGESTIONS FOR FURTHER READING

Richard J. Baron, "Medicine Cut Off From Its Roots: Context Matters in Medical Education," *Health Affairs* 27, no. 5 (2008): 1357–1361.

Abraham Flexner, *Medical Education in the United States and Canada*, The Carnegie Foundation, 1910 (http://www.carnegiefoundation.org/eLibrary/docs/flexner report.pdf), excerpt reprinted in the *Bulletin of the World Health Organization* 80, no. 7 (2002): 594–602 (www.who.org).

James Le Fanu, M.D., *The Rise and Fall of Modern Medicine* (New York: Carroll amp; Graf, 1999).

Medical Economics (monthly) Medical Economics Publishing: Montvale, New Jersey.

"Medical Education," annual special issue of the *Journal of the American Medical Association.*

Richard Shryock, *Medical Licensing in America, 1650–1965* (Baltimore: Johns Hopkins University Press, 1967).

Paul Starr, *The Social Transformation of American Medicine* (New York: Basic Books, 1982).

Rosemary Stevens, *American Medicine and the Public Interest* (New Haven, Conn.: Yale University Press, 1971).

SUMMARY

1. About 16,000 M.D.s graduated from 126 medical schools in the United States in 2008. Since the bulk of the physician supply consists of those who have already been, and will continue to be, in practice for many years, any changes in the number of new graduates will only slowly affect the supply of services. The "physician boom" of the 1970s will move through the health care system, creating strains and opportunities until the year 2020. The supply of physicians stayed roughly constant at around 1.4 physicians per 1,000 population from the start of modern medical education in the 1920s until 1965, but has risen rapidly since then to 3.0 physicians per 1,000 population today.

2. **Control over physician supply and licensure in the United States is actually exercised by control over medical education**, a system that grew out of the Flexner Report of 1910 to the Carnegie Commission, supported by the AMA. Three factors contributed to the development of medical licensure based on graduate training at that time: (a) advances in medical technology (surgery, anesthesia, radiology) that were powerful aids to healing but could also be harmful if used improperly; (b) a scientific knowledge base that gave university-educated physicians a real advantage over physicians who only learned by apprenticeships; and (c) a reformist political climate favoring regulation, combined with evidence that many doctors were not competently trained before entering practice.

3. **Competition** for clients in medical care is dominated by quality, not price. Physicians have used quality concerns and licensure laws to foreclose competition by graduates of foreign medical schools, osteopaths, chiropractors, and other health practitioners.

4. **Control over supply** by professional associations has increased the **profits** of physicians relative to other workers. While the physician-to-population ratio stayed constant from 1930 to 1960, demand was actually increasing due to new medical advances and an increasingly affluent society, creating a physician shortage. The AMA was unwilling to increase the number of physicians (which would have meant lower incomes), but public opinion was sufficiently strong to force the opening of new medical schools and revisions in immigration laws to make it easier for foreign doctors to practice in the United States. As the increase in new graduates during the 1970s and 1980s relieved this pressure, the size of entering medical school classes was reduced and immigration was again restricted. Since 1980, graduate rates have stayed constant even as population and per capita income have grown, increasing demand and pushing physician incomes upward.

5. **Group practice**, increasing the scale of physician operations, requires more coordination and uses more ancillary help, but increases output per physician and uses physicians' informational advantages by having them monitor the quality of one

another's practices. The ability to trade patients more efficiently is a major function of such economic organizations. However, such coordination increases transaction costs and limits the autonomy of individual physicians because they must now operate as part of a team.

6. **Price discrimination**, charging higher prices where demand is less elastic (due to insurance, high income, lack of information or alternatives) is common in medicine, although much of the motivation seems to be purely charitable and is officially sanctioned by the public. Even though there are many physicians in a city, each one is unique and patients are reluctant to switch. The reduced price sensitivity that arises from such "monopolistic competition" allows price differentials to endure.

7. The potential for kickback payments on referrals and profits from related business may hamper the ability of physicians to act as the patient's **agent**. Ownership of pharmacies and sale of drugs by physicians is prohibited in the United States (but not in Japan, where patients are prescribed more drugs for each visit and many physicians make a third of their income that way). Ownership of laboratories, physical therapy clinics, and diagnostic radiology facilities has been shown to lead to abuses of trust (excessive ordering of tests, excess charges) and is increasingly being discouraged and regulated by government payers.

8. Physicians in some areas perform a specific operation, such as tonsillectomies, at a rate six times that of physicians in another area, even though both areas seem to be similar in all respects. Such unexplained **practice variations** call into question the idea that there is some well-defined need for medical care that can be objectively agreed upon by most physicians. Since such variations have been shown to occur, governments have begun studies to examine more carefully how differences in treatment are related to outcomes, thus developing standard protocols known as **clinical pathways** and **practice standards**.

9. **Markets for health insurance** are more competitive than for the underlying service, medical care, because insurance is a homogenous product (dollars are used to pay bills) with little quality variation, which is bought in advance on a geographically dispersed national market and often purchased by well-informed corporate benefits managers.

10. **Insurance distorts the market for medical care** because use of third-party payment breaks the link between buyer and seller. Insurance acts like a price reduction or subsidy, making consumers less price sensitive, fostering competition on the basis of quality rather than price, and necessitating special contracts to reimburse providers who do not collect much money directly from the patients they serve. **Insurance rules are the dominant regulatory force in health care because they control the flow of money.**

PROBLEMS

1. {*licensure*} Does licensure raise the quality of medical care, or does it just raise the profitability of medical practice?

2. {*competition*} Why are the markets for health insurance so much more price competitive than the markets for medical care?

3. {*incidence*} Who pays the costs of medical education: the student, the patients, the insurance companies, or the taxpayers?

4. {*demand curves, derived demand*} Draw the demand and supply curves for two medical professions, one with licensure and one without (e.g., physicians compared to hospital administrators).

    a. Which would show the greater percentage increase in incomes for an equivalent shift in demand?

    b. What would be the effect of the government giving scholarships of $10,000 per year to all students entering the licensed profession compared with the effect of giving scholarships to all students entering the unlicensed profession?

    c. What would be the effect of these scholarships on tuition at the licensed and unlicensed professional schools? On the number of students applying?

    d. Would it make a difference if, instead of giving scholarships to everyone, the government gave them to only 5,000 students?

5. {*price controls*} Some states have mandated Medicare "assignment." Assignment means that the doctor agrees to treat a patient and accept the fee Medicare sends as payment in full. Doctors not accepting assignment bill the patient (almost always for more than Medicare would pay) and the patient pays the doctor, sends in the bill, and gets reimbursed by Medicare. Typically 20 percent to 60 percent of physicians in an area accept Medicare assignment because patients prefer it and payment is assured. Other physicians want to bill for the extra money. The number of doctors accepting assignment depends on the rates Medicare is currently paying, local market conditions, how "full" the doctor's practice is, and so on. Draw demand and supply curves to show the effects of passing a state law mandating that all physicians accept Medicare assignment. What happens to price, quantity, demand, and supply? Distinguish between short-term and long-term effects. Describe other effects you might expect.

6. {*competition*} Several politicians have proposed that the United States become more restrictive regarding immigration, allowing fewer foreign-educated physicians to undergo training or establish practices in the United States. Would this increase or decrease the earning power of U.S.-educated physicians? Which specialties would be most affected?

7. {*licensure*} The state of New Jersey was unwilling to allow physicians to become licensed in 1850. Which factors changed to make the state willing to enact and enforce licensure restrictions in 1950?

8. {*licensure, property rights*} How did the reformers in the medical profession who wanted to impose higher standards obtain the consent of physicians who were educated under the old system? Did power get translated into money in the process?

9. {*supply*} What controls the supply of physicians in the United States? Distinguish between short- and long-term and between proximate and fundamental factors (i.e., the actual decision-making individuals and organizations versus the underlying economic and political forces).

10. {*anti-trust*} Has the AMA ever been sued for restraint of trade? If so, did it win or lose?

11. {*competition*} Are chiropractors substitutes or complements for physicians in the production of medical services? What about podiatrists? Psychologists? Osteopaths? Homeopaths? Which professions are more competitive and which are more cooperative? Why?

12. {*dynamics*} How long does it take to become a doctor? How long does a doctor usually practice medicine? How long does it take for the supply of doctors to adjust to a change in the number of patients or a change in the availability of technology?

13. {*dynamics, geographical span*} Is the time required for a city to adjust doctor supply different than the time required for a state to adjust doctor supply? The time required for the country as a whole to adjust doctor supply? What is the relevant geographic unit for measuring the market for physician services?

14. {*productivity*} Is the productivity of a medical practice determined primarily by the amount of capital employed or the number of people employed?

15. {*trade*} Do physicians pay each other for patients? If so, explain how.

16. {*industrial organization*} Why do physicians choose to practice together in groups? Is assembling physicians into groups any different from assembling employees into a manufacturing firm, or lawyers into a legal firm, or baseball players into a team?

17. {*economies of scale*} What advantages does a large physician group have over a solo physician? What disadvantages?

18. {*input compensation*} Is it possible for a physician to use ancillary inputs to increase profits without paying for those inputs? If so, give several different examples.

19. {*price discrimination*} When physicians choose to give a discount on fees, does it raise or lower their income? Will a profit-maximizing physician charge higher prices for services or groups of patients for which demand is more elastic or less elastic? Explain why, providing a numerical calculation to illustrate your point and giving several examples.

20. {*price controls*} Let's assume that the state of Idaho decides that Medicaid will pay only 75 percent of what private insurance pays in order to save money and balance the state budget. Will this cause a shortage? What kind of evidence would you look for?

21. {*transaction costs*} Why are kickbacks illegal?

22. {*practice variations*} Which factors determine the number of knee surgeries in a state? Will the same factors determine the number of hip surgeries? Colon surgeries? Hospital admissions as a result of asthma?

23. {*price discrimination*} The Saga of the Doctor and the Wannabe:

A. Dr. Jones is the only doctor in Calexico. It is a town of Anglos, who mostly own farms and local businesses or who work in schools and government, and Chicanos who mostly work on the farms growing lettuce. Dr. Jones obviously has a monopoly on medical care in Calexico. Rodrigo is a field worker. Everyone who knows him says he is very smart and muy simpatico (very empathetic) and knows a lot about what makes people sick. His grandmother was a Curandera, or herb doctor, and taught him a lot. He also learned from other native curers and read medical books. He earned straight A's in school until he had to drop out and work in the fields to help support his family. At night and on weekends he acts as the "doctor" to many poor families. He asks them to pay what they can to help him and his invalid mother.

One day in May a man who was seeing Rodrigo for "faintness" dies. A Chicana who was in labor and being cared for by Dr. Jones also dies. A big fight follows. Rodrigo says, "Dr. Jones gets rich by charging big fees, while he butchers our people." Dr. Jones says, "This illiterate Mexican tries to pass himself off as a doctor and kept this man from coming to me for treatment that could have saved his life." Dr. Jones also states, "I am the greatest friend the Chicano community has. I charge them less than half of what I charge my other patients because I know they can't afford more." *Comment briefly on Dr. Jones pricing and its relationship to his desire to help Chicanos.*

B. The fight between Dr. Jones and Rodrigo is getting worse and threatens this once peaceful agricultural community. Anglo and Chicano are openly hostile to each other, but within each camp there is also dissension. Some Chicanos say, "Dr. Jones did help a lot of our people, and when they couldn't pay, he didn't send the bill collector or take their car, as the department store or bank would have done. Besides, although the mother died, he saved the baby—if not for him, both could have died." Some Anglos say, "That young upstart Rodrigo may be right. I've been going to Dr. Jones for eight years, he's made a bundle off of me, and my arthritis isn't any better." At the urging of the mayor, Dr. Jones and Rodrigo get together to talk about the problem. Afterward, each has a much different point of view. Rodrigo states, "Dr. Jones is an honest and hardworking doctor who has the best interests of the community at heart. He actually loses money taking care of Chicanos and should be paid more. I will work with him in every case I can." Dr. Jones says, "Rodrigo is an exceptionally talented young man who knows more than any layperson, and even some doctors I have met, about the practice of medicine. We are in complete agreement about the tremendous need for better medical care in Calexico and will work together to solve this problem. Many Chicano patients who cannot afford to see me on a regular basis can be treated just as well by Rodrigo after I have done any initial diagnosis and evaluation, and I will send them to him. Together we can provide better medical care for all." *Explain why this togetherness occurred among two people, each of whom had claimed the previous night that the other was a killer. In your answer, assume that each was motivated solely by economic considerations. Why does Rodrigo say that Dr. Jones should raise his prices?*

C. One year later, Dr. Jones announces, "Working with Rodrigo has opened my eyes to the plight of Chicanos and the reluctance of Anglos to accept them as equal members of society. Furthermore, as I become older I face the inevitable diminution of my ability to meet the needs of our community, and as a doctor I face the responsibility of ensuring that Calexico can continue to receive good medical care. Therefore, I have formed La Raza de Calexico Scholarship Fund. Rodrigo will work as a staff member at my clinic part time while he completes college and his medical education. He will, of course, continue to help the Chicanos who have always come to him, but he will also treat Anglo patients. This exceptional person should not work as a field hand when he can so ably act to meet the medical needs of all citizens in Calexico. We have just signed a contract that will make him my junior partner the day he graduates from medical school and that will turn over my full practice to him when I retire." *Given that both of them had a good deal with their cooperative arrangement, why take this further step?*

D. In 1994 Rodrigo said, "I can only be grateful to Dr. Jones and his unselfish commitment to helping Chicanos like myself." In 2000, after graduating from medical school, he condemns Dr. Jones as "a racist exploiter who sought to take advantage of me and the whole Chicano community to help himself alone" and seeks to void the 1994 contract and have Dr. Jones expelled from the county medical society. *Why would he do that?*

ENDNOTES

1. Enrollments and other data are taken from the annual "Medical Education" issue of *Journal of the American Medical Association.*

2. J. Ganem, J. Krakower, and R. Beran, "Review of U.S. Medical School Finances, 1993–1994," *Journal of the American Medical Association*, 274, no. 9 (September 6, 1995): 723–730; Sherry A. Gleid, Ashwin Prabhu, Norman Edelman, "The Cost of Primary Care Doctors," NBER working paper #14568, December 2008.

3. American Association of Medical Colleges, *AAMC Data Book 2002*, tables E1, E4. It is worth noting that whereas the average doctor under age 35 was at least $200,000 in debt, just 10 percent of that debt was for student loans, while 90 percent was for home mortgage, indicating that tuition was not financially burdensome relative to current and expected income; see Lawrence Farber, "How Financially Secure Are Young Doctors?" *Medical Economics* (August 24, 1998): 34–43.

4. Richard Shryock, *Medical Licensing in America, 1650–1965* (Baltimore: Johns Hopkins University Press, 1967); Rosemary Stevens, *American Medicine and the Public Interest* (New Haven, Conn.: Yale University Press, 1971).

5. Rashi Fein, *The Doctor Shortage: An Economic Diagnosis* (Washington: Brookings Institute, 1967).

6. Edward Berkowitz and Wendy Wolf, *Group Health Association: A Portrait of a Health Maintenance Organization* (Philadelphia: Temple University Press, 1988).

7. Erwin Blackstone, "The AMA and the Osteopaths: A Study of the Power of Organized Medicine," *Antitrust Bulletin* (Summer 1977); Jeff Forster, "Remember When Osteopathy Was Called a Cult?" *Medical Economics* (April 27, 1998): 220.

8. Elton Rayack, "The Physicians Service Industry," Chapter 6 in Walter Adams, ed., *The Structure of American Industry*, 5th edition (New York: Macmillan, 1982): 407–408.

9. U.S. Department of Health and Human Services, *Fifth Report to the President and Congress on the Status of Health Personnel in the United States* (Washington, D.C.: U.S. Government Printing Office, 1984).

10. U.S. Department of Health and Human Services, Office of Graduate Medical Education, *Report of the Graduate Medical Education National Advisory Committee to the Secretary, DHHS.* Pub No. 81-651 (Washington, D.C.: U.S. Government Printing Office, 1981). This became widely known as the "GMENAC Report."

11. Richard A. Cooper, Thomas E. Getzen, Heather J. McKee, and Prakash Laud, "Economic and Demographic Trends Signal an Impending Physician Shortage," *Health Affairs* 21, no. 1 (January 2002): 1140–1154.

12. American Medical Association, *Physician Characteristics and Distribution in the U.S., 2002–2003* (Chicago: AMA, 2004).

13. *Health, United States, 2002*, Tables 103, 104 (www.cdc.gov/nchs); Peter Hilsenrath and Fernando Wilson, "Osteopathic Medicine and Physician Supply in the United States," *Journal of Health Care Finance* 35, no. 1 (2008): 34–43.

14. Richard A. Cooper, Thomas E. Getzen, Heather J. McKee, and Prakash Laud, "Economic and Demographic Trends Signal an Impending Physician Shortage," *Health Affairs* 21, no. 1, (January 2002): 1140–1154; Richard Cooper, Thomas Getzen, and Prakash Laud, "Economic Expansion Is a Major Determinant of Physician Supply and Utilization," *Health Services Research* 38, no. 2 (2003): 675–696.

15. Frederick Wolinsky and William Marder, *The Organization of Medical Practice and the Practice of Medicine* (Ann Arbor, Mich.: Health Administration Press, 1985).

16. Uwe Reinhardt, *Physician Productivity and the Demand for Health Manpower* (Cambridge, Mass.: Ballinger, 1974).

17. R. A. Cooper et al., "Current and Projected Workforce of Nonphysician Clinicians," *Journal of the American Medical Association* 280, no. 9 (1988): 788–794; B. G. Druss et al., "Trends in Care by Nonphysician Clinicians in the United States," *New England Journal of Medicine* 348, no. 2 (January 9, 2003): 130–137.

18. Joseph Newhouse, *The Economics of Medical Care* (Reading, Mass.: Addison-Wesley, 1978), 40.

19. Thomas Getzen, "A 'Brand Name' Firm Theory of Medical Group Practice," *Journal of Industrial Economics* 33, no. 2 (1984): 199–215.

20. Helen Clapesattle, *The Doctors Mayo* (Minneapolis: University of Minnesota Press, 1941).

21. Sandy Lutz, "Troubled Times for Psych Hospitals," *Modern Healthcare* 21, no. 50 (December 16, 1991): 26–27, 30–33; and "NME Totals Costs of Psych Woes," *Modern Healthcare* 23, no. 43 (October 25, 1993): 20.

22. Troyen A. Brennan et al., "Health Industry Practices That Create Conflicts of Interest," *Journal of the American Medical Association* 295 (2006): 429–433.

23. Jean M. Mitchell and Jonathan H. Sunshine, "Consequences of Physician's Ownership of Health Care Facilities—Joint Ventures in Radiology," *New England Journal of Medicine* 327 (1992): 1497–1501.

24. Physicians are allowed to buy stocks and make other forms of investments in laboratories, hospitals and medical businesses, but they cannot be partners or get special treatment different from nonphysicians who are not in a position to refer patients.

25. Reuben Kessel, "Price Discrimination in Medicine," *Journal of Law and Economics* 1, no. 2 (October 1958): 20–53.

26. The same process of overcharging for less price-sensitive ancillary items is found when purchasing an automobile, as the dealer puts a larger mark-up on radios, air bags, floor mats, and so on.

27. American Child Health Association, *Physical Defects: The Pathway to Correction* (New York: Author, 1934), pp. 80–96, as cited in David Eddy, "Variations in Physician Practice: The Role of Uncertainty," *Health Affairs* 3, no. 2 (Summer 1984): 74–89.

28. John Wennberg, J. L. Freeman, and W. J. Culp, "Are Hospital Services Rationed in New Haven or Over-Utilised in Boston?" *Lancet I* (May 23, 1987): 1185–1188; John Wennberg, Klim McPherson, and Philip Caper, "Will Payment Based on Diagnosis-Related Groups Control Hospital Costs?" *New England Journal of Medicine* 311, no. 5 (1984): 295–303.

29. Writing Group for the Women's Health Initiative Investigators, "Risks and Benefits of Estrogen Plus Progestin in Healthy Post-menopausal Women," *Journal of the American Medical Association* 288, no. 3 (July 17, 2002): 321–333, (http://jama.ama-assn.org/issues/v288n3/fpdf/joc21036.pdf).

30. David Kindig, *Purchasing Population Health: Paying for Results* (Ann Arbor: University of Michigan Press, 1997).

31. Charles Phelps, "Information Diffusion and Best Practice Adoption," Chapter 5 in A. J. Culyer and J. P. Newhouse, *Handbook of Health Economics* (Amsterdam: Elsevier, 2000), 223–264.

32. David Dranove, *From Marcus Welby to Managed Care, The Economic Evolution of American Health Care* (Princeton, N.J.: Princeton University Press, 2000). Of interest to a health economist, the title of the first Dr. Kildare movie was *Interns Can't Take Money*. The young Dr. Kildare saves the life of a gangster, but as a doctor in training, he is not allowed to be paid for his services. The gangster, not bound by social rules, gives him a small fortune ($1,000), which the impoverished young doctor, acting nobly, returns.

CHAPTER 8

HOSPITALS

QUESTIONS

1. How do hospitals get paid? What do they pay for?
2. Why don't philanthropists donate as much to hospitals as they used to?
3. Does it make a difference to hospitals that 95 percent of their funds come from third-party insurance rather than patients?
4. Who pays for medical research?
5. Does cost-shifting help the poor or the rich?
6. Does tax exemption help hospitals serve the public welfare?
7. Who owns a nonprofit hospital? Who gets the profits?
8. If hospitals are not-for-profit, what do they compete for?
9. Does reimbursement increase employment? Does it drive up costs?
10. Are hospitals still charitable institutions, or have they become instruments of corporate control?

8.1 FROM CHARITABLE INSTITUTIONS TO CORPORATE CHAINS: DEVELOPMENT OF THE MODERN HOSPITAL

The hospital as an institution for the care of the sick has a long and noble history. During the twentieth century, the hospital became the dominant organizational force in health care and the biggest user of health care funds. As the twenty-first century proceeds, hospitals are being replaced or transformed into larger and more complex "health systems" that encompass different modes of care (inpatient, ambulatory centers, home health, nursing homes) spanning multiple sites.[1]

As long as people have gotten sick, society has needed a place to care for them, both to provide special support and to isolate the ill from the rest of the community. In prescientific times, cure was often identified with casting out evil, and hospitals were religious structures. In classical Greece (600 B.C. to 1 A.D.), temples known as *asclepia* took in the sick, especially those who were poor and lacked resources to be cared for at home.[2] Cities used taxes to support hospitals and dispensaries staffed by physicians, who also received fees from those who could afford to pay. The Romans, who created their large-scale hierarchical organizations to rule a vast empire, found it necessary to provide hospitals for the slaves and gladiators who served on plantations or in the military, respectively. The word "hospital" was first used in the twelfth century to refer to a facility run by the church that housed and cared for the sick, the disabled, and the insane, as well as provided lodging for pilgrims and other travelers, orphans, and the poor. Only those who had no homes stayed in hospitals, because everyone else, even if ill, preferred to remain with their families. Economic changes and the great epidemics that came with the expansion of trade greatly increased the need for institutional care. By the end of the thirteenth century, 19,000 hospitals were scattered across Europe. The shift from religious care to scientific cures took place gradually over the next 600 years, but came even more rapidly toward the end of the nineteenth century. Florence Nightingale's work with injured and sick British soldiers during the Crimean War became the basis for her two books, *Notes on Hospitals* (1858) and *Notes on Nursing* (1859), which significantly changed the shape of the hospital and which are still influential today.[3]

Hospitals were founded in 1527 in Mexico and 1635 in Canada, but it was not until 1751 that a hospital was founded in the American colonies. The Pennsylvania Hospital, still a major hospital today, was created by a bill passed in the Assembly with the support of Benjamin Franklin, which obligated the governor to provide £2,000 to match £2,000 in public donations for construction.[4] Philadelphia already had an almshouse and quarantine hospitals (temporary housing for sailors and others with contagious diseases), but the new building was slated to be a more grand and permanent edifice that would promote science as well as provide care. The six physicians who worked twice a week without pay were selected because they were outstanding and were mostly trained abroad. Other notable early American hospitals were the New York hospital chartered by King George III in 1771 to provide care for the sick poor and instruction to medical students of the Columbia Medical School, and the Massachusetts General Hospital built in 1821 at a cost of more than $100,000, an imposing structure superior to the European hospitals of that time and the first to have indoor plumbing. American hospitals were based on the model of the British and Continental voluntary hospitals. However, the American hospitals were more likely to have paying patients who tended to be charged extra to subsidize care for the poor.[5]

These three important hospitals still exist, but the economics of hospital operations have changed drastically. In the eighteenth and nineteenth centuries, most funding came from donations, with patient fees playing a minor role, and insurance reimbursement was nonexistent. The major category of expenditure was food, and the work of the staff was supplemented by making patients labor alongside employees cleaning, cooking, and nursing. Today "hotel costs" (room, meals) account for less than 10 percent of hospital expenditures, and it is impossible to imagine making patients work alongside doctors and nurses. The colonial hospitals were similar to most modern hospitals in that they were nonprofit institutions run by volunteer governing boards, with medical care directed and conducted by physician staff members who were not paid by the hospital but were in private practice as independent businesses in the community.

The development of the modern hospital, like the development of medical specialties, was driven by the creation of new technology. With anesthesia and antiseptics making safe surgery possible, a clean and controlled operating suite with skilled assistants became a necessity. The discovery of X-rays made it necessary to acquire access to radiographic equipment. Advances in clinical pathology and chemistry made the laboratory vital for diagnosis. Major capital investment was required to obtain access to all these new technologies. A solo physician practicing alone could not make full use of this new equipment or manage all the specialized technicians who operated it. It was necessary to bring all the patients of many physicians together under one roof, to obtain funding and make effective use of the new technology, and to hire a manager to coordinate the efforts of medical and ancillary staff. An organizational revolution had to take place.[6] Within the custodial institutions that had existed for centuries serving the disabled poor there arose a new type of hospital, a modern organization with sophisticated and expensive equipment to provide scientific cures where middle-class patients wanted to be treated and were willing to pay. The large and uncertain monetary requirements caused a corresponding financial revolution (insurance reimbursement), which further increased demand and made possible the massive flow of funds required to support a technologically sophisticated system of intensive care costing thousands of dollars for each patient.

8.2 HOSPITAL FINANCING: REVENUES

From the founding of The Pennsylvania Hospital in 1751 until the beginnings of Blue Cross in 1929, the primary source of hospital funding was philanthropy from the community, supplemented by patient fees. Since 1940, hospital revenues have grown rapidly, but philanthropy and patient fees have decreased drastically as a percentage of the total. Now the largest sources of payment are Medicare, which provides government funding for the 60 percent of patient days used by the elderly, and health insurance firms shopping for low prices and good information systems to control costs. Around 1960, the dominant payers were nonprofit Blue Cross plans. At that time, these plans were affiliated with various hospital associations. They were designed to reimburse the full cost of patient care, thus allowing hospitals to break even while taking care of the indigent and undertaking whichever new treatments, diagnostic technology, or research they wanted. By 1995, several Blue Cross plans had fallen into bankruptcy. The survivors all started managed care plans to compete with (or complement) their traditional insurance plans. Some, such as the giant Blue Cross of California, have turned themselves into billion-dollar private for-profit firms.[7]

A new financing system had to be created, and re-created again and again, to provide all the new technology and services that Americans wanted. By 2010, 250 times more money was transferred from the pockets of the public into hospital expenses than had been paid at the end of World War II, with an average increase of more than 10 percent a year. Revenue growth slowed substantially in the mid 1990s as managed care took hold, with an increasing share of revenues coming from outpatient services or new business ventures (ambulance, nutrition counseling, home health care). Since 2000, revenue growth has once again accelerated. In 2007, the average community hospital's revenues were around $128 million, receiving over $10,000 for each patient admitted. About 38 percent of revenues came from ambulatory outpatient services. Table 8.1 lists the current sources of hospital revenues.[8]

The first thing to note from Table 8.1 is that it is unlikely and implausible that hospital behavior will be significantly shaped by consumers' decisions based on prices in this environment, as they would be in most markets, because more than 95 percent of revenues come from someone other than the recipient of services.[9] The second important fact to note is that the "someone else" is likely to be the government, which accounts for almost 60 percent of all revenues. The next thing to realize is that these are complex contracts for hundreds of thousands, even millions of dollars. Although we may talk about "patient revenues" or the "price" of a laboratory test, to actually bring in revenues a hospital chief financial officer (CFO) has to enter an intricate legal relationship with Medicare or a joint venture with a group of radiologists, or structure a risk-sharing arrangement with a consortium of community physicians. Such deals are quite different from retail sales added up at the cash register.

Sources of Revenues

Although a complete picture of hospital revenues is beyond the scope of this book (and indeed beyond the grasp of most economists and accountants and even experienced hospital

TABLE 8.1	Hospital Characteristics, 2007
5,708	Total number of hospitals
4,897	Community hospitals
164	Average number of beds
67%	Occupancy rate
11.4	Admissions per 100 population
5.5 days	Average length of stay
68	ER visits per day
270	Outpatient visits per day
932	Employees
243	RNs
$339	Average cost per outpatient visit
38%	Percent of revenues from outpatients
$1,694	Average cost per adjusted patient day
$128 million	Revenue per hospital
7.4%	Average profit margin

Sources of Funds		Uses of Funds	
Patients self-pay	3%	Labor	53%
Private insurance	36%	Professional fees	5%
Philanthropy, other private	5%	Supplies, other	34%
Medicare	29%	Depreciation and interest	8%
Medicaid	20%		100%
Other government	7%		
	100%		

Source: American Hospital Association, Hospital Statistics 2009, Table 3.

TABLE 8.2

Major Types of Hospital Reimbursement

Philanthropy and grants
Global budgets
Charges
Per diem
Cost reimbursement
DRGs (per admission)
Capitation
Managed care contracts

financial managers—the details, exceptions, exclusions, covenants, and formulas go on forever), an overview of the major ways that revenues flow into hospitals is helpful in grasping the financial incentives they face (see Table 8.2).

Philanthropy and Grants   Grants are funds that are donated for a specific purpose: to conduct cancer research, build a new operating pavilion, provide outreach programs for prenatal care, and so on. Donors want to make sure that funds are used for the purpose intended, but there is little direct pressure to compete on price or to control costs. The program director spends the budget and, if sufficiently good results are achieved in public-relations terms, another grant usually will be forthcoming sometime in the future. This revenue flows from the belief of the donor that the task facing the hospital is important and socially valuable, and is not to make profits or even necessarily to show measurable effects. All nonprofit organizations must begin with a charitable grant. Tax appropriations are a form of grant, with the donor being the government. Tax breaks in the form of relief from property taxes and user fees are even more important to many hospitals these days and have become increasingly controversial.[10]

Global Budgets   A hospital operating under a global budget is getting a grant for all its costs. This form of payment is typical for state mental hospitals, military hospitals, and hospitals run by the Department of Veterans Affairs and other government entities, as well as a few specialized private institutions. Since a global budget is fixed, there are few incentives either to attract more patients or to reduce costs. In Canada, England, and much of the developed world outside the United States, global budgets are the most common form of hospital payment.

Charges   Hospital charges are known as "list prices" in most industries. A hospital, like a flower shop, can set its charges at whatever level it likes. It is rare for a patient, or an insurance company, to actually pay what is "charged." However, these paper charges often form the basis for reimbursement under a system of "discounted charges" (e.g., 60 percent of list price) or under a cost reimbursement system that will be described shortly.

Per Diem   Latin for "per day," per diem payments were common when hospitals originated and are increasingly favored in managed care contracts today. Originally, per diems were charges set by the hospital and usually exceeded costs to help subsidize nonpaying patients. Today per diems are often negotiated with managed care firms under very competitive conditions and are sometimes set below average costs per day in order for a hospital to maintain or increase its market share.

Cost Reimbursement   Cost reimbursement sets the payment level equal to the hospital's audited costs. "Days" and "discharges" are poor measures of the hospital's "product" since they do not account for variations in quality, severity of illness, or use of new technology. Because the hospital's output is so difficult to define and measure, it may be more equitable and easier to reimburse for incurred costs, rather than try to set appropriate prices. The Blue Cross (BC) plans, organized under the aegis of the American Hospital Association, wrote manuals describing how nonprofit hospitals can break even by setting charges to cover costs (including costs for treating nonpaying patients and setting aside money for a prudent reserve) and designed a method of cost reimbursement to break even. This method is known as **ratio of cost to charges applied to charges (RCCAC)**. The RCCAC method is complex in practice but simple in concept: estimate the cost per dollar billed in each department (Emergency, Laboratory, OR, Oncology) and then apply that to all of the bills paid by each type of insurance (Blue Cross, Medicare, Medicaid, etc.) so as to send each insurer one big bill at the end of the year.

When Medicare was created in 1965, it adopted the RCCAC methodology; therefore, this form of cost reimbursement became the dominant method by which funds flowed into hospitals from the 1960s until the mid-1980s. The RCCAC methodology is still used to determine most hospital unit costs today. The RCCAC is calculated separately for each revenue-producing hospital department using this formula:

$$\text{RCCAC Method } BC\ Payment = \frac{\text{Total Department Costs}_{\text{all payers}}}{\text{Total Department Charges}_{\text{all payers}}} \times BC\ Charges$$

Thus, if radiology costs are $6 million and total charges to all payers (i.e., for every insurance company and self-paying patient) are $10 million, the cost-to-charges ratio would be .60, and if BC patients have a total of $3 million in charges, BC would send the hospital a check for .60 × $3 million = $1.8 million as payment for its share of the costs. Although the reimbursement calculation uses charges, the amount paid does not depend on the level of charges. If the hospital doubles its charges (to $20 million), its ratio of cost-to-charges is cut in half (to 0.30), and even though the BC charges are doubled (to $6 million), the reimbursement stays the same.

The complicated RCCAC formula is needed because costs must be divided among different payers who are responsible for the costs of different patients. If there were only one payer, it would pay all costs, and cost reimbursement would be like an open-ended grant. With many payers, however, some way must be found to allocate the costs across patients, and the RCCAC method uses the hospital's billed charges to do so. The method worked very well for a number of years to reimburse hospitals for all their costs. Indeed, it worked so well that costs rose explosively. Costs rose so much that cutbacks became inevitable, causing arguments between hospitals and Medicare over money. Medicare removed the return on invested capital as an "allowable cost" for reimbursement. Extra payments to increase nursing employment and wages were dropped. Charity care and bad debts (resulting from patients who were expected to pay but did not) became a source of contention. Medicare initially accommodated the needs of hospitals by covering as a part of overhead the cost of caring for patients who did not pay. In a subsequent interpretation of the rules, Medicare in effect said, "Since we pay all our bills in full and on time, we are not responsible for those who don't." When charity care and bad debt are not counted as overhead costs distributed across all payers, these charges get included in the RCCAC formula as if they would be paid by someone. This makes the cost-to-charges ratio smaller so that Medicare pays less. This helps the Medicare budget, but not the hospital, which must then increase charges to other payers to make up the difference.

DRGs—Diagnostically Related Groups Diagnostically related group (DRG) payments are fixed payments made based on the patient's diagnosis at discharge. DRG payments cover the complete hospital stay, including all ancillary services (but not surgery and other physician fees). To create this prospective payment system for Medicare payments, the government split all illnesses into 473 DRGs and estimated the cost per case within each group (similar to the resource-based relative value scale [RBRVS] payment system for physician services discussed in Section 6.1). Adjustments are made for these factors: local wages in the area in which the hospital is located, extremely long or short stays, hospitals with large teaching programs, and hospitals with a large proportion of indigent patients. In essence, DRGs are administered prices set by the government at what the government believes is a fair rate. It is called a prospective payment system because the DRG rates are set in advance, unlike the previous retrospective cost reimbursement payments that were continually adjusted to match any change in costs so that the final amount was never set until long after the year ended. Under a charge system, the sellers (hospitals) have the power to set rates arbitrarily—subject to the power of the market to refuse to buy. Under a retrospective cost system, there is no set rate; instead, there is reimbursement of actual costs incurred, perhaps subject to some review. With a DRG prospective payment system, the buyer (Medicare) has all the rate-setting power. In the first year of operation (1983), Medicare did little to force rates down, but in the years since, reimbursement has become progressively tighter; therefore, Medicare patients have become less and less profitable to treat. Once Medicare's DRG system was in place, it was adopted by many other payers.[11]

Capitation Capitation means payment "per person," so that for example a hospital would get paid $120 per month for each person within a group (covered by the plan), and the payment would remain the same amount regardless of how many patients were admitted from the group or how many days they stayed in the hospital (see Chapter 5). Capitation is a relatively rare form of payment for hospitals, since a large and well-defined number of patients must be pooled to reduce risks and make actuarial projections. Once an organization

CASE RATES ADJUSTED FOR SPECIAL SITUATIONS*

Case-mix classification systems are used to determine the amounts that Medicare pays for the hospital inpatient care its beneficiaries receive. These systems include diagnosis-related groups (DRGs) for acute care hospitals, case-mix groups (CMGs) for inpatient rehabilitation facilities (IRFs), and long-term care (LTC)–DRGs (LTC-DRGs) for long-term care hospitals (LTCHs). Payment rates are established prospectively and are expressed on a case or discharge basis, depending primarily on a patient's diagnoses, procedures, and other clinical indicators. To avoid overpayments that may promote early discharge and underpayments that may jeopardize access, Medicare pays additional or reduced amounts in the following situations:

- Short-stay outliers
- Transfers and readmissions
- Patients who die
- High-cost outliers

The total net payment for these situations is budget-neutral—that is, the net amount for these situations translates into a corresponding decrease in the amount available for care rendered under all other circumstances.

Short-Stay Outliers

Some patients have significantly shorter stays than average for their case-mix group. Typically, a short stay costs remarkably less than the corresponding case rate. If the full rate were paid, hospitals would have financial incentives to discharge patients prematurely and would strongly prefer patients who could be discharged quickly to other care settings. In general, Medicare relies on per diem methods to reimburse short stays to align costs and payments more closely. An extra amount may be paid for the first day to acknowledge the disproportionately higher costs associated with the earliest portion of the stay.

For example, for LTCH patients staying no more than five-sixths of the *geometric* average length of stay for the appropriate LTC-DRG, the payment amount equals the lowest of: (1) 120 percent of the estimated cost of the case, (2) 120 percent of the LTC-DRG per diem rate multiplied by the patient's length of stay, or (3) the full LTC-DRG rate. The closer the stay is to the threshold, the more likely the full rate will be the lowest of the three amounts.

For IRF patients who are discharged within three days after being hospitalized, Medicare pays a CMG rate established specifically for short-stay patients. This rate equals about 17 percent of the amount paid for the typical long-stay patient who receives a full course of treatment.

Transfers and Readmissions

A patient may be discharged to another care setting and subsequently readmitted to the discharging hospital. If the intervening period is relatively short and two separate case rates were paid (one each for the discharge and readmission), hospitals would have financial incentives to shift patients around solely to maximize net income. The incentives would be especially alluring if the discharging and receiving facilities were under common ownership or located on the same campus. Medicare makes reduced payments to dilute these incentives.

(Continued)

CASE RATES ADJUSTED FOR SPECIAL SITUATIONS (CONTINUED)

For instance, if an LTCH patient is discharged to an acute care hospital and readmitted to the discharging hospital within nine days, the discharge and readmission is defined as one stay and one LTC-DRG rate is paid to the discharging hospital. The threshold is 27 days for IRFs and 45 days for skilled nursing facilities. In addition, there is a 5 percent cap on the proportion of Medicare patients that hospitals within hospitals, distinct-part skilled nursing facilities, and other co-located facilities may discharge and readmit annually. If the cap is exceeded, each corresponding onsite discharge and readmission is paid as one discharge, including those occurring before the cap was surpassed.

Medicare also pays a reduced amount for an IRF patient whose length of stay exceeds three days but is below the average for his or her CMG and who is discharged to another rehabilitation facility. The reduction assumes that care in one inpatient setting is substituted for care in another inpatient setting. No reduction applies, however, if a patient is discharged to a home health agency on the assumption that this pattern represents a normal progression of care. Payment is based on a per diem rate that includes an extra 50 percent for the first day. Thus, if a patient stays six days and the applicable per diem rate is $900, the payment would be $5,850 = (6 \times $900) + (0.50 \times $900)$.

Patients transferred between acute care hospitals are paid similarly. Medicare pays the transferring hospital on a per diem basis up to the full DRG rate, whereas the receiving hospital that ultimately discharges the patient is paid the full DRG rate. For 10 specific DRGs, an acute care hospital is paid on a per diem basis up to the full DRG rate for Medicare patients who are transferred to a skilled nursing facility or other post-acute-care setting, including an extra amount for the first hospital day.

Patients Who Die

A reduced amount is paid for certain patients who die while hospitalized. For IRFs, there are four distinct CMGs for Medicare patients who stay longer than three days but die before treatment is completed. The case rate varies with the patient's length of stay and whether he or she was hospitalized for an orthopedic condition. Similarly, Medicare pays acute care hospitals a distinct case rate for neonates who die before discharge or are transferred to another facility.

High-Cost Outliers

Additional payments are made for Medicare patients who are extraordinarily costly to treat. The extra amount is determined by multiplying the excess of the estimated cost of treating the patient over a cost threshold by a marginal cost factor. The cost of treating the patient is estimated by multiplying the amount billed for covered services by the facility's cost-to-charges ratio. The threshold equals the DRG rate plus a predetermined "fixed-loss" amount (e.g., $24,450 for LTCHs and $33,560 for acute care hospitals for fiscal year 2003), which reflects the loss a hospital incurs before outlier payments begin. The marginal cost factor is generally 80 percent. Thus, if a hospital's cost-to-charge ratio is 65 percent and billed charges equal $80,000, the estimated cost would be $52,000 = $80,000 \times 0.65$. If the cost outlier threshold is $42,000, the outlier payment would be $8,000 = 0.80 \times ($52,000 - $42,000)$. If the DRG rate is $23,000, the total payment would equal $31,000 = $23,000 + $8,000$.

*This box section on case rate adjustment was prepared by Paul L. Grimaldi, Ph.D., health finance consultant and lecturer, ©2003.

agrees to accept payment on a capitation basis, it in effect becomes a risk-bearing insurer. Usually, when it is said that a hospital is setting up a capitation arrangement, what is really meant is that some larger organization, such as the corporation that controls a number of hospitals, is creating an insurance company/health maintenance organization (HMO) to provide services on a capitated basis. Once the contract extends to multiple institutions and different kinds of care, the hospital becomes a "health system" rather than a traditional community hospital.

Managed Care Contracts   Blue Cross and most private insurance companies are shifting to managed care contracts with hospitals (see Chapter 5). In these arrangements, payment is usually made on the basis of per diems, discounted charges, or a negotiated fee schedule. The crucial difference that sets managed care contracts apart from cost reimbursement or payment of charges is the role of the care manager. Rather than just paying the bills, the insurance company has a specialized **utilization review** (**UR**) nurse or physician critically examine each case to determine, for example, whether hospitalization was justified, a lower cost alternative (such as outpatient surgery) was available, and adequate documentation was provided for all laboratory tests. By negotiating discounts, discouraging use, and denying payment for disallowed or undocumented charges, managed care firms can usually obtain medical care for their clients at a lower cost than traditional indemnity or cost reimbursement insurers and, therefore, are taking over the market. Being constantly questioned and audited has not been easy or pleasant for the doctors who admit patients or for those working in hospital financial departments. Patients also dislike having to justify and obtain approval for every additional service or extra day in the hospital, but they are willing to put up with it if premiums are sufficiently reduced.

8.3   HOSPITAL FINANCING: EXPENSES

Hospitals are personal care institutions, and labor accounts for the bulk of their costs (see Table 8.1). In the early days, food and housing took up most of a hospital's budget, but today such "hotel functions" are relatively minor in comparison with the provision of medical care. Similar to 1750, physician care today is paid for separately and therefore is largely not included in the hospital budget. Few physicians are employees of the hospital, although the services of contracted pathologists, radiologists, and emergency room doctors do show up under the category "professional fees." It might be thought that the acquisition of lithotripters, magnetic resonance imaging (MRI) scanners, and other expensive medical technology would make "equipment" a large category, yet the wages of the skilled people required to operate each new piece of equipment usually runs two or three times the cost of the machinery itself. Much of the category "other" takes the form of services and thus also involves labor hired in the local market. When payroll, professional fees, and local services are added together, about 75 percent of a hospital's costs are labor. This fact makes it politically difficult to cut costs, since the only way to do so is to cut people, by reducing wages or laying off employees. Energy, raw materials, and other goods traded in competitive national and international markets are relatively unimportant in the hospital budget. Access to capital, however, has significantly shaped the growth of health care systems (see Chapter 12).

8.4   FINANCIAL MANAGEMENT AND COST SHIFTING

Revenues must exceed expenses for an organization to survive, but there is no reason that the individuals for whom expenditures are incurred must be the same as the individuals from whom revenues are obtained. Whereas individual matching of benefits and payments is common in most consumer markets, in health care this almost never takes place. For the early hospitals, donations by the wealthy members of the community and general tax funds (paid mostly by landowners) were used to provide services to the sick and poor people with disabilities. Funding and benefits were matched at the level of the community, not the individual. It was considered fair that those who benefited most from the economy should give the most to help those in need. Paying patients who could afford hospitalization were usually charged a bit extra to help support the hospital's charitable mission. In effect, the excess of charges above costs constituted a "hospital tax" on the working-class and upper-class people who happened to get sick.

When hospitals took care of the poor who could not help themselves, it was obvious and necessary that the burden of financing would fall primarily on a different group of people who did have money: philanthropists and taxpayers. As technology advanced and hospital services became more desirable to all people, it was inevitable that there would be a great increase in hospital expenditures and that there would be more overlap between the people who paid and the people who received care. Insurance, pooling funds from the many so that a few could receive care, was a significant extension of financing that furthered the ability of the market to transfer the burden of payment away from the individual who was sick. One of the expenses that was factored into private insurance premiums was charity care; thus, insured patients were also paying for those who had no insurance.

The process of using revenues from one group of clients to subsidize another group is known in health care as **cost shifting**. Under philanthropic funding, all revenues are cost shifted—they are intended as donations to benefit others, not the giver. With insurance and cost reimbursement, the flows are more complex, but it is clear that somebody else is paying for the nonpaying patients (bad debt, charity care) since they do not bring any revenues into the hospital. Several other functions, such as medical education, research, and community outreach, are usually supported through cost shifting, because they bring in very little revenue, certainly less than what they cost to provide.

Financial managers in the early days assumed that the hospital would be a losing proposition and that their job was to find additional revenues from donors, grants, or tax rebates to cover the deficit. Indemnity insurance brought in more funds but did not change the underlying rules. Hospitals were still nonprofit entities, but many now made an excess that could be used to fund growth or extra services. As cost reimbursement came to dominate payment systems, the financial manager's task became more complex but easier. A fully reimbursed hospital was guaranteed to break even and thus could do all the research, education, and outreach it wanted because all costs were fully covered retrospectively. Medicare and Medicaid fundamentally changed the economic status of the hospital by providing coverage for what had previously been charity. As of 1970, the typical hospital faced a reimbursement situation similar to this: at the top, commercially insured patients paid full charges, bringing in about 20 percent more revenue per day than the cost-based Blue Cross and Medicare patients; the indigent Medicaid rate was usually lower; uninsured working patients paid what they could; and charity cases brought in no revenues directly, but did help bolster the hospital's image and its cost reimbursement.

Cost shifting applied to certain services as well as to certain patient groups. Hospitals needed to perform autopsies to help improve the quality of care, but obviously could not bill the patient. Clinical pathologists found it easy to support this scientific need by charging separately for laboratory tests that previously had been included as part of the regular hospital per diem for services. Billing for lab tests met with so little resistance that charges were pushed up and up, and by the 1970s it was not uncommon for a lab to charge ten times what a test cost and to be a major source of excess revenues for subsidizing other parts of the hospital, such as the emergency room, which was a chronic loser. Research programs must conduct extensive tests, keep patients in the hospital for extra days, and perform experimental surgeries that may turn out to be totally useless to perfect techniques and make new discoveries. Since these bills are paid just like any other patient care, research costs are shifted to the insurance company. Also, the bill for a day in the intensive care unit (ICU) is based on the average; thus, the easy cases (since they actually cost less) provide an implicit subsidy for the complex cases and research. Medical education is expensive and usually conducted along with the research that keeps faculties on the cutting edge. Teaching salaries and research equipment are included when calculating the basis for cost reimbursement. Cost per day in a major university hospital is often two to three times that in a small community hospital. Since insurance pays whether the patient gets a broken arm fixed in a local hospital at $1,100 or a university hospital at $3,600, insurance (or rather the employed workers from whom premiums are taken) are paying for most of the research and education expenses.

Cost shifting and cross subsidies are pervasive and long-standing features of medical care reimbursement. In general, hospitals have had public support for taking revenues from a variety of sources and using them to fund not just basic care, but also outreach to indigent people, community prevention programs, research, teaching, and other activities that were seen as being in the public interest. A number of forces have interacted over the past 20 years to cause this consensus on the purpose and funding of hospitals to crumble.

Net income to support research, education, or growth could be obtained either by increasing income or reducing expenses. Growth is difficult to accomplish without increasing expenditures, and thus it is unlikely that managers will concentrate on cuts. Furthermore, there was a general perception in the 1960s and 1970s that health care workers were already underpaid compared with other workers, and there is always a resistance to laying people off. Thus, in the era after 1965, "financial management" came to mean "revenue maximization." The new cost reimbursement rules were very complex and often ambiguous. This left some room for the creative accountant to reclassify, amend, and adjust so that more dollars flowed in. Such financial gamesmanship, along with the inherent expansionary tendencies of cost reimbursement, fueled rapid growth in expenses. Although the number of patients grew only slightly (less than 1 percent a year), the number of employees per patient (full-time equivalent (FTE) per occupied bed) increased from 2.3 in 1960 to 2.5 in 1965, 2.9 in 1970, 3.8 in 1980, 5.5 in 1990, and 8.4 in 2007.[12] Cost control was out, and revenue maximization was in.

The tremendous and unanticipated rise in expenditures for Medicare and Medicaid forced the government to try to modify the reimbursement system to cut costs. Payments for returns on equity capital to investors in for-profit hospitals were eliminated, as was a differential payment for nursing and a number of other minor elements. Yet the basic forces that led to explosive cost increases still remained. Also, although the government could change the rules, hospital financial managers had gained experience in working around the rules and could call on the assistance of consultants from major accounting firms to help them find the most remunerative interpretation or allocation basis. After a series of legislative cost controls attempting to maintain the solvency of the Medicare program failed to work, unpopular premium and tax increases had to be pushed through Congress. Medicare, forced into a corner, began to refuse to pay for the cost of charity care. Medicare claimed that it needed to be a "prudent buyer" and therefore reneged on the fundamental cost-shifting premise.

On one hand, Medicare's decision not to fund charity care and bad debt made sense. The bills of all Medicare patients were being paid in full and on time. Acting as an insurer of people 65 and older, this new interpretation certainly fulfilled its financial obligation to hospitals. On the other hand, hospitals had always charged everybody extra to make up for losses on charity care. Furthermore, it appeared that if anyone should be taking responsibility for the poor, it should be the government. Medicare, by taking a narrow interpretation of its contractual responsibilities, broke up the larger social contract based on cost shifting that had been fundamental to hospitals as caring community institutions. As Medicare ratcheted down its rates, hospitals had to look elsewhere to make up the difference. Whereas charges to commercial insurance companies had been 10 to 15 percent above average cost, the breakdown of cost shifting pushed these "overcharges" up to 20 to 30 percent above cost. The private insurance companies howled in protest as they were forced to pick up what previously had been paid for by general tax funds. The university hospitals, with large indigent populations and big research programs, were in even worse shape than the community hospitals. They had a much smaller fraction of revenues coming from commercial insurance and, to make up for losses, had to raise their commercial rates 50 to 100 percent. The federal and state governments argued that the provision of Medicare and Medicaid had reduced the hospitals' burden of bad debt and charity care, but the large number of people seeking care who were still uninsured made hospitals skeptical.

Small price differentials and a shared sense of purpose made a social contract sufficient to enable cross subsidies in hospitals to continue. Big differentials and a hostile, "I'll pay for mine, and you pay for yours" attitude ruined this consensus. Market forces came into play. The outrageously high prices for tests done in hospital laboratories created a profit opportunity for commercial companies, which started providing services through independent doctor-entrepreneurs, cut prices in half, and still had large profit margins. Specialized psychiatric hospitals that treated only mild cases of mental disorder sprang up, able to make money at a per diem far below that of the inner city psychiatric wards filled with violent and chronically disturbed individuals and staffed by residents more interested in research and understanding the causes of mental illness than in cost-effectiveness of care. Whenever prices are distorted by cross subsidy, there is an opportunity for a firm to make extraordinary profits by **cream skimming**, providing only the services that are overpriced, not the ones that are more costly and subsidized. Tradition and expressions of disapproval were able to limit the extent to which profits were drained from the system by cream skimming prior to 1970. Since then, however, the margins have become too large, and the ideology of health care too fragmented, to keep the old system afloat.

Founded initially on the premise that government and the wealthy would provide for the poor and support research, the social contract of hospitals was so pervasive and unexamined that it is likely that the people who initially brought it under attack had no idea what those efforts might lead to. However, it has subsequently become clear that hospital financial managers, by taking advantage of the system, and Medicare, by refusing to take responsibility for all of America's needy, contributed to the demise of cost shifting. Rapidly rising per diem costs and distortional cross subsidies eventually led to stringent managed care systems in which an insured employee group contracts to pay only for the services its members use. The public understands that it is not possible to "pay your own way" for hospital care and that risk pooling through insurance is required. The collapse of cost shifting forces us now to confront the question of who will pay for the poor and who will pay for medical research. Although there is a general recognition that caring for the poor and paying for research will cost something, the public seriously underestimates how large that bill will be because of the cost shifting that has gone on for so many years. Most of the income in the United States is earned by employed people between the ages of 30 and 60. This generally healthy group, whose wealth is increasing, makes up less than a third of the population. Paying for the other two-thirds, and for all the medical advances working people want, will require transfers of billions and billions of dollars. We are in the process of giving up on the old system of transferring funds, but have not been able to find and agree on a new one.[13]

8.5 HOW DO HOSPITALS COMPETE?

The flow of revenues into a hospital follows the flow of patients. In some cases, such as emergency room or outpatient clinic visits, patients themselves decide where to go, and for these types of care, hospitals compete directly by trying to attract patients. However, for most care the decision regarding hospitalization is made by the physician. The agency relationship changes the nature of the transaction, so that the patient follows the advice of the physician and, therefore, the hospitals compete for doctors. If the ability to decide on hospitalization is taken out of the doctor's hands by the insurance company, as it sometimes is under managed care (see Chapter 5), then hospitals must compete for contracts and appeal to payers, which usually forces a hospital to put more emphasis on lowering prices. The important point is that the hospital must compete for the contracting party that has the power to make the revenues come to them, not necessarily for the patient.

Quality is the most important aspect of medical care, and hospitals such as Johns Hopkins and Massachusetts General have an edge over the competition because of their reputation for outstanding care and scientific prowess. Regardless of whether the final decision-making power lies in the hands of the patient, the physician, or the payer, all of them must be satisfied, and quality is usually the most important concern. It is difficult to convince patients to go to a hospital they are not familiar with, for doctors to give up control by transferring patients to a specialized facility where they are not on the medical staff, and for insurers to pay extra for admission to a facility where they do not have a contract guaranteeing discounts, yet each of these accommodations becomes easier to make when some accepted expert authority has rated this unfamiliar hospital as "the best."

Competing for Patients

The types of care for which patients make their own decisions are those in which they are able to judge important aspects of quality and in which they pay a large share of cost directly out of their own pockets. Maternity care is a good example. Many mothers want to have their babies close to home, have strong preferences regarding patient services (natural childbirth, religious orientation, attitude of staff), and can get good information for comparing hospitals by talking to other mothers in the neighborhood. Since the need for care is known months in advance, potential parents can do the kind of comparison shopping that is impossible to do after accidents or heart attacks. Also, the fact that births are expected means that they are not "risks" in the insurance sense and, therefore, frequently are reimbursed on a shared or fixed-price basis that leaves much of the marginal cost to the parents. For these reasons, hospitals must actively compete for patients on the basis of price and service. Casual investigation reveals a number of special deals, from free baby clothes, gourmet meals, and a postpartum vacation to cut-rate "fixed-price packages," not unlike the competition for selling cars and houses. Outpatient clinics, where patients are more likely to self-refer and where cost sharing is usually higher, also use marketing strategies such as nice waiting rooms, receptionists who call to make or remind patients about appointments, free transportation to the clinic, and deductible or copayment waivers. The rise of "preferred provider" plans (see Chapter 5) that provide full coverage only for a limited group of hospitals has also increased the importance of direct marketing to patients.

Increasing competition by making more information on price and quality available to patients has generated considerable interest. However, most of the "report card" efforts directed at consumers have shown little impact. Indeed, it appears that patients are more sensitive to superficial differences in amenities (good food, attentive staff, pleasant surroundings) than to significant differences in mortality rates, surgical qualifications, or charges.[14]

Competing for Physicians

The agency relationship and control over admissions means that most hospital competition is over doctors rather than over patients. Recruitment incentives are a very visible sign of such competition. Income guarantees (e.g., if you come to hospital X, and your income in the first year is less than $125,000, we will make up the difference), relocation assistance, and promises of referrals from other doctors on the medical staff are common contractual provisions. Sometimes there is even a "signing bonus" similar to what a professional athlete might receive. As Mark Pauly's "doctor's workshop" model suggests, hospitals also compete by helping physicians earn more money in their private practices by providing free or subsidized office space; providing secretarial, phone, and billing services; setting aside 10 beds for nephrology or another specialty so that the specialist will always be able to admit a patient; and so on.[15] Reducing practice costs or work effort is a limited competitive tool. Far more important is that the hospital help a physician build his or her practice through the hospital's reputation for quality and the technological sophistication of services offered.[16] A cardiologist is able to attract more patients if he or she is the only cardiologist in town who has access to a catheterization lab that does stents, or percutaneous transluminal coronary angioplasty (PTCA), or a newer development in vein obstruction removal. In some instances, such competition can lead to a sort of "**medical arms race**," in which nearby hospitals each try to be the first with the most and respond strategically. For example, if one hospital gets an MRI scanner, the other one gets one that is bigger; if one gets a lithotripter, the other gets one that has more settings and finer resolution; and so on. It is possible that competing on the basis of which hospital has the most new technology can lead to inefficiencies and escalating costs, with the two scanners and two lithotripters empty half the time because there are only enough patients in the market to keep one piece of equipment operating at full capacity. This points out one of the major problems of hospital markets structured on the basis of competing for physicians to increase patient flow. A hospital has an incentive to subsidize office space to attract physicians, but not to reduce charges to patients, change billing practices, or make trade-offs that lead to overall reductions in the cost of medical care. The competition for physicians does not necessarily push hospitals toward an efficient use of inputs or mix of services.

Competing for Contracts

The scale on which medical practice is conducted is increasing. When organized on the basis of atomistic transactions between individuals, the choice of hospital falls to the doctors acting as agents for the patients under their care. However, it has become more and more common for a payer to make contracts directly with hospitals, negotiating a fixed or discounted price, and limiting patients to hospitals with which the payer has a contract. Payers can direct patient flow even when contracts are not fully binding. Although Medicare has a contract with every hospital, it will allow heart transplants only in certain approved facilities, and in a request for proposals to become an approved provider, price is a factor. Health maintenance organizations (HMOs) can be even more aggressive, sometimes threatening to transfer a

TABLE 8.3	Competition between Hospitals
Hospitals Compete for	**On the Basis of Quality and**
Patients	Amenities, out-of-pocket $$
Doctors	Technology, practice assistance
Contracts	Price, information systems

large group of patients to a rival facility unless negotiations result in a substantial discount or making approval conditional on assurances that the HMO will receive the lowest price the hospital gives to any contractor.

Although managed care contracting at this level is a relatively recent development, structurally it bears a resemblance to the original social contract between the hospital and the community and to the agreements under which hospitals receive tax subsidies and other favorable treatment from the government. In each of these contracts, there are two parties: the hospital and a representative of consumers as a group (community, insurance plan, taxpayers). Such large-scale arrangements are inevitably less accommodating to the needs of individual patients and the professional autonomy of physicians. However, any attempt to implement public accountability and successful cost control involves compromises. Trade-offs are necessary in any system that takes its broader social responsibilities seriously and are the core concept for creating economic efficiency in health care (see Table 8.3).

Measuring Competitive Success

How can it be determined which hospitals are more successful in the competition for patients? A firm that has failed by going out of business is clearly not successful, and economists have used "survivor analysis" to measure competitive success by counting the number of new entrants or exits (bankruptcy, takeover) within different categories. Survivor analysis has been used to show that hospitals with fewer than 100 or more than 500 beds appear to be inefficient and less able to compete.[17] Such analysis has also shown that for-profit hospitals are not necessarily more efficient or better competitors than nonprofits (the number of for-profit hospitals has fluctuated, but these hospitals accounted for around 10 to 20 percent of total bed supply throughout the twentieth century, indicating competitive performance that is about average). A hospital that has grown relative to its competitors is clearly more successful, and such traditional measures as total assets, market share, and geographic spread have been used as indicators. With 90 percent of hospitals operated by either voluntary (charitable and/or religious) or government organizations, profits are less useful as a measure of success than they are in other industries. However, the excess of revenues over expenditures is available to fund growth and is necessary to avoid bankruptcy, and thus it can be a useful indicator. In the current environment, with many hospitals trying to form chains or acquire physician practices to cover a larger area and offer a full line of services for managed care contracting, strong earnings and large financial reserves clearly provide a competitive advantage.

What has proven almost impossible to measure is the success of a hospital in achieving its goals as a provider of health care to the community. Although charity care, participation in outreach programs, and mortality rates are often monitored and commented on, there is general agreement that these are incomplete and inadequate measures at best, and are frequently misleading. Attempts are being made to assess community benefit in more comprehensive and objective ways, but there is as yet no reason to believe that these will be any more convincing than previous efforts.[18] Economists and other policy makers are in the awkward position of recognizing that they know which dimensions are most important (quality, compassion, technological advances), but they do not how to gauge them numerically or even how to make a fair comparison between hospitals.

Measuring the Competitiveness of Markets

Competition can be a significant factor in forcing hospitals to become more efficient and provide better services.[19] However, a single hospital in a rural area or a chain that controls almost all the hospitals in an urban market is not constrained by competition. The potential loss of consumer welfare due to a merger or acquisition that reduces the amount of competition is the central concern of the Federal Trade Commission (FTC) and a source of much litigation under antitrust law. This litigation provides many consulting projects for economists called in to testify as expert witnesses on how competitive a particular market is or will be. Competition is usually measured by the number of hospitals or concentration of market share in a geographic area (e.g., within a 15-mile radius; within a city, county, or metropolitan statistical area) or by the overlap between hospital services (how many patients use several hospitals). Although the complexities of antitrust law and the economic assessment of competition policy are beyond the scope of this text, it is worth noting that all hospitals are multiproduct firms. The relevant market for services such as liver transplant, residential psychiatric care, and abortion, therefore, covers a large area because patients are willing to travel hundreds of miles for treatment, whereas the market for other services such as kidney dialysis, outpatient psychiatry, and prenatal care depend on patients living nearby, and hence is much smaller. After decades of being exempt or ignored, hospitals have come under increasing scrutiny by the FTC, and antitrust enforcement is now considered an important alternative to regulation as a means of controlling costs.

8.6   ORGANIZATION: WHO CONTROLS THE HOSPITAL AND FOR WHAT ENDS?

The standard model firm in a microeconomics textbook is an organization created by the owners, who invest time and money, to make a profit. To do so, the firm must meet the needs of customers who pay for the firm's products and the needs of employees and other vendors who get paid by the firm to supply inputs. By the fundamental theorem of exchange, each party must benefit for the organization to continue to exist. The customers get consumers' surplus from purchasing products they prefer in terms of price or quality to those of other firms; the employees get jobs they prefer in terms of wages or conditions; and the owners take home as profits the value added by organizing a firm. The owners are known as "residual claimants" because they get what is left over, profits (or losses), a net residual difference between revenues and expenses. A firm operates as a rational economic organization because the owners who make the decisions must bear the consequences, whether good (profits) or bad (losses). The linkages among owners, employees, and customers usually have some slack in the real world, which gets assumed away in textbook models of perfect competition. Corporate "agency theory" (see Section 12.4) deals with the implications of raising capital through the stock market, which separates ownership (stockholders) from control (managers).[20] To the extent that managers are not perfect agents of the owners, they may dissipate or capture some of the firm's profits by purchasing inputs from favored relatives, having big offices, not taking enough risks, or not working hard enough. Such deviations from profit maximization may change the firm's behavior, as can taxes, regulations, social conditions, ideology, culture, and political constraints.

Hospitals differ from the standard firm in three significant ways:

- Patients do not pay because of insurance or charity.
- Ownership is usually unclear because of nonprofit voluntary or governmental organization.
- Medical care is largely controlled by doctors, who neither pay nor receive any money from the hospital and, therefore, have no direct connection from a financial perspective.

Doctors are neither customers nor employees nor owners, but in practice they are the dominant voice in hospital operations; therefore, they sometimes look like they are all three. This structure—combining power, money, and service with no direct line of control or financial accountability—is a unique form of economic organization that makes it difficult to model or predict the behavior of hospitals. A hospital does not do anything without directions from a physician; only physicians are allowed to admit patients, perform surgery, or prescribe drugs. The hospital organizes a medical staff, but some claim that the reality is the other way around: that the medical staff organizes a hospital as its workshop. This is the basis of Mark Pauly's model of the hospital as the doctor's workshop, which hypothesizes that the hospital will behave to maximize the profits of the doctors who are on staff, rather than to maximize the profits of the organization (see Chapter 6).[21] Joseph Newhouse has pointed out that hospitals are nonprofit organizations with no owners who can claim the profits, and he suggests that hospitals and other nonprofit organizations are run for the benefit of managers.[22] Managers want their hospitals to be the biggest and the best, which, not incidentally, justifies the highest managerial salaries and hence maximizes some combination of quantity and quality of services rather than profits or doctors' incomes. Employees are also important stakeholders, but because their importance derives from being input suppliers, their influence in hospitals is not much different from their influence in other organizations. Most hospital mission statements claim that their primary concern is patient care, yet this sort of general assertion does not address the method by which prices are set, the trade-off between one group of patients and another (e.g., surgery or immunization, abortion or family planning clinics), or the trade-offs between employees and doctors. The American Hospital Association maintains that hospitals are, in essence, public institutions whose purpose is to benefit the community. From a financing perspective, this makes sense, because most of the capital investment in a voluntary hospital comes from the community in the form of charitable donations and taxes. The problem is: how is community benefit defined and who, exactly, exercises control?[23] The board, although in theory representing the community, is often deferential to the medical staff and depends on the information provided by the administration to make decisions (see Table 8.4 and Chapter 12).

Despite a considerable amount of theoretical and empirical work by economists and a clear recognition that insurance, nonprofit status, and medical control over admissions and treatment make hospitals different, no truly satisfactory theory of the hospital as a distinct type of organization has been developed. Research has shown that nonprofit hospitals are more likely to serve the urban poor and provide unprofitable services (immunization, prenatal care, emergency rooms, drug detoxification), whereas for-profits are more likely to charge higher prices, locate facilities in growing suburbs where patients have higher incomes and better insurance, and emphasize high-margin procedures (diagnostic radiology, invasive cardiology).[24] However, the differences are usually small. In part, this may result from the fact that competition and the pressure to survive forces a hospital to maximize revenues and minimize costs much like a for-profit firm. The greater the amount of debt,

TABLE 8.4

Who Gets the Profits from a
Nonprofit Hospital?

Doctors?
Administrators?
Employees?
Patients?
Community?

the more pressure a hospital faces, and any deviation from profit-maximizing behavior becomes a threat to survival. The lack of substantial differences might also result from social expectations that force for-profit hospitals to meet the standards of community benefit and medical professionalism to attract patients. An area with mostly nonprofit hospitals seems to have for-profits behaving more like nonprofits, and conversely in an area dominated by for-profit hospitals the nonprofits appear more overtly commercial. Although all general acute hospitals seem to behave in similar ways, it is possible to discern a continuum, with for-profits at one end being more aggressive and quick to respond to incentives, government hospitals at the other end being a bit more inflexible and committed to public service, and voluntary nonprofits occupying the broad middle ground. The large hospitals that do most of the teaching and research are almost always nonprofit institutions. The range of behavior resulting from differences in hospital ownership category is fairly narrow, and it is outweighed by differences related to mission, size, teaching status, and local factors.

SUGGESTIONS FOR FURTHER READING

American Hospital Association, Hospital Statistics and Hospital Guide is published annually.
David M. Cutler, ed., The Changing Hospital Industry: Comparing Not-for-Profit and For-Profit Institutions (Chicago: University of Chicago Press, 2000).
Modern Healthcare and Hospitals and Health Networks are biweekly magazines covering the hospital industry in depth.
Rosemary Stevens, In Sickness and In Wealth: American Hospitals in the Twentieth Century (New York: Basic Books, 1989).
Burton Weisbrod, The Nonprofit Economy (Cambridge Mass.: Harvard University Press, 1988), and "Rewarding Performance That Is Hard to Measure: The Private Non-Profit Sector," Science (May 5, 1989): 541–546.

SUMMARY

1. The Pennsylvania Hospital, founded in 1751, was the first hospital in the United States. Like most **early hospitals**, it was **funded primarily by charitable donations and government** tax appropriations and **housed the sick and poor** people with disabilities, although some paying patients were admitted.

2. The development of **new technology** created the need for a central facility where the **capital cost** of equipment could be shared by many doctors and where dangerous surgical procedures could be performed in a more controlled and supportive environment.

3. More than **95 percent of all hospital revenues come from third parties**, with more than half coming from **government** through the Medicare and Medicaid programs. Patients pay so little of the hospital bill that **charges are almost irrelevant in decision making**. Although cost-based reimbursement using the ratio-of-cost-to-charges-applied-to-charges RCCAC formula developed by Blue Cross plans under the aegis of the American Hospital Association was the major form of payment from 1965 to 1985, since then the prospective DRG per case payments and a variety of managed care plans have become the main sources of revenues. Approximately one-third of

hospital revenues come from outpatient services, and an increasing amount comes from home health, long-term care, and other related services.

4.   Hospitals obtain revenues in a variety of ways, including **philanthropy** and grants, **global budgets**, billed **charges**, per day **(per diem)** payments, **DRG** per case payments, **cost reimbursement**, and **managed care contracts**.

5.   **Labor** is the largest category of health care expenditure. When employees of local service firms are included, personnel accounts for more than 75 percent of a hospital's costs. Therefore, the only way to cut costs is to reduce wages or reduce employment, neither of which is politically popular. **Doctors are usually independent contractors** paid separately by the patient and thus do not show up as a large item on hospital budgets, even though they play a dominant role in providing and directing care.

6.   **Cost shifting** is the process of charging one group (e.g., commercially insured patients) more to cover the loss due to undercharging another group (indigent patients, Medicaid). The pervasiveness of cost shifting and insurance coverage gave financial managers far more room to raise revenues as a means of supporting the hospital and little incentive to find efficiencies that would reduce costs. **Cream skimming** is the action of taking on only the profitable patients for whom services are priced considerably above unit costs, while avoiding the loss-making patients with heavy care needs. Changes in Medicare reimbursement and the advent of managed care firms that shop to obtain hospital services at the lowest possible price have eroded the ability of hospitals to cross subsidize and have made it difficult to support research, teaching, and charity care.

7.   **Hospitals compete for physicians**, because physicians control the flow of patients (and hence, revenues). Unlike most businesses, hospitals do not compete directly for "customers" because their customers (a) do not pay their own bills and (b) do not make their own choices, but are directed by physicians who act as their agents. Only for some patient-initiated or relatively uninsured services is direct competition important for patients (plastic surgery, childbirth). Larger scale and cost pressures are causing hospitals to compete for contracts, trying to attract employees, HMOs, or insurance companies directly. To do so, they must compete more and more on the basis of price rather than quality.

8.   Hospitals differ from most firms in that they are largely paid for by third parties, are often **nonprofit organizations** directed by volunteer boards rather than owners and **dominated by doctors, independent professionals** who work for themselves with no direct financial ties to the hospital. Despite much research and lots of theoretical expectations, there appear to be only slight differences among voluntary not-for-profit, government, and private for-profit hospitals. In general, for-profits appear to be somewhat less likely to take on charity care, research, teaching, and outreach and to react more quickly to changes in reimbursement regulations, with government hospitals at the other extreme and voluntary hospitals falling in the middle, but any differences are small and occur only occasionally.

PROBLEMS

1.   {*industrial organization*} Which technological, organizational, and financial innovations caused the rise of hospitals in the twentieth century?

2.   {*incidence*} Who pays for most of the care in hospitals? Are the people who pay the bills the same as the people who receive the care?

3. {*flow of funds*} Which input accounts for the largest portion of hospital costs? Which input is responsible for most of the growth in hospital cost per patient day?

4. {*payment methodology*} Both Hospital A and Hospital B are paid by Medicare using the DRG methodology. Assume that the reimbursement for the average Medicare patient (case weight of 1.0) is $2,600. Hospital A has an average case-mix index of 1.32 and admits 24 patients who stay in the hospital a total of 192 days, whereas Hospital B has an average case-mix index of 0.95 and admits 35 patients who stay in the hospital a total of 238 days. Which hospital gets paid more? Which hospital gets paid more per case? Which hospital gets paid more per diem? Which hospital gets paid more for an appendectomy (case weight of 0.85)?

5. {*flow of funds*} Over the past 100 years, the major source of hospital revenues has changed three times. Name these types of payments, and explain why each one gave way to the next.

6. {*payment*} If a hospital decides to raise prices because it needs more money, what effect does this have on the following:
   a. Patients who pay their own bills?
   b. Patients whose bills are paid by an insurance company?
   c. Hospitals with insurance contracts that reimburse on the basis of costs?
   d. Hospitals with previously negotiated per diem contracts with HMOs?

7. {*cost shifting*} Is the mark-up (ratio of prices to direct per unit costs) relatively constant across different types of hospitals? Are mark-ups the same for different services or departments within a hospital?

8. {*cost shifting*} How do hospitals pay for medical research?

9. {*ownership*} Are doctors usually employees, owners, or managers of hospitals?

10. {*ownership*} Who owns most hospitals? Who gets the profit when a nonprofit hospital makes money? Can nonprofit hospitals be bought and sold?

11. {*rate of return, incidence*} How does a philanthropist who donates funds to a hospital get "returns on capital"? Are these returns measured as a dollar amount, as an annualized percentage rate, or by some other method?

12. {*competition*} Wills Eye Hospital in Philadelphia is a 114-bed hospital specializing in ophthalmologic surgery. Who do you think competes with Wills Eye?

13. {*competition*} Describe the factors you would expect to be most important in competition for patients for each of the following services. For which services is price more important? Location? Quality? Would hospitals compete for patients or for doctors?
   a. Heart transplants
   b. Maternity
   c. Immunization
   d. Depression
   e. Chemotherapy
   f. Plastic surgery
   g. AIDS

14. {*cost shifting*} What does it mean for Medicare to act as a "prudent buyer" of hospital services? Does doing so strengthen or weaken Medicare as a social insurance program?

15. *{cost shifting}* What adjustments would a hospital have to make if it began to serve a larger number of indigent patients? Would most of the adjustments come on the revenue side or the expenditure side?

16. *{cost shifting}* Who benefits from cost shifting: the poor or the rich? Do any health care workers benefit from cost shifting?

ENDNOTES

1. Paul Starr, *The Social Transformation of American Medicine* (New York: Basic Books, 1992); Rosemary Stevens, *In Sickness and in Wealth: American Hospitals in the Twentieth Century* (New York: Basic Books, 1989).
2. George Rosen, *A History of Public Health, New York* (New York: MD Publications, 1958).
3. Florence Nightingale, *Notes on Nursing: What It Is, and What It Is Not* (New York: Appleton-Century, 1938).
4. Charles Lawrence, *History of the Philadelphia Almshouses and Hospitals from the Beginning of the Eighteenth to the Ending of the Nineteenth Centuries* (Philadelphia: C. Lawrence, 1905).
5. Marshall K. Raffel and Norma K. Raffel, *The U.S. Health System: Origins and Functions*, 4th ed. (Albany, N.Y.: Delmar, 1994).
6. An illustrative case study is found in the history of the Mayo clinic. See Helen Clapesattle, *The Doctors Mayo* (Minneapolis: University of Minnesota Press, 1941); Gunther W. Nagel, *The Mayo Legacy* (Springfield, Ill.: Charles C. Thomas, 1966); and compare with an annual report of the Mayo Clinic (now operating in Arizona and Florida as well as Minnesota) in the 1990s.
7. J. Hermann, "Blue Cross of California goes for the Gold-Wellpoint Health Networks," *Health Systems Review* 26, no. 3 (May/June 1993): 14–19; T. Kertesz, "California Blue Cross Tries Again With Bigger Foundation Plan," *Modern Healthcare* 25, no. 16 (April 17, 1995): 2–3.
8. American Hospital Association, *Hospital Statistics* (Chicago: American Hospital Association, 2002).
9. Prices paid by patients are even less important than Table 8.1 would suggest, since much of the 3 percent is actually deductibles, copayments, and other charges that are in effect insurance premiums or taxes and not directly related to the prices of the services chosen.
10. Some legislators argue that hospitals are no longer providing the charitable public services for which they were founded, and hence do not deserve help, and that public funds should be redirected toward community programs or inner-city hospitals. The City of Philadelphia, for example, has forced local hospitals to pay millions of dollars under its PILOTs/SILOTs program (Payments/Services In Lieu of Taxes). A hospital is assessed an amount equal to its tax liability, and then must document provision of services provided without compensation of an equal amount or pay the city the difference.
11. State Medicaid plans used the DRG system but generally paid few dollars for each patient. In time, this underpayment led to complaints and a series of lawsuits. Temple University Hospital sued the state of Pennsylvania under the "Boren Amendment" to the Social Security Act, which obligated states to make payments sufficient to cover the cost of efficiently provided services. The hospital eventually won—creating a precedent that hospitals around the country quickly followed (and that forced state budgets into deficits). Hence, although in concept a charge system gives all the power to the seller, and an administered price system (like DRGs) gives all the power to the buyer, in reality both sides are at least to some extent constrained by the political process and public opinion.
12. American Hospital Association, *Hospital Statistics*, various years.
13. Henry J. Aaron and Robert D. Reischauer, "The Medicare Reform Debate: What Is the Next Step?" *Health Affairs* 14, no. 4 (Winter 1995): 8–30.
14. Dana Goldman and John Romley, "Hospitals as Hotels: The Role of Patient Amenities in Hospital Demand," NBER working paper #14619, December 2008; Mark W. Legnini et al., "Where Does Performance Measurement Go from Here?" *Health Affairs* 19, no. 3 (2000): 173–177; P. S. Romano and H. Zhou, "Do Well-Publicized Risk-Adjusted Outcomes Reports Affect Hospital Volume? *Medical Care* 42, no. 4 (2004): 367–377; Michael Rothberg et al., "Choosing the Best Hospital: The Limitations of Public Quality Reporting," *Health Affairs* 27, no. 6 (2008): 1680–1687.
15. Mark Pauly and Michael Redisch, "The Not-for-profit Hospital as a Physicians Cooperative," *American Economic Review* 63 (1973): 87–99; Mark V. Pauly, *The Doctor's Workshop* (Philadelphia: University of Pennsylvania Press, 1980).
16. H. Luft, J. Robinson, D. Garnick, S. Maerki, and S. McPhee, "The Role of Specialized Clinical Services in the Competition Among Hospitals," *Inquiry* 23, no. 1 (1986): 83–94.
17. Carson W. Bays, "The Determinants of Hospital Size: A Survivor Analysis," *Applied Economics* 18 (1986): 359–377.

18. Robert Sigmond and J. David Seay, "Community Benefit Standards for Hospitals: Perception and Performance," *Frontiers of Health Services Management* (Spring 1989).

19. Jean M. Abraham, Martin S. Gaynor, and William B. Vogt, "Entry and Competition in Local Hospital Markets," NBER working paper #11649, September 2005.

20. Michael C. Jensen and William H. Meckling, "Theory of the Firm: Managerial Behavior, Agency Costs and Ownership Structure," *Journal of Financial Economics* 3 (1976): 305–360.

21. Mark V. Pauly, *Doctors and Their Workshops: Economic Models of Physician Behavior* (Chicago: University of Chicago Press, 1980).

22. Joseph Newhouse, "How Do Hospitals Make Choices?" in *The Economics of Medical Care* (Reading, Mass.: Addison-Wesley, 1978), 68–73.

23. Robert Sigmond and J. David Seay, "Community Benefit Standards for Hospitals: Perceptions and Performance," in "The Future of Tax-Exempt Status for Hospitals" issue of *Frontiers of Health Services Management* (Spring 1989).

24. E. R. Becker and Frank Sloan, "Hospital Ownership and Performance," *Economic Inquiry* 23, no. 1 (1985): 21–36; Deborah Freund et al., "Analysis of Length-Of-Stay Differences Between Investor-Owned and Voluntary Hospitals," *Inquiry* 22, no. 1 (1985): 33–44; Mark Schlesinger, Theodore Marmor, and R. Smithey, "Non-Profit and For-Profit Medical Care," *Journal of Health Politics, Policy and Law* 12, no. 3 (1987): 427–457; Sujoy Chakravarty, Martin Gaynor, Steven Klepper, and William B. Vogt, "Does the Profit Motive Make Jack Nimble? Ownership Form and the Evolution of the U.S. Hospital Industry," NBER working paper #11705, October 2005; Jill R. Horwitz and Austin Nichols, "What Do Nonprofits Maximize? Nonprofit Hospital Service Provision and Market Ownership Mix," NBER working paper #13246, July 2007; Jill Horwitz, "Making Profits and Providing Care: Comparing Nonprofit, For-profit and Government Hospitals," *Health Affairs* 24, no. 3 (2005): 790–801; J. Silverman and J. Skinner, "Medicare Upcoding and Hospital Ownership," *Journal of Health Economics* 23, no. 2 (2004): 369–389; Hsien-Ming Lien, Shin-Yi Chou, and Jin-Tan Liu, "Hospital Ownership and Performance: Evidence from Stoke and Cardiac Treatment in Taiwan," *Journal of Health Economics* 27 (2008): 1208–1223.

CHAPTER 9

MANAGEMENT AND REGULATION OF HOSPITAL COSTS

QUESTIONS

1. Why do some hospitals cost more than others?

2. The number of patients and the number of days each patient spends in the hospital has gone down. Why have hospital costs continued to increase faster than other health care costs?

3. Are large hospitals expensive because they suffer from diseconomies of scale, or because they admit the most difficult-to-treat patients?

4. Why would a hospital want to buy a new magnetic resonance imaging (MRI) scanner if it expects the MRI to be busy only half the time and the hospital next door already has such a machine?

5. Will computers and other new technology improve efficiency and hence reduce costs, or will they improve quality and hence raise costs?

6. Has regulation cut costs or cut competition?

9.1 WHY DO SOME HOSPITALS COST MORE THAN OTHERS?

The cost of a day in the hospital can be as little as $400 or more than $4,500. Which factors could account for such a wide variation? It is not surprising if a day in the hospital costs $4,500 for a critically wounded trauma patient in an intensive care unit (ICU) and just $400 for a patient resting after breaking a leg while skiing.[1] The ICU patient is much sicker and requires more complex services. It is also understandable that staying in one of the nation's top research and teaching hospitals under the care of famous doctors can cost more than staying in a small rural facility with limited equipment and staff.[2] The hospital bill can be a misleading guide to costs. One hospital may charge more but give every patient a discount, while another sticks to list prices. One hospital could charge $400 for the bed, with extra charges for medication, laboratory tests, physical therapy, and so on, while another hospital charges $900 for the bed and all other services, making it less expensive (see Table 9.1).

It is often assumed that a hospital with a lower cost per patient day is more efficient, but such a conclusion is only justified if the comparison hospital provides the same services

TABLE 9.1	Reasons for Differences in Hospital Costs

Severity of patient's illness
Quality of care
Intensity of services (e.g., number of nursing hours or lab tests)
Cost shifting to pay for research and teaching
Differences in billing
Prices of labor and other inputs
Efficiency

to similar patients under similar conditions. Unless this ceteris paribus (all other things constant) assumption is valid, which it rarely is, efforts must be made to adjust for all the other factors listed in Table 9.1 to compare costs. Of course, patients and their insurance companies prefer a cheaper stay in the hospital to a more expensive stay if all other factors are constant. If not, the more relevant question is: Is a hospital that costs 10 percent more (or 20 percent, or 400 percent) really worth that much more? Although this relative value question is more meaningful, it is also much more difficult to answer, and the answer depends on the patient's values as well as calculations of technical efficiency. Therefore, it is useful to look first at the simpler and more standard question of variations in costs for the same unit of service.

9.2 HOW MANAGEMENT CONTROLS COSTS

Short-Run versus Long-Run Cost Functions

What can management do to change the costs of production? If a hospital receives fewer admissions than expected this morning and wants to reduce its costs by the afternoon, not much can be done. People have already shown up for work, meals have been prepared, ambulances and wheelchair transport have been arranged, and so on; therefore, *in the short run almost all costs are fixed.* Thus any reduction in the number of patients will cause the average cost per patient to be higher than usual. If the reduction in admissions continues and management is given enough time to respond, the hospital may shut down a wing, refrain from hiring, and perhaps lay off some employees. This is but one case demonstrating a general rule: as more time is allowed for adjustment, more changes can be made, and as more changes are made, costs per unit become lower.

In the very long run, almost all costs become variable. The director can train new management, hire clinical staff, rewrite treatment protocols, replace the existing building with a new one, pave some grounds for parking, and even move the facility to a more accessible site near a freeway. This ability to plan and choose the optimal scale and combination of inputs allows management to minimize the costs of production for any desired level of output. If management expects to average only 100 patients per day, it would build a smaller hospital, hire fewer people, and incur lower fixed costs. If management expects 175 patients a day, it would build a medium-sized hospital. If 300 patients a day are expected, management would build a large hospital with a dedicated computer system, pneumatic transport tubes to speed laboratory samples between floors, and other equipment (Figure 9.1).

For any expected level of output, management would choose a building size and number of permanent employees that would minimize costs. In geometric terms, the long-run average cost curve (LRAC) is an "envelope" that traces a minimum, just touching all the

FIGURE 9.1   Cost per Unit Varies with Plant Size

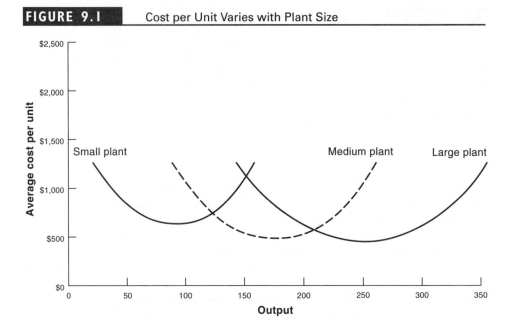

possible short-run average cost curves (SRAC), as shown in Figure 9.2. No SRAC can fall below the LRAC because if a short-run cost function with lower costs exists, management would choose that production configuration instead and incorporate it into the long-run function. Whether a particular cost is fixed or variable is determined by the time frame for decision making. Decisions regarding temporary agency nurses can be made on a day-to-day basis and thus are fixed for only 24 hours or so. Permanent employees take a while to train or to terminate when no longer needed, and thus are fixed for at least several months. Reducing the number of vice presidents is so traumatic that it may take several years. Construction is a fixed cost once completed, but it is a variable cost during the planning stage.

FIGURE 9.2   Long-Run Average Cost Curve

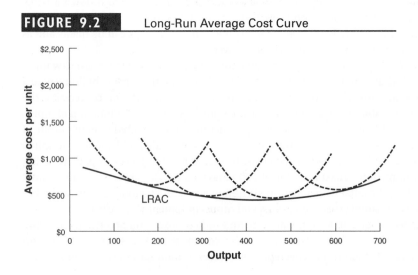

FIGURE 9.3	How Organizations Deal with Change

	Planned (known)	Random (uncertain)
Short Run	Scheduling Weekly budget Part-timers	Overtime, temps Inventory Maintain excess capacity
Long Run	Capital budgeting Change plant size Facility conversion	Hold financial reserves Encroachment by or on competitors Bankruptcy

Uncertainty and Budgeting

A director must deal with two kinds of variation in the level of output: foreseeable and unknown. Expansion to accommodate a growing population in the suburbs, eliminating maternity beds in response to declining fertility, and opening a cardiac rehabilitation unit to serve an aging community are all examples of foreseeable long-run changes. The lower number of hospital admissions on Saturday and Sunday, on Christmas and New Year's day, and during August are examples of foreseeable short-run changes. Adjustment to foreseeable changes can be planned in advance. For example, hiring and training can be accomplished efficiently over a reasonable period of time, and space and building modifications can be accomplished on a schedule, so that the path and pace of adjustment reflect conscious decisions by management to minimize costs. Random variations, on the other hand, must be accommodated in the operations of the organization but are not known in advance. For example, there may be 16 surgeries on Monday, 12 on Tuesday, 22 on Wednesday, 13 on Thursday, 18 on Friday, and 15 on Saturday, and there may be twice as much work for the admitting office to do on Wednesday as on Tuesday with the same amount of staff and equipment. Staff members are likely to do only what is necessary on a particular day, and perhaps even work late, while putting off until the next day some routine tasks, such as filing charts, checking documentation, and entering data into forms. Long-run unknown changes in output might occur because a new factory is built nearby, resulting in many new families moving to the area; an epidemic such as AIDS increases the demand for care; or a competing hospital is built, reducing demand. Such major changes often force a hospital to change its long-run strategy (see Figure 9.3).

How do managers control costs? Primarily through the use of a budget, a plan stated in dollars.[3] A budget that does not change with volume is called a **fixed budget** (also known as a standard budget), and a budget that changes with volume is called a **flexible budget**. Typically, a hospital or medical group practice creates an **operating budget** that projects all anticipated expenses for the next year. For example, if labor expenses rose 7 percent in 2001 and 9 percent in 2002, management may project an increase of 8 percent in labor costs for 2003. Managers usually define short-run changes as those that occur during the current budget period. Long-run changes and plans are incorporated in a **strategic budget** (also known as a **long-run capital budget**) that focuses on trends in the number of patients and capital renovations and expansions (new buildings and equipment, adding partners). These budgets often are accompanied by financial projections, or **pro forma financial statements** of incomes, assets, and fund balances for a period of three, five, or even twenty years in summary format. Only infrequently are detailed budgets prepared for more than one year in advance. Most managers define *long-run* changes as those that occur more than one year in the future, but some managers designate changes that occur during the next two to five years as *intermediate-run* changes. In any such analysis the terms are relative, making definitions somewhat arbitrary. The important points to gain from economic theory are that short-run adjustment is always more costly than long-run adjustment and that as the time perspective changes, so does the focus of management attention on cost control.

Known short-run variations are dealt with by making limited changes in the number of staff scheduled. For example, fewer nurses work on Sundays and at 3:00 A.M. However, the percentage change in staff is less than the percentage change in patient load, because all units must still have a head nurse, technical support, and so on, even though they are only partially full. Changes in plant capacity are prohibitively expensive in the short run. Although 50 beds may be empty in the hospital on Sunday night, not all of them would be in unit 7-East. To close that unit down, many patients would have to be transferred out of that unit on Sunday and transferred back in on Monday when patient occupancy increased again. The savings from not having a head nurse on 7-East on Sunday would be more than offset by all the transfers; thus, it would actually cost more to shut down one unit for the sake of "efficiency." Therefore, most units are underutilized on weekends and most staff members usually have an easy day.

A *known long-run change*, such as a declining trend in admissions due to the closure of a local manufacturing plant, calls for a permanent reduction in capacity. Unit 7-East can be converted into storage or nursing home beds, or leased to a group of physical therapists. Furthermore, staffing should be reduced proportionately to the long-run decline in patients, so that every employee carries a regular workload, rather than making partial staff adjustments on nights and weekends.

Random short-run fluctuations are dealt with primarily by building in some excess reserve capacity, making the staff work faster or slower, and allocating less immediate tasks to the slower days. Suppose that the number of surgeries are as suggested earlier: 16 on Monday, 12 on Tuesday, 22 on Wednesday, 13 on Thursday, 18 on Friday, and 15 on Saturday. The manager does not care about the cost of care on Monday or Tuesday, but wants to minimize the cost for the week as a whole. There is no reason to reprimand a manager for having too many nurses on duty Thursday, because there was no way to tell whether admissions would be light until the shift started. Also, although management might be able to get staff members to work extra hard and put in overtime on Wednesday to accommodate the influx of patients, they will not stay if they are abused with continual overloads. They will quit and go to work at another hospital, raising labor costs at the first hospital, because the manager would have to use temporary employees and retrain new staff members frequently. If the hospital has a range of 10 to 25 admissions per day, with an average of 16, it can staff for 16 admissions plus a bit of reserve. However, if another hospital had less random variation and always had 14 to 18 admissions per day, it could match staffing more exactly to the number of patients, would need less reserve capacity, and have a lower average cost per unit for the same average number of patients. This is only one example of the general principle that dealing with uncertainty is costly, and the greater the range of uncertainty, the greater the cost.

Unforeseen long-run changes in output really provide the test of the organization's ability to control costs. Here, tactical attention to detail is not enough—the hospital must make a strategic gamble based on a specific expectation of the future (e.g., population will grow older and increase demand, or people will move to Florida, reducing demand; a major competitor will go bankrupt, giving the hospital a great opportunity, or perhaps the competitor will go all out trying to survive by stealing the hospital's patients). The hospital could build in flexibility by making investments to cover both alternatives, but would then incur higher costs per unit regardless of which alternative happens.

9.3 CONFLICT BETWEEN ECONOMIC THEORY AND ACCOUNTING MEASURES OF PER UNIT COST

Timing

In Table 9.2, the cost per surgical operation is examined from two perspectives: direct accounting costs and a full economic cost that includes the hidden cost of dealing with disruptions (staff burnout, mistakes, overtime). In this example, the budgeted fixed costs are $5,000 per day and the variable costs are $300 per operation. The direct cost on Monday, when the expected number of patients (16) are operated on, is $5,000 + (16 × $300) = $9,800; therefore, the cost per operation is $9,800 ÷ 16 = $613. On Wednesday, if more patients (22) were operated on than the staff expected, the calculated average cost per operation is $11,600 ÷ 22 = $527. It appears that the hospital benefited from its mistake in planning for too small a number of patients. Why not increase the advantage by planning for only 15 operations instead of 16? Everyone would work even harder and faster, and if that is not good enough, the hospital could just plan for 12 or 10 or 6 operations and keep pushing the staff to become more and more efficient. Taking the example to an extreme highlights the flaw in the reasoning. The accounting measure does not accurately capture all costs. Let's consider what really happens. To work so hard on Wednesday, the staff must put off some of their routine tasks until Thursday, and they also expect extra consideration from management on Friday when they ask to go home early. Once these costs of catching up afterward are factored in, the surge of patients on Wednesday is seen to have been very costly, not cheap. If everything went according to plan, 16 operations each day would cost $9,800, for an average cost per operation of $613. Yet extra operations mean disrupting the plan. To accommodate the costs of making sudden adjustments, an "adjustment cost" must be added (assumed here to be $100 × [actual-expected operations]^2). For deviating from the plan by one operation, the added cost of adjustment is $100; for two, $400; for three, $900; and so on.[4] The actual economic costs (with adjustments) are $15,200 for 22 operations, an average of $681 per operation rather than $613. Of course, it would be cheaper if a hospital could get patients to come in at evenly spaced intervals, exactly 16 each day, all between the hours of 9:00 A.M. and 4:00 P.M. so that workload could be exactly matched to staff and equipment. Yet illness does not go according to plan, and the flow of admissions is never

TABLE 9.2 Accounting versus Economic Cost per Unit with Short-Run Fluctuations

	Mon	Tues	Wed	Thurs	Fri	Sat	Average
Surgeries	16	12	22	13	18	15	16
Direct cost	$9,800	$8,600	$11,600	$8,900	$10,400	$9,500	$9,800
Accounting "cost" per operation	613	717	527	685	578	633	613
Adjustment cost	—	1,600	3,600	900	400	100	
Total cost	9,800	10,200	15,200	9,800	10,800	9,600	10,900
Economic "cost" per operation (AC curve)	613	850	691	754	600	640	681

Note: Accounting per costs per surgery are lower for days with many surgeries, even though economic costs are higher. In this hypothetical example, a hospital has planned for 16 surgeries each day, and has fixed costs of $5,000 plus $300 per surgery. Deviations from the plan disrupt operations, reducing efficiency by a cost of $100 × (deviation squared) (i.e., being 1 surgery above or below the planned amount reduces efficiency by $100, 2 surgeries off by $400, 3 by $900, and so on).

smooth. Health care managers have learned that such disruptions are costly and that every deviation from the planned level of operation raises costs.

In accountants' terms, the per unit cost in row three of Table 9.2 is calculated on a cash basis (when spent), rather than allocating costs to different days on an accrual basis (when actually earned or obligated). In practice, accrual and all other adjustments made to the cost accounting system are inevitably incomplete and imperfect. The advantage of using economic theory is that the contradiction of the general principle—short-run costs must logically always exceed long-run costs—lets us know immediately that something was wrong with the analysis and that these cost-accounting figures, no matter how precise they may have seemed, did not reflect reality. It also explains why the budgeted $613 per operation was less than the actual expenses of $681: random fluctuations forced the payment of overtime, hiring of temps, rush ordering of exhausted supplies, and all other daily crises that managers are hired to work out.

Careful examination of Table 9.2 shows that cost per operation was not minimized on Monday, when the expected number of patients were operated on, but that the cost per operation was actually lower on Friday, when more than the expected number patients came in, even after including adjustment costs (see Figure 9.4). Why is it not more efficient to increase output or downsize the facility so that the lowest cost per unit comes at the expected level of output? The reason is that the manager must minimize not the cost on the day when output hits the expected level, but the average cost per unit over all the days, with their randomly varying levels of output. If the average number of operations had been 18 instead of 16, 24 operations might have occurred on the heavy Wednesday, exceeding capacity limits so greatly that an additional $2,800 in costs would have been incurred. Having extra reserve capacity is expensive, but not as expensive as not having it when you need it. In general, managers need to be able to accommodate the usual fluctuations in volume without major disruptions—to have flexibility that minimizes cost over a range. It is possible to have a highly routine production process that is very efficient at a set level of output but would become very inefficient if it had to be speeded up or slowed down. Such fixed-output mass production may work well for manufacturing cars or light bulbs, but it is not well adapted to services such as medical care, where constant adjustments and varying demand are the norm. Managers are willing to pay a bit extra in fixed costs to increase flexibility (see Figure 9.5). Building a facility that is very efficient when exactly the expected number of patients shows up, but that cannot easily accommodate changes in the level of demand (represented by the dark line), is less efficient in the long run than a more flexible facility (represented

FIGURE 9.4   Accounting versus Economic Costs

| FIGURE 9.5 | A Specialized Plant Has Lower Cost within a Narrow Range, but the Flexible Plant Has Wider Range |

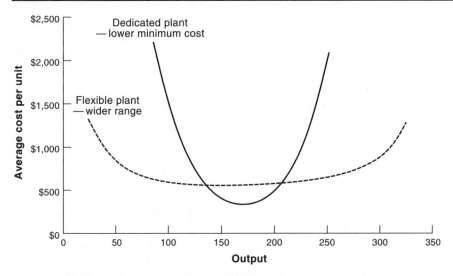

by the dashed line) that has slightly higher costs at the expected level of output but is able to maintain average costs per unit at a low level over a wider range.

Whose Costs?

The displacement of costs in time is only one accounting mistake that can be made. Attempts to increase efficiency lead to many management practices that are clearly wrong yet persist for years because of an inability to count all costs. For example, many public clinics provide services free to indigent patients. They try hard to produce these services at the lowest cost to maximize the number of clients they can serve (and to keep taxes down). One way public clinics produce services at lower costs is to bring patients in early and keep them waiting so that the doctor's flow of work is never delayed because a patient is late or an appointment is broken. Such "block booking" or "clinic appointments" maximize the number of patients that can be seen by the physician, but they make patients unhappy because they have to spend many hours waiting. If the cost of the patient's time is included, it becomes apparent that block booking is not efficient; it only seems so because the clinic budget counts only direct costs.

How can economists tell that block booking is inefficient? Because if block booking were truly efficient, some paying patients would choose to patronize doctors who block booked, putting up with extra long waits to save a little money (i.e., choosing to pay $30 for a block-booked visit rather than $35 for care by appointment). The fact that doctors cannot attract patients by block booking demonstrates that the extra patient waiting time is more valuable than the small $5 savings in the doctor's time. Indigent patients either must put up with inefficiency because they cannot obtain the convenience of an appointment by paying just the marginal $5 cost differential or must forgo free care entirely and pay the whole $35 private market price to obtain care by appointment. One might argue that the indigent patient has a lower cost of time and thus is more willing to put up with longer waits than most paying patients; however, the fact that even physicians in low-income neighborhoods have to provide appointments suggests that it is the large gap between marginal amenity cost ($5) and average per visit cost ($35), not lower value per hour of patient time, that allows free clinics to continue block booking.

Time, pain, and other nonmarket costs borne by patients do not show up on the hospital bill. Yet it is precisely these issues—suffering, fear of death, a need for caring and respect—that distinguish the economics of medical care. These intangible issues are one reason this textbook began with a broader perspective on optimization using the techniques of cost-benefit analysis (Chapter 3) rather than a narrow look at minimizing cash outlays. Some of the common mistakes made in accounting for the true costs of medical care are as follows:

- Provider costs are misallocated (displaced in time, overhead, or wrong department).
- Patient costs are not counted (wait time, transportation, family care).
- Emotional costs are not counted (pride, fear, pain, lack of respect).

9.4   ECONOMIES OF SCALE

Hospitals exist to allow a large number of doctors to share expensive capital equipment and cooperate in the care of many patients. Since many of these costs are fixed, hospitals should show economies of scale (i.e., average cost per patient day falling as more patients are treated).[5] It appears that basic hospital services for routine care are most efficiently delivered when organized and staffed in units of 20 to 40 beds, usually known as a floor or wing. The need to accommodate random fluctuations in the number of admissions and to preserve a buffer of empty beds for emergencies creates economies of scale. Admissions to a 40-bed hospital might fluctuate by ±10; therefore, only 30 beds could be occupied on average. In a 400-bed hospital, excess admissions to one unit are likely to offset a lack of admissions in another; therefore, the overall fluctuation might be ±25, which is larger in absolute numbers but much smaller as a percentage. Thus, percentage occupancy rates can be higher, and per unit costs lower, in a large facility that is more able to smooth out patient flow. The greater division of labor in a large hospital that allows staff to become more specialized and efficient at a particular function also creates economies of scale.

There is good evidence that economies of scale are important in hospital services. Hospitals with fewer than 100 beds are usually too small to offer a full range of services; are unable to fully utilize operating suites, computed tomography (CT) scanners, and other diagnostic equipment; and cannot allow staff to specialize. Very small hospitals clearly have higher costs per day, although this is somewhat obscured because they tend to offer fewer expensive and technologically advanced services. A better indication that hospitals with fewer than 100 beds suffer from a lack of economies of scale is that a disproportionate number of them have gone bankrupt or been absorbed by larger institutions over the past 20 years. Only in rural areas have small general hospitals been able to thrive, and even their numbers are falling as better highways and helicopter transport have reduced the time required to travel to large urban medical centers.

Diseconomies of scale arise from the difficulties of coordinating and managing larger institutions. Relatively few hospitals have more than 500 beds, evidence that costly administrative and transportation difficulties arise when this number of beds is exceeded. Patients increasingly complain about "getting lost in the system" and being part of a "factory" rather than a caring institution. Table 9.3 shows that cost per day rises long

TABLE 9.3

Average Cost per Adjusted Patient Day by Hospital Size

6–24 beds	$1,364
25–49	1,234
50–99	1,063
100–199	1,343
200–299	1,677
300–399	1,788
400–499	2,061
500 or more	2,188

Source: American Hospital Association, Hospital Statistics 2009, Table 2.

before the 500-bed size limit is reached. How can such large hospitals continue to exist in a competitive environment?

The Hospital Is a Multiproduct Firm

Hospitals are complex institutions, and different parts of a hospital actually produce very different products. The "average" is made up of units for routine care along with some very specialized units, such as heart transplant, oncology, and respiratory intensive care. Although it might take only 20 beds to create an efficient-size cardiac-care unit, only a large hospital has enough cardiac admissions to fill such a specialized unit. Most 400-bed university hospitals are, in fact, composites, with perhaps 100 beds providing general care, with 20 dedicated to oncology, 15 to nephrology and kidney transplant, 20 to cardiology, 40 to pediatrics, and so on. Thus, although the efficient size of a unit that produces one product is just 20 beds, the more specialized types of care a hospital provides, the larger it must be to reach efficient scale. Indeed, a hospital large enough to produce heart transplants and nuclear medicine efficiently is too large to produce routine care for broken bones and pneumonia and, therefore, suffers from diseconomies of scale with regard to these less-specialized services.

One solution to the conflict between economies and diseconomies of scale is to treat patients with uncomplicated illnesses at local community hospitals of relatively modest size (100 to 150 beds) with few specialized services, while referring patients whose treatment demands sophisticated technology and expertise to large "tertiary" institutions usually affiliated with universities. However, just as increasing hospital size causes diseconomies of scale by making management communication and coordination more difficult, so too does the process of transferring patients back and forth between community and specialty hospitals. The savings from triaging patients so that their illnesses are treated in the most efficient size hospital are to some extent offset and eventually reversed by the increase in the number of transfers required, since each transfer requires some extra documentation, management oversight, duplication of tests, and so on.

Contracting Out

Some services show economies of scale even at sizes far larger than any hospital in existence. Laboratory testing, for example, has become so automated that costs are minimized in facilities that process hundreds of thousands of tests per day. The cost of equipment, information systems, and technical expertise that constitute a good laboratory is largely a fixed cost; therefore, overhead per unit continues to decline even when millions of samples are being processed. To take advantage of such economies of scale, many hospitals are contracting out such services. Rather than having their own laboratories for conducting routine tests, they use a reference laboratory that may service hundreds of hospitals. Food services, security, and even emergency rooms are now contracted out to allow hospitals access to economies of scale through contractual relationships.

9.5   QUALITY AND COST

Technology: Cutting Costs or Enhancing Quality?

What does it mean when someone says that technological improvements have made the production process better? It may mean that the identical product can now be produced at a lower cost per unit. It may also mean that a better product can be produced, regardless of cost. Medicine has been dominated by the latter type of technological change. The tremendous

TABLE 9.4	Total Spending May Rise Even as Greater Efficiency Reduces Costs per Unit
1980	**2010**
Medication cost $150 Post-MI mortality = 70%	Medication cost $75 Post-MI mortality = 29%
Surgery cost $25,000 Post-MI mortality = 68%	Surgery cost $15,000 Post-MI mortality = 14%
Decision: Take medication for $150	Decision: Have surgery for $15,000

value of any increase in cure rates is one factor biasing researchers toward discoveries that have the effect of increasing costs. Yet quality enhancements have occurred rapidly in other areas of technology, such as computing, while still reducing unit costs. Why have such developments been so notably absent in medicine? Quite simply, it has been much more profitable to discover a new cure than to find a method to cut costs.

Insurance and cost reimbursement virtually eliminated price competition in hospital care. Without it, there was no incentive for research laboratories to seek innovations that reduced costs or for hospitals to switch to cheaper versions of existing equipment. The process of trading off a small reduction in speed or accuracy for a large reduction in price that occurs in most markets has rarely taken place in health care.

Improved Efficiency May Raise Total Spending

It is important to recognize that improved production efficiency always causes the "real" cost function to fall, even though the amount spent and cost per unit may rise because making quality and quantity more available and affordable may make people spend more. This is illustrated in Table 9.4 Suppose, for example, that in 1980 a person had a heart attack (myocardial infarction, or MI) and faced the choice of (a) taking medication costing $150 that gave a 30 percent chance of having a fatal MI within five years (70 percent mortality), or (b) undergoing a new, experimental operation costing $25,000 that gave a slightly better chance of survival, with 68 percent mortality. It would be rational for one to take the medication rather than to give up $24,850 additional dollars for such a slight improvement in one's chances. Let's also suppose that in 2010, much better medication more than doubled the chance of survival, with only 29 percent mortality, and cost only $75. In addition, research and practice improved surgery to the point where it had only a 14 percent five-year mortality and a reduced cost of $15,000. The 2010 option of giving up $14,925 to cut the risk of dying in half is very attractive. Thus, even though technological advances reduced the cost of both options, the amount spent on medical care would rise. Improvements in medical production frequently create this type of response. Even though 1980s medicine can be produced now for less than it cost in 1980, patients choose to spend more to get high-quality modern medicine that would have been impossible or prohibitively expensive to obtain in 1980.

Quality costs money, and the drive for higher quality is one of the defining characteristics of modern medicine. Although we cannot always agree on what quality is, we know that more quality is always preferred to less and that the cost–quality trade-off is usually more important in understanding the economics of medical practice than the cost–volume trade-off. Before making a comparison on the basis of cost per unit, it is first necessary to ask, "What is the product?" If the product is defined as "a day in the hospital," a top-flight research center may seem very expensive. If the product is "an increase in my chance of survival to age 75," the same institution's $2,500 per day charges might seem like a bargain.

9.6 CONTROLLING HOSPITAL COSTS THROUGH REGULATION

Hospital costs have risen steadily throughout the post–World War II era, from $9 per day in 1946, to $74 in 1970, then rising 300 percent in the next 10 years to $244 in 1980, to $682 in 1990, $1,148 in 2000, and over $1,800 today.[6] Hospital costs have grown about 10 percent a year over the past 50 years. Even after adjusting for inflation, the increase in cost per day is still an astounding 3,660 percent from 1950 to 2005 (an average of 5 percent above inflation each year). By and large, the public has wanted the additional care and new technology and has not been displeased with the billions of dollars expended. However, after the passage of Medicare and Medicaid in 1965, costs became a problem for public policy for two reasons: (1) the influx of government money caused costs to rise much more rapidly than before and (2) the costs were now being paid by the government (i.e., taxpayers) rather than the mutually agreed-upon private transactions of individuals or employer-paid insurance, and thus caused state and federal budget deficits (see Table 9.5 and Figure 9.6).

In the immediate postwar period, the Hill–Burton Act of 1946 funded the building of more hospitals, and the Health Professions Educational Assistance Act of 1963 increased the number of doctors. The early 1960s were boom years when it seemed that the economy would continue to grow robustly "forever." This desire to continue spending enabled Congress to create Medicare and Medicaid as entitlement programs in 1965. However, by 1975, the United States was trapped in a global recession, federal and state expenditures had escalated far beyond even the most outlandish budget projections, and the need for cost-cutting was clear. It was thought that system efficiencies could be generated through better planning; therefore, a number of initiatives were funded to promote "regional medical programs" and create planning boards for oversight. Evaluations showing that planning alone could not affect costs, and the obvious excess capacity created by the Hill–Burton construction boom led to the idea that a forced reduction in the growth of hospital beds could reduce the rate of growth in hospital costs.

Certificate-of-need (**CON**) legislation required that a planning body conduct a study and approve any capital project that would increase the number of hospital beds in the region.[7] In an insightful study of the economics of hospital regulation, David Salkever and Thomas Bice showed that although CON legislation reduced the number of new beds built, hospitals increased the amount of capital equipment for each bed; thus, capital spending continued to rise at the same rate.[8] In discussing their findings, Salkever and Bice argued that "CON regulation is like pushing on a balloon"—forcing costs down in one dimension caused them to bulge in another dimension. Similar dynamics have been demonstrated in other studies of many regulatory initiatives over the years; the type of cost subject to regulation declines, but any savings are negated by an overflow in another area so that total health care costs are unchanged (see Table 9.6). An unintended side effect of CON and most other regulations is that they create barriers that make it harder for new organizations to enter the market, thus protecting existing hospitals and retarding the evolution of the health care system toward more efficient configurations. Studies of CON in operation confirmed the economists' version of the golden rule ("them that has the gold makes the rules"): almost every well-established, wealthy, and politically connected hospital that applied for certification eventually got it, while denials fell disproportionately on outsiders that threatened the status quo or weaker institutions that lacked a constituency (see discussion of CONs in Chapter 10, Section 4). The death knell for CON came in the form of a Supreme Court ruling that discriminatory reimbursement of a hospital chain that refused to apply for a CON (which the chain knew would be denied because of opposition from existing local hospitals)

TABLE 9.5	Hospital Costs per Patient Day, 1950–2007	
Year	Cost per Day	Cost per Day (2007 $)
1946	$ 9	$ 73
1950	14	103
1955	21	134
1960	29	167
1965	40	215
1970	74	321
1971	83	344
1972	95	377
1973	102	384
1974	113	390
1975	133	419
1976	153	456
1977	173	485
1978	194	508
1979	216	522
1980	244	541
1981	284	576
1982	327	625
1983	368	676
1984	410	726
1985	460	791
1986	499	839
1987	537	879
1988	581	920
1989	631	962
1990	682	1,002
1991	745	1,057
1992	816	1,132
1993	875	1,186
1994	930	1,235
1995	967	1,258
1996	1,005	1,283
1997	1,032	1,296
1998	1,065	1,323
1999	1,101	1,348
2000	1,148	1,375
2001	1,216	1,423
2002	1,289	1,482
2003	1,379	1,553
2004	1,450	1,587
2005	1,522	1,613
2006	1,611	1,654
2007	1,694	1,694

Hospital cost per adjusted patient day in nominal current dollars and inflation adjusted to 2007 dollars using gdp deflator.

Source: AHA.

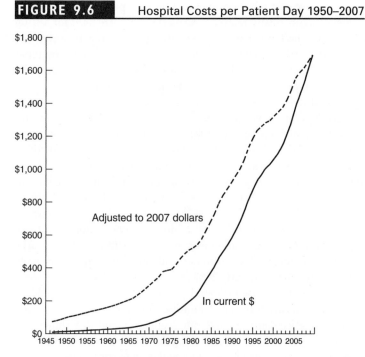

FIGURE 9.6 Hospital Costs per Patient Day 1950–2007

constituted an illegal restraint of trade under antitrust laws and harmed consumers by restricting competition.

The attempt to impose controls over other dimensions moved on to utilization review (UR), a process to eliminate unnecessary surgery and other services by having a panel of doctors and nurses in a professional standards review organization (PSRO) review patients' charts to find cases of inappropriate care. The PSRO or other agency would be empowered to order the doctor to change improper behavior and, failing that, to deny payment. In practice, the process proved cumbersome and ineffective, although the current managed care review, which does appear to work better (see Chapter 5), developed from the experience with UR. Rapid inflation and an unwillingness to accept the lessons of history led the Nixon administration to impose **price controls** in 1971. Although removed for most sectors of the economy in 1973, they were maintained in hospitals for an extra year. Rate setting through **budgetary review** was a much more labor-intensive process, involving the line-by-line examination of spending plans. A notable example was the legislation passed in the state of Washington in 1973 when a severe local recession crimped the state's ability to raise tax revenues. The legislation lasted, albeit in weaker and weaker form, for 10 years. Perhaps the most far-reaching cost-control regulation was the replacement of Medicare's

TABLE 9.6 Types of Regulation to Control Hospital Costs

Certificate of need (CON)
Utilization review (UR, PSRO)
Budgetary review
Price controls (ESPN)
Administered prices (DRGs, PPS, BBA)

open-ended system of retrospective cost reimbursement by the **prospective payment system (PPS)** in 1984, in which **diagnostically related groups (DRGs)** were used for setting federally administered prices per discharge covering the entire patient stay. However, the demonstrable reductions in cost per inpatient admission were more than offset by rapid increases in outpatient charges; therefore, overall Medicare costs continued to rise as rapidly as before—another example of a regulation pushing on one side of the balloon.

The **Balanced Budget Act of 1997 (BBA)** was much more successful in cutting costs, at least in the short run. It directly reduced Medicare payments to physicians, hospitals, and home health agencies by reducing the hospital update factor (annual base payment increase percentage), reducing payments for graduate medical education, limiting the growth in total Medicare physician payments to a "sustainable growth rate" linked to the annual rate of growth in GDP, establishing a prospective payment system for home health benefits, and allowing HMOs to compete for Medicare beneficiaries through the "Medicare+Choice" program. Payments for home health, which had been the most rapidly growing part of Medicare, fell from $16 billion in 1996 to less than $8 billion in 1999.[9] Altogether, these reductions were able to save more than $100 billion over five years. However, as the curbs put in place by BBA really began to bite, protests from hospitals and physician groups grew louder and politicians more sympathetic. By early 2003, a consensus had arisen that some release from the stringent constraints imposed on Medicare payment increases would be implemented soon. Since then, Medicare costs have again risen rapidly.

The experience with CONs, price controls, state rate regulation, and PPS shows that whatever successes might be attributed to cost-control regulation have been limited and short lived.[10] The failure of this kind of government price regulation to control costs should not come as a surprise, since the central difficulty in medical care transactions is the inability to specify what the product is. Special market adaptations, such as nonprofit status and the agency relationships between physicians and patients, are signals that any attempts to set prices or to quantify quality and other important attributes are likely to be exercises in futility. A government official in a state capital, or in Washington, D.C., is not going to be able to specify a detailed contract in advance to purchase something that the participants have trouble measuring even after the fact (e.g., how good the obstetrical care really was for a low-birthweight baby left with disabilities). It would be easy to cut spending on Medicare and Medicaid in a number of ways (set global budget caps, eliminate services, deny eligibility), but there is not sufficient public consensus or political willpower to do so. Managed care and new regulations may bring some relief, but the macroeconomic cost pressures we examine in Chapters 13 to 18 will eventually force the public to face these hard choices—and force politicians to deal with the fallout.

SUGGESTIONS FOR FURTHER READING

William O. Cleverley and Andrew E. Cameron, *Essentials of Health Care Finance*, 5th ed. (Gaithersburg, Md.: Aspen, 2002).

Steven A. Finkler and David M. Ward, *Cost Accounting for Health Care Organizations*, 2nd ed. (Gaithersburg, Md.: Aspen, 1999).

Healthcare Financial Management, monthly journal of the Healthcare Financial Management Association (www.HFMA.org).

SUMMARY

1.   Managers plan to produce efficiently; therefore, any deviation from the plan (more or fewer patients, shifting wage rates) tends to increase average cost per unit, particularly in the short run. Since management can more fully adapt operations over the long

run, the short-run average cost curve always lies at or above the long-run average cost curve. The primary way **managers control hospital costs is through the budget process**. Often extra capacity and flexibility is built in so that uncertainty and changes are not so difficult to deal with.

2. **Economies of scale** are said to exist when increasing the level of output causes the average cost per unit to fall. Gains from the **specialization of labor and spreading the fixed costs of capital equipment** over more volume are the major factors creating economies of scale. **Diseconomies of scale**, in which rising costs per unit eventually set in, are primarily due to the **difficulty of managing and coordinating larger operations**. Hospitals appear to show economies of scale up to a size of about 120 beds and diseconomies of scale after reaching a size of about 500 beds. For simple services, small hospitals appear to be relatively efficient, but only a large hospital has enough patients of a particular type (e.g., brain cancer) to run a specialized service at an efficient volume. Thus, a hospital may be both too big to deliver some services efficiently and too small to deliver others efficiently.

3. **Cost per day in the hospital varies for many reasons**: differences in quality and type of services offered, cost shifting to pay for research and teaching, billing practices, severity of patient illness, prices of labor and other inputs, and differences in production efficiency. **Hospitals are multiproduct firms**, providing many types of care; thus, comparisons of cost per day or per case may not be very meaningful indicators of how efficiently a hospital is producing care.

4. **Accounting costs often do not measure true economic costs**. A larger-than-expected number of patients may make average costs appear lower, but actually the overcrowding and staff stress tend to increase costs. Patient time, pain, and worry are other costs often not counted.

5. **Technology** has tended to increase total spending in health care because generous insurance payments and cost reimbursement have given little incentive to develop cost-reducing techniques or to give up a little quality for a large reduction in cost. An increase in capability to improve health often makes more spending worthwhile.

6. Although able to switch cost from one part of health care to another (pushing on a balloon), **regulation** has not succeeded in controlling the overall cost of health care. CON regulations to control construction and prospective price setting (PPS, DRGs) have forced hospitals to respond in a number of ways, but total spending has continued to soar. Government is financially responsible for most of a hospital's patients (66 percent of inpatient days are paid for by Medicare and Medicaid), but is unable or unwilling to pay the price, forcing the health care system toward a crisis point. The cost shifting under which the rich cared for the poor and the healthy contributed to pay for the sick has begun to crack under the strain of unequal payments and a burgeoning federal deficit.

PROBLEMS

1. {*economies of scale*} What major factors create economies of scale in hospitals? Diseconomies of scale? Are most hospitals of optimal size, too small, or too large?

2. {*case mix, cost shifting*} Why do university teaching hospitals cost so much more per day of care than local community hospitals?

3. {*economies of scale*} Misericordia Hospital had a 20 percent increase in admissions from 1995 to 2000. Total patient care costs went from $50 million to $61 million.

Does Misericordia show evidence of economies of scale or diseconomies of scale? Could other factors besides the number of admissions affect the costs of care?

4. {*economies of scale*} The number of patients at Harbordale Hospital increased from 120 to 144 from Monday to Tuesday. The hospital's costs increased $720,000 to $722,000 as temporary nurses were called in to deal with the heavy patient load. Does Harbordale Hospital show economies or diseconomies of scale? Which hospital is better managed for cost control: Harbordale or Misericordia (in Problem 3)? Which is more costly, short-run adjustment between Monday and Tuesday or long-run adjustment between 1995 and 2000?

5. {*marginal cost, accounting*} What is the cost of an extra admission to a hospital? Does it make a difference whether the admission is for an emergency service or for a scheduled service? Who bears the costs of additional emergency admission? Is there any difference in who bears the cost of a 50 percent increase in emergency room admission in the short run and the long run?

6. {*compensation*} Should hospital managers be rewarded for dealing with random fluctuations in demand, or for dealing with planned changes in demand?

7. {*efficiency, case mix*} Costs per day are usually lower in community hospitals than in university hospitals. Does this mean that transferring patients from university hospitals to community hospitals would increase efficiency?

8. {*substitution*} Why do people spend so long waiting to be treated in an emergency room? Would it be more efficient if there were sufficient doctors available so that people could be treated right away?

9. {*economies of scale, discrimination*} Many rural counties have fewer hospital beds than urban and suburban counties, even when rural counties experience more accidents and injuries for which immediate access to care is crucial. Does this disparity indicate systematic discrimination against rural counties?

10. {*transaction costs*} Why would a hospital that just expanded its home health care agency to service the patients of other hospitals in the region close down its clinical laboratory and purchase lab services from a neighboring hospital?

11. {*quality*} Why have quality improvements in health care caused costs to rise, while quality improvements in computers have caused costs to fall?

12. {*technological change*} Automation has vastly increased the efficiency and accuracy of laboratory testing. The cost per test has fallen by more than 75 percent in many cases. Do you think that the total cost of laboratory testing has fallen by more or less than 75 percent? Why?

13. {*price controls*} What would you expect to be the effect of a set of regulations limiting hospital revenues to an increase of 1 percent a year on the following?

a. Number of nurses hired
b. Number of doctors
c. Quality of care
d. Advertising budgets
e. Emergency room staffing
f. New construction
g. Depreciation

Would there be a difference if the regulation applied to just one hospital rather than to all hospitals? Would there be a difference between short-run and long-run effects?

14.   {*regulation*} CON regulation effectively limited the number of new hospital beds constructed in a region. Who would favor CON? Who would be against CON? When hospitals in a state with CON regulation renovate old buildings, would you expect the cost per bed to be more or less than in a state without CON regulation?

ENDNOTES

1.   E. R. Becker and B. Steinwald, "The Determinants of Hospital Case-Mix Complexity," *Health Services Research* 16, no. 1 (1981): 439–458.

2.   Frank Sloan, Roger Feldman, and Bruce Steinwald, "The Effects of Teaching on Hospital Costs," *Journal of Health Economics* 2, no. 1 (1983): 1–28; Howard Berman and Louis Weeks, *The Financial Management of Hospitals*, 5th edition (Ann Arbor, Mich.: Health Administration Press, 1990).

3.   Howard Berman and Louis Weeks, *The Financial Management of Hospitals*, 5th Edition, Ann Arbor, Mich.: Health Administration Press, 1990.

4.   The adjustment calculation used here is arbitrary and intended for illustrative purposes only, rather than an estimation of actual cost penalties. The important point is that being over or under the optimal level of planned output causes a disproportionate increase in per unit costs.

5.   T. W. Granneman, R. S. Brown, and M. V. Pauly, "Estimating Hospital Costs: A Multiple-Output Analysis," *Journal of Health Economics* 5, no. 2 (1986): 107–127; T. G. Cowing, A. G. Holtman, and S. Powers, "Hospital Cost Analysis: A Survey and Evaluation of Recent Studies," *Advances in Health Economics and Health Services Research* 4 (1983) 257–303.

6.   American Hospital Association, *Hospital Statistics* (Chicago: American Hospital Association, various years).

7.   CON, UR, PSROs, DRGs, and other regulations have all taken many different forms in different state or national programs over time. The brief discussion here refers to general conclusions about that type of regulation, rather than any particular specific program. The interested reader should consult one of the many comprehensive reviews that have been written, such as those in Paul Joskow, *Controlling Hospital Costs: The Role of Government Regulation* (Cambridge, Mass.: MIT Press, 1981); D. Abernathy and D. A. Pearson, *Regulating Hospital Costs: The Development of Public Policy* (Ann Arbor, Mich.: Health Administration Press, 1979); or the relevant chapters of Michael Rosko and Robert W. Broyles, *The Economics of Health Care: A Reference Handbook* (New York: Greenwood Press, 1988); or Sherman Folland, Allen Goodman, and Miron Stano, *The Economics of Health and Health Care*, 5th ed. (New York: Prentice Hall, 2006).

8.   David Salkever and Thomas Bice, *Hospital Certificate-of-Need Controls: Impact on Investment, Costs and Use* (Washington, D.C.: American Enterprise Institute, 1979).

9.   Nelda McCall et al., "Medicare Home Health Before and After the BBS," *Health Affairs* 20, no. 3 (May 2001): 189–198; Charles N. Kahn and Hanns Kuttner, "Budget Bills and Medicare Policy: the Politics of the BBA," *Health Affairs* 18, no. 1 (January 1999): 37–47.

10.   David Dranove and Kenneth Cone, "Do State Rate-Setting Regulations Really Lower Hospital Expenses?" *Journal of Health Economics* 4 (1985): 159–165; C. L. Eby and D. Cohodes, "What Do We Know About Rate-Setting?" *Journal of Health Politics, Policy and Law* 10, no. 2 (1985): 299–327.

CHAPTER 10

LONG-TERM CARE

QUESTIONS

1. Do the elderly pay to be cured, or to be cared for?

2. Who provides most long-term care for the disabled elderly? Who is the largest insurer?

3. What do nursing home owners compete for? Do they want patients who are more sick or less sick?

4. How can substituting nursing homes for hospitals increase the total cost of care if the cost per day is lower at nursing homes?

5. Have government payments and regulations raised or lowered the quality of care?

6. How can Medicaid payments create an excess and a shortage of patients at the same time?

7. Do certificate-of-need (CON) rules reduce costs or reduce access?

8. Are retirement communities "managed care" for the aging? Is there "managed death"?

9. As people live longer, does that mean that they are healthier and thus spend less on medical care, or more disabled and spend more?

Of the $226 billion paid for **long-term care (LTC)** in 2010, most is spent for institutional services in nursing homes. Yet for every person in a nursing home, there are two equally disabled people living in the community who are cared for by family and friends. Hence, more care comes from unpaid labor and acts of obligation and love, rather than patient fees or third-party payments.[1] LTC revolves around *care* rather than cure, around quality of life rather than treatment of disease. LTC needs are defined by a person's ability to function, the ability to conduct activities of daily life. Most LTC patients continue to require assistance for the rest of their lives. Food, housing, comfort, and social relationships are more important than diagnostic tests and surgical procedures. Although doctors, hospitals, nurses, drugs, and all the other elements of modern medicine are employed in LTC, they are actively involved in only a small portion of the care that patients receive. LTC is not "medical" in the same way that most acute care is. These differences—long-term chronic disabilities rather than short-term diseases capable of being cured, predominantly human caring rather than medical science, and a reliance on unpaid acts of love and obligation rather than services purchased in the market—tend to make LTC transactions somewhat different from acute medical care transactions and from the ordinary two-party transactions for most economic goods and services.

The challenge of meeting both medical and social needs has left LTC public policy in a confused state, with legislators uncertain about which aspects of care should be funded through social welfare programs and which should be funded as part of the health care system. The response to people with chronic illness and disability is an LTC system in which boundaries are often unclear and many fundamental issues are unresolved. This chapter presents a few aspects of the many and multifaceted economic entities that make up the fragmented LTC sector.

10.1   DEVELOPMENT OF THE LONG-TERM CARE MARKET

The original hospitals were LTC facilities. They served destitute patients who could not work and could no longer live at home. Most people had family members who took care of them at home when they became sick, old, or infirm, and the wealthy called upon the services of paid home nurses; therefore, only a small group of disabled and indigent paupers were forced to reside in hospitals. After the scientific revolutions of the nineteenth century, curative medicine was increasingly separated from caring for the disabled. By the start of World War II, the distinction between acute medical care and LTC was clearly demarcated in the minds of the public and in the flow of funds. It was hoped that poorhouses and "almshouse hospitality" would disappear as infectious diseases were cured and the desperately poor were elevated by a rising economy. To a large extent, sanitation and Social Security did cause the old system to fade, but some problems were troublingly persistent. No cure was found for mental illness, and more people were confined to state hospitals. These institutions made limited attempts at cure, but often served more to relieve the community of a burden rather than to improve the patients' quality of life. Rising incomes meant that fewer and fewer elderly people were left truly destitute, but there were always some who had no friends, no family, and no place to go except to a county "home" once they could no longer work. Although people with severe mental illness and homeless elderly people had persistent needs, they were small in number and almost ignored in planning for the overall health care system. In 1940, nursing home expenditures constituted less than 1 percent of the nation's total health spending.

The number of elderly people rose rapidly in the postwar era, from 10 million in 1940 to 17 million in 1965 and 40 million in 2010. This burgeoning group of elderly Americans is relatively healthy, thanks to years of good nutrition and sanitation, and relatively wealthy, thanks to pensions and years of saving. After the 1960s, a sizable population could look forward to living for many years after working, with no need to depend on their children for financial support. This emerging group of retirees constituted a distinct market. They wanted to enjoy their "golden years" and often looked to each other for social activity. Retirement communities sprang up in Florida, California, and Arizona that catered to this growing group of middle-class elderly people. Retirement communities were specially designed to appeal to the elderly, featuring single-story dwellings without steps, limited traffic, and social centers for bridge games, dancing, and crafts. Many of these communities discouraged or excluded families with children. This market response to the special needs of the elderly occurred without any reference to medicine or LTC.

Nursing home patients constituted another small group within the elderly population that was destined to grow rapidly during the postwar era. The fraction of total health expenditures devoted to nursing homes, which was less than 1 percent in 1940, more than doubled by 1950, doubled again by 1960, and nearly doubled again by 1970, but was increasingly constrained after that (see Table 10.1). The fraction of total health spending devoted to nursing homes peaked at 8 percent around 1980 and has fallen steadily since then, while the

TABLE 10.1 Changes in the LTC Market

	1940	1950	1960	1970	1980	1990	2000	2010
Persons aged 65+	9,540,000	12,400,000	16,600,000	20,100,000	25,710,000	30,390,000	34,778,000	40,229,000
% of population	7.2%	8.1%	9.2%	9.8%	11.3%	12.2%	12.6%	13.0%
Nursing home $ (millions)	$28	$178	$980	$4,867	$19,989	$54,810	$92,947	$151,200
% of total health $$	0.7%	1.5%	3.6%	6.5%	8.0%	7.9%	7.1%	5.8%
Home health $ (millions)	—	—	$37	$143	$1,347	$11,056	$32,426	$74,600
% of total health $	—	—	0.1%	0.2%	0.5%	1.2%	2.4%	2.8%

TABLE 10.2

Percentage of Population in a
Nursing Home, by Age

Under 65	0.1%
65–74	1.1%
75–84	4.3%
85+	18.3%

Source: CDC, NCHS, Health United
States, 2002.

number of active retirees living in segregated housing with special amenities continues to soar. Distinguishing the active senior citizens from the institutionalized patients is easy at the extremes, but there is a range in between for which neat separation is impossible. The simple dichotomy of "at home" versus "in a nursing home" has been replaced by a range of organizational settings, from high-intensity facilities that are almost like hospitals, to a variety of intermediate care and assisted-living facilities, to houses identical to those occupied by young families. The picture is further clouded by the provision of visiting nurse services, Meals on Wheels, home intravenous (IV) and physical therapy, and other supplemental services that make it possible to provide a wide range of care in the homes where people live before they become disabled.

Although some disabled younger people receive LTC, the majority of people who receive LTC are above age 65, and the rate of institutionalization increases with advancing age (Table 10.2). Residents in nursing homes are disproportionately female (74 percent) and poor. Older males who are disabled are more likely to be married and hence receive assistance from a spouse or adult child. Traditionally, care of disabled elders has been provided by adult daughters, who were expected to take on the task of caring for one or more parents or parents-in-law after their own children were raised. This informal system was adequate in the 1950s, when most women married and had children early and did not have careers. In the 1990s, with the majority of women in the labor force, and childbearing frequently delayed so that children did not leave home until the mother was in her fifties, finding time to care for a 78-year-old parent was much more difficult. The "shadow price" (forgone wage opportunity) of unpaid middle-aged women has become much greater. At the same time, demand has risen. In the immediate postwar 1950s era, fewer parents lived past age 70. In addition, families were larger; therefore, middle-aged women were likely to have several sisters to help share the burden. As family size shrank and longevity increased, there were more elderly disabled parents per potential caregiver daughter. The stress and family complications became greater. As the supply of unpaid labor fell and demand rose, what formerly had been care provided within the household became care purchased in the marketplace.[2]

The services provided by family members are invisible in the national income (gross domestic product GDP) accounts: no one is billed, no one is paid, and from one point of view, no transaction has taken place. Yet from another point of view, one that pre-dates the existence of money, the obligations of parents to care for children, of neighbors to care for the sick, and of any person present to ease the pain of dying are fundamental transactions that define society. In LTC, the boundary between market and nonmarket activities is blurred. The fact that nursing home admissions or expenditures double does not mean that twice as many disabled people are getting care or that they are getting more or better services. Some of that increase is simply the movement from the realm of household production and family obligation into monetarized commerce.

10.2 DEFINING LTC: TYPES OF CARE

A person's potential need for LTC can be analyzed as occurring in three dimensions: physical illness (medical diagnoses), functional disability (ability to perform activities of daily living, ADLs, and instrumental activities of daily living, IADLs, see Section 10.5, and psycho-socioeconomic deficits (family support, see Table 10.3). LTC can be provided either at

TABLE 10.3	Dimensions of LTC Need		
	Medical Need	**Functional Need**	**Social Need**
Acute hospital	********	—	—
Rehab hospital	***	***	—
Nursing home	*	********	********
CCRC	—	—	*
Skilled home care	********	***	*
Personal home care	*	***	***
Family/community	*	*	*

******** High
*** Medium
* Low
— Varies or not applicable

home or in an institutional setting. Institutional settings can be ranked by the intensity of medical intervention: acute hospitals, long-term hospitals providing rehabilitation and psychiatric treatment, nursing homes (skilled, intermediate), and assisted living or board-and-care homes. Placement depends on the interaction among medical, social, economic, and functional needs rather than any single dimension. A postoperative patient who only needs regular bathing and hourly medication could be cared for at home if there is sufficient support from the family. A patient without actively involved family members may be a candidate for nursing home placement, and if there are no available nursing home beds, the patient might continue to stay in the hospital for many days.[3]

Home health care is growing rapidly in two different directions.[4] On the one hand, medical treatments that used to be performed in the hospital are being performed in the patient's home, paralleling the trend away from the hospital evidenced by shorter lengths of stay, the growth of ambulatory surgery, and the development of outpatient rehabilitation. For home medical care to be effective, the physician and nurse must be able to count on a high degree of family support to assist in monitoring the patient, administering medication, and performing basic nursing functions such as feeding, bathing, and changing clothes. On the other hand, personal home care is provided to otherwise healthy but homebound individuals whose lack of relatives at home is compensated for by having unskilled aides do ordinary cleaning, cooking, and other household tasks. Meals on Wheels, a publicly funded program that delivers hot meals to the homebound, is a good example. Although the services are quite different, the terminology and provision can become confusing, since a single provider may do both. A visiting nurse could stop at one house to change an IV antibiotic and proceed to the next house where the only service provided is to help someone into a wheelchair.

A person who has good friends, good health, and no functional limitations can have an active life in the community. As elderly people begin to need more care and protection, their likelihood of being placed in a nursing home depends most of all on the presence of social support. For example, most married people with Alzheimer's disease can continue to live at home and be cared for by their spouses at least through the early phases of the disease. Those who have children, but no spouse, are less likely to be able to remain at home, and those with no family nearby are likely to be institutionalized. The extent of disability is the second most important factor. Eventually, almost every family who cares for a person with Alzheimer's becomes overwhelmed by the necessity to provide constant attention, as well as by the pain and alienation of caring for someone who may not know or appreciate any of the things being done. Mental dysfunction is a significant cause in more than half of all LTC

TABLE 10.4

Breakdown of Nursing
Home Costs

Physician Services	1%
RNs (estimated)	8%
Other Wages & Salaries	46%
Employee Benefits	11%
Food	4%
Drugs	3%
Other Supplies	6%
Contract Services	8%
Utilities	2%
Equipment	2%
Interest	4%
Depreciation	4%
Rent, etc.	1%

Source: CMS National Nursing Home
Input Price Index Market Basket, 2005
http://www.cms.hhs.gov/Medicare
ProgramRatesStats/downloads/
mktbskt-snf.pdf

institutionalization. Medical needs, although often critical in precipitating a crisis, are relatively less important than social, housing, and functional needs in determining the use of LTC.

The goal of acute care is to increase the level of functioning and reduce the risk of dying. In contrast, most LTC is supportive. Attempts are made to slow the patient's decline and stabilize functioning, but only rarely is an attempt made to achieve a definitive cure, and it is expected that the person will remain dependent. Since acute medical care is focused on cure, the quality of the meals, the room, and social functions are incidentals and contribute little to the total cost of a hospital stay. Most of the cost of LTC, on the other hand, is for helping people with their daily lives, not treatment. Drugs are supposed to help the patient get through the day, not to get better, and curative procedures account for a relatively minor fraction of total expenditures. A physician may show up at a nursing home only once a month. In studies of nursing home costs, physician services account for only 1 percent of costs, whereas wages, salaries, and benefits, mostly for unskilled labor, account for 66 percent. A breakdown of nursing home inputs by category (Table 10.4) shows that most LTC expenses result from providing supported living rather than medical care.

10.3 MEDICAID: NURSING HOMES AS A TWO-PART MARKET

The nursing home market was radically transformed, almost created anew, by the passage of Medicare, Title XVII, and Medicaid, Title XIX, of the Social Security Amendments of 1965. When Medicare was drafted to provide health insurance for the elderly, Medicaid was somewhat of an afterthought. Medicare explicitly did not pay for the kind of supportive care provided by most nursing homes.[5] It was presumed that housing, nutrition, and personal assistance were individual or family responsibilities. Inability to provide for oneself indicated a need for charity or welfare assistance, not medical insurance.[6] Originally, Medicaid was intended mostly to expand and consolidate insurance coverage of medical services for indigent women and children who received Aid to Families with Dependent Children (AFDC—now TANF, Temporary Assistance to Needy Families). Since it was directed toward a dependent indigent population, Medicaid did pay for social support such as that provided in nursing homes. Therefore, elderly people who were poor, or who became poor after spending down or giving away their savings, could obtain government insurance payments for institutional LTC. Soon Medicaid was funneling billions of dollars each year into nursing homes. Medicaid now accounts for 52 percent of total nursing home funding, with Medicare paying 8 percent (mostly for skilled medical nursing care and therapy), as illustrated in Figure 10.1. Medicaid is a joint state/federal program, with poor states getting as much as 80 percent of their total Medicaid funding from the federal government, whereas wealthy states get only 50 percent. States are required to cover basic medical services for people who are on public

FIGURE 10.1 Nursing Home Sources and Uses of Funds

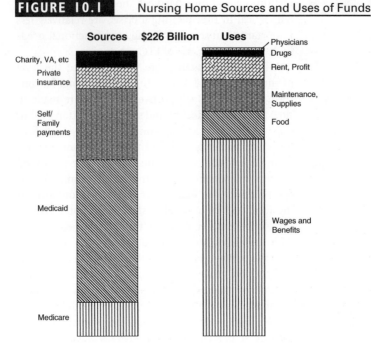

assistance and/or meet federal poverty definitions but have discretion to increase benefits and eligibility above these limits. (Please note that any brief description of Medicaid must be qualified, because there are more than fifty state Medicaid payment systems with numerous clauses, exceptions, and special programs.)

Although nursing homes were only a minor consideration in the creation of the Medicaid program, LTC payments soon soared out of control, more than doubling every five years. Governors and state budget officials discovered that Medicaid, even with federal matching funds, was an onerous financial burden. In most years since 1965, Medicaid has been the most rapidly growing category of state spending. The surge of Medicaid money into what had been a tiny market caused a rapid increase in prices and a shortage of spaces for millions of new patients. As prices rose, state financial burdens increased. Any new nursing homes built were quickly filled with more of the waiting Medicaid-eligible people, adding millions to state budget outlays. States responded to this financial drain in two ways: capping the price they would pay for each day of nursing home care and halting the construction of new nursing homes. The methods of price control varied, but usually regulations were based on costs incurred or on a set percentage increase over prior years (see Section 10.5). Control over the number of beds was established by requiring that nursing home owners obtain a certificate of need (CON) before building or expanding facilities (see Section 10.4 and discussion of hospital CONs in Section 9.6).

With these two moves, price controls and capacity constraints, government created a unique market for nursing home beds. This market's distinctive feature is a constant excess demand, but an excess of below-market-price Medicaid patients only. Consider Figure 10.2. On the upper-left side is private market demand, with a normal, downward-sloping demand schedule. The upper-right panel shows Medicaid demand. Since price is fixed by government regulation, there is no change in price as quantity increases; therefore, the demand "curve" is a right angle. Nursing homes can get as many patients they want at the state-regulated price, until there are no more Medicaid-eligible patients in the area. The lower-left panel

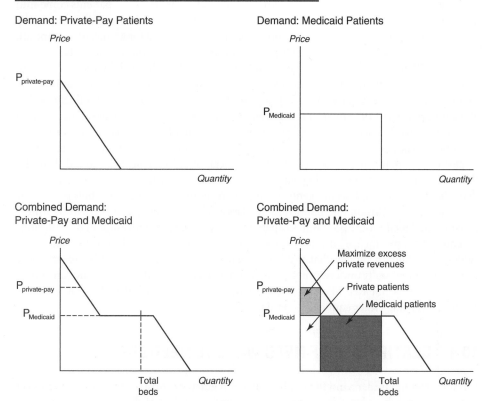

FIGURE 10.2   Two-Part Nursing Home Market

shows the combined private and Medicaid demand. Only private-pay patients can be served above the fixed Medicaid price; thus, the initial portion of the demand curve is composed solely of private patients and is downward sloping. Once the Medicaid price is reached, the demand curve flattens out, because the nursing home can get more patients without reducing price. If a nursing home became too large, it would eventually exhaust the excess Medicaid demand and have to attract additional private patients with even lower prices, as shown by the bottom third, downward-sloping segment. Increasing the number of beds sufficient to force nursing home owners to dip into the demand of those only willing to pay an amount less than Medicaid pays is usually unintentional, since expansion typically ceases before all Medicaid patients are served. The two-part market faced by the nursing home owner is shown in more detail in the lower-right panel of Figure 10.2.[7] The vertical line represents the total bed capacity of the nursing home, the maximum number of patients that can be cared for. To maximize profits, the owner first sets a price for private-pay patients P_{pp} that maximizes the total amount of excess revenues above the Medicaid rate (i.e., the dashed rectangle $Q_{pp} \times (P_{pp} - P_{medicaid})$) and then fills the remaining beds from the waiting list of Medicaid patients who pay the state-regulated price $P_{Medicaid}$ (the shaded rectangle $(Q_{max} - Q_{pp}) \times P_{Medicaid}$).

The two-part market structure causes nursing home utilization to have an unusual U-shaped relationship to income. Although most normal goods show demand steadily rising as income rises, in this market, utilization is high at low incomes (where patients readily qualify for Medicaid), drops for middle incomes (where lack of coverage reduces demand), and rises at high incomes (where wealthy people can afford $50,000 or more per year for care).

The real world is, of course, more complicated than the straight lines drawn in Figure 10.2. Often a nursing home will only admit private-pay patients. Many patients come into a nursing home with considerable assets, but over the years **spend down** all their savings by paying for care, and only then become poor enough to be eligible for Medicaid (a common guideline is less than $2,000 in financial assets and $564 per month in income for a single person).[8] There are stories of couples becoming divorced solely to allow the spouse who is disabled to qualify for Medicaid so that the one who is still living at home can keep the savings accounts. Elderly couples are protected to some extent by federal guidelines that allow the spouse at home to keep the house, car, and some additional assets. Elderly single people may give their assets to their children in anticipation of entering a nursing home. This must be planned with care, however, since most states include recently transferred assets as part of personal funds to be used before Medicaid reimbursement is allowed. Families that would never consider "going on welfare" use asset transfers to make aging parents dependent on state funds as indigents. With 50 percent of all nursing home bills paid for by Medicaid, the conclusion that many middle-class and wealthy people are benefiting from a program designed for the poor is inescapable.[9] The fact that a certain amount of subterfuge is required ("convenience" divorces, paper-only transfers of ownership of cars and land, "giving" to children money that the parent still controls) only makes this process more distasteful and morally undermining.[10] Medicaid is an entrenched part of the nursing home market, but it is not well liked by taxpayers or beneficiaries, and it is difficult to justify Medicaid as being either equitable or ethical.

10.4 CERTIFICATE OF NEED: WHOSE NEEDS?

It is important to understand the implications of regulatory constraints on the LTC market and to examine whose interests are served by creating a situation of chronic excess demand in which frail and sick patients must wait months for a bed. For example, the surge of Medicaid money into nursing home care after 1965 meant that there would be a shortage of beds for the years it would take until the market could catch up. In addition, imposing a construction moratorium through the CON process increased the shortage and made it permanent.

Money and Quality

It would seem that pushing more money into nursing homes during the late 1960s would have improved the quality of care provided. However, for perfectly reasonable economic reasons, conditions actually became worse in many nursing homes. For instance, a nursing home owner does not choose furniture or service based on what can be afforded but on what will maximize profits. With a long line of Medicaid patients waiting to get in, it was not necessary to keep up the appearance of the nursing home to attract new patients, nor was it necessary to provide good nursing service or good food to keep patients there. Since every bed was always filled from the waiting list, profits were maximized by reducing costs (e.g., providing fewer hours of nursing, employing less-skilled nurses, making fewer repairs, providing less maintenance). The flood of Medicaid money washed away any incentive to provide high-quality care to attract more patients.

Competing for Certificates of Need, Not for Patients

With chronic excess demand guaranteeing full occupancy from the first day, new nursing homes were sure money-makers. If placed in nice locations to attract a sizable share of private-pay patients, even more money could be made. CON regulations slowed, but did not entirely stop, the construction of new nursing homes. Since a CON was now required, what would determine who could build these facilities, and where would they be placed? State officials faced a dilemma. If the beds were built in a nice area, they would generate higher profits and would not cost the state as much money, since only a few beds would be taken by Medicaid patients. On the other hand, placing a nursing home in a poorer area of high need would do more to relieve the shortage of Medicaid beds but would cost the state more money. The conflict between patient needs and state budget pressures made it necessary to compromise. It is unlikely that CON regulation actually did much to change or improve the location of new nursing home beds.

Who gets to build?   Certainly the state might favor faith-based groups that donated money to help care for patients. Being political, however, the state might favor nursing home owners who donated money to help elect a congressperson or senator. With chronic excess demand, the CON itself became valuable property. In effect, one could "buy" patients by obtaining a CON from the government. Once a nursing home owner had a CON, the supply of Medicaid patients was ensured, and the owner would not have to do any marketing or make any quality improvements to attract patients. Competition was thus shifted away from the market into the political regulatory arena.

Windfall profits accrued to anyone who was able to obtain a CON for new construction or who already owned a nursing home. This did not mean, though, that the next owner would make excess profits. When the facility was sold, the new owner had to pay for the building and implicitly for the CON—a piece of paper whose value was roughly equal to the expected future profits of the facility. The new owner, after paying $10 million for a $5 million building to get the CON, would have high fixed costs and find it hard to make a profit unless he or she reduced operating costs and hence reduced quality.

Who pays?   CON restrictions succeeded in reducing state Medicaid budgets and providing excess profits to nursing home owners. The question then became: if both owners and regulators benefited, who got hurt? The answer is that patients and their families paid, directly or indirectly, to generate those financial gains. Without competition among nursing homes, patients were often forced to take whatever bed they could get. Instead of conducting market research to meet patient needs, nursing home operators sensibly devoted their dollars to lobbying for continued regulation. Restrictions on supply also meant higher prices for private-pay patients. The biggest cost of CON regulation is all the hours of unpaid labor and disruption imposed on families who could not get their loved ones into a needed nursing home bed or who had to wait months to do so. In the highest need category (people with dementia, people with multiple impairments in performing ADLs), more than 90 percent are in nursing homes in states where there is no shortage of beds, but only 50 percent of similarly impaired patients are in nursing homes in states that continue to impose tight limits on bed supply.[11] What happens to the other 40 percent? Who cares for them and at what personal sacrifice? Just because family labor and unnecessary declines in quality of life are not charged for in the market does not make them less costly.

Evidence on the Effects of CON

The primary purpose of CON from the beginning has been to limit the growth of states' Medicaid expenditures. The crisis atmosphere generated after Medicaid suddenly flooded the market has eased over time and the reflexive need to use regulations to impose order on a market out of control faded. The shortage of beds created by restricting supply became more of an issue. Long waiting lists and the protests of families whose lives were disrupted by having to provide unpaid caregiving put pressure on states to relax or eliminate their CON rules. The differences between states that have continued to use CON and those that have stopped illustrate some of the effects of artificial controls on supply. The length of time a patient has to wait for a bed has fallen in states where CON has been repealed. Also, the large disparity in waiting time between private-pay and Medicaid patients has been reduced or eliminated as shortages have disappeared. It often has been assumed that nursing homes with a high percentage of Medicaid patients are less successful in attracting private-pay patients and are thus of lower-than-average quality. A study comparing states with and without CON showed that higher percentages of Medicaid reimbursement were indeed associated with lower quality in states where CON caused a chronic shortage of beds.[12] However, this was not the case in the states without CON. As free entry made more beds available, nursing homes had to compete for Medicaid patients by providing better quality. Since 1990, the supply situation has continued to ease, and more and more states show declines in occupancy. With empty beds, competition for all types of patients has intensified.

10.5 CASE-MIX REIMBURSEMENT

Even with an adequate supply of beds, the fact that the state pays only a single fixed rate per day for nursing home care means that some patients may be denied care. A patient who is very sick or whose disruptive mental condition requires frequent attention costs more than a patient who is healthy and lucid. With revenue per day fixed, a nursing home can increase profits by accepting only less costly patients who need very little care. To provide nursing homes with incentives to admit more severely ill patients, some states have developed **case-mix reimbursement** systems that increase payments based on an index of need. Whereas the starting point for acute medical case-mix reimbursement is the diagnosis (see Section 8.2 for a discussion of diagnostically related group (DRG) reimbursement in hospitals), in LTC the starting point is the patient's level of functioning. Most frequently, this is measured in terms of the number of **ADLs** (activities of daily living) for which the individual needs assistance (dressing, grooming, bathing, eating, mobility, transferring, walking, toileting; see Table 10.5) as well as the level of assistance required.[13] In New York state, the association between number of ADLs and cost of care was used to create a number of **resource utilization groups (RUGS)**.

The U.S. General Accounting Office issued a report in 1990 showing that the problem that "heavy care" patients have in obtaining a nursing home bed is substantially reduced in states with systems that adjust reimbursement according to case mix. However, the adjustment is always imperfect, and even with differential payment rates, nursing homes may find it profitable to accept some patients while turning others away. Minnesota created a system with eleven levels of reimbursement from A (patients with 0 to 3 ADLs and no special problems) to K (patients with 7 to 8 ADLs who require special nursing). To the extent that differences in payment rate correctly adjust for differences in cost, a nursing home would have no reason to selectively admit one group rather than another. However, researchers at the University of Minnesota estimated that categories H and J were significantly overcompensated, while categories C and F were significantly undercompensated.[14] The total number of days of care remained basically the same from 1986 (the first year of the case-mix reimbursement system) to 1990, but nursing homes admitted more patients in the overcompensated categories over time and admitted fewer patients in the undercompensated categories (Table 10.6). Even though some of the change may have been due to "gaming" of the regulatory system by reclassifying patients into more profitable categories, part of the change appears to have been a result of selective admissions policies. The lesson of this study is that nursing homes, even nonprofit nursing homes, will respond to any remaining inaccuracies in case-mix reimbursement.

TABLE 10.5	Activities of Daily Living (ADL) Evaluation Form

For each area of functioning listed below, check the description that applies.*

Bathing—either sponge bath, tub bath, or shower

☐	☐	☐
Receives no assistance (gets in and out of tub by self if tub is usual means of bathing)	Receives assistance in bathing only one part of the body (such as the back or a leg)	Receives assistance in bathing more than one part of the body (or not bathed)

Dressing— gets clothes from closets and drawers, including underclothes, outer garments, and using fasteners (including braces, if worn)

☐	☐	☐
Gets clothes and gets completely dressed without assistance	Gets clothes and gets dressed without assistance except for assistance in tying shoes	Receives assistance in getting clothes or in getting dressed, or stays partly or completely undressed

Toileting— going to the "toilet room" for bowel and urine elimination; cleaning self after elimination and arranging clothes

☐	☐	☐
Goes to "toilet room," cleans self, and arranges clothes without assistance (may use object for support such as cane, walker, or wheelchair)	Receives assistance in going to "toilet room" or in cleansing self or in arranging clothes after elimination or in use of night bed pan or commode	Doesn't go to room termed "toilet" for the elimination process

Transfer—

☐	☐	☐
Moves in and out of bed as well as in and out of chair without assistance	Moves in and out of bed or chair with assistance	Doesn't get out of bed

Continence—

☐	☐	☐
Controls urination and bowel movement completely by self	Has occasional "accidents"	Supervision helps keep urine or bowel control; catheter is used or is incontinent

Feeding—

☐	☐	☐
Feeds self without assistance	Feeds self except for getting assistance in cutting meat or buttering bread	Receives assistance in feeding or is fed partly or completely by using tubes or intravenous fluids

* The word *assistance* means supervision, direction, or personal assistance.

Source: Adapted from Katz et al., "Studies of Illness in the Aged. The Index of ADL: A Standardized Measure of Biological and Psychosocial Function," *Journal of the American Medical Association* 185 (1963): 94*ff*.

10.6 SUBSTITUTION

The lack of extra payment for patients who need extra care may mean that they cannot be transferred to a nursing home and hence must remain in a high-cost acute care hospital bed for additional **administratively necessary days (ANDs)**. Some hospitals have even purchased nursing homes primarily to make it easier to discharge their post-acute-care

TABLE 10.6   Nursing Homes Admit More of the Patients Who are Relatively More Profitable

	(Care Level)	Case Index	Revenue	Estimated Cost	Profit	Days of Care 1986	Days of Care 1990	Change %
A	(0–3 ADLs)	1.00	$47.50	$43.64	9%	3,008,098	2,781,037	−8%
B	(0–3 ADLs with behavior problem)	1.30	$51.40	$55.31	−7%	1,236,058	1,066,884	−14%
C	(0–3 ADLs with special nursing)	1.64	$55.83	$68.09	−18%	193,084	76,229	−61%
D	(4–6 ADLs)	1.95	$59.86	$66.96	−11%	1,466,417	1,457,940	−1%
E	(4–6 ADLs and behavior problem)	2.27	$64.01	$61.40	4%	1,252,917	1,071,265	−14%
F	(4–6 ADLs and special nursing)	2.29	$64.28	$89.53	−28%	249,083	105,049	−58%
G	(7–8 ADLs and heavy feeding)	2.56	$67.79	$66.00	3%	1,791,836	2,471,990	38%
H	(7–8 ADLs, heavy feeding & behavior)	3.07	$74.42	$60.66	23%	1,225,666	1,370,201	12%
I	(7–8 ADLs and very heavy feeding)	3.25	$76.76	$79.85	−4%	1,812,752	954,488	−19%
J	(7–8 ADLs, feeding & severe neurology)	3.53	$80.39	$62.79	28%	1,688,881	2,345,085	39%
K	(7–8 ADLs and special nursing)	4.12	$88.06	$89.86	−2%	1,364,042	835,112	−39%
Average			$66.39	$67.64	−0.3%	14,658,834	14,535,280	−0.8%

Source: J. A. Nyman and R. A. Connor, "Do Case-Mix Adjusted Nursing Home Reimbursements Actually Reflect Costs? Minnesota's Experience," *Journal of Health Economics* 13, no. 2 (1994): 145–162.

patients. Yet opportunities for system-wide savings are often passed up because different parties are paying different bills. For instance, Medicare (federal) pays most hospital bills, whereas Medicaid (state) pays most nursing home bills. A state may be unwilling to pay for additional nursing home days, even though each additional hospital day is much more expensive, because the cost of hospital days is borne by the federal government rather than the state.

A larger and more general problem in trying to use service substitution to reduce costs is controlling who gets the additional days of nursing home care. Increased bed supply and changes in reimbursement that make it easier to transfer patients from hospitals to nursing homes also make it easier for new patients to obtain care. The cost of providing care to these new patients tends to outweigh the savings obtained by switching some patients from hospitals to nursing homes. A large experiment attempted to demonstrate cost savings by "channeling" patients at high risk for repeat hospitalization into less expensive nursing homes, home health care, and social services.[15] The channeling project was not able to generate savings, because only a few hospitalizations could be avoided. Counseling patients was itself expensive and, for the most part, resulted in new patients using additional services rather than old patients moving from hospitals to cheaper LTC substitutes.

It was once thought that expanded home health care and ambulatory surgery would save money for Medicare by reducing hospitalization. Part A (hospital) expenses have indeed declined in recent years, but Part B (professional services) expenses have increased by a much greater amount. For example, cataract surgery, IV antibiotics, and physical therapy are cheaper when performed on an outpatient basis, but once the need for a hospital admission was eliminated, so many new patients utilized these services that the total cost of treatment more than doubled.

10.7   FINANCIAL REIMBURSEMENT CYCLES

There is a recurrent cycle of scarcity, generosity, and abuse that occurs in the financing of medical services. This is well illustrated by home health care, which just moved through a surge of uncontrolled spending and is now being restrained. There are typically four stages of reimbursement (see Table 10.7), beginning with charitable assistance, moving through cost reimbursement and complex administered price systems, and ending with firm controls over total budgets. This extended cycle is seen in the development of financing for hospitals, ambulatory surgery, nursing homes and, more recently, home health care. Before the spread of insurance coverage, most medical organizations were nonprofit and the need for more services (and more funding) was broadly recognized. Requests for payment were based on trust. It was assumed that the fees were less than the cost of care or that any excess was being used to subsidize needy people. The amount of funding was limited primarily by the availability of donors. For home health care, this situation held for a number of years. The dominant providers were community and regional visiting nurse services, charitable agencies that employed salaried nurses to visit the disabled homebound. As such, home health care was a minor and unprofitable niche within the health care system, accounting for less than 0.3 percent of national medical expenditures.

As the length of stay in hospitals began to shorten, patients were discharged "quicker and sicker," raising the need for skilled assistance at home. Reimbursement on the traditional "what you ask for" basis was made, mostly to visiting nurse services. Soon, Medicare was paying 25 to 30 percent of the bills, with Medicaid picking up another 5 to 10 percent. Entrepreneurs spotted a new guaranteed stream of funding and developed for-profit businesses that were tightly managed, paid nurses well (and made them see more patients per hour), and raised charges to build the bottom line and expand rapidly. By 1980, home health care had become a $2 billion business, accounting for about 1 percent of total health expenditures, rising to $10 billion (1.6 percent of national health expenditures in 1989).

The second stage of the reimbursement cycle commences when the payer attempts to replace traditional fees with a more precise determination of what services actually cost. This impulse is driven by two opposing claims: (1) from the providers, that the existing payments are not sufficient to cover their costs and will not allow expansion to provide services to all patients who need care, and (2) from the payers, a suspicion that fees are too large and provide excess profits and incentive to create new providers where none are needed. So begins the debate and the implementation of reimbursement based on costs rather than fees.

TABLE 10.7	Stages in The Reimbursement Cycle
Stage 1	**"What you ask for"** —Trusting charity providers to charge appropriately
Stage 2	**Cost reimbursement**—Leads to expansion, manipulation of cost reports
Stage 3	**Complex administered prices**—PPSs put in place to reduce costs get "gamed" by providers seeking even more reimbursement
Stage 4	**Global budget control**—Setting reimbursement increases to match increases in the tax base

Cost reimbursement appears simple—and then the accountants move in. What exactly is "cost" anyway? Shouldn't owners be paid for the use of their buildings and other capital rather than only for operating expenses? Isn't it important to pay owners extra to ensure that patients who are more difficult to treat (those with dementia or AIDS) are able to obtain service? Shouldn't every new home health care agency that opens receive enough cost reimbursement to make sure that it stays in operation? Although these positions are defensible, such cost reimbursement is much different from the way capital markets respond to investors opening new restaurants and predictably leads to a massive increase in capacity. The facile comment regarding accountants should not be taken as disparaging. The accountants who work for health care providers are doing their jobs—which in this situation is to maximize reimbursement so that providers can grow and do more. Over time, the accounting system becomes more highly regulated and more complex, but no more satisfactory. No matter how costs are counted, there always will be disputes (overtime wages, capital arbitrage, sunk costs) and continual expansion (since more costs mean more reimbursement). Eventually, the cost reimbursement system becomes unsustainable, and the era of cost control arrives. For home health care, this turning point was reached in the early 1990s.

After the pathologies of open-ended cost reimbursement have become apparent, attempts are made to set payment limits in advance, usually based on an objective indicator such as patient diagnosis. This method was adopted by hospitals (via DRGs), physicians (via the resource-based relative value scale, RBRVS), and nursing homes (via RUGS). These payments were more difficult to arrange in home health care because the extent of disability and social isolation, not medical need, drives care. Also, unlike surgery or nursing home admission, home health visits were actively welcomed by the homebound elderly and even by elderly people who just needed someone to change their sheets, make a meal, and chat for a while. In some cases, agencies appear to have driven demand by calling elderly patients and asking "Would you like someone to visit you at home? Medicare will pay for it." Abuse of the system became rampant. Payments, which rose 17 percent a year from 1980 to 1989, rose by 40 percent in 1990, 35 percent in 1991, and 37 percent in 1992. This exploitation of the system was unsustainable and led to the inevitable retrenchment with multimillion dollar lawsuits for fraudulent billing and improper referrals.[16] Several years were required to bring the system under control. In 1996, Medicare and Medicaid were still paying $20 billion for home health care, more than half of all home health care expenses. Whereas Medicaid expenditures continued to rise slightly, by 2000 Medicare had cut payments by 50 percent to just $9 billion. Forcing patients and private insurance to pay directly for more visits restored some balance to the system.

October 2000 marked the implementation of the newest Medicare home health financing reform, a fixed predetermined payment rate per 60-day episode.[17] The payment rate depends on an assessment of the patient's overall need for care as classified into one of 80 home health resource groups (HHRGs). Doctors must certify (and recertify) a patient as qualifying for care when the first visit is made, but the number of visits made within a 60-day episode has no effect on total payments. It appears that home health care reimbursement has entered the third stage of the reimbursement cycle, because it is semifixed and largely divorced from the cost accounting procedures of providers.

The endpoint of cost control comes when the payer decides to match payments to the availability of funding, not to the number of patients or visits, or to diagnoses. This has already happened for Medicare payment of physicians under the rubric of sustainable growth rate (SGR), a mechanism for linking the increase in total payments each year to the increase in gross domestic product (and hence to the tax revenues available). Such a rigid and mechanical approach to funding, of course, brings its own problems, leading to further amendments, enlargements, reforms, and revolutions. In this regard, it is not so much the end as the start of a new cycle.

What is important in this discussion is not the specifics of home health care or federal payment regulations, but the fact that the *financial reimbursement cycle* is repeated over and over again as a strategic game between payers and providers in different contexts: hospitals, physicians, nursing homes, home health (and recently, inpatient rehabilitation facilities that in 2002 implemented an IRF PPS system for rehabilitation of hip replacements, stroke, etc.).[18] One side wants to control costs, while the other side wants to increase revenues. The rules are not abstract truths or arbitrary legal dictums written in stone, but are themselves part of the game. Expanded funding in a new area, such as home health care, inevitably means excesses and a certain amount of fraud. Such excesses will, to a greater or lesser extent, be corrected over time.

10.8   THE EFFECTS OF AGING ON COST AND UTILIZATION

Age and Health Care Spending

It is widely assumed that aging increases the need for, and the use of, medical services. This assumption, at least in its simplest form, is not well supported. As an economist, you would quickly point out the constraints imposed by a limited life span. Treating disease in a patient who is expected to die of other causes within five years is less valuable than treating a young patient likely to live another 50 years. When scarce medical resources have to be allocated, most people, even the elderly, support favoring the young. Scarcity imposes another constraint that may limit use: elderly people who cannot afford care. In 1953, older people in the United States spent about 1.3 times as much ($108 versus $85) on medical care as the middle-aged.[19] This is more, but not a lot more. With the advent of Medicare, older people spent more than three times as much on medical care as the under-65 in 1970, five times as much in 1987, then dropping to less than four in 2004 (see Table 10.8 and Figure 10.3).[20] The reason so much more money is spent on medical care for the elderly today than 50 years ago is because the system has made more money available, not because today's elderly are sicker. Comparisons made with other countries confirm that income and insurance, not aging, have caused expenditures to rise.[21]

Close examination of the data shows that today's elderly are healthier and less likely to be disabled than in prior years. Much of the growth in spending has been for the oldest old, and for LTC rather than for curative medicine or surgery.[22] The data suggest that the number of elderly is growing and cumulative disability is increasing, but that health status at age 65, at age 75, and even at age 85 is markedly improving. Spending on medical care

TABLE 10.8	Per Capita Personal Health Expenditures by Age Group, 1953–2004							
	1953	1963	1970	1977	1987	1996	2000	2004
All persons	$69	$143	$291	$616	$1,664	$3,153	$3,803	$5,276
Under age 65	$65	127	234	452	1,088	2,115	2,650	3,953
Age 65 and older	$108	299	809	1,962	5,830	10,285	11,778	14,797
ratio: over/under	1.7	2.4	3.5	4.3	5.4	4.9	4.4	3.7

Adjusted to 2002 dollars. *Source*: Cutler and Meara, 1997, 2004; Hartman, 2009.

FIGURE 10.3   Health Care Spending in the Old and Young, 1953–2004

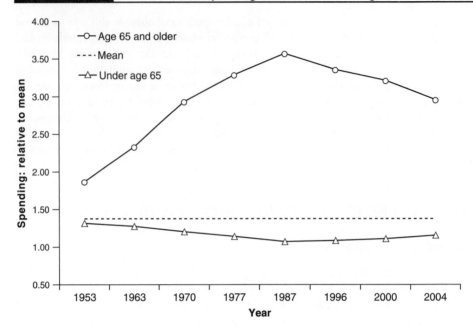

is significantly higher for the last year of life—but that final year, by definition, only occurs once in each lifetime. Furthermore, heroic efforts to save life that seem necessary at age 30, and perhaps justified at age 70, look intrusive and wasteful at age 90. Thus, the actual pattern of spending for medical intervention peaks at about age 75 and begins to decline after that as family and physicians become more willing to accept the dictates of nature. Total health spending continues to rise with advancing age only because more is spent for nursing home, hospice, home health, and related supportive care.

Defining Boundaries: Is Long-Term Care "Medical"?

The Medicare program is immensely popular (and immensely expensive) because it serves every elderly person regardless of need and therefore provides an upper-middle-class standard of care to all by using taxpayers' money. Attempts to forge an equally popular LTC program have failed. Although numerous cultural and political factors are involved, a major reason is that most of the features that characterize medical care (randomly occurring illness, reliance on physicians when quality can be a life-and-death issue, rapid technological innovation) are missing in LTC. Instead, much of the cost of LTC is for housing, food, social amenities—things normally identified as personal responsibilities or lifestyle choices rather than medical care. The boundaries between medical care, social services, and living expenses often become ambiguous. Distinctions between professional services and unpaid family help are often similarly unclear. The divergence between medical care and LTC suggests that the types of health insurance financing developed for medical care may not be appropriate for financing the costs of assisted daily living characteristic of most LTC.

What difference does it make whether LTC is called *medical* or not? In a word, money. Distinguishing services as *medical* makes it more likely that they will be covered by insurance, more likely that the people providing services will be licensed, and more likely that quality will be regulated and that choices by consumers in the marketplace will be supplanted by

TABLE 10.9	Reasons that LTC Insurance Is Not Popular

1   Incidence of LTC is less random than acute illness.

2   Insurance must be purchased so far in advance of anticipated need that savings become a good alternative to insurance.

3   Medicaid is always there, providing a stop-loss against large expenditures.

4   To get benefits paid, purchaser must often be admitted to nursing home. Unlike treatment for acute illness, the person would usually rather make treatment more rather than less difficult to obtain.

5   Benefits mostly reduce expenditures by heirs and Medicaid, rather than helping the patients who pay the premiums.

professional standards. LTC has more in common with social insurance programs such as disability, workers' compensation, pensions, and Social Security than it does with medicine. Yet the tremendous cost of expanding entitlements and the lack of taxpayer support has caused many advocates to try to find ways to "medicalize" LTC to increase the flow of funds to professionals and institutions.

LTC Insurance

Although most medical care is paid for through third-party insurance, private LTC insurance did not even come into existence until the 1980s and still pays for less than 4 percent of nursing home and home health care bills. There are several major reasons LTC insurance is not as attractive to consumers as insurance for acute medical care, which are summarized in Table 10.9. The incidence of disability requiring LTC is not so much random as delayed. If we live long enough, almost all of us will need some form of LTC. Yet if we wait until age 70 to purchase LTC insurance the premiums will be very high since the likelihood of needing that insurance is so great. A more prudent course would be to plan in advance. However, people who purchase LTC insurance at age 40 will have to wait many years to obtain benefits. Financially, they may do almost as well if they put aside savings to be used for LTC if the need arises, letting interest accrue over the intervening years. In addition, people may die without entering a nursing home, and hence the money used for LTC premiums could instead be passed on to their heirs. If one did end up needing a lot of LTC and ran out of savings, there would always be Medicaid to fall back on. Why should people pay premiums for 30 years when the government would pay if they really needed help?

A final barrier to LTC insurance is the nature of the benefit: payment for a nursing home stay. Unlike payment for acute medical treatment, which is expected to improve health or reduce the risk of premature death, payment for nursing home care just makes it easier to be taken from home and be placed in an institution. It is hard to get excited about paying thousands of dollars to merely slow the rate of decline and extend the number of years spent living with disability. On reflection, it becomes clear that the greatest beneficiaries of LTC insurance are not the patients, but their children and the Medicaid program. Children benefit because they may find it easier to send a disabled parent to a nursing home if the charges are paid for by insurance. In addition, children protect their inheritance by having the risk of caring for a disabled parent insured. Medicaid also benefits because nursing home charges are paid for by premiums rather than state and federal tax monies. Expansion of private LTC insurance will be limited until (a) benefits are modified so that they help patients continue to live at home rather than making it easier to be admitted to a nursing home; (b) payments are made in advance with favorable tax treatment by employers, as is the case with most group medical insurance; and (c) policies are coordinated with Medicaid so that they yield financial benefits to patients, their spouses, and heirs, instead of offsetting government expenditures.

Continuing Care Retirement Communities and the Wealthy Elderly

Elderly people with enough money to afford LTC insurance have not been particularly interested in purchasing it. However, the wealthy elderly have flocked to retirement communities and other market alternatives. Among the most successful have been life care communities or **continuing care retirement communities (CCRCs)**. In essence, these residential developments combine an LTC insurance health maintenance organization (HMO) with a retirement community, guaranteeing people a pleasant place to live and nursing care for the remainder of their lives.[23] In most retirement communities, new entrants (usually married couples in their 70s) pay a substantial fixed fee upon entry ($75,000 to $250,000) for their apartments and then a monthly fee ($600 to $2000 a month) for maintenance, housekeeping, social services, and some or all meals. Home health nurses are provided when needed. As a person becomes disabled, he or she can enter a nursing home on the premises. Residents do not own their apartments, but do have the right to live in them until they die or are admitted to the nursing facility. Major advantages of CCRCs are the controlled environment geared toward the elderly, the possibilities of creating a new circle of friends even as health declines, and the ability to continue seeing these friends daily even after entering the nursing facility. CCRCs range from modestly nice to quite luxurious. The nursing facilities tend to be less institutional than those in most nursing homes. Even severely impaired people may still have table linens, candles with dinner, and a homelike atmosphere.

The large entry fee and sizable monthly payments generate two problems: (1) the possibility of bankruptcy or fraud on the part of the owner and (2) lack of affordability. The first CCRCs depended almost entirely on entry fees and had very low monthly rates. Many were "sponsored" but not financially supported by religious denominations. After taking the up-front fee (sometimes, the entire savings and estate of the couple), CCRCs were obligated to provide care for life. The facilities ought to have invested the money wisely so that interest income could have been used to pay for maintenance and nursing home care. Unfortunately, the actuarial estimates were often quite far from the mark. Financial projections assumed that apartments could be turned over and resold every ten years or so, but the people who chose to enter lived much longer than usual for their ages (a form of adverse selection). In many cases, the husband began to need nursing home care (which cost extra) while the wife continued to live for many years (occupying a large apartment that could not be resold). Some religious leaders were uncomfortable about raising monthly fees when millions of dollars in investments were in the bank, even though the future obligations for nursing home care and maintenance were greater than what could be covered by the interest. Necessary financial reserves were depleted over time when monthly rates were not raised promptly. These factors alone would have been sufficient to cause problems, but were compounded in case after case when unscrupulous CCRC operators paid themselves excessive sales fees or salaries, or simply embezzled funds. Immediately after a facility opened, there would be millions of dollars in entry fees in the bank. The loss or mismanagement of these funds would not become evident until years later, when buildings needed repair or residents needed nursing home care. By then, the money was sometimes literally out of the country. Numerous reforms have been instituted to maintain the financial integrity of CCRCs. Now, if a religious denomination agrees to sponsor a facility, it must legally guarantee future expenses. Reserves must be routinely reported, and financial viability, including coverage of medical and nursing home expenses, must be demonstrated. The risky "pay everything up front" financing has been supplanted so that more costs are covered by monthly fees, and often the nursing home care component is paid for separately and subject to standard underwriting practices (e.g., waiting periods, extra fees, exclusions for those entering with preexisting conditions such as cancer or Alzheimer's disease).

TABLE 10.10 Average Income and Wealth for Different Age Categories

	Income		Wealth	
	Median	**Average**	**Median**	**Average**
All Families	$47,300	$84,300	$120,300	$556,300
Under 35	37,400	51,700	11,800	106,000
35 to 44	56,600	83,700	86,600	325,600
45 to 54	64,200	112,400	182,500	661,200
55 to 64	54,600	111,200	253,700	935,800
65 to 74	39,000	92,400	239,400	1,015,200
75 and older	22,800	45,700	213,500	638,200

Source: Survey of Consumer Finances, Federal Reserve Bulletin, page A1-35, February 2009.

More and more elderly people can afford the cost of entering a CCRC. Definitions of "wealthy" are to some extent always subjective, but by any measure, the wealth of the elderly has risen dramatically both in absolute terms and relative to the wealth of the younger population. In the 1950s, many elderly were poor, still struggling with the aftermath of the depression. In contrast, young families faced bright economic prospects, and relatively few children lived in poverty. By 1990, Social Security, marital patterns, and other factors had reversed the incidence of poverty. The elderly were much better off than their children. Favorable tax and transfer treatment, along with years of savings, have made people 65 to 74 the wealthiest group in America, with a net worth of $1,015,200 in 2007, and people 55 to 64 almost equal in net worth at $915,800 (see Table 10.10).[24] This does not mean, however, that there are no subgroups of the elderly with high poverty rates (the single black elderly are notably poor, as are the oldest old, above age 85), but it does mean that many can afford to buy care and protection in the market using their own substantial assets rather than depending on government programs. Married couples reaching age 65 have higher average incomes than the rest of the population, and twice as many financial assets. At least half of them can readily afford a CCRC or other market-based LTC financing mechanism. Public protection of the poor will always be necessary. What is important to change is the perception that all or even most of the elderly are "poor."

The market for supportive services among the elderly is affected not only by demand but also by supply. In this regard, it is important to remember that most care is actually provided by unpaid family and friends. Estimates by Darius Lakdawalla and Tomas Philipson suggest that the increase in the number of healthy older people able to care for others, and particularly the increase in the percentage of the elderly who are male (and thus likely to be married to the more numerous females), will reduce the number of elderly people placed in institutions.[25] It is the lack of someone at home to care for the person, not just disability, that drives up the rate of nursing home admissions.

SUGGESTIONS FOR FURTHER READING

Connie J. Evashwick, ed. *The Continuum of Long-Term Care* (Albany, N.Y.: Delmar Publishers, 2005).

Micah Hartman et al., "U.S. Health Spending by Age," *Health Affairs* 27, no. 1 (2008): w1–w12.

Darius Lakdawalla and Tomas Philipson, "The Rise in Old-Age Longevity and the Market for Long-Term Care." *American Economic Review* 92, no. 1 (March 2002): 295–306.

National Center for Health Statistics, *Trends in Health and Aging*, (http://www.cdc.gov/nchs/). AARP (www.aarp.org).

National Institute on Aging, *An Aging World: 2001*, (www.census.gov/prod/2001pubs/p95-01-1.pdf).

William Scanlon, "A Theory of the Nursing Home Market," *Inquiry* 17, no. 1 (1980): 25–41.

Urban Institute, *Long-Term Care: Consumers, Providers and Financing, a Chartbook*, (www.urban.org/pdfs/ LTC'Chartbook.pdf).

SUMMARY

1. Most LTC expenditures are for nursing home care, but most care of the disabled elderly is **provided by unpaid family members** and friends.

2. As the number of elderly rose and the **shadow price of labor** by adult daughters increased, more and more LTC was shifted from unpaid household production to commercial market purchases of care.

3. Nursing home economics is dominated by a **split two-part market**. Private-pay patients tend to pay more and sometimes receive better care. Medicaid patients must demonstrate to the state that they qualify by being poor. The state pays their bills, but will not pay as much; therefore, there is a chronic excess of Medicaid patients trying to get into beds that nursing home owners would prefer to fill with private-pay patients.

4. CON **regulations** were intended to slow down the construction of new nursing homes after the passage of Medicaid in 1965 greatly increased demand and hence the tax burden on the states. CON has exacerbated the shortage of nursing homes and caused patients to wait months for a bed. **Competing for CONs** has helped regulators and nursing home owners, but has not helped the patients who are forced to wait months for a bed or accept substandard care.

5. In a shortage situation, patients most in need of nursing home care are more likely to be denied a bed, because their care tends to be more costly. To alleviate this problem, some states have replaced the flat-rate per diem with a rate that is **case-mix adjusted** for differences in need. Such systems help match reimbursement with cost, but can never be perfect.

6. **Substituting** lower-cost LTC for hospital care (or home health care for nursing home care) sounds good, but usually increases total system costs because so many new patients are brought in.

7. Payment for home health care, like that of most other medical services, proceeded through a *financial reimbursement cycle* with four stages:

    a. **Fees** paid to trusted voluntary organizations

    b. **Cost reimbursements**

    c. Complex **administered prices**

    d. Total cost control through global **budgets** adjusted to match growth in GDP

    This reimbursement cycle is driven by the strategic behavior of providers who push the boundaries and "game" the system to maximize revenues.

8. LTC primarily provides assistance to people with disabilities to help them perform activities of daily living, and financing is appropriately done through social insurance. "**Medicalizing**" LTC enables providers to tap new sources of funding, allows workers to justify licensure, probably increases quality, and clearly increases total costs. It has become clear that **increases in income and insurance**, not increases in disease and disability, **have allowed medical care expenditures to rise**. The cost of medical care for the elderly is now five times higher than the cost of medical care for the middle-aged, whereas in 1950 the cost of medical care for the elderly was less than two times the cost of medical care for the middle-aged.

9. People in the United States are living longer. Although this means that there will be more and **more elderly people**, the average person age 75 **will be healthier**, more likely to live at home, and more likely to be able to care for a spouse or friend so that he or she too can live at home rather than being admitted to a nursing home.

PROBLEMS

1. How much is the average cost per day of a nursing home stay? On a typical day in the United States, are there more patients in hospitals or nursing homes? Which type of care is growing more rapidly? What is the most rapidly growing form of LTC?

2. {*incidence, social insurance*} Who provides most of the care for elderly people who need assistance with the daily tasks of living? How do these helpers get paid?

3. {*case-mix selection*} Does the administrator of a hospital want to admit patients who are more sick than average or less sick than average? Does the administrator of an LTC facility want to admit patients who are sicker than average or healthier than average? Why do LTC administrators face financial incentives that are different from those that hospital administrators face?

4. {*competition*} Hospitals compete for doctors and the newest technology. How do nursing homes compete? Does price play more or less of a role? What about technology?

5. {*supply controls*} Draw a set of supply and demand diagrams illustrating how CON legislation could cause waiting lists and increase the price of care.

6. {*labor markets*} Several major trends have characterized labor markets in the United States over the past 80 years: wages have increased, life expectancy has increased, and women's participation in the labor force has increased. Discuss how each of these has affected the market for LTC services. Which has been more important in determining the shape of LTC markets: changes in labor market factors or changes in medical technology?

7. {*substitution*} Use supply and demand diagrams to show what would happen if additional LTC insurance allows more substitution of nursing home care for hospital care. According to your diagram, do LTC expenditures increase or decrease? Do hospital expenditures increase or decrease? Do total expenditures (LTC + hospital) increase or decrease?

8. {*rent seeking*} If there is competition for CONs, what is the price of a CON? Who gets paid? Is the CON worth more than is paid for it? If so, who obtains these gains from trade?

9. {*shortages, discrimination*} Would a shortage of beds created by regulation make it easier or more difficult for a nursing home administrator to racially discriminate among patients for admission? Draw supply and demand graphs to illustrate.

10. {*risk*} Are the risks in LTC insurance different from the risks in hospital insurance?

11. {*substitution*} Does the federal/state-funded Medicaid program expand or contract the market for private LTC insurance? Who would benefit from a federal subsidy of private LTC insurance plans?

12. {*productivity, outcomes*} To measure the productivity of medical care, economists attempt to measure outcomes of treatment: increases in longevity, fewer sick days, increased earnings. Which measures would you use to compare the productivity of two nursing homes?

13. {*Medicaid, two-part market, tax incidence*} If you were elderly, would you be in favor of or against a proposal to increase the amount paid per day under Medicaid? Which factors would your response depend on?

14. {*management, vertical integration*} In what ways is a CCRC like an HMO? In what ways is a CCRC different? Are payments made on a similar or different basis? Which is more subject to adverse selection? To moral hazard? Which relies most on gatekeepers? On financial incentives to physicians?

15. {*incidence*} Which socioeconomic groups in the United States benefit most from extensive government funding of LTC? Is the flow of funds progressive or regressive?

16. {*risk aversion, Medigap insurance*} Virtually all elderly people in the United States qualify for Medicare. Almost 70 percent also purchase Medigap insurance, which covers copayments, deductibles, and often home health care and pharmaceuticals. Which insurance, Medicare or Medigap, provides the largest "welfare gain from risk pooling" (see Chapters 4 and 5). Does Medigap insurance increase or decrease the cost of Medicare?

ENDNOTES

1. Peter S. Arno, Carol Levine, and Margaret M. Memmott, "The Economic Value of Informal Caregiving," *Health Affairs* 18, no. 2 (March 1999): 182–188.

2. A. E. Benjamin, "An Historical Perspective on Home Care," *Milbank Quarterly* 71, no. 1 (1993): 129–166.

3. Robert L. Kane, Joseph G. Ouslander, and Itamar B. Abras, *Essentials of Clinical Geriatrics* (New York: McGraw-Hill, 1989), 30–44.

4. Susan Hughes, "Home Health Care," in Connie J. Evashwick, ed., *The Continuum of Long-Term Care* (Albany, N.Y.: Delmar Publishers, 1996), 61–81.

5. Brian Burwell, William H. Crown, Carol O'Shaunessy, and Richard Price, "Financing Long-Term Care," Chapter 13 in Connie Evashwick, ed., *The Continuum of Long-Term Care* (Albany, N.Y.: Delmar Publishers, 1996), 199.

6. William Aaronson, "Financing the Continuum of Care: A Disintegrating Past and an Integrating Future," Chapter 14 in Connie Evashwick, ed., *The Continuum of Long-Term Care* (Albany, N.Y.: Delmar Publishers, 1996), 225.

7. William P. Scanlon, "A Theory of the Nursing Home Market," *Inquiry* 17, no. 1 (1980): 25–41.

8. Korbin Liu, Pamela Doty, and Kenneth Manton, "Medicaid Spend-down in Nursing Homes," *The Gerontologist* 30, no. 10 (1990): 7; H. Temkin-Greener, M. Meiner, E. Petty, and J. Szydlowski, "Spending Down to Medicaid in the Nursing Home and in the Community," *Medical Care* 31, no. 8 (1993): 663–679.

9. Brian Burwell, *Middle-Class Welfare: Medicaid Estate Planning for Long-Term Care Coverage* (Lexington, Mass.: Systemetrics, 1991).

10. S. Moses, "The Fallacy of Impoverishment," *The Gerontologist* 30, no. 1 (1990): 21–25.

11. U.S. General Accounting Office, *Nursing Homes: Admission Problems for Medicaid Recipients and Attempts to Solve Them*, GAO Report #GAO/HRD-90-135, USGPO: Washington, D.C., September 1990.

12. John Nyman, "The Demand for Nursing Home Care," *Journal of Health Economics* 8, no. 2 (1989); and "Excess Demand, the Percentage of Nursing Home Patients, and the Quality of Nursing Home Care," *Journal of Human Resources* 23, no. 1 (1988): 76–92.

13. S. Katz, A. B. Ford, R. W. Moskowitz, B. A. Jackson, and M. W. Jaffee, "Studies of Illness in the Aged. The Index of ADL: A Standardized Measure of Biological and Psychosocial Function," *Journal of the American Medical Association* 185 (1963): 94ff.

14. J. A. Nyman and R. A. Connor, "Do Case-Mix Adjusted Nursing Home Reimbursements Actually Reflect Costs? Minnesota's Experience," *Journal of Health Economics* 13, no. 2 (1994): 145–162.

15. P. Kemper, "The Evaluation of the National Long-Term Care Demonstration," *Health Services Research* 23, no. 1 (special issue) (1988).

16. George Anders and Laurie McGinley, "How Do You Tame a Wild U.S. Program? Slowly and Reluctantly. Medicare Home Health Visits Are a Boon for Entrepreneurs; Costs Explode 30% a Year," *Wall Street Journal*, 6 March 1996, sec. A, p. 1ff.

17. Paul L. Grimaldi, "Medicare's New Home Health Prospective Payment System Explained," *Health Care Financial Management* 11 (November 2000): 46–56.

18. Nereraj Sood, Melinda Buntin, Jose Escarce, "Does How Much and How You Pay Matter? Evidence from the Inpatient Rehabilitation Care Prospective Payment System," *Journal of Health Economics* 27 (2008): 1046–1059.

19. David M. Cutler and Ellen Meara, "The Medical Costs of the Young and Old: A Forty-year Perspective," National Bureau of Economic Research Working Paper #6114, Cambridge, Mass. (July 1997).

20. The relative reduction since 1987 is even more pronounced among the oldest old aged 85+, who spent 6.9 times as much in 1987 but just 5.7 times as much in 2004. See Micah Hartman et al., "U.S. Health Spending by Age," *Health Affairs* 27, no. 1 (2008): w1–w12; James Lubitz et al., "Three Decades of Health Care Use By the Elderly, 1965–1998," *Health Affairs* 20, no. 2 (March 2001): 19–21.

21. Thomas E. Getzen, "Population Aging and the Growth of Health Expenditures," *Journal of Gerontology: Social Sciences* 47, no. 3 (1992): S98–104.

22. Brenda C. Spillman and James Lubitz, "The Effect of Longevity on Spending for Acute and Long-term Care," *New England Journal of Medicine* 342 (May 11, 2000): 1409–1415.

23. H. S. Ruchlin, "Continuing Care Retirement Communities: An Analysis of Financial Viability and Health Care Coverage," *The Gerontologist* 28, no. 2 (1988): 156–162.

24. B. K. Bucks, A. B. Kennickell, T. L. Mach and K. B. Moore, "Changes in U.S. Family Finances from 2004 to 2007: Evidence from the Survey of Consumer Finances," *Federal Reserve Bulletin* (2008), pp. A8–38, http://www.federalreserve.gov/pubs/bulletin/.

25. Darius Lakdawalla and Tomas Philipson, "The Rise in Old-age Longevity and the Market for Long-term Care," *American Economic Review* 92, no. 1 (March 2002): 295–306.

CHAPTER 11

PHARMACEUTICALS

QUESTIONS

1. Which are most important in the pharmaceutical industry: fixed costs or variable costs?

2. How many drugs do Americans take? Who pays for them?

3. What events led to the regulation of prescription drugs by the Food and Drug Administration (FDA)?

4. Are patents a cost or an asset?

5. Why is so much more spent on marketing drugs than on marketing surgery or psychotherapy?

6. How profitable is the drug industry?

7. Do patents raise or lower the productivity of research?

8. Do generic drugs replace or compete with brand-name drugs?

9. How are prescription costs "managed" by insurance companies?

10. Do pharmaceutical companies compete for patients, prescriptions, or payments?

In any given week, more than 80 percent of U.S. adults use some form of medication, with 50 percent taking a drug prescribed by a doctor.[1] Twelve prescriptions per year are filled for the average American. It is this "ethical" prescription pharmaceutical market that we examine in this chapter. Sales of creams, ointments, vitamins, herbal supplements, headache pills, digestive aids, and other over-the-counter (OTC) medications, which can be obtained without a prescription, amount to around $40 billion—a large sum, but only a fraction of the $256 billion spent on prescription drugs in 2010.[2] The cost structure (large sunk costs for research, development, and marketing, then almost zero variable cost per pill no matter how high the price) makes the economics of pharmaceuticals dramatically different from most medicine care and more like software, books, DVDs, and other "information goods." Pharmaceuticals can be easily packaged, stored, and shipped overseas, which is a primary reason that this part of health production is truly international. U.S. companies make more than a third of their sales overseas, and several major U.S. suppliers are based in Europe and Asia (see "Pharmaceuticals" in Chapter 17).

Pharmaceuticals make up 10 percent of national health expenditures but are a much larger part of the free cash flow in health care. The reason is that the industry is so concentrated and profitable—consisting of a dozen companies earning billions of dollars. With many prices far above marginal cost, drug companies are vulnerable to criticism, and repeated calls have been made for price controls. However, it is evident even to critics that pharmaceuticals have been one of the major technological success stories of the twentieth century, with new drugs extending life span and productivity at much lower cost than surgery and hospitalization. The profits earned by shareholders, while perhaps excessive in some cases, have been the incentive for expanding corporate research and development (R & D), which has increased from $2 billion in 1980 to more than $40 billion in 2005. The gains in health directly attributable to profit-driven pharmaceutical innovation are collectively worth far more than all sunk costs and shareholder dividends.

11.1 PHARMACEUTICAL REVENUES: SOURCES OF FINANCING

As with all health care services, funding for pharmaceutical products comes from a variety of sources, including patients, employers and private insurance, and federal and state governments (see Table 11.1). The process of obtaining a drug begins with the patient visiting a physician. After making a diagnosis, the physician may give the patient a prescription for a specific drug and directions for its use. Although all drugs are approved for sale by the **Food and Drug Administration (FDA)** based on specific indications, physicians can prescribe drugs as they think appropriate. Moreover, when writing a prescription, physicians usually do not have to provide a specific indication for the medication. The prescription may be written using the scientific name of the drug or a brand name made up by the manufacturer that first patented the drug.

The patient usually takes the prescription to the local pharmacy, where a licensed pharmacist fills the prescription. Pharmacists provide additional information about how to take the drug and its potential side effects. If the drug has been in use for a long time, the original patent period may have expired and there is apt to be a chemically and biologically equivalent FDA-approved **generic drug** that is cheaper than the original brand-name version. The pharmacist will usually substitute the cheaper version unless the prescription explicitly requires the brand name (65 percent of all prescriptions were filled with generics in 2006). The average prescription has a retail cost of about $70: $120 for brand names and $34 for generics (Table 11.2).[3]

In 1970, 82 percent of all drug costs were paid by patients out of pocket. The little bit of drug insurance that was available operated retrospectively through "major medical" benefits, requiring the patient to submit bills and wait for payment, or through government programs for the indigent. This situation was totally reversed by 2010, when only 19 percent of prescription costs were paid out of pocket. Shifting payments to insurance and providing a "drug card" that could be used at the local pharmacy required the development of a new

TABLE 11.1	Sources of Funds for Pharmaceuticals Products
2010 Total	$825 per person, 10% of National Health Expenditures
Out of pocket	16%
Private insurance	39%
Medicare	27%
Medicaid	12%
Other public programs	6%

Source: CMS National Health Account Projections.

TABLE 11.2	Pharmaceutical Sales, R&D, and Profits

Major Brand Pharmaceutical Manufacturers

	Total 2001 Revenues	U.S.	R&D	*Profit*	A Major Drug	U.S. Sales
Pfizer	$32,084	$17,631	$4,847	*$7,752*	Lipitor	$4,423
GlaxoSmithKline	29,847	15,474	5,496	*4,498*	Flonase	–NA–
Merck	47,716	12,519	2,456	*7,282*	Zocor	$4,690
Johnson & Johnson	33,004	10,922	3,591	*5,668*	Procrit	$2,335
Bristol-Myers Squibb	19,423	10,505	2,259	*2,570*	Glucophage	$2,655
Lilly	11,543	7,627	2,235	*2,809*	Prozac	$1,659
Wyeth	14,129	6,983	1,869	*2,285*	Effexor	$1,098
Pharmacia	19,302	6,512	2,949	*1,291*	Celebrex	$2,447
Schering-Plough	9,802	5,059	1,312	*1,943*	Claritin	$2,716
Abbott	16,285	3,770	1,578	*1,550*	Depakote	$869
Total U.S. sales, including generics		175,000 ($ millions)				

Generic Manufacturers

Teva	$2,077			*$278*	Fluoxetine (Prozac)	
Ivax Corp	1,215			*236*	Onxol (Taxol)	
Watson Pharmaceuticals	1,161			*116*	Diliatizem (Cardizem)	
Andrx	740			*73*	Loratadine (Claritin)	
Barr Laboratories	510			*63*	Oral contraceptives	

Biotechnology Firms

Amgen	$4,016		967	*$1,120*	Epogen	$2,109
Biogen	1,043		366	*273*	Avonex	$972
Genentech	2,082		613	*404*	Humulin	$1,061
Incyte	219		183	*(188)*		
Millenium	246		510	*(192)*		

Source: Standard & Poors Industry Profile, Pharmaceuticals, 2002; CMS Health Care Industry Update—Pharmaceuticals, 2003.

form of contractual intermediary—the PBM, which took care of all claims and rebates that had to be processed. PBMs expanded rapidly and were responsible for more than half of all prescriptions filled by 2002.

Most patients have insurance and pay only the copayment, which currently averages $11 for generics and $25–$45 for brand names. Some insurance plans require the patient to pay a percentage of the price (coinsurance) rather than a specified amount, and other insurance plans require the patient to pay in full when the prescription is filled and send a copy of the bill for full or partial reimbursement later. These alternatives are more confusing and more cumbersome, which is one reason the market has shifted over time to the copayment system run by carve-out managed care organizations called **pharmacy benefit managers (PBMs)**. PBMs are subcontractors used by insurance companies to develop benefit plans, administer claims, and manage relationships with pharmaceutical companies (manufacturers) and retail pharmacies that operate behind the scenes and so are mostly invisible to patients. PBMs do not have any direct control over physicians' prescribing behavior. However, by creating a formulary (list of preferred drugs) and setting differential copayments (see the discussion of three-tiered benefits in Section 5.5), PBMs indirectly influence physicians' choices through patients' pocketbooks. In addition, PBMs have become sophisticated about calling physicians and suggesting product substitutions.

Inpatient Pharmaceuticals

The process of receiving a drug as an inpatient in a hospital differs significantly from the process used for outpatients. Again, it begins with a physician writing a prescription, but the prescription goes directly to the hospital pharmacy. The prescription is filled by the staff pharmacist and administered to the patient by the nursing staff. All medications are carefully noted on the patient's hospital chart.

Payment for an inpatient's drug depends on how the hospital is reimbursed for its services. Under Medicare, the hospital receives a flat, fixed payment based on patient diagnosis and the average cost of treating a patient with that diagnosis (DRG, as described in Section 8.2). A component of this payment is based on average drug utilization, but the hospital does not receive payment linked directly to drug utilization. A number of states have adopted all-payer DRG reimbursements that extend this form of payment to all patients. If the hospital is being paid on a per diem rate, average drug utilization generally is incorporated into the daily rate. Again, the hospital does not receive any payment directly associated with drug utilization. Only in cases where the hospital is paid on a "charges" basis is drug utilization itemized and billed directly to the patient or third-party payer. Thus, in many cases, the hospital bears the full marginal cost of the drug.

Because hospitals often bear the marginal cost of the drugs they administer to patients, they have a strong financial incentive to minimize the overall pharmaceutical budget. In pursuit of this objective, hospitals often establish their own formulary of drugs they keep in stock and from which physicians may prescribe. By negotiating with pharmaceutical companies over including particular drugs in the formulary, hospitals are able to utilize their market power to obtain discounts on drugs that have close competitors. However, a hospital must balance these economic decisions against antagonizing the physicians on the hospital medical staff, on whom the hospital must rely for admissions.

11.2 USES OF FUNDS

When a person goes to a local pharmacy to fill a prescription, the retailer gets 20 to 25 percent of the $70 (average price) total to cover the costs of labor, overhead, and profit.[4] Most of the remainder, 70 to 80 percent, goes to the pharmaceutical company that manufactured the drug. A small amount, 2 to 3 percent, goes to a wholesaler that obtains drugs from many manufacturers, then warehouses and delivers them to a variety of retail pharmacies. The flow of funds is complicated because most payments come from insurance companies (which must be compensated for risk bearing) and go through PBMs (which must get compensated for claims processing and negotiating). This flow of funds also depends in part on the negotiating power of each party. A diagram of this flow is presented in Figure 11.1, which has been simplified to reduce clutter and make the flow of funds more understandable. In addition, the amounts are approximate because only partial or incomplete survey estimates are available for many aspects of the industry. Patients using their own money are not involved in this complex set of transfers—and they lose! Patients without insurance pay list rather than discounted prices, which are 5 to 45 percent higher than what HMOs, insurance companies, and Medicaid plans pay for the identical prescription filled at the same pharmacy.[5]

FIGURE 11.1	Flow of Pharmaceutical Funds

Retail Pharmacies

There are 55,000 local pharmacies, with more than half in three large chains (CVS, Walgreens, and Rite-Aid).[6] Increased competitive pressure and the need for sophisticated information systems for insurance billing, ordering, marketing to consumers, and preventing drug interactions have caused the number of pharmacies to fall and an increasing number of them to be located in chain stores. Patients with chronic illnesses who take large quantities of medicines on a continuing basis have increasingly turned to mail-order and Internet pharmacies with even lower prices and distribution costs. Mail order now accounts for about 15 percent of retail drug sales. Most retail pharmacies purchase inventories from wholesalers that buy both generic and brand-name drugs from the manufacturers. Because of the many drugs available, most local pharmacies do not carry a large inventory of each drug but rely on computerized inventory systems to get daily deliveries from the wholesaler. Wholesalers and pharmacists usually cannot switch patients from one product to another (except for generic products). As a result, they are unable to exert market power against the manufacturer, but instead must pay the full, list price of the drug—often called the **average wholesale price (AWP)**. Hospitals purchasing drugs for inpatient use may buy directly from the manufacturers, but usually purchase from wholesalers.

Wholesalers

Three companies (McKesson, Cardinal, and AmerisourceBergen) account for more than 80 percent of the wholesaling business.[7] Their jobs are limited to warehousing and distribution—they play no role in the acquisition of patients or insurance financing. Thus, the physical movement of drugs—buying and selling on the wholesale side—is totally separate from the complex flow of funds on the patient/retail side. As such, moving drugs is fairly cheap and accounts for only a fraction of total costs despite the large volume of items being shipped around.

Insurance Companies and PBMs

The financial side of the pharmaceutical business is made up of insurance companies and PBMs, some of which may not be entirely distinguishable from one another because large insurers (such as Aetna, CIGNA, Wellpoint) have their own PBMs. Managed care has had a major impact on the way the pharmaceutical industry conducts business. PBMs consolidate the purchasing power of multiple insurance companies and employer health benefits plans covering millions of people, and thus can force manufacturers to give sizable discounts. The three big PBMs (Express Scripts, Medco, AdvancePCS) have a majority of the business and are relatively independent, although they have equity ties both to insurance entities and to pharmaceutical manufacturers. More than half of the total pharmaceutical dollars now flow through PBMs, leaving perhaps one-quarter to one-sixth still flowing through unmanaged insurance payment systems.

The PBM gets fees from the insurance company for handling claims (and may even be a capitated, risk-bearing provider of benefits), but gets most of its funding from pharmaceutical manufacturer discounts. Aggregate purchasing power is exercised in the form of mandatory rebates. Although the prescription passes through the wholesaler at list (AWP) price with a retail markup, the PBM negotiates with the manufacturer, and a rebate of 5 to 15 percent is paid directly to the PBM. Medicaid gets a special superdiscount of 15.1 percent based on the best available price given to any nongovernment buyer, which returned $5 billion to state budgets in 2002.[8] The various transfers and rebates make it difficult to determine exactly who gets what in dollar terms. Health insurance premiums paid by employers and patients include prescription coverage, but the amount attributable to pharmaceuticals (with or without overhead) cannot be determined without using a set of arbitrary allocations. Rebates should be counted as revenue to the PBM but are not routinely reported. Thus, the percentages in Figure 11.1 should be considered approximations rather than exact measures.

Pharmaceutical Firms

About $286 billion dollars in 2007 went to the pharmaceutical manufacturing companies, accounting for the bulk (80 percent) of all drug costs. The top brand name blockbuster drugs (e.g., Lipitor, Zocor, Prevacid, Procrit, Plavix, Advair, Epogen, Nexium, Zoloft, Zyprexa) have more than $3 billion in annual sales, and a single drug can make or break a company (see Table 11.2). The largest pharmaceutical companies (Merck, Johnson & Johnson, Pfizer, GlaxoSmithKline) each have more than $30 billion in sales, and the top ten pharmaceutical companies account for 60 percent of all prescription dollars.[9]* Conversely,

---

*Standard & Poor's Corporation generously made available access to a number of its proprietary industry reports.

TABLE 11.3

Uses of Funds for
Pharmaceutical Products

Cost of goods	30%
Research & development	13%
Sales, marketing, admin	31%
Taxes	6%
Net income	20%

Source: CMS Health Care Industry
Update—Pharmaceuticals, 2003.

although generics account for 65 percent of all prescription volume and are four of the ten most frequently prescribed drugs in terms of units, they account for only 21 percent of total sales in dollars. Only one generic firm, Teva, had prescription sales of $2 billion or more—and it has begun to develop brand-name drugs.

Funds that flow into pharmaceutical firms are used in a variety of ways. For example, they are used to support R&D efforts as firms seek to develop newer and better drugs before their competitors. These funds are also used to support the marketing and promotional efforts needed to get physicians to prescribe their drug rather than a competitor's drug. In addition, some of these funds are used to cover the costs of manufacturing, distribution, and administration that go along with any production process, and a portion of these funds are profits, which are either given to stockholders in the form of dividends or reinvested in the company in the form of retained earnings. A breakout of the uses of funds is shown in Table 11.3.

Manufacturing the drugs takes about one-quarter of pharmaceutical companies' resources. Most studies have shown that there are constant returns to scale in the manufacturing of pharmaceutical products; that is, the average manufacturing cost is independent of the amount produced. In part this is because most drugs are manufactured in small batches rather than in a continual process. Production in small batches is a result of the need to maintain high quality standards. Although large batches are generally more economical to manufacture, there is a greater variance in the quality of the product and a greater chance that some of the units will have either too much or too little of the active ingredients. With pharmaceutical products, such deviations could be deadly; hence, small manufacturing batches are the norm. However, the initial development of the sophisticated extraction and production process is itself very costly and constitutes a large fixed (sunk) cost, which gives rise to economies of scale.

Advertising and promotional activities account for 20 to 35 percent of the pharmaceutical dollar. These activities primarily consist of detailing, sampling, and journal advertising. Of these, detailing and sampling are the most important. Detailing involves a representative of the pharmaceutical firm calling on an individual physician. During this meeting, the representative will discuss one or two products with the physician. For each drug discussed, the representative gives the physician the results of recent tests, explains how the drug works, what the potential side effects are, and discusses the advantages of this drug over competitors' drugs. The representative may give the physician literature on the drug, as well as free samples to pass on to patients. In addition, the detailer answers questions the physician might have about the drug or its use. The information presented and literature given to the physician must meet with strict FDA guidelines. Empirical studies have shown that detailing can have a large impact on a physician's prescribing behavior and on the elasticity of demand for individual products. As a result of these studies, a number of politicians have charged that the promotional activities of the industry are wasteful and excessive and have called for increased regulation of the industry. Whether such actions are justified, and their overall social impact, are the subject of ongoing research and debate.

R&D accounts for 10 to 25 percent of the total pharmaceutical dollar. Viewing R&D in this manner, however, is somewhat inappropriate because it gives the impression that R&D activities are funded by current sales, a notion perpetuated by current accounting practices and the drug industry itself. It is more appropriate to view R&D expenditures as investments in intangible capital rather than a current period expense (see Chapter 12). Viewing R&D in this manner reveals that current cash flows are the result of past R&D expenditures and that the primary incentive for current R&D efforts is the future cash flows expected from these investments. When viewed this way, it is clear that policies and environmental changes that jeopardize future cash flows adversely affect current R&D incentives.

Profits account for 10 to 25 percent of the pharmaceutical dollar. Pharmaceutical firms are consistently ranked as the most profitable industry by *Fortune* magazine, and have been for many years. In 2002, profitability was reported as 18.5 percent of sales. Banking was ranked as the second most profitable industry at 13.5 percent of sales. The median profitability of all industries was reported to be 3.3 percent.[10] Looking at the profits per dollar of sales, however, may not be the correct way to examine the issue. It is necessary to examine the implied rate of return on capital invested in the pharmaceutical industry to determine whether returns are excessive. Doing so requires a complicated set of adjustments, in part because of the need to capitalize R&D expenditures. Depending on how R&D is treated, on the cost of capital used for the industry, and on the time period examined, researchers have arrived at differing conclusions.

Cost Structure

The ***economics of the pharmaceutical industry are dominated by fixed costs.*** Discovery, R&D, regulatory approval, and market introduction all are sunk costs when the first pill is sold. The cost of manufacturing an additional unit is a fraction of the price, usually less than 20 percent, and sometimes amounts to mere pennies on the dollar. After fixed costs are recovered, each additional unit sold is almost pure profit. This makes it worthwhile to put millions, even billions, into marketing. The pharmaceutical industry is an exemplar of the post-modern "information economy," where a label is worth much more than the cost of the product on which it is placed. Other industries in which most costs are fixed, such as information technology (software, Web sites), media (movies, CDs, books), and luxury goods (clothes, perfume) tend to use mega-marketing techniques for the same reason—the gross margins (revenue less variable cost) are so attractive.[11]

Such a disproportionate cost structure does not apply to the other parts of the pharmacy industry: retail drug stores, wholesalers, insurance companies, and PBMs. Although there are some economies of scale, costs rise almost proportionately (perhaps 80 percent) with volume. Since there are substantial incremental variable costs per unit, it is not worth pushing so hard for more sales or putting so much money into marketing. Hence, behavior in these parts of the industry resembles that of more traditional firms.

11.3 HISTORY AND REGULATION OF PHARMACEUTICALS

The pharmaceutical industry has existed in its current form since the 1930s. Before then, local pharmacists (or chemists) mixed potions and elixirs from bulk chemicals using either standardized formulas or their own concoctions. Today, the modern U.S. pharmaceutical industry comprises more than 1,200 firms that produce a wide range of products for disease treatment and prevention, although the industry is dominated by a much smaller number (about 20) very large firms. Recently, the pharmaceutical industry has drawn considerable attention for its pricing and promotional policies. Some politicians have alleged that the industry charges excessive prices and spends too much money promoting products to physicians. These allegations have resulted in calls to regulate prices in the pharmaceutical industry.

The regulation of the pharmaceutical industry and its products evolved during the twentieth century in response to increased potency, effectiveness, and toxicity of drugs. Until the late 1800s, most "pharmaceutical preparations" had an immediate effect of making the patient feel better, although in most instances they did little to cure the underlying disease. This meant that patients could directly evaluate the benefits of the drug and did not need extensive guidance from health care professionals in choosing which products to use.

The first "modern" pharmaceutical product, diphtheria antitoxin, was developed in the mid-1890s and dramatically reduced the incidence of diphtheria. However, because this new drug did not have an immediate effect on the patient (it prevented the person from becoming sick), it was much more difficult for the patient to evaluate the drug's benefit. (Would he or she have gotten sick without the drug?) Also, although the benefits were not readily apparent to the patient, some of the dangerous side effects were all too obvious. Thus, health care professionals with specialized knowledge about drugs became involved in helping patients decide which products to use.

The first regulation of pharmaceutical products was the Biologics Control Act of 1902. This legislation was a direct response to contaminated diphtheria antitoxin that fatally infected 13 children. This incident contributed to overall concerns about the safety of the food and drug supply that were being raised in the popular press and in books, such as Upton Sinclair's *The Jungle*. These events were quickly followed by the passage of the Pure Food and Drug Act of 1906. Although the act focused primarily on the food supply, it required drug manufacturers to provide adequate labeling. The manufacturers either had to use a standardized formula for making the product or provide a complete list of their product's contents.

These companies were not producing pharmaceuticals the way today's integrated firms do. Mostly, they were producing bulk and specialty chemicals for sale to packaging firms and local pharmacies. They were contract producers, with firms providing similar lists of products and competing on the basis of price and service, not science.[12] Moreover, despite the production of many "drugs," few diseases could actually be cured or controlled by drugs. The 1902 and 1906 acts reduced the number of competitors, making the remaining firms larger and more profitable. Then the start of World War I brought an unexpected and inadvertent windfall. Germany, at that time the leader in chemical and pharmaceutical research, held most scientific and process patents. U.S. firms paid license fees for use of these patents but rarely did their own research. When the United States entered the war against Germany, the existing patents were voided or transferred to U.S. firms, and the production of specialty chemicals greatly increased (because obviously the nation could not depend on an enemy to provide medications). U.S. firms came out of the war flush with profits, with a portfolio of patents taken from German firms such as Bayer and IG Farben, and vastly increased their technological capabilities. During the 1920s and 1930s, pharmaceutical firms built a new strategy, forging alliances with physicians and being identified with "ethical" (prescribed) medications rather than industrial chemical suppliers and secret tonics for home use.[13] Prior to 1930, most drug profits came from these tonics and "patent medicines" (which did not really have a patent) using secret formulas (usually heavy on alcohol and opiates) with fancy names and labels (Lydia's Little Liquid Drops, Dr. Johnson's Miracle Feelgood) marketed to people at "medicine shows" held in rural areas or general stores in town. After 1940, profits increasingly came from purified medicines, which were made under strict supervision using scientific methods and prescribed and administered by doctors.

In 1931, the regulatory aspects of the federal Bureau of Chemistry became known as the FDA, which today is responsible for evaluating new products and overseeing their manufacture (see Table 11.4). In this era before antibiotics, the discovery of broad-spectrum sulfa drugs was a major breakthrough. Although saving many lives, however, they also

TABLE 11.4	Major Legislation Affecting Pharmaceuticals

1902	Biologics Control Act
1906	Pure Food and Drug Act
1938	Food, Drugs, and Cosmetics Act
1962	Harris-Kefauver Drug Act Amendments
1984	Hatch-Waxman Drug Price Competition and Patent Restoration Act
1992	Prescription Drug User Fee Act
2001	TRIPS: Agreement on Trade-Related Aspects of Intellectual Property Rights (World Trade Organization)

precipitated a major public disaster. Produced as a yellow powder, sulfa was awkward to ingest in large quantities. The Massengill Company decided to provide a liquid formulation, but the powder would not dissolve in water or alcohol. Eventually the company produced Elixir Sulfanilamide by dissolving sulfa in ethylene glycol. However, this solvent, commonly referred to as antifreeze, is quite poisonous. In 1937 more than a hundred people who drank the new product convulsed from pain and suffered agonizing deaths. Outraged, the public called for sanctions—but could find no law the company had broken. Massengill, an old and proud company, was mortified and anxious to make amends. Killing people with a toxic product was not yet against the law; therefore, the company pled guilty to "mislabeling" (technically "elixir" was supposed to mean "in alcohol") and paid a fine of $26,100, the largest such fine ever paid up to that time. Reaction to the incident led to major legislation.[14]

The Food, Drug, and Cosmetics Act of 1938 established several important provisions. First, it required pre-registration of all new drugs with the FDA, giving the agency the opportunity to test the drug before marketing. The act also gave the FDA the mandate of preventing unsafe drugs from *entering* the market. The new law, however, specifically excluded drugs that were administered by "trained professionals" for testing purposes. Second, it increased the amount of information that had to be included on the label of any drug sold without a prescription. This information included statements of recommended uses and potential dangers. Drugs sold "by prescription only" were not held to these same labeling standards.

Through these labeling provisions, the Food, Drug, and Cosmetics Act created the first real distinction between prescription and over-the-counter (OTC) drugs. Although previously any nonnarcotic could be sold as either prescription or OTC, after 1938 nearly all new drugs were classified as prescription only. This was an unintended effect of the law; the original intent was not to restrict self-medication, but simply to place the use of the most dangerous drugs under professional supervision. Manufacturers, however, soon realized that *restricting sales of a product to prescription only reduced the elasticity of demand*, since the physician writing the prescription was not directly paying for the drug and the patient paying for the drug rarely challenged the physician's authority. The lower price elasticity allowed the firm to charge a higher price, since the patient and pharmacist could not substitute a cheaper product once the prescription was written. Moreover, requiring a prescription gave the appearance that the drug was more potent or effective. Finally, the medical profession strongly supported these restrictions, in part because the profession directly benefited from forcing patients to see a physician before receiving treatment.

During the 1940s, three key changes dramatically altered the pharmaceutical industry. First, new techniques for discovering and isolating potentially beneficial substances were developed in the process of discovering streptomycin. Second, the U.S. Patent Office ruled that the chemical modifications made to streptomycin, which enabled it to be isolated and purified, created a new product. Moreover, the process that developed this product and the product itself were deemed patentable. Third, instead of licensing patents to competitors, as had been done in the past, pharmaceutical firms began to exercise their patent rights to control the production, distribution, and price of the product. Together, these changes ushered in the era of the modern pharmaceutical firm. These firms are R&D driven and use patents to maintain prices above short-run marginal cost and reap the rewards of R&D activities.

The 1950s and early 1960s represented a heyday of drug development, as one firm after another introduced "wonder drugs." Many states passed "anti-substitution" laws, which further reduced the elasticity of demand by requiring pharmacists to fill the prescriptions as written rather than substituting cheaper generic products. However, questions began to arise about the effectiveness of some of these new drugs and whether the prices were too high.

In 1959, Senator Estes Kefauver's Antitrust and Monopoly Subcommittee began hearings on whether too many drugs that were minor variations of existing drugs were being introduced to extend the patent life of a product line, a concern that has a familiar ring today. However, it was the thalidomide incident in 1961–1962 that triggered passage of the 1962 Harris-Kefauver Drug Amendments and brought this heyday of drug development to a screeching halt.

Thalidomide was a drug used to treat nausea during pregnancy. Although it had not yet received FDA approval, it was being widely distributed to physicians for "experimental purposes" when it was discovered that it caused major birth defects in some babies born to women who had taken the drug. This inflamed the fears that drug companies, in their rush to market new drugs and earn large profits, were "egregiously exposing humans to potentially harmful drugs during clinical trials."[15] As a result of this fear, Congress passed legislation that greatly increased the burden on pharmaceutical firms not only to show that their products were safe, but also to show that they were effective when used in the manner directed. In addition, the testing procedures used to establish these results were put under the oversight of the FDA. The 1962 amendments also required pharmaceutical firms to follow "good manufacturing and laboratory practices," as defined by the FDA, and gave the FDA the authority to inspect manufacturing plants. Finally, the 1962 amendments extended these testing requirements to both generic (identical) and similar (me-too) drugs. Previously, these drugs could avoid premarket testing through certification from the FDA that they were in effect the same as the original drug.

These amendments dramatically increased the costs of and time required for new drug development and, as a result, slowed the rate of new drug introductions. The average number of new drug introductions fell from 51 per year between 1956 and 1961 to only 20 per year between 1962 and 1967. Although these restrictions increased the development cost for pioneering drug firms, they also reduced competition once patents expired by creating larger barriers to entry for the producers of generic products. Over the years, considerable debate erupted over whether these restrictions were excessive, whether they increased or decreased consumer welfare, and whether they increased or decreased the profitability of pharmaceutical firms. What is clear, however, is that after the passage of the 1962 amendments, the length of time between the discovery or synthesis of a new drug and its market introduction increased dramatically. In 1960, the average drug development time was 35 months; by 1980 this had increased to 145 months. These amendments also had a chilling effect on the introduction of generic products, since generic manufacturers had to duplicate all the research conducted by the pioneering firm to gain approval for their own new drug application.

In 1984, Congress passed the Drug Price Competition and Patent Term Restoration Act (known as the Hatch-Waxman Act after its sponsors), which attempted to remedy some of the problems created by the 1962 amendments. First, the act established the Abbreviated New Drug Application (ANDA), which allowed a generic manufacturer to show that its drug was "bioequivalent" to the pioneer manufacturer's product, rather than repeat all the safety and efficacy studies. Since 1984, hundreds of products have been introduced under the ANDA provisions. Second, the act established a formula for increasing the patent life of a new product to restore some of the time (up to five years) lost due to the premarket regulatory process.

The 1997 FDA Modernization Act made a number of changes to speed the approval of new drugs. It also allowed seriously ill patients easier access to experimental compounds, provided new incentives for development of pediatric medicines, and expanded the ability of pharmaceutical companies to provide information about off-label (unapproved) uses of drugs.

The World Trade Organization (WTO) brought drug patents into the global trading system through the Agreement on Trade-Related Aspects of Intellectual Property Rights (TRIPS) adopted at the November 2001 meeting in Doha, Qatar. The TRIPS agreement establishes minimum international obligations, including a patent term of 20 years and a period of exclusivity for clinical data. This agreement has been adopted by 140 countries and represents a major step forward. In negotiations, exceptions were provided to allow countries to take special measures to protect public health, thus creating special mechanisms to provide AIDS medications to developing countries at low cost.

Regulation of the pharmaceutical industry has evolved over the past hundred years by responding to the perceived needs for consumer protection and industry development, attempting to balance the benefits and costs of regulation. What began as a requirement for adequate labeling, ensuring that the public was protected from adulterated or misrepresented products, grew into a system in which consumers no longer make choices about the drugs they receive but rely on their physicians (and sometimes even third-party payers) to make these choices for them. Along the way, the entire industry was transformed from one that simply manufactured bulk products to one that spent $40 billion dollars actively searching for new products in 2005.

11.4 RESEARCH AND DEVELOPMENT

The pharmaceutical industry consists of many small companies, each producing only one or two products, and about 25 large global corporations that have broader product lines. Even in the largest corporations, however, one or two blockbuster drugs are responsible for most revenues. Competition for the development of these key products, through R&D activities, is fierce. The success or failure of even a single product could mean the success or failure of the corporation. As a result, R&D activities drive competition in the pharmaceutical industry. The cost of developing a new drug ranges from $150 million to $1.5 billion, and the process can take up to ten years. Once developed, patents protect the new product from competition. Patents give the innovator the exclusive right to manufacture and sell that product, once approved, for up to 22 years from the time of discovery. Pharmaceutical firms spent an amount equal to 17.7 percent of sales on R&D in 2001, more than four times the 4 percent of sales spent by the average nonpharmaceutical firm and significantly more than the 11.9 percent pharmaceutical companies spent on R&D in 1980.[16] To understand competition in this industry, one must be familiar with the R&D process and its role in the industry.

The R&D of a new product takes place in several distinct steps, with the pharmaceutical company making decisions on whether to continue the project or abandon it at each step. The first step is either the discovery stage or the synthesis stage, reflecting two very different approaches to new drug development. In the discovery stage, natural chemical compounds having desirable properties are isolated from biological samples. Alternatively, in the synthesis stage, a new synthetic compound is created in the laboratory based on the results of previous research or computer models. Once the new compound has been isolated, regardless of its source, it is generally immediately patented and then screened for pharmacological activity and toxicity, first in vitro (i.e., in test tubes with tissue cultures) and then in animals. This preclinical phase can take up to three years, and literally thousands of compounds are examined and rejected for each one that moves on to the next stage of testing. Once a promising compound has been found, the firm files an **Investigational New Drug (IND)** application with the FDA and, unless rejected, the firm can begin testing in humans within 30 days of filing the application. There were 1,817 INDs filed in 2001, somewhat below the average for the previous decade.[17]

Clinical trials (i.e., human testing) are generally conducted in three distinct phases (see Figure 11.2). **Phase I** testing is usually performed on a small number of healthy patients, although cancer drugs are typically tested on patients who are terminally ill because a high level of toxicity is generally necessary to kill the cancer cells. The objective of these studies is to obtain preliminary information on the toxicity and tolerable dosage range in humans. Generally, the drug is given sequentially to sets of three patients at each dosage level until a preset toxicity threshold is crossed (the acceptable toxicity level depends greatly on the nature of the disease the drug is intended to treat and the availability of alternative therapies) or until a predetermined dose is reached. During Phase I trials, data are also collected on the drug's absorption, metabolic effects, and how the body eliminates the drug. These trials generally last slightly more than a year. Although signs of efficacy are always encouraging, they are not necessary for moving on to the Phase II trials because the sample size is so small.

In **Phase II**, the drug is administered to a limited number of patients whom the drug is intended to benefit (generally 30–300 patients). The first evidence of efficacy is obtained at this stage, even though the general focus of the trial is still on safety. The trial also begins to examine the cumulative effects of the drug. On average, these trials last about two years. If the safety profile continues to look good and there are signs of beneficial effects, the drug is moved into the final stage of human testing.

The final stage of clinical testing, the **Phase III** trials, are intended to establish the efficacy claims of the manufacturer. Large samples, frequently thousands of patients, are exposed to the new drug. Often, these trials are double blind, where neither the patient nor the treating physician knows whether a specific patient is taking the experimental drug or the control drug (perhaps a placebo). In addition to looking for evidence of efficacy, researchers continue to look at the safety profile of the drug and begin to look for potential adverse

FIGURE 11.2 Stages of Drug Testing

		Number of compounds at each stage
Discovery	Screen compounds to find a drug	5,000–10,000
Preclinical	Laboratory and animal testing	250
IND—Investigational New Drug		
Stage I	20–80 volunteers, safety and dosage	20
Stage II	100–300 patients, test efficacy, side effects	13
Stage III	Large randomized trial of clinical effectiveness	9
NDA—Application	File New Drug Application	2
FDA Approval	Launch new drug	1

|← —————— **Up to 15 Years** —————— →|

Total: 3 to 15 years, cost of $100 million–$1,500 million to bring one new drug to market.

reactions to the drug.[18] To obtain information on the long-term effects of the drug, these Phase III clinical trials can go on for several years and on average last nearly three years.

When the clinical trials are under way, pharmaceutical firms typically continue their long-term animal testing, looking for possible adverse genetic and/or reproductive effects. Once the firm believes that it has sufficient information to show that the product is both safe and effective, it files a **New Drug Application (NDA)** with the FDA. Once the NDA is filed, the FDA has 60 days to determine whether there is sufficient information in the NDA for the agency to conduct a substantive review. Although the FDA is supposed to render a decision within six months, the Office of Technology Assessment estimated that for drugs approved in 1990, the average time from application to approval was nearly 30 months. Part of this delay was the result of additional testing required by the FDA before granting approval. A section of the FDA Modernization Act of 1997 extended the 1993 Prescription Drug User Fee Act, allowing the FDA to charge companies for applications and to use the money (more than $100 million per year) to hire extra personnel. This reduced the time required for approval to 16 months in 2001.

On average, only one out of five drugs for which an IND is filed with the FDA ultimately obtains FDA approval for use. As a result of the lengthy testing and approval process, a total of more than ten years generally elapses from the time the firm first began spending money on researching a new product until a successful drug is introduced to the market. Because of this lengthy period of time, it is very important to take into account the opportunity cost of these expenditures when assessing the costs of drug development. In perhaps the most comprehensive analysis to date, DiMasi and colleagues estimated that the capitalized out-of-pocket costs to pharmaceutical firms at the point of market approval averaged $231 million (1987 pretax dollars).[19] This figure includes the cost of projects abandoned along the way. Thus, each individual marketed drug represents a substantial investment of resources for the firm. These investments are made in the anticipation of obtaining future profits on the manufacture and sale of the drug. The estimated average cost of a drug development project in 2002 was approximately $800 million. Others have examined the profitability of these investments, and one study found that only the top 20 percent of the drugs tested had large enough returns to cover the cost of R&D.[20]

A portfolio of patents, and the creativity and expertise of the scientists that generated them, are major assets to the pharmaceutical firm. Mergers are often carried out to obtain a set of patents, to fill out a product line, or to create synergies in research. Whereas marketing benefits from increased size, it appears that economies of scale and scope are quite limited in research.[21] Indeed, some of the most innovative work is performed in small boutique biotechnology firms composed of a few scientists moonlighting from a university laboratory, suggesting diseconomies of scale. The causes and antecedents of successful research are difficult to determine. It does appear, however, that some firms and research groups are just better at it than others, and are able to obtain more new products and conceptual breakthroughs with the same level of resources.

11.5 PHARMACOECONOMICS AND TECHNOLOGY ASSESSMENT

Are new drugs worth the high prices drug companies charge to cover their R&D and marketing costs? Drug discovery in general is obviously beneficial, but should we really pay $2 per pill (or $250 or $1,500 per prescription) for a particular drug? Could the company get by with charging only $1.50 per pill? Conversely, from the company's point of view, since blockbuster drugs are rare and must cover the cost of many failed R&D efforts, could the company reasonably charge $2.50 per pill? An entire discipline with its own scientific journals, conferences, and university professorships has developed to answer these questions. Known variously as **pharmacoeconomics**, disease management, outcomes research, and health technology assessment, this discipline attempts to determine the following:

- How much of a gain in health (outcome) will this drug provide?
- How much will people value that gain?
- Do other drugs provide similar effectiveness in treating this disease?
- How many people will benefit from this drug?
- Will some people benefit more than others?
- Will some people value the drug more than others?

A number of countries with national health systems have gone beyond asking questions and have empanelled experts to help the government make decisions about pharmaceutical reimbursement. Leading the field is the U.K.'s National Institute for Clinical Effectiveness (NICE).[22] Established in 1999, NICE convenes groups of experts on request from the Department of Health to examine specific illness or therapies, then reviews medical studies and models costs and benefits to determine clinical effectiveness. Once the review is complete, a report is issued that is instrumental in determining payment policies. Other official review agencies include the Australian Pharmaceutical Benefits Advisory Committee (PBAC), Canadian Agency for Drugs and Technology in Health (CATH), and German Institute for Quality and Efficiency in Health Care (IQWIG). A drug may be approved at full price, considered so ineffective that it should not be reimbursed at all, sent out for further review, or placed in some intermediate category. For example, a *reference price* may be set that is equal to the current price of an equivalent drug already being used for that disease. Even in the United States, where administrative pharmaceutical price controls do not exist, drug companies have found it useful to employ health economists to estimate the potential size of the market for a new drug and to create an economic justification to help sell the drug to price-conscious buyers with limited budgets (Medicaid, hospital pharmacies, and increasingly, PBMs), and to follow the activities of NICE and other national advisory bodies. Indeed, so many economists are now looking at the value of drugs that some doctors and pharmacists think that this is all there is to health economics, and may use the term "health economics" as a synonym for pharmacy value studies without considering all the other issues covered in the chapters of this textbook.

Most health economists in pharmaceutical companies are employed in the marketing department. Even though committed to objective social and medical science, their job is to sell drugs and to help the company sell the largest amount of drugs at the highest price possible (actually, to maximize the present value of future cash flows, which is a bit more complex). To obtain greater expertise and credibility, corporate health economists often work with or fund studies conducted at universities. However, as most economists would predict, studies funded by pharmaceutical companies are consistently more favorable to the products of those companies (and unfavorable to competitors) than those done independently, leading to increased calls that all conflicts of interest be publicly identified.[23] It is not realistic to expect that funding will have no effect on judgment, even for scientists.

11.6   INDUSTRY STRUCTURE AND COMPETITION

The market for pharmaceutical products can be divided into three segments based on the type of buyer: **individual** patients, **group** purchasers (hospitals, PBMs), and **government**.

In the traditional retail market, physicians prescribe drugs and consumers and/or insurers pay for them. Because these actions are separate, individual patients have little influence over what the physician prescribes and, as a result, this market segment is not very price sensitive. The second market segment, which has been growing in importance, is the group purchasers. In this market, drugs are purchased directly by PBMs and hospitals, and a physician's choice of which drug to use is constrained by the use of a formulary and ordering directives. Because PBMs and hospitals can shift a large number of patients from one product to another, they have some market power and are more sensitive to prices. Exercising this market power enables them to obtain discounts from drug manufacturers. The third market segment consists of the largest purchasers of pharmaceutical products: state and federal government. Governments make and interpret the rules, potentially giving them absolute control over the market.

Medicare D: An Experiment in Rational Choice

Passed in 2003 and implemented in 2006, Part D (D for drugs) was the largest expansion of Medicare since its inception. The Bush administration wanted not only to provide benefits for the elderly (for which presumably the elderly might show some gratitude when voting in the next election) but also to move the health care system toward more market-oriented, consumer-directed health insurance (see Section 5.2) that emphasized individual ownership and choice. Whereas regular Medicare is a social insurance program run by the government (but administered by private contractors), Part D was designed explicitly to rely on private insurance plans (although provided with sizable government subsidies) chosen by individuals who would manage and pay for their own care. The legislation attempted to create a natural experiment in consumer-directed individual private market health insurance, and to that end specifically denied the government any ability to negotiate prices. The government, though, did set minimum standards for coverage and rules for marketing and consumer information.

Since the majority of the elderly already had coverage through existing plans (employee retiree insurance, Medicaid, Medicare HMOs, group or individual Medigap policies) a number of political and practical compromises were required to implement the plan. Most notably, in order to meet budget constraints the legislation introduced a gap in the benefit structure: patients had to pay a deductible and 25 percent of costs up to $750, then were 95 percent covered after their out-of-pocket costs exceeded $3,600, leaving a "donut hole" in between, where consumers had to pay 100 percent. More important for the social experiment in rational choice, 72 percent of beneficiaries were automatically enrolled in existing retiree benefit plans, Medicaid/Medicare, and such, and so did not exercise any choice of plan.

Among those seniors who were confronted with a choice of plans, early results suggest that their choices were "sort of" rational. The large government subsidy made Part D such a good deal that almost everyone eligible should have enrolled, but many did not. Instead, it seems as if seniors looked at their last year's drug expenses and compared that dollar amount with what personal costs (premium plus out of pocket) would have been under the plans offered to them—and almost entirely ignored the insurance benefit of protection against higher costs.[24] The process here is familiar to those who study "behavioral economics," a growing field that examines people's real-world choices for inconsistencies with rational choice theory. Confronted with a complex problem, consumers come up with a simple decision rule ("would I have saved money under this plan last year?") rather than evaluate the expected value of a full range of choices under uncertainty. Thus the evidence from this experiment with regard to consumer choice must be considered somewhat mixed: consumers do make choices among health insurance plans, but they avoid and oversimplify the complexities and contingencies involved. Unfortunately, much of medical care falls into the category of contingent and complex decisions that may not be so amenable to direct consumer choice (see "Uncertainty" in Section 6.5).

Market Segmentation: Types of Buyers

Competition for sales differs significantly across these segments. In the traditional retail market for individual patients, where consumers (patients) are price insensitive, competition takes place among products on the basis of product quality and detailing. **Detailing** is a form of marketing that is unique to the pharmaceutical industry. A salesperson, or detailer, provides a physician with detailed information on the approved uses of a product. Even though much of the demand for a drug may be for treating a disease for which the drug is not yet (or ever) approved by the FDA, detailers are prohibited from discussing such **off-label** uses of the product.[25] Studies have consistently shown that detailers greatly influence a physician's choice of drugs. Moreover, once a physician becomes familiar with a particular product, its method of action, and its potential side effects, he or she may be reluctant to try a new product unless it offers either a substantial advantage in efficacy or a decrease in side effects. Price tends not to be an important criterion for consumers.[26] Because competition in this market is usually based on product quality, effectiveness, and detailing, generics have not been able to make significant inroads in this market.

To date, government purchasers have chosen not to exercise fully their **monopsony** market power on a drug-by-drug basis. Medicare part D explicitly disallows governmental price negotiations, and Medicaid has adopted a standardized discount policy that pharmaceutical firms can either accept or reject. Under this policy, the government is rebated an amount equal to 15.1 percent of the average wholesale price for Medicaid purchases, or equal to the best deal given by the drug company on a particular product. Similar provisions have been established for other government contracts. In exchange for agreeing to these discounts, Medicaid agreed not to establish restrictive formularies. Thus, although pharmaceutical firms must cut their prices to sell to this market, they are essentially free to detail physicians on their products and do not face stiff competition from generic products.

The growth, and most of the change, has come in the "managed" segment. HMOs, PBMs, and hospitals paying directly for drugs can influence physicians' prescribing patterns through a formulary. These group purchasers are the ones most interested in, and able to assess, price and cost-effectiveness. This is the segment in which generics have had the most impact, because they are chemically identical to brand-name products and are sold at a much lower price (up to 60 percent less). When the patent expired on Eli Lilly's blockbuster drug Prozac, 70 percent of prescriptions were switched to generic substitutes within a single month.[27] Unless a drug has demonstrated clear superiority through health economics outcomes research studies, price-sensitive managers choose the cheaper product. Most large pharmaceutical companies have developed sales, marketing, and research groups aimed at addressing the concerns of the managed market. In addition, pharmaceutical companies are beginning to explore new contractual relationships to increase sales and lock in specific customers.

Contractual Responses to Pharmacy Benefits Management

Managed care greatly increases the elasticity of demand. Organized payers with sophisticated information and outcome assessment methods are able to switch large numbers of patients from one drug to another in response to small changes in relative prices. Pharmaceutical firms can respond in several ways to this shift in market power.

The first response is by making **price reductions**. Pharmaceutical firms can compete with one another through successive reductions in the prices of their competing products. Since much of the costs of drug development and manufacturing are sunk, short-term competition can significantly reduce prices. During the past few years there has been increased price competition, particularly in pharmaceutical categories in which several branded products exist, such as antihypertensives and cholesterol reducers. Price reductions reduce profitability and thus are not popular with pharmaceutical firms. These firms argue that continued reductions would reduce funding for research and eventually lead to fewer new drugs.

A second response to the increased elasticity of demand is the development of new ways to establish **product differentiation**. Outcomes research, pharmacoeconomics, and disease management are several ways pharmaceutical firms try to differentiate their products from their competitors and develop "value" messages about their products. Fundamentally, these are attempts by the industry not only to demonstrate the safety and efficacy of their products, but also to translate the efficacy of treatment into measures that consumers value. For example, rather than simply showing that a cholesterol drug can reduce LDL cholesterol by x percent, pharmaceutical firms have undertaken studies to show what that percent reduction means in terms of reduced coronary events (e.g., heart attacks, strokes) and to show that reducing these events reduces future health care expenditures and improves the quality of patients' lives. New metrics, such as cost per life year saved and cost per quality adjusted life year (QALY) saved, have been developed to provide more descriptive information to physicians and consumers to help them make decisions (see Chapter 3). Nearly every major pharmaceutical firm has begun to develop expertise in this area, and several new scientific journals have been founded to publish the results of these kinds of studies.

A third response involves developing **contractual relationships** that serve to "lock in" customers to a specific product line. These are often called "disease management programs." Possible arrangements include the following:

- Providing discounts for specific drugs based on specific performance measures (i.e., reduced prices, but only if the purchaser provides the manufacturer with increased market share)
- Establishing cost-sharing arrangements or warranties on specific products
- Developing capitated contracts, whereby a pharmaceutical company agrees to provide all the drugs needed for a fixed (per member per month) charge for a managed care population (e.g., specific drugs, drug classes, or even large bundles of drugs)
- Developing complete disease management programs, whereby the pharmaceutical firm assumes some of the financial risk for the total costs of treatment, not just the pharmaceutical costs

Value and Cost

The structure of the pharmaceutical industry is dictated by a single fact: the large and important costs are all sunk costs. The value of a drug depends on how useful it is in treating disease, not how many years it took to conduct clinical trials or perfect the production process, or on the number of failed projects the company had to fund in order to get a winner. Research and testing to bring the pill to market costs so much more than manufacturing that there is essentially no rational connection between price and cost, however measured. Instead, value and price depend on therapeutic effectiveness.[28]

Medical "value" is worthless economically unless potential buyers know how effective a drug is. Treatment capability must be turned into effective demand. This means marketing. Given the large gross margin (profit per unit) caused by the combination of high sunk research costs and low per unit variable production costs, it is inevitable that marketing will be much more important and expensive than physical distribution—as it is for products with a similar cost structure, such as software, movies, CDs, and perfume. Most of this marketing is directed toward doctors, since they are the ones who write prescriptions. For each practicing physician, pharmaceutical companies spent more than $2,500 on meals, events, and scientific meetings (some conducted in very nice resorts) in 2002.[29] Spending on personal visits by industry representatives and free samples was more than $10,000 per doctor. The size of the expenditure on marketing indicates how valuable the power to influence doctors is in terms of company profits.

Marketing creates additional divergence between price and "unit cost" because the value of each pill increases as it becomes better and better known as a brand-name drug. Although clinical value may not depend on marketing, economic value does. Once the drug is launched in the market, any distinction between the value added from increased therapeutic effectiveness and the value added from increased marketing is not meaningful. (How much of a blockbuster movie's profits are derived from star power? From plot? From the cool 30-second video advertisement that drew everyone into standing in line to see it the first weekend?) Even the drastic difference in price between brand name and generic versions (20, 40, 50, or even 80 percent) probably underestimates the value added by marketing. Perfectly good drugs have languished almost unused for years because they were not being advertised and detailed to doctors.

Once marketing launches a drug, the brand name is worth something even if the drug has been superseded by superior competitors (kind of like old sports stars still being used to sell athletic shoes). The brand-name version will often continue to sell at the old high price even after the patent has expired in order to capture the consumer surplus of customers who are not price sensitive. Also, competition from generic manufacturers has created incentives for research-based, brand-name companies to introduce and subsequently patent minor changes in their most important products. These changes might include introducing a sustained release or once-a-day formulation, or changing the route of administration from injection to inhaler or pill. AstraZeneca made such an effort to shift users of Prilosec, its blockbuster antiulcer drug, to a new improved version, Nexium, which retained the distinctive purple coloration of the original and incorporated minor modifications protected by new patents to limit the impact from generic competitors.

The Prilosec/Nexium example illustrates an important aspect of the pharmaceutical market: competition is between treatments for a specific disease (in this case, ulcers). Most drugs do not compete with one another because they are used for different illnesses. The real market is "treatments for disease X" and thus is much narrower than "all prescription drugs." Firms focus their research and marketing efforts on a particular set of diseases (cardiovascular, neurological, gastric), making the effective market share (and market power) of the top firm, or top three firms, more concentrated than it appears to be when reviewing industry-wide statistics.

The Role of Middlemen: Distribution versus Marketing

Wholesalers distribute drugs. They buy in bulk from pharmaceutical manufacturers and distribute on demand to retail pharmacies and hospitals. The customer is not involved in this back-office physical distribution network, and it is a commodity business with low margins. Conversely, the PBM never touches the physical product, but controls the flow

---

STEPPING UP IN PRICE: PROVIGIL TO NUVIGIL

Provigil is a drug used to treat narcolepsy. Although only a modest seller ($950 million in 2008) it accounts for almost half the total sales of Cephalon, the company that makes it. Provigil will go off patent and be subject to generic competition in 2012. In order to meet that challenge, the company is planning to bring out a longer acting version, Nuvigil, which has a patent that extends to 2023. In order to switch consumers to the new drug rather than losing them to cheaper generic competition, Cephalon is following a strategy of aggressive price increases. The price per pill for Provigil stayed relatively steady around $5.00 after the drug's introduction in 1999 until being bumped above $6.00 in 2004 and to $8.71 in 2008.[30] Cephalon has stated to investors that it plans to keep pushing the price upward to generate extra revenues (see Chapter 2 for discussion of *long-run* versus *short-run price elasticity* and *marginal revenue*) so that the new branded substitute can be priced significantly lower on a per dose basis when it is introduced in 2010—gathering a dedicated block of users before generic competition comes in.

Patients who take the drug for its official FDA-approved uses and have health insurance will not experience much of the price increases, but Provigil is frequently taken off-label as a "lifestyle" drug to help patients stay awake during work or leisure activities rather than for diagnosed narcolepsy or related conditions (Cephalon agreed to pay a fine of $444 million in September 2008 to settle federal and state allegations that it illegally promoted off-label uses). Optional lifestyle use is not medically necessary, and hence even though a patient has obtained a prescription from a doctor, the bills are not covered by insurance. For patients without insurance, or for the many who use Provigil off-label, the price increases are substantial.

---

of customers and money, and for performing this market aggregating function, is paid handsomely. The essential element here is control. Assume that a drug cures a horrible disease and thus is worth more than $1,000 to the patient, but production cost is only $1. This difference is up for grabs. If there is lots of competition, prices may get forced down toward $1.50, providing just enough for the costs of manufacture, distribution, and a small profit. If patents or market power keep competition out, then profits of $100 or $500 or even $999 per customer are possible. It is that possibility which makes marketing so valuable.

Consider how different the case of diamonds is. The product itself (not the label) is valuable; therefore, anyone involved in transport and transfer must be trustworthy and highly compensated—it is worth a lot of money to keep from losing a few diamonds. Jewelry stores can advise, but they cannot prescribe, 2 carats, extremely fine yellow-white, or Lucida™ cut. Thus, in the case of diamonds, wholesaling and physical distribution is relatively profitable, and although marketing is a decent business, the large number of competitors keeps margins small relative to the cost of operating a jewelry store.

The essential question is control—who "owns" the business. To a large extent, the business of patients is controlled (owned) by the doctors who write the prescriptions for them. However, these doctors are prohibited by law and ethics from taking any of that $999 in surplus value. If there is only one treatment for an illness and it is protected by a patent, the company with the patent in effect "owns" the business. The main question becomes how much business (total sales) there will be. A company will detail doctors to push them to prescribe more, but it does not have to worry about competing drugs. If there are two or more treatments for an illness, the situation becomes more complex. In theory, the choice should be made by the patient, balancing therapeutic effectiveness, cost, and side effects. In that case, marketing will focus directly on the patient (**direct-to-consumer** (**DTC**) advertising). However, patients often do not have enough information or confidence to make complex choices and tend to rely on their doctors to advise them. Thus, the marketing effort (detailing, scientific meetings at nice resorts) is directed at the doctor.

Insurance companies pay for most drugs, and they may be able to induce some patients to switch from treatment B to treatment A by making the copayment for B much larger. The insurance company may even insist that it will provide reimbursement for drug A, and only A, if that drug is a chemically equivalent to B. In this case, the insurer/PBM captures some of the surplus. Notice how little market power and how little excess profit the pharmacy is able to get. Even though pharmacies are the point of contact where the patient obtains the drug, they have to fill the prescription as written by the doctor or as modified by the insurer (generic substitution, tiered copayments) and are not allowed to try to shift patients from A to B. Pharmacies are almost as neutral and powerless as wholesalers—they simply distribute pills from the manufacturer to the patient. It is much more difficult and costly at the individual retail end, which is why retail accounts for 20 to 25 percent of costs and wholesale only 2 to 3 percent, but there is not a lot of excess profit to be obtained here. Actually, one of the most lucrative parts of the retail pharmacy business is all the other stuff (candy, bandages) that pharmacies sell at above-average markups to people who come in to fill their prescriptions. That is, the pharmacy does not "own" the prescription business (because there are so many retail pharmacy competitors and wholesale prices are fixed), but it does own the idle shopping time of the patient who is waiting to have his or her prescription filled—and can exploit that to sell high-markup magazines, mints, and other items.

Research Productivity

Research is a sunk cost for drugs already on the market. These drugs would still be manufactured even if prices were reduced to the level of marginal cost, but then no new research would be undertaken. The high prices are the incentives for investing millions of dollars in the hope of making a discovery. Almost every economist and politician accepts this simple premise connecting research expenditures and innovation to the promise of future profits. However, some issues remain. How much profit is necessary to provide an incentive? If a company can make $1 billion on a new drug at a price of $30, will allowing the company to make $2 billion at a price of $60 double the productivity of its research labs—or increase it only by 10 percent? Although there is no question that higher profits lead to more research, the magnitude of the gains and the real importance to patients is still an open and relevant issue. Research indicates that increases and decreases in R&D funding are more tied to short-run changes in past profits than to the changes in expected future profits that theory would predict.[32] More disturbing, it is not clear whether more R&D spending leads to the development of more innovative new drugs. Much of the expenditure goes for imitative "me-too" drugs to fight off the competitive threat from generics and chemically related drugs that other companies have made sufficiently different (by adding some side molecules or by using a new production process) to engineer around existing patents and claim their own brand names. Whereas 46 percent of all new drug approvals in 1991 were for new molecular entities (NMEs), by 2001 only 35 percent of approvals were for new molecules. Furthermore, only seven of these 24 NMEs were ranked by the FDA as priority drugs promising important advances entitled to expedited review, compared with 19 in 1999.[33] During the 1990s, research spending grew from $10 billion to $30 billion, yet the number of important new drugs brought to market fell, and the number of INDs submitted by pharmaceutical companies to the FDA declined from 2,116 to 1,872. Investment banking

CLARITIN: DIRECT-TO-CONSUMER ADVERTISING, OVER-THE-COUNTER MEDICATION, AND PRICING

Claritin had a tortuous transition from laboratory to market. Schering-Plough submitted a new drug application (NDA) for the compound (scientific name, loratadine) in 1980, but did not obtain approval until 1993, by which time there were only five years left on the basic patent.[31] The FDA felt little pressure to approve what was classified as a "me-too" drug that promised little clinical advance over existing prescription and OTC antihistamine remedies for allergy and hay fever. However, when FDA rules regarding **direct-to-consumers (DTC)** advertising were relaxed in 1997, Schering-Plough spent $322 million promoting Claritin to the public. Ads featuring clear skies and happy faces (with pollen-carrying flowers in the background) were seen on TV shows, billboards, bus stops, and leaflets handed out on street corners. Sales of Claritin ballooned to more than $2.6 billion in 2000.

In clinical trials, 46 percent of allergy sufferers showed improvement with Claritin, compared with 35 percent who showed improvement when given a placebo. Tests indicated that Schering-Plough's old drug, Chlor-Trimeton, now sold cheaply over the counter, was equally or perhaps more effective in relieving symptoms—and may not have been much more sleep-inducing when used in a low dose. Was it really worth paying six times as much for the new version? The question rarely arose because prescriptions were covered by insurance. Wellpoint, a large health insurance company, sued in 1998 to force Claritin and similar allergy drugs to be sold over the counter without prescription, claiming that they clearly were safer than the existing OTC medications such as Chlor-Trimeton. If Claritin were declared safe enough to be used without a prescription, then it would no longer qualify for insurance reimbursement, consumers would have to pay out of pocket, and demand would become much more price sensitive. Despite concerted efforts by Schering-Plough and other pharmaceutical firms, the insurance companies made a persuasive case. In November 2002 the FDA approved Claritin for OTC use. Schering-Plough's stock dropped precipitously as the price of Claritin had to be cut, and cut again, to compete in the more wide-open OTC market, and as Johnson & Johnson and Wyeth geared up production of generic versions of loratadine to sell at less than $20.

firm Lehman Brothers expected global drug firms to launch only 47 new drugs in 2002, down a third from 1997.[34] The number of new drug approvals by the FDA has steadily fallen from 39 in 1997 to 27 in 2000 and down to just 18 in 2006. *The Wall Street Journal*, Standard and Poor's industry surveys, *Modern Healthcare* magazine, and most reputable analysts agree that the major financial problem facing the industry is a lack of important new drugs in the pipeline.[35] More than 10 years of increased R&D spending have not provided impressive results, making it hard to argue that having a bit more profit to pour into laboratories would make a big difference in the rate of therapeutic advances or drug discovery.

It may be that research productivity is in a stage of secular decline. Some analysts suggest that "discovery" methods have been played out, with most significant compounds already investigated and under patent, so that any surge of new drugs will have to come from "synthesis" and rational drug design, perhaps following from the increased understanding of fundamental disease processes brought about by deciphering the human genome. Most analysts opine that a real therapeutic benefit from such breakthroughs is at least 10 (maybe 15, 25, or 35?) years in the future. Someday there will be designer drugs customized for each patient—not a pill for high cholesterol and another for gastric reflux, but a pill for the current health condition (and preventive needs) of Mr. ABC at age 36, who has decided to run a marathon and move to Tampa. The gains from that set of advances will be amazing—and a long time in coming.

11.7 TRENDS: FORM FOLLOWS FUNCTION (AND MONEY)

The structure of the pharmaceutical market is wondrously strange and revealing. It was an unintended consequence of the labeling provision in the Food, Drug, and Cosmetics Act of 1938 that made "prescription" drugs so inelastic with respect to price, adding to the power of physicians and the profits of pharmaceutical companies. This triangle (patient as payer, physician as prescriber, pharmaceutical company as producer) was first strengthened, then undermined, by the expansion of insurance. At first, prices became even more irrelevant with third-party payment. Pharmaceutical profits soared, making still more expensive physician detailing worthwhile. Then the vast sums of money being spent made it worthwhile for insurers to set up sophisticated systems to (a) save more by increasing price elasticity with formularies and differential copayments and (b) use this countervailing market power to extract discounts from producers. As the prescribing power of physicians and the pricing power of drug companies declined, the gap was filled with appeals to patients through DTC marketing, empowering them to ask for a new drug by name. Claritin was the drug made famous (and its parent company Schering-Plough rich) through advertising. The revenge of the payer came when insurance companies made the case that if consumers could be trusted to use advertising information to ask for a drug, they could be trusted to choose it over the counter without a prescription. Empowered consumers, acting on their own—and with their own dollars at stake—drove prices rapidly downward. Furthermore, since pharmaceuticals are among the most international of markets and the economies of China and India are growing more massive than any other country, it is unlikely that U.S. or EU companies will continue to dominate research or trade in drugs to the same extent in the future.

Research creates a wedge between price and marginal cost, but it is marketing that consolidates big margins. With regard to pricing power, the demand side may prove more powerful than supply. Strategic growth and mergers have made market share more concentrated within each therapeutic category, despite the limited evidence for economies of scale in research. Moreover, it appears that much of the significant research in the coming decades will be conducted within small biotech firms. Changes in legal structures have played a role in this, as the courts have ruled that new organisms created in the laboratory may be patented. Much of the most basic research has shifted from the large firms in the industry to smaller, high-risk ventures. As these products move out of the laboratory and into clinical testing, biotech firms usually take on partners from the traditional pharmaceutical industry, are bought out by established firms, or develop licensing agreements. The growing split between discovery and development/marketing may presage a growing split in the sources of capital: venture capital for high-risk discovery in biotech firms, and reliance on the vast pools of equity capital extracted from the success of old drugs for the financing of methodical development, approval, and marketing efforts.

SUGGESTIONS FOR FURTHER READING

Geeta Anand, "Support System: Through Charities, Drug Makers Help People—and Themselves," *The Wall Street Journal*, December 1, 2005, page 1.

Stirling Bryan, Jestyn Williams, and Shirley McIver, "Seeing the NICE Side of Cost-Effectiveness Analysis: A Qualitative Investigation of the Use of CEA in NICE Technology Appraisals," *Health Economics* 16 (2007): 179–193.

Iain M. Cockburn and Rebecca M. Henderson, "Scale and Scope in Drug Development: Unpack the Advantages of Size in Pharmaceutical Research," *Journal of Health Economics* 20, no. 6 (November 2001): 1003–1057.

David H. Kreling, David A. Mott, and Joseph P. Wiederholt, *Prescription Drug Trends, a Chartbook Update* (November 2001); and *Prescription Drug Trends* (September 2000), Kaiser Family Foundation, www.kff.org

Daniel McFadden, "Free Markets and Fettered Consumers," *American Economic Review* 96, no. 1 (March 2006): 5–29.

NICE: National Institute for Clinical Effectiveness http://www.nice.org.uk

Prescription Drug Trends, Kaiser Family Foundation, www.kff.org

Standard & Poor's Industry Surveys—Healthcare: Pharmaceuticals (June 27, 2002) Standard & Poor's, www.standardandpoors.com

2008 Industry Profile, PhRMA (Pharmaceutical Research and Manufacturers of America), www.phrma.org

SUMMARY

1. The average American fills 12 prescriptions a year. Pharmaceuticals were a **$256 billion industry** in 2010, for which government (41 percent) and private insurance (40 percent) paid most of the bills. Of all the funds flowing in, about 70 percent go to pharmaceutical companies, 20 percent to retail pharmacies, and 10 percent to PBMs and insurers—much of that in the form of rebates from manufacturers.

2. Once an industry that made most of its profits from household potions and elixirs, the pharmaceutical industry has been revolutionized by **science, regulation**, and **insurance**. Pharmacology is among the most successful of technologies, having greatly improved human welfare and generated enormous profits—18.7 percent of sales in 2001, more than any other industry in the Fortune 500. A single successful drug can earn more than $5 billion in a year, and make or break the company.

3. **R&D** of new products is a risky, lengthy, and costly process. Only one in a thousand compounds initially studied eventually makes it to the market. On average, the time from discovery to successful market introduction is more than ten years, at a total cost of $800 million. The most costly parts of the process are the clinical trials needed to establish safety and efficacy claims, which can take up to five years and involve thousands of patients.

4. **Patent protection** means that the price of a drug is determined by its value to consumers, not the cost of production. The hope of making large profits from discovering the next blockbuster product keeps pharmaceutical firms investing in R&D and fuels progress in the pharmaceutical industry.

5. The **dominant** economic feature of the pharmaceutical industry is the large **sunk costs**, first for R&D and then for the physician detailing and marketing blitz required to launch sales. The marginal cost of producing additional pills is small; therefore most of the price is pure profit once these large fixed costs are covered. The ability to control the flow of funds determines who will hold onto most of these profits; the brand-name manufacturer with a patent, the generic competitor, the government, the physician, the PBM, the insurance company, or the patient.

6. **Generics** (chemically identical compounds made by other firms) have increased in importance since the legal changes in 1984 enabled easier approval. Generic drugs sell for much less than branded products ($25 versus $75) and have been increasingly successful as the **price-sensitive** managed care PBM market has grown.

7. Pharmaceutical manufacturers have begun to respond to changes in their markets brought about by managed care and generic competition. These changes include the use of discounts, development of **pharmacoeconomics** and disease management, and the development of various forms of risk-sharing contracts.

PROBLEMS

1. What determines the price of a drug?

2. Why are fixed costs more important for pharmaceuticals than physical therapy? How does this affect marketing expenditures?

3. What events led to the formation of the FDA? Does regulation change because of successes or because of failures?

4. Do patents raise or lower the productivity of research?

5. How are prescription costs "managed" by insurance companies?

6. {*flow of funds*} What fraction of the total cost of pharmaceuticals is paid for directly by patients? Does this mean that price is more, or less, important than for other types of medical care?

7. {*research, incidence*} How is most pharmaceutical research paid for? What is the most costly aspect of pharmaceutical research?

8. {*market segmentation*} How many distinct market segments exist in the pharmaceutical industry? How do these segments differ?

9. {*competition*} On what basis do pharmaceutical firms compete in each market segment? Is price a more important factor for the choice of which doctor to see or for which drug is prescribed?

10. {*insurance coverage*} The major form of health insurance coverage for the elderly is Medicare, and the elderly are much heavier users of pharmaceuticals than other groups. It would seem reasonable to expect that Medicare is the largest source of payment for drugs. Is it?

11. {*marginal costs, revenues*} Do hospitals have more of an incentive to control the costs of surgical implants, anesthesiologists' fees, or pharmaceuticals? In which case do they bear the highest fraction of marginal cost? In which case do they receive the highest fraction of marginal revenue?

12. {*patents*} How would a change in the length of the patent period affect the structure of the pharmaceutical industry?

13. {*competition*} Marketing accounts for a much larger portion of the cost of pharmaceuticals than the cost of other forms of care. Why? To whom are most pharmaceutical marketing efforts targeted?

14. {*capital investment*} If $50 million is invested in a drug that subsequently fails to gain approval from the FDA, what is the rate of return on this investment? Are pharmaceutical firms more, or less, capital intensive than hospitals? Than doctor's office practices?

15. {*antitrust*} Since FDA regulations limit the entry of new drugs into the market, do they constitute an "unfair restraint of trade" that reduces competition and raises prices to consumers?

16. {*price elasticity*} When a brand-name drug loses patent protection after 17 years and competing generic products enter the market, will the price of the brand-name drug increase or decrease? (*Hint*: What changes occur in the brand-name drug's demand curve?)

17. {*risk*} Which form of investment is more risky: developing a new drug or building a new nursing home? Which type of publicly traded for-profit firm would you expect to show greater variability in earnings, a pharmaceutical firm or a nursing home chain? (*Hint*: See Chapter 12).

ENDNOTES

1.   David W. Kaufman et al., "Recent Patterns of Medication Use in the Ambulatory Adult Population of the United States," *Journal of the American Medical Association* 287, no. 3 (January 16, 2002): 337–344.

2.   "Drugs," *The Economist* (June 3, 2000), 106.

3.   David H. Kreling, David A. Mott, and Joseph P. Wiederholt, *Prescription Drug Trends, a Chartbook Update* (November 2001); and *Prescription Drug Trends* (September 2000), Kaiser Family Foundation. (www.kff.org).

4.   *Prescription Drug Trends* (2000), Exhibit 3.2.

5.   John K. Iglehart, "Medicare and Prescription Drugs," *New England Journal of Medicine* 344, no. 13 (March 29, 2001): 1010–1015; *Prescription Drug Trends*, Exhibit 1.4.

6.   *Prescription Drug Trends* (2000), Exhibits 4.13, 4.15.

7.   *Prescription Drug Trends* (2000), Exhibit 4.9.

8.   *2002 Industry Profile*, PhRMA (Pharmaceutical Research and Manufacturers of America), (www.phrma.org). Estimate projected from 1999 PhRMA estimate for 1999 increased by the percentage increase in pharmaceutical spending from 1999 to 2002 from U.S. National Health Accounts.

9.   *Standard & Poor's Industry Surveys—Healthcare: Pharmaceuticals* (June 27, 2002), Standard & Poor's (www.standardandpoors.com).

10. "Industry Rankings," *Fortune* (April 15, 2002), F26.

11. "The prize for finding a blockbuster luxury product is much the same as in the pharmaceuticals industry, magical margins" (quote from) "Luxury Goods," *The Economist* (March 23, 2002), 65.

12. Jonathan Leibenau, *Medical Science and Medical Industry: The Formation of the American Pharmaceutical Industry* (London: Macmillan, 1987), 34, 79.

13. Edward Kremers and George Urdang, *History of Pharmacy*, 2nd ed. (Philadelphia: Lippincott, 1951).

14. Peter Temin, *Taking Your Medicine: Drug Regulation in the U.S.* (Boston: Harvard University Press, 1980).

15. S. Peltzman, "An Evaluation of Consumer Protection Legislation: The 1962 Drug Amendments," *Journal of Political Economy* (September 1973), 1050–1051.

16. *Standard & Poor's Industry Surveys: Health–Pharmaceuticals* (June 27, 2002), Standard & Poor's (www.standardandpoors.com).

17. *Standard & Poor's*, op.cit., page 5.

18. Despite the relatively large sample sizes, many important adverse reactions can be missed during the Phase III studies because they have a low probability of occurring. For example, a 1:10,000 adverse reaction causing death could easily go unnoticed in a Phase III trial on several thousand patients, even though it could cause 30,000 deaths if the drug were released to all 300 million citizens. As a result, when a new drug is released, the FDA requires the pharmaceutical firm to conduct extensive postmarketing surveillance for any adverse reactions and to immediately report all deaths of people taking the drug, regardless of whether there appears to be a direct link between the death and the drug usage.

19. J. A. DiMasi, R. W. Hansen, H. G. Grabowski, and L. Lasagna, "Cost of Innovation in the Pharmaceutical Industry," *Journal of Health Economics* 10 (1991): 107–42.

20. Henry J. Grabowski and John Vernon, "A New Look at the Returns and Risks to Pharmaceutical R&D," *Management Science* 36 (July 1990): 804–821.

21. Iain M. Cockburn and Rebecca M. Henderson, "Scale and Scope in Drug Development: Unpack the Advantages of Size in Pharmaceutical Research," *Journal of Health Economics* 20, no. 6 (November 2001): 1033–1057.

22. Stirling Byan, Jestyn Williams, and Shirley McIver, "Seeing the NICE Side of Cost-Effectiveness Analysis: A Qualitative Investigation of the Use of CEA in NICE Technology Appraisals," *Health Economics* 16 (2007): 179–193.

23. Niteesh K. Choudhry, Henry Thomas Stelfox, and Allan S. Detsky, "Relationships Between Authors of Clinical Practice Guidelines and the Pharmaceutical Industry," *Journal of the American Medical Association* 287, no. 5 (February 6, 2002): 612–617; H. T. Stelfox, G. Chua, K. O'Rourke, A. S. Detsky, "Conflict of Interest in the Debate Over Calcium Channel Antagonists," *New England Journal of Medicine* 338 (1998): 101–106; F. Davidoff et al., "Sponsorship, Authorship, and Accountability," *Journal of the American Medical Association* 286, no. 10 (September 12, 2001): 1232–1234.

24. Florian Heiss, Daniel McFadden, and Joachim Winter, "Mind the Gap: Consumer Perceptions and Choices of Medicare Part D Prescription Drug Plans," NBER #13627, December 2007.

25. As discussed earlier, although a product is approved by the Food and Drug Administration for a specific use or indication and some drugs may have multiple indications, physicians are permitted to prescribe the product as they see fit. At the same time, physicians and drug companies are always exploring potentially new (or related) uses for the drug. The results of these studies are often published in the literature long before a new indication is obtained from the FDA. As a result of these publications, many drugs are prescribed for conditions outside of their indications. This practice is called off-label prescribing.

26. Alan T. Sorenson, "An Empirical Model of Heterogenous Consumer Search for Retail Prescription Drugs," NBER working paper 8548 (2001), National Bureau of Economic Research: Cambridge, Mass. (www.nber.org).

27. Cinda Becker, "Drugmakers Fight for Good Name," *Modern Healthcare* (August 27, 2001): 28–33; Standard & Poor's, op. cit., 3.

28. Z. John Lu, and William S. Comanor, "Strategic Pricing of New Pharmaceuticals," *The Review of Economics and Statistics* (1998): 108–118.

29. Scott Hensley, "AMA, Prescription Drug Makers Agree Ethics Policy Needs Better Implementation," *The Wall Street Journal* (January 21, 2002).

30. Jonathan D. Rockoff, "How a Drug Maker Tries to Outwit Generics," *The Wall Street Journal*, November 17, 2008.

31. Stephen S. Hall, "The Claritin Effect: Prescription for Profit," *New York Times*, Magazine Section (March 11, 2001), 40 ff.; Laura Benko, "Ugly Wait at the Counter: Insurer Pushes to Make Allergy Drugs Nonprescription," *Modern Healthcare* (August 6, 2001), 22–23; Cynthia A. Jackevicius et al., "Use of Ezetimibe in the U.S. and Canada," *New England Journal of Medicine* 358, no. 17 (April 24, 2008): 1819–1828.

32. F. M. Scherer, "The Link Between Gross Profitability and Pharmaceutical R&D Spending," *Health Affairs* 20, no. 5 (September 2001): 216–221.

33. Standard & Poor's, op. cit., pp. 3, 5.

34. "Bloom and Blight," *The Economist* (October 26, 2002), 60.

35. Gardner Harris, "For Drug Makers, Good Times Yield to a New Profit Crunch," *The Wall Street Journal* (April 18, 2002), sec. A, p. 1; Standard & Poor's, *op. cit.*, p. 5.

CHAPTER 12

CAPITAL FINANCING AND OWNERSHIP OF HEALTH CARE PROVIDERS

QUESTIONS

1. How much is a year of medical education worth?
2. What are the major financial risks facing an insurance company or HMO?
3. Which faces greater risk of bankruptcy: a nursing home company or a pharmaceutical company? Which has the more diversified "portfolio" of assets?
4. Does financial innovation in health care improve productivity and consumer welfare the way technological innovation does?
5. Why did hospitals borrow so much and load up their balance sheets with debt during the 1980s?
6. Do changes in Medicare change the value of hospitals? Do they change the value of the hospitals' bonds?
7. Who owns a nonprofit hospital? Who gets the profits?
8. Is an HMO more concerned about fixed capital or working capital? Does this make it easier or harder to finance rapid growth?

12.1 WHAT IS CAPITAL FINANCING?

For any for-profit or nonprofit organization, whether in health care, farming, or computer services, the total inflow of money must exceed the cumulative outflow or the organization ceases to exist. The funds may come in the form of loans, gifts, equity capital, sales, or reimbursements—but if the amount that has gone out ever exceeds the amount that has come in, the organization can no longer pay its bills and bankruptcy occurs. This poses significant issues at each point in the life cycle of an organization from beginning to end:

1. **Start-up** financing must come from somewhere before operations can begin.
2. **Regular operations** must generate funds: revenues must be greater than expenses.
3. **Ending residual** funds (or debts) must be transferred or cleared.

These three elements are interrelated but distinct. Corporate finance textbooks deal more with the start-up (debt and equity) and ending residual (mergers and acquisitions, bankruptcy) phases but do not say much about ordinary business operations. In contrast, health officials often talk about financing as if it were only a matter of getting the operating revenues to stay above expenses and usually leave start-up and ending issues aside. The CFO (chief financial officer) of an organization must deal with both, although the relative allocation of effort differs markedly across industries.[1] In a public health center, the CFO spends most of his or her time on transactions: filing for reimbursement, negotiating rates, paying bills, and overseeing all of the daily operational tasks common to the accounting department. A real estate CFO will only occasionally think about how rents are collected or utility bills paid but focuses constantly on buying and selling properties, the interest rates on loans, and the ability to raise equity capital by selling shares in the market.

Physicians may or may not think of their careers in financial terms. People are often attracted to medicine at an early age and consider it a job in which they can help people, deal with the latest scientific advances, and not worry too much about money. On the other hand, aspiring doctors also know that medical school takes a long time, costs a lot, and provides better than average incomes. Junior physicians worry about paying back school loans and how difficult it is to start a practice, so many of them work on salary for a clinic or a hospital for a while to accumulate funds. Conversely, senior physicians are often trying to extract capitalized value from their successful practices and patient goodwill as they get older and no longer want to work so many hours. In medicine, unlike real estate or banking, finance is not the main interest. Yet without financing a doctor cannot set up a practice or keep the door open any easier than a bank or shopping mall can. The development of financial institutions and intermediaries such as guaranteed loans, tax-exempt municipal bonds, insurance and reinsurance, and the use of venture capital to finance biotechnology research has been crucial to the growth of modern medicine. Careful review of a few simple financial terms and equations can help us understand certain aspects of the practice of medicine. Students wanting more background than can be provided in this very brief review should consult one of the standard finance texts such as Brealey and Myers' *Principles of Corporate Finance* or Louis Gapenski's *Understanding Health Care Finance*.

12.2   VALUE AND RATE OF RETURN

The Time Value of Money

Is it worthwhile to spend all those years studying hard and paying a high tuition in order to become a doctor? As economists, we have to conclude from the fact that people choose to do so that it must seem worthwhile to them—but that is also true of people who study poetry or art history, or take a few dance lessons or join a gym just to look better. What about in strictly financial terms, leaving aside all of the other considerations (which may be more important but can here usefully be ignored)? Most people think that becoming a doctor is financially worthwhile because physician incomes are higher than average ($200,000 versus $42,000), but a number of other factors must be accounted for even in a strictly financial analysis: tuition paid, long hours, years of unpaid study and practice, the fact that medical students are above-average to begin with and would probably earn more anyway, the chance of flunking out or graduating and being hit by a bus two weeks later, and so on. To begin, it is helpful to start with a simple example: a hypothetical therapist who is graduating in May with a B.S. and will earn $40,000, but could spend the extra year at school necessary to obtain an M.S. in order to earn a higher annual salary of $46,000. Is this worthwhile? More specifically, what is the rate of return on the M.S. degree compared to the B.S.?

In order to get the higher salary, the therapist will not be able to work next year (opportunity cost) but will gain a higher salary ($46,000 – $40,000). The approximate rate of return is found by considering "gains" divided by "costs."

(approximate) Rate of Return = Gains ÷ Costs = $6,000/$40,000 = 0.15 or 15%

Another way of stating this is to say that if one put $40,000 in an investment paying a 15 percent rate of return, then one would receive $6,000 each year. This is an approximation with many simplifying assumptions to make the calculation easy. In reality, the therapist will not make an extra $6,000 forever but only as long as he keeps working; we forgot about tuition; the work may be harder; everyone, whether B.S. or M.S., will have salary increasing over time; taxes will take away part of the raise; and so on. Nonetheless, it is a pretty good first approximation. Now we can work toward making the approximation a bit more exact (nothing in finance or economics is truly precise or known with certainty—except, as Keynes observed, that we must all pay taxes and eventually die).

Interest Rates and Present Value

If the therapist put $40,000 in a bank account with a 6 percent annualized rate of interest, at the end of the year the balance would be ($40,000) × (1.06) = $42,400. After five years, it would be $40,000 × (1.06) × (1.06) × (1.06) × (1.06) × (1.06) = $53,529. Repeat multiplication or compounding means that the five-year return is not five times 6 percent (that would be 30 percent) but actually 1.3382 times the original amount, or 33.82 percent.

In finance class, you probably learned that getting $53,529 five years from now was equivalent to getting $40,000 today if the interest rate is 6 percent. Stated succinctly, the **present value** of $53,529 in five years at 6 percent is $40,000. This means that the present value of a single dollar received in five years (at 6 percent interest) is $40,000/$53,529 = $0.75 (more precisely, $0.747258), which is equivalent to 1/1.3382 or 1 divided by 1.06 five times. The present value of each dollar next year at 8 percent is $1/1.08 = $0.9259, and the present value of each dollar in five years at 8 percent is (letting you do the division five times on your own calculator) $0.68. The present value of each dollar received 40 years from now at 8 percent is less than $0.05, which is why we often ignore the financial consequences of money far into the future.

Note, however, that the present value of a dollar received in 40 years evaluated at 6 percent is more than twice as large ($0.09722), and at 3 percent it is substantially larger ($0.3066). At the 15 percent rate of return the therapist is getting on his education, the present value of a dollar in 40 years is less than one-half penny ($0.00373)—so one could say that from a financial point of view, if rates are that high, things happening 40 years from now only matter 1/300th as much as they do today.

The discount (reduction in value) is obviously less if the waiting period is shorter. Thus although the present value of a dollar received in 40 years at 6 percent is $0.10, for a wait of 10 years the value of a dollar has fallen only to $0.55. Differences in interest rates matter more the longer the period. The difference between 6 percent and 8 percent is large in 40 years and gigantic after a century. The difference between annual rates of 6 percent and 15 percent is substantial even over a single year, but may not make much difference to someone borrowing money for just a week or two.

Which rate should be used to calculate present value? It depends (see your finance textbook for more discussion). The "appropriate" rate of return for a month is different from the rate for a year, the rate for a month with 28 days is different from the rate for a month with 31 days, and it may also vary from one year to the next. The present value is determined by applying the appropriate discount for each period. For example, if the interest rate in the first year is 6 percent, then 15 percent in the second year, and 8 percent in the third year, the present value is $1 \div [(1.06) \times (1.15) \times (1.08)] = \$0.7596$ today for each dollar received in three years.

What is the gain from obtaining an M.S. degree described above worth? Cash flows that are the same in each period ($6,000) and last forever are called a **perpetuity**, and if the same interest rate is used for discounting each period, a single equation links present value, annual payment, and interest rate.

Present Value of a Perpetuity = ($ amount)/(interest rate) = $6,000/0.15 = $40,000

This is just a formal restatement of the remark made above "that if one put $40,000 in an investment paying a 15 percent rate of return, then one would receive $6,000 each year." But is 15 percent the appropriate rate of return? If instead of getting an education, one put money in a bank at 6 percent, it would take $6,000 ÷ .06 = $100,000 on deposit to earn $6,000 each year. Is the value of an extra $6,000 per year in salary worth $40,000 or $100,000? How can the therapist correctly evaluate the financial impact of going to school relative to alternative investments of his time?

IRR: The Internal Rate of Return

The first calculation in the example above told us that spending a year getting an M.S. provides approximately a 15 percent rate of return, which seems substantially better than the 6 percent return the bank would provide if he spent the year working and deposited all paychecks into a savings account. Comparisons based on rates of return are often used by financial analysts because they are quick and easy to understand, and they also avoid the forced choice of one (or two or three) interest rates for discounting to find present value. Such calculations are called the "internal" rate of return (IRR) because they require that the analyst know only the cash flows of the project itself and not external considerations such as the market interest rate(s), what the potential risks are, future tax rates, and other factors affecting the decision as to which discount rate might be appropriate. IRR calculations are more objective and purely financial because they stay away from judgments and external considerations. For any given set of cash flows, every financial analyst would calculate the same IRR. If asked to determine "true" value, each would have to apply external assumptions, and to the extent that those analysts' assumptions varied, so would their estimates of value.

The calculation of IRR is easy for a perpetuity, but if the cash flows are not the same in each period (and in most business they are not) there is no simple formula to determine IRR. Fortunately we have computers with spreadsheets, and we can make use of the more general definition of IRR as the interest rate that, when used to discount a set of cash flows, makes the net present value neither positive nor negative, but just equal to 0.

Internal Rate of Return (IRR) = *the interest rate at which Net Present Value = 0*

For the typical project that requires initial investment to gain future rewards, if the first interest rate assumption makes the PV > 0 (positive), then keep raising the interest rate in the spreadsheet until PV = 0. If the initial interest rate estimate makes PV negative, then reduce the interest rate. There are several problems at the end of the chapter to give you exercise in finding IRRs. For now, consider the simple example used above with investment

SPREADSHEET TIMELINE FOR NPV AND INTERNAL RATE OF RETURN

Calculating net present value was a laborious task before spreadsheets became common, and doing the many trial-and-error calculations required to determine internal rate of return so daunting that most classes taught theory or shortcuts rather than practical applications. The advent of cheap computing has radically transformed the day-to-day work of financial analysis, making it possible to determine the NPV and IRR of even the most complicated sets of cash flows within a few minutes. The most important, and most difficult step, is to set out all of the cash flows in an organized way. To do so, a timeline is used, conventionally running left to right, such as in Table 12.1. The top row shows the periods (for this example, it can be assumed that they are years). The left-border column(s) are used for labels and formulas. The first column after that is year 0 or today. Year 1 is a year from now, and so on. The second row shows the present value of a dollar in that period. A dollar today has a present value of 1.000, a dollar in year 1 has a present value of $1.000 \div (1 + \text{interest rate})$. The present value of a dollar in year 2 is (PV year 1) $\div (1 + \text{interest rate})$. Year 3 is (PV year 2) $\div (1 + \text{interest rate})$, and so on, for as many periods as are needed. The easiest way to accomplish this calculation is to write the formula for PV year 1 and copy it across the row (remembering to use a fixed reference to the cell A1 with the interest rate). In the third row, put the net cash flow (CF). (If one wanted to be more detailed, one could use separate rows for cash in, cash out, and then net; or multiple rows for different types of revenues and expenses, but here we will keep it simple and just use one net cash flow entry for each year). In this example, there is a net investment of ($1,000) today, and net operating cash flow (revenues minus expenses) of $250, $300, $400, and $450, respectively, in years 1 to 4. In the next row, multiply the present value of $1 times the net cash flow for the year to get the present value of cash flows in each year. Finally, sum across that row to obtain the NPV of $195.14.

That was a bit tiresome—but, having set up the spreadsheet timeline for NPV once, it can be used over and over and over. To change the interest rate, simply type a new interest rate (in cell A1 if you used the indicated format) and immediately the new NPV is calculated. Want to find NPV for a different set of cash flows? Just type the new cash in and cash out into the appropriate cells. Want to find NPV for 10, 20, 250 years? Just

---

TABLE 12.1 Spreadsheet Timeline for NPV and IRR

6%	Year 0	Year 1	Year 2	Year 3	Year 4
PV of $1 @	1.000	0.943	0.890	0.840	0.792
Net CF	$ (1,000)	250	300	400	450
PV of CF	$(1,000.00)	$235.85	$267.00	$335.85	$356.44
NPV (sum)	$ 195.14				

Formulas	(Copy cells across to the right for as many columns as needed to get to the end)		
(Type in interest rate)	0	+ (cell to left) + 1	... + (cell to left) +1
PV of $1	1.000	+ (cell to left)/(1 + A1)	...+ (cell to left)/(1 + A1)
Net CF	(Cash In − Cash Out)	(Net CF year 1)	...(Net CF year n)
PV of CF in year	Multiply cell above by PV of $1	Multiply by PV $1 in year 1 ...	Multiply by PV $1 in year n
Net present value	= (sum across row above all the way to the last year)		

(Continued)

SPREADSHEET TIMELINE FOR NPV AND IRR (CONTINUED)

copy the formulas across (it takes a single set of mouse clicks—less than 10 seconds once you get the hang of it).

Oh yes, finding IRR—that is now a snap. If the NPV is positive, raise the interest rate until NPV is just zero (or near enough). If the NPV is negative, reduce the interest rate until NPV becomes positive. Usually you can get to within three or four decimal points in a few tries, and rarely more than a dozen (which, given the speed of most computers, takes less than a minute). Try it with the example above, and you should converge on 8.6 percent pretty quickly.

---

of $40,000 and returns of $6,000 each year. A discount rate of 12 percent yields an estimated value $6,000 ÷ 0.12 or $50,000 minus the ($40,000) initial cost and thus a positive NPV. A discount rate of 18 percent yields $6,000 ÷ 0.18 or $33,333 minus ($40,000) and thus a negative NPV. At 15 percent the estimated value of $40,000 minus the ($40,000) initial cost makes NPV = 0, so 15 percent is the correct rate of return. By a similar process of trial and error using the NPV timeline spreadsheet, we could determine that the IRR for the investment in the M.S. degree taking account of tuition at $12,000 (half of which is paid back by the therapist's employer after three years on the job), books costing $500, and the fact that he is already 40 years old and expects to spend only another 18 years working, not forever, is 11 percent.

Internal rates of return provide a shorthand measure of how financially desirable a project is. If the rough measurement makes it seem worthwhile, then other elements such as taxes, working conditions, probability of getting laid off, and the prestige and satisfaction obtained with a higher degree can be factored in.

Human Capital: Medical Education as an Investment

We can use the **human capital** approach to evaluate whether going to medical school is a sacrifice, a sound investment, or both.[2] The returns on medical education are estimated from the increased annual earnings, relative to a person's opportunity cost, that flow from the decision to go to medical school. The costs are all the things that are given up, which include tuition, but mostly the forgone earnings and leisure from working 80 hours a week without pay in medical school or for below-market wages during residency. Real returns (after adjustment for inflation) on financial assets have historically been about 1 to 3 percent for savings accounts and treasury bonds and 3 to 6 percent for stocks, which are a bit riskier. Economic studies of the rates of return for high school and college education have typically shown substantially better returns, 8 to 10 percent or more.

Empirical studies of rate of return on education become complex in practice, since one must adjust for the superior earning power of above-average students, the costs of the excess hours worked by physicians, and so forth. Also important is the fact that the returns from a medical education are much less risky than from a bachelor of arts (B.A.), master of business administration (M.B.A.), or doctor of law (J.D.) degree, and thus should be adjusted accordingly (see the discussion of risk and expected returns below). In addition, becoming a medical doctor confers prestige and other valuable privileges. Empirical studies in labor economics have reached a consensus on some major conclusions, although many details are still subject to disagreement. The return on investment from a college education clearly exceeds the market rate of return on financial assets, and the premium for being a college graduate is rising. The return on investment from graduation from medical school,

TABLE 12.2		Returns on Investment for a Professional Education			
(Length of training)	**Business** (2 years)	**Law** (3 years)	**Dentistry** (4 years)	**Primary Medicine** (4 years)	**Specialty Medicine** (4 years)
Tuition	$34,452	$32,317	$70,620	$74,504	$74,504
Annual income (age 40)	$135,579	$139,616	$133,050	$132,592	$219,733
Hours worked (age 40)	2,448	1,959	1,781	2,565	2,707
Internal Rate of Return	*26%*	*23%*	*22%*	*16%*	*18%*

Source: Weeks and Wallace[5], 2002.

with real returns of 10 to 20 percent, is higher than that for graduation from college (see Table 12.2).[3] Returns on other graduate degrees, such as a doctor of philosophy (Ph.D.) degree in biology or sociology, are much lower, and in some fields the returns are effectively zero. Returns on residency training follow incomes: they are high for surgical specialties (40 percent), intermediate for internal medicine (20 percent), and low for pediatrics (2 percent).

Risk

One of the benefits of medical education is the certainty that one will always have a job. Although the average income for lawyers might be similar to that of doctors, the variance is greater. Lawyers with salaries over $1 million are offset by other J.D.s who are barely getting by or have given up the practice of law entirely. Business incomes, particularly for entrepreneurs, are even more variable and extreme. Some are multimillionaires, while some are self-employed (and making less than minimum wage). Every investment carries risk to some degree or another. To calculate the internal rates of return using the spreadsheet timeline above, we first had to enter the cash flows for each future period—but we will never actually know what those cash flows are until after the fact. The precision of the calculations should not blind us to the reality that they are based on estimates, "best guesses" about what will (or might) happen in the future.

Some areas of medicine are relatively stable and provide low-risk earnings (physician, hospital administration). Others, like biotechnology, have extremely high risks. Discovery of a new cure is worth hundreds of millions of dollars, but most biotechnology ventures end up disappointing their investors by producing little revenue and no profits. Rather than the stocks, bonds, and retained earnings used to finance large established companies, biotech firms get most of their funding from risk-taking specialists known as "venture capitalists" (VC) and the human capital of the doctors and scientists who believe enough in their own ideas to work very hard for very little money but many stock options. Biotech is too risky for bank loans, and investors must be quite knowledgeable and experienced in this specialized field to assess the likelihood that a real drug will ever get produced, or how much it could be worth. If a biotech start-up produces a potentially useful new drug within five years, the venture capitalists will "cash out" by selling the rights to a large pharmaceutical firm or to the public through an initial public offering (IPO). If the start-up has not found a product within five years, it will usually be shut down and the investment written off.

Suppose that a hypothetical VC obtains $95 million dollars from its backers (usually wealthy individuals or pension funds) and adds $5 million of its own funds to invest $100 million in exciting new projects. It chooses ten projects, investing $10 million in each one. At the end of five years one of the projects has a great drug that is sold to a pharmaceutical company for $140 million, another project seems promising and is sold for $60 million, two of the projects have some promise and are sold for $10 million each (i.e., breakeven),

SPREADSHEET FOR EXPECTED NPV AND RISKY RETURNS

An NPV or IRR is certain only if one is certain of all future cash flows. Usually, the current (year 0) prices can be known with reasonable certainty. Future cash flows are almost always treated as risky unless they are interest payments on U.S. Treasury bonds or equivalents. The analyst must consider three things:

    a.   What are the possible future outcomes (scenarios)?

    b.   What are the cash flows for each outcome?

    c.   What is the probability of each outcome?

Frequently an analyst will consider several scenarios (most likely, good, bad) and determine the cash flows expected in each case. Then the analyst will estimate the likelihood that each scenario will occur. After that, finding NPV and IRR is simply a matter of calculation.

    In the example below, the most likely case is the same as in Table 12.1, whereas in the good scenario net operating cash flows are better ($300, $350, $450, and $500, respectively, in years 1 to 4) and in the bad scenario they are worse ($100 for each year; see Table 12.3). The analyst judges that the most likely scenario will happen 60 percent of the time, the good outcome 10 percent of the time, and the bad scenario the remaining 30 percent. The "expected cash flow" in year 0 is ($1,000) because regardless of the scenario, $1,000 must be paid for the investment. In year 1, the expected cash flow is (60% × $250) + (10% × $300) + (30% × $100) = $210. This is a weighted average, with the weights being the likelihood for each scenario. Similarly for year 2, expected cash flow is (60% × $300) + (10% × $350) + (30% × $100) = $245, and so on for years 3 and 4. In setting up the spreadsheet, one needs to type in the formula for weighted average only once and copy it across (remembering to use fixed cell references for the probability weights).

TABLE 12.3   Spreadsheet Timeline for *Expected* NPV and Risky Rates of Return

6%		Year 0	Year 1	Year 2	Year 3	Year 4
PV of $1 @		1.000	0.943	0.890	0.840	0.792
	Probability					
Net CF (middle)	60%	(1,000)	250	300	400	450
Net CF (good)	10%	(1,000)	300	350	450	500
Net CF (bad)	30%	(1,000)	100	100	100	100
Expected CF	*100 %*	*(1,000)*	*210*	*245*	*315*	*350*
PV of eCF		(1,000)	$198.11	$218.05	$264.48	$277.23
NPV (sum)		$ (42)				

Formulas	*(Copy cells across to the right for as many columns as needed to get to the end)*
(Type in interest rate)	
PV of $1	1.000 + *(cell to left)/(1 + A1)*
Expected CF	*Weighted average = (B3*C3) + (B4*C4) + (B5*C5)*
PV of eCF in year	*Multiply cell above by PV of multiply by PV$1 in year 1*
Expected NPV	*= (sum across row above all the way to the last year)*

(Continued)

SPREADSHEET FOR EXPECTED NPV AND RISKY RETURNS (CONTINUED)

This spreadsheet may seem like a bit much work to set up, but it only has to be done one time. With a single keystroke, the interest rate is changed. This makes it easy to determine expected IRR (here, since expected NPV is negative at 6%, the interest rate must be reduced to get NPV to zero, and that occurs at an interest rate of about 4.3%, which is thus determined to be the expected IRR). A few keystrokes and copying are all that is required to add on two or four or forty more years, or to change the probabilities of each scenario or the cash flows that will occur in each scenario. More scenarios can be created by adding rows (remembering that probability must always sum to 100 percent) but in practice most analysts stay with less than a dozen. The venture capital example discussed previously has ten rows, but cash flows in only two columns, year 0 (initial investment) and year 5 (when projects are sold off).

It is worth noting how important the probability weights are: the expected NPV goes from positive to negative with a small shift in the likelihood of the good or bad scenario. This sensitivity is even more extreme when "bad" is something like a hurricane—or bankruptcy or a malpractice suit—as it often is in the real world. The job of the analyst is not so much to predict the future as to point out to management what the financial implications of different futures might be, and how sensitive the financial strength of the organization is to both likely and extreme outcomes.

---

and six of the projects are terminated and thus valued at $0. At the end of five years, the $100 million invested has become $220 million. The internal rate of return is $220/$100 − 1.00 = 1.20 or 120 percent. Note that you must subtract 1.00 to account for the return of the original investment (i.e., if you invest $100 and get $103 back, that is a 3 percent IRR, not 103 percent). Note also that is a five-year return, so it is necessary to convert to an annualized rate of return by using the NPV timeline spreadsheet. There, you can see that turning $100 into $220 is an annualized rate of approximately 17 percent per year for five years.[4]

Valuing Assets

Finance is conceptually simple because **the only thing that ultimately matters is cash flow.** All other elements are considered only to help make estimates of cash flow better. The analyst only needs to know the cash flows in each period, and then makes the appropriate calculations to discount for when (*time*) and if (*risk*) the cash flows will occur. Although valuation is simple in theory, it is difficult and subject to large errors in practice, and it relies heavily on the judgment and expertise of the analyst.

What is an **asset**? Since cash flow is all that matters, from a financial point of view any item— a share of stock, a hospital building, a computer, or anything else—is an asset only to the extent that it provides future cash flow. The value of an MRI scanner is how much additional cash it can bring in before it is sold for scrap. Since the M.S. degree added to the future income of the therapist, is it an asset? Of course, but a medical education is just part of what makes a physician valuable. The most important assets of a physician's practice are intangible—not the building or the X-ray machine or the surgical instruments, but the skill and reputation of the doctors practicing there. Patients will continue going to a practice where they feel the physicians are well qualified and caring. If patients stopped coming the stream of revenues would dry up, reducing the value of the practice to zero. Is reputation an asset? Just ask Tiger Woods how much his name is worth (or ask Kobe Bryant how much the value of his reputation has gone up and down over the years). Think how much a brand like "Coke" or "Tylenol" or "Nexium" or "Viagra" or "the Mayo Clinic" is worth. When a biotech firm is sold, the most valuable assets are the patents to the new drug and the information about how it works and how to make it, not the actual chemicals or any equipment.

12.3   UNCORRELATED (INDEPENDENT) AND CORRELATED (SYSTEM) RISKS

Venture capitalists are a form of financial intermediary, pooling funds from a group of investors and using them to purchase a bundle of several projects. Putting ten biotech projects together averages out some of the risks: the expected value is the same, but the variance is reduced. In that way, VCs perform a function similar to insurance companies that pool the funds (premiums) of a large group of people to share risks so that no single person is bankrupted by catastrophic expense (see Chapter 4). Of course insurance companies pool losses, whereas venture capitalists pool projects that have net gains (or at least, they hope they have gains). Financial intermediation is not cheap. A VC firm changes a management fee up front and then takes a big slice of the profits. (Note, however, that the VC is also usually investing a chunk of its own funds in the pool.) The projects chosen must be really good prospects in order to pay the VC so much off the top and still provide the 15 to 25 percent gains that investors in such risky pools expect. The VC is providing two functions: (1) expert project selection and (2) bundling funds together. A VC is like a mutual fund, which collects money from many individuals and invests in stocks chosen by the fund manager, except that the number of investors is much smaller (maybe 10 or 20 instead of thousands) and the VC invests in start-up companies rather than traded stocks.

Mutual funds help investors by diversifying risks. Rather than purchasing $10,000 worth of shares in one stock, an investor purchases $10,000 worth of shares in the "fund," which holds hundreds of stocks. Much financial theory is devoted to the analysis of such portfolio diversification. Rather than reviewing that extensive body of knowledge here, it is better to refer those who wish to know more to a finance textbook; for those who do not want to read finance theory, it is important to understand clearly why grandmother's admonition "not to put all your eggs in one basket" is sound financial advice. Portfolio diversification works to the extent that the risks of each stock are independent on one another. If Moleculetech happens to go up because a clinical trial was favorable, that does not affect the likelihood that Exxon or Biolyne will go up or down. Risks that are independent are also said to be uncorrelated. However, the CFO and the chief biologist for Moleculetech will both get rich, or not, depending upon the outcome of the same clinical trial—and thus their financial risks are highly (almost 100 percent) correlated. Perfect correlation exists between two shares of stock in the same company: if the price goes up, it goes up the same for both.

Some risks affect almost all stocks, so there is a high degree of correlation. If interest rates rise, the value of most stocks will decline because investors will start to sell stocks to buy the bonds that now pay more per year, and also because the present value of future earnings is reduced when the discount rate is higher (see Section 12.2 and the NPV timeline spreadsheet above). Similarly, if the economy heads toward a recession, profits are likely to be lower for most companies, and the entire stock market will tend down. Having bought a mutual fund with a thousand stocks rather than a single company stock does not help the investor minimize these systemic risks. Macroeconomic shifts affect all stocks, and thus the risk and cannot be reduced by diversification.[5]

A risk may be correlated for a certain type of asset but not others. A hurricane might pose significant losses to all property insurance companies operating in Florida but not affect automobile insurers. A rise in the price of steel would affect automobile and appliance manufacturers but not movie companies or book publishers. The main macroeconomic risks (falling GDP or rising interest rates) actually have little effect on most health care stocks. People go to the hospital whether times are good or bad, and the future of a Moleculetech is going to depend more on the results of a clinical trial than on the state of the economy. The major risks in health care often come from government action, as when Medicare Part D was enacted (affecting all drug companies) or cuts to Medicaid (affect all hospitals with high concentrations of poor patients) or changes in the RBRVS payment system (affected all physicians).

Which Is Riskier: Nursing Homes or Drug Companies?

The financial concepts of independent (uncorrelated) and systemic (correlated) risks can usefully be applied to the various kinds of health care organizations examined in previous chapters. Since it cost hundreds of millions of dollars to develop a new drug, and since most new drugs fail to even reach the marketplace much less make any profits, it would seem that the pharmaceutical industry is very risky. The nursing home industry serves a growing number of elderly people with a product that does not require a lot of innovation or marketing to sell. Most nursing homes operate nearly full most of the time. Thus it would seem that the nursing home industry is quite stable and low risk.

First appearances can be deceiving, and the market evidence contradicts the propositions in the paragraph above. Pharmaceutical companies almost never go bankrupt and usually rank among the most consistently profitable industry groups in the S&P 500, whereas almost every publicly traded LTC company went bankrupt or became financially distressed during the 1990s. Why such discrepancy between first appearances and financial reality? Pharmaceutical companies are in fact diversified firms with many products: drugs for heart disease, drugs for cancer, drugs for skin conditions, and on and on. The portfolio of products means that in any given year at least some drugs are profitable and make up for the ones that fail. Overall the demand for drugs is stable and growing—higher interest rates or a looming recession may keep people from buying new cars or remodeling their homes but not from purchasing blood pressure medication, particularly now that most drugs are insured. An individual biotech company is a highly risky enterprise with a high likelihood of failure, but that failure is not correlated with the risk of biotech firm B or with the general stock market. It is specific to the particular drug the firm is investigating. However, the fact that most biotech firms are small start-up companies with few tangible assets does increase their relative risk. Big pharmaceutical firms are pretty resilient, and only occasionally suffer setbacks.

Nursing homes, in contrast, all suffered together when the government cut Medicare and Medicaid reimbursements under the Balanced Budget Act of 1997. A single entry in the federal register caused Genesis, Manor Care, Beverly Enterprises, and the other major firms in this industry to suffer massive and unexpected losses. What had been a growth industry became a shambles of distressed assets almost overnight. The budget cuts pushed down revenues per bed everywhere, and expenses per bed could not be reduced fast enough to stave off disaster.

Assessing Business Risk

In the example above, a change in government policy hurt the nursing home in two ways: it reduced revenues, and that in turn reduced the value of the assets (value being the capitalized sum of future earnings an asset can generate). Financial analysts use a number of ways to assess the value and risks of a business. From an investor's point of view, the single most important issue is how much is earned for each dollar invested (called "return on equity" or ROE) and often analyzed using the "DuPont Equation."[6] This is appropriate for corporate finance based on the assumption that the most important objective (or even the only objective) is maximization of shareholder wealth. In health care, such an assumption is rarely justified. A physician is often both the owner and the chief employee of the practice, not just an investor. Hospitals are often nonprofit organizations with the community at large as the only "shareholder" of their equity fund balance. Clinics run by the city or county or the Veterans Administration have CFOs that apply business principles but are units of government with public, not private, returns on investment. Even publicly traded for-profit HMOs, hospital chains, and pharmaceutical companies are often held to a higher standard (or other standards) than pure shareholder wealth maximization. Therefore a more conceptual and generalized approach to the assessment of business risk is more appropriate than a narrow focus on ROE. A conceptual structure used by managers in both for-profit and nonprofit enterprises is formulated as:

Business Risk = (Revenue Risk) × (Operating Expense Leverage) × (Financial Leverage)

The overall financial risk to the organization is separated into components:

a. How variable are revenues? Is there growth?
b. Do expenses adjust a lot or only a little as revenue changes?
c. Are the assets financed mostly with equity or debt? What kind of debt?

The first issue to face is how much revenue the organization will bring in. Is it stable, growing, or shrinking? Will revenue trend close to forecast, or will it be subject to lots of random fluctuations and variability? Is the generation of revenue under the control of management, perhaps because the organization can easily raise prices, serve more patients, or call upon donors? Having some handle on the range of risks in revenue, the organization must understand how readily it can adjust to unanticipated ups and downs. Will expenses automatically decline proportionately if there is a drop in revenue (as happens with variable costs when volume declines)? Can some expenses be easily cut or deferred for a while (R&D, maintenance, vanity projects, new product launch)? Operating leverage is often dominated by the fixed to variable cost ratio. Whereas a clinical laboratory or a physical therapy practice may find that many of its costs go up and down as patient volume rises or falls, nursing homes, hospitals, and pharmaceutical companies with large fixed costs tend to have inflexible expenses, so they make good profits when revenues surge and are sunk if revenues unexpectedly dip. To the extent that a hospital treats its labor force as permanent, it will have high operating leverage; management that is willing to quickly adjust nursing and other employment up and down to match patient flow is more flexible—but may be perceived as ruthless cost-cutters rather than friendly patrons.

Revenues and expenses, the first two components, determine the cash flow from operations.[7] They establish the degree of risk in the business before any financial engineering to change the debt-to-equity structure takes place. Typically, businesses with a low degree of operational risk (utilities, real estate, nursing homes) take on more debt to increase leverage and raise the rate of return on equity, while businesses with a high degree of inherent risk (biotech, restaurants, moviemaking) must rely almost entirely on equity and thus have low leverage. Most corporate finance concentrates on the structuring of debt and equity. Although this issue has become increasingly important for hospitals, and was central to the problems of LTC companies with lots of highly leveraged debt-heavy real-estate, it is relatively unimportant for physician practices (self-financed), pharmaceutical firms (equity financed with excess retained earnings) and insurance companies (more likely to be net creditors than debtors).

12.4 OWNERSHIP AND AGENCY

The original health care firm was the solo physician, taking care of patients and collecting fees. Even the author of the Hippocratic Oath was a businessperson.[8] Today's physicians, like Hippocrates, operate within an ethical context. The financial structure of ancient Greek medicine was fairly simple, since there were no stocks and bonds. There were risks and rewards, and a form of debt and equity in the set of personal obligations that went with being part of an organized profession. The Oath talks about the physician's obligations (personal and financial) to the one who taught him (today, we might talk about medical school debts and junior partnerships), and the most valuable asset was the physician's reputation and that of the medical profession. Indeed, one of the goals of the Hippocratic Oath was to increase the value of this reputational equity. It is instructive to begin with this prototype, which is not so different from the single physician entering practice today, to see the elements that led toward increasingly powerful financial structures and complex intermediaries.

Equity and Debt

A physician who starts a practice is an entrepreneur risking time and effort in the hope of doing well.[9] In common parlance, this is called "sweat equity." Some cash will be required. In most cases, this will come from government subsidized guaranteed student loans and from the parents who are proud of their daughter, the doctor. First come the tuition and living expenses during medical school, and then the expenses (rent, equipment, payroll) of furnishing a practice. The typical practice starts small and grows, paying for most of its expansion as more and more patients come in paying more and more fees (retained earnings).

In terms of finance, this physician practice is a 100 percent equity-financed sole proprietorship. Any profits go to the physician who started the practice and works there. Her employees may get paid better as the practice does better, but that is at her discretion. She, as **the owner, is the residual claimant to all of the money left after expenses are paid**. As the practice grows, she may want to add equipment or build a new office, and she approaches a bank for a loan. She is doing so because she expects the returns on the new computer system (increase in future cash flows) to be greater than the cost—perhaps a 15 percent return on funds borrowed at just 7 percent interest. Financial leverage is being used to increase the returns on equity (her hard work and M.D. degree). Of course if the computer system doesn't work, then she as the residual claimant is the one who suffers.

If the practice continues to grow, she will add other doctors. Initially, they will be on salary rather than sharing profit, both because (a) they do not want to take a risk, but want to be guaranteed they will earn enough to live if they move there to work, and (b) she does not want to share the profits from her years of hard work and practice-building until the new doctors prove that they are worthwhile partners. As long as these additional doctors continue to work on salary, or even on some percent of billings (if they were salespeople, we would call it a commission), the financial structure is still that of a sole proprietorship, even if she decides to buy the building and finances it with debt using a bank loan.

Once she finds a compatible doctor who wants to stick with the practice, the practice will undergo a legal change and become a **partnership**. Now there are multiple residual claimants to the profits, and this poses several challenges. The new doctor may be young and willing to work nights, while the founding doctor is close to retirement and wants more time off. She may feel that she is owed a bigger share since she built the practice up and bought all of the equipment. The potentials for conflicts are endless, but commonly people who want to work together find a way to do so. As there are more and more partners, it becomes more necessary to use legal contracts and to regularize the role of partners: defining shares, relating pay to number of services each doctor bills for, making new doctors "buy in" over a period of years, and so on (see "Group Practice" in Section 7.4).

The clinic may decide to move aggressively into new technology by becoming a center for diagnostic imaging. The equipment is expensive and the task of running an operation with 40 exam rooms and hundreds of technicians is complex, so the medical group partnership decides to get help from an outside firm, DioTech. Also, the local bank has told the doctors they are not comfortable lending them more money because then the doctors would have too much debt relative to the value of their building and other liquid (i.e., easy to sell and convert into cash) assets, so any additional millions are a "maybe" and would carry a much higher interest rate. The imaging center will be set up separate from the medical group as an independent **corporation**. A corporation is a legal entity, like a person or a partnership, but with limited liability. Only the assets of the corporation can be taken if it goes bankrupt. The doctors and DioTech will both be residual claimants to the profits of the imaging center (according to some specified contract), but usually most of the financing is put up by the outside company.

DioTech may have been a project funded by some venture capitalists to build and operate imaging centers and is now ready for its IPO (initial public offering). Once DioTech decides to "**go public**" and have stock traded on NASDAQ, NYSE, or other exchange, all of its financial statements including quarterly and annual reports are made openly available on the Web at http://idea.sec.gov. Investors from around the world send in their money to buy shares and thus get fractional equity ownership. Some do not even know what business DioTech is in, only that it is supposed to be a hot stock. The better informed ones are hoping DioTech will get bought up by a large firm such as MegaMed and thus provide them with shares in a well-known established company or a quick profit by selling.

Who Owns the Business? Who Owns the Patient? Agency Issues

At this point it is appropriate to ask, who really owns this imaging center? The medical group, or at least the senior partners, usually have an active role in management and get a share of the profits, but profits also go the shareholders who have never been near the clinic. It should be apparent that "running the business," "making money off the business," and "owning the business" are no longer the same, as they were in the simple solo proprietorship with which Dr. Smith started. For a large publicly traded company like the hypothetical MegaMed (or a real company like Universal Healthcare or Johnson & Johnson) over half of the "owners" are people whose money is in pension or mutual funds and do not even know that they are receiving the profits of this business. The original equity was put up by the initial proprietor, Dr. Smith, and she had a triple role of working, managing, and investing. These roles become increasingly distinct as the organization gets larger. As the medical group gets larger, some differentiation of roles is likely to occur with one or more senior physicians taking a leadership role, but each doctor is still doing some of each. Even in the joint venture the outside firm is putting in both management and operational expertise as well as money. A real bridge is crossed when a business goes public and the majority of investors are people who are not actually part of the company. In financial theory, the **separation of ownership from control** is the subject of agency theory.[10] The managers of the business are supposed to make decisions on behalf of the shareholders, using their expertise and efforts to maximize shareholder wealth—but instead they may decide to take it easy, hire their friends, buy fancy corporate jets, or even engage in sweetheart deals that enrich the CEO and members of the board by draining money from the company. Agency theory was discussed in Chapter 6 with regard to physicians (agents) making decisions on behalf of patients (principals). In corporate finance, most of the attention is on managers making decisions on behalf of shareholders, or other owners. For example, will the doctors do their best for DioTech? Will DioTech provide the physicians a fair share of the lucrative fees obtained from the hundreds of scans the center performs each day? What is "fair" in the distribution of a business profits?

In a legal sense, a "fair" distribution of profits is whatever the parties agree to. DioTech may feel that the medical group would never have made millions in the imaging business if it were not for their expertise and the $20 million in construction and equipment they provided. Smith Medical Group may feel that DioTech would not be making millions without their patients. Similar conflicts may have arisen when Dr. Smith first thought about taking on a partner. Also, the answers change as business conditions change. For example, if there are five different publicly traded firms all offering to serve as joint venture partners in developing imaging centers (as there are now) then the medical group will have choices, get a competitive offer, and keep the bulk of the profits. Conversely, 20 years ago, DioTech may have been the pioneer taking all the risks and been the only game in town, leaving the medical group no choice but to accept a contract in which half the profits were permanently ceded to DioTech. More recently, Middletown HMO may be the payer for most of the patients coming to the clinic, and thus they can say "these patients are ours" and siphon off most of the profits by agreeing to let "their" patients be treated at the clinic only in return for reduced rates.

Current controversies over executive pay show that agency conflicts are quite serious. How much does the CEO deserve to get? Clearly, somebody has to run the company, and if he does a good job, he should benefit. Yet the CEO can award himself stock options and benefit just because the market goes up (carrying lazy MegaMed along with it). Even more egregious, the CEO can simply stack the board of directors with friends and ask them to vote him a bonus of $50 million, or to provide an interest-free loan that he will never pay back. If the shareholders are not paying attention, then there are few consequences for such behavior. Even if the shareholders do think something is wrong, often the best they can do is simply sell their shares and hope the next company they invest in is better managed. This shows how difficult it is to determine who really "owns" a company.

Since the separation of ownership and control can create such problems, why is publicly traded stock used as equity? It is done simply because the efficiencies gained more than outweigh the inefficiencies. How many single proprietors can come up with billions of dollars? And if they can, wouldn't they be wise to diversify putting some of their money into other companies rather than letting their entire wealth ride just on their own company? The doctor with a great idea usually needs investors to make it a reality. Consider why patients allow the inefficiencies that come with having a doctor make decisions for them about what medicines to take, whether or not to have an operation, and whether an artificial knee is a better solution than ligament repair. Making decisions on one's own is too costly for most patients because they would have to spend many hours learning the relevant medical facts, and because they would make more mistakes than a trained specialist. Most investors also need professional help to make good decisions.

The Role of Financial Intermediaries

Turning over functions to a specialist who can do them for less is central to the role of financial intermediation. Consider Dr. Smith's loan from the bank. The bank acts as an intermediary taking money from depositors and loaning to businesses. Why don't the depositors just loan their own money to Dr. Smith and get 8 percent instead of the 5 percent the bank pays them? By pooling the funds of many depositors, the bank is able to average out good and bad loans.

The bank has expertise in credit assessment, choosing what businesses to loan to and which to avoid. The bank is also able to transfer funds from depositors to borrowers at much less cost than the parties could do on their own—masses of legal and accounting transactions are done at low cost with standardized forms and computers.

Major brokerage firms and stock markets make it possible to raise large amounts of equity financing at low cost. They are far enough away from operations that they do not have to provide management expertise, just financial expertise. Modern business transactions go through hundreds of intermediaries, allowing each one to prosper by making all the other parties in the chain better off (another example of the fundamental theorem of exchange first discussed in Chapter 1). At each stage, the costs are reduced by concentrating expertise and using economies of scale to find the cheapest form of credit. When a hospital borrows $100 million, those bonds are transferred from investment banks who sell them to mutual funds that hold them on behalf of investors. The hospital is also likely to deal with brokerage firms that allow them to buy or sell swap options that effectively convert some of their fixed rate 30-year, 5 percent tax-exempt bonds into lower-cost variable rates that fluctuate weekly with the market. Money flows efficiently with rapid smoothness throughout the system at low cost—except occasionally, when a "kink" or stoppage suddenly occurs that makes each link in the chain worried about getting payment from the next link (insurance, credit card, hospital, bondholder, bank, hedge fund, pension fund, mutual fund, etc.), which can make the flow less "liquid" or even set off a chain reaction (as occurred in 2008/2009) in which the flow is so disrupted that everyone stops trading for no apparent reason, rather like a chance accident causing a traffic jam with massive tie-ups and multiple collisions as sometimes suddenly occurs on a busy freeway.

Health Insurers as Financial Intermediaries

Health insurers are financial intermediaries, taking in cash (premiums) and then paying it out several months later (claims). Whereas the public thinks about insurance primarily in terms of the cost of covering claims, the earnings of an insurer often depend more on the investment returns from the money it holds. The residual left after medical costs and administrative expenses are paid is often less than 5 percent, and may be near 0 percent. In a good year, the return on investments is much larger. That is one reason insurance companies are regulated as financial firms, with capital requirements related to liquidity (ability to pay) and investment risk, more than with regard to medical payments.

12.5   CAPITAL FINANCING: HOSPITALS

A frequent saying among hospital board members is "no margin, no mission," meaning that unless the hospital can keep expenses lower than revenues (margin), it will not be able to carry out its objectives (mission). Revenues must also be sufficiently above operating costs to compensate those who have invested capital. If a hospital borrows $10 million for construction, it must pay back the principal over time and pay interest on the loan each year. For a philanthropist making a donation, the returns on capital take the form of social services rather than interest or dividends. Having a nonprofit organization that is supposed to lose money each year, with the difference made up out of endowment or contributions, tends to blur the line between capital and operating funds. However, the conceptual requirement for a return on capital is clear. The philanthropist could always invest the money in financial assets and make a donation each year from the resulting interest if that were a more efficient way to achieve the charitable purpose than providing a lump-sum capital donation.

The start-up capital for most hospitals came from a combination of philanthropy and local government funds. Land and buildings were often donated. At the beginning of the twentieth century, there were also a number of doctors' hospitals, usually started in a portion of the doctor's house or in a converted dwelling nearby. The capital financing for these small, private hospitals came from the doctor's own savings or from family members. Hospitals grew because they were successful in attracting funds or because they were successful in attracting paying patients and could build up reserves (which would be called "retained earnings" at a for-profit organization).

During World War II, millions of servicemen experienced the benefits of modern medical technology firsthand. The power of antibiotics and new surgical techniques to heal impressed many people, especially those from rural areas. This created a desire to spread hospitals across the land.[11] Yet only a few hospitals had been able to build up reserves during the Great Depression or World War II, and organizations that had conserved money wanted to expand their own operations, not help rural communities. The success of the New Deal and the victories of the military made it seem natural to mobilize government resources to meet this need. In 1946 the Hill-Burton Act was passed, making construction funds available to new hospitals in areas that had fewer than four beds per 1,000 people. As a form of repayment, hospitals receiving these funds were to give an equal or greater value in free care to indigent people. City and suburban hospitals were envious of the easy access rural areas had to capital and, because power tends to accrue to those who already have it (i.e., existing hospitals) and not necessarily to those who need it, subsequent changes were made to allow Hill-Burton funds to be used for expansion and renovation projects, as well as new construction.

Hill-Burton, retained earnings, and philanthropic fund drives provided most capital financing until the enactment of Medicare and Medicaid in 1965. Hospitals, which had chronically suffered operating losses, suddenly had steady revenue streams guaranteed by the government. They could meet the demand for new construction by borrowing against that promise, and they proceeded to do so. Borrowing increased from less than $100 million in 1960 to $200 million in 1970, $1,215 million in 1975, and $2.6 billion in 1977.[12] Three factors combined to make debt quickly become the dominant form of hospital capital:

- Guaranteed revenues from Medicare and Medicaid that assured investor repayment
- Tax exemption as municipal bonds made it cheap for nonprofit hospitals to borrow
- Cost reimbursement for interest expenses

Medicare and Medicaid totally changed the financial picture of hospitals, from social organizations that had to beg for money each year, to solidly funded services backed by the government. For a time, it was virtually impossible for most hospitals to go bankrupt and hence for investors not to get repaid. States and localities created "health care financing authorities" that allowed nonprofit hospitals to qualify as municipal borrowers so that investors did not have to pay federal, state, and local taxes on the interest they received. This reduced the cost of borrowing by a third, making it possible for a hospital to issue bonds at 5 percent and invest at 7 percent while waiting to use the money for construction. Such arbitrage generated millions of dollars for astute hospital financial managers before being outlawed. The shift to cost reimbursement also favored borrowing. A hospital that used its own reserves to construct a new building could get reimbursed for depreciation, but the hospital that issued debt to do the same thing got reimbursed for interest expenses as well as depreciation.

THE ALLEGHENY BANKRUPTCY*

Allegheny General Hospital was one of the largest hospitals in the Pittsburgh, Pennsylvania, area.[13] It provided a broad range of services, had high occupancy, and generated large cash flows. In 1987, it merged with the cash-poor Medical College of Pennsylvania in Philadelphia to form Allegheny Health and Education Research Foundation (AHERF). The merger seemed to benefit both organizations: Allegheny General Hospital had the medical school affiliation it needed to enhance its image, and the Medical College of Pennsylvania had the cash it needed.

Medical schools represent significant fixed costs, however. Shortly after the merger, AHERF began to look to purchase other hospitals in the Philadelphia market over which these fixed costs could be spread. From 1990 to 1996, AHERF went on a hospital-buying spree. It acquired a children's hospital, another Philadelphia medical college, and a number of community hospitals in the Philadelphia and Pittsburgh markets. All along the way, AHERF was leveraging the strong cash flows from its Allegheny General Hospital to buy up financially troubled hospitals.

During the 1990s, many hospitals, fearful of the advent of managed care, began purchasing physician practices to make sure that they would not lose admissions. AHERF was aggressive in doing so, trying to increase market share and rapidly increasing the price paid for practices in the Philadelphia area. In the end, much money was spent, and few new admissions were gained as hospitals simply started paying extra for what they had received previously without payment—the doctors' business.

AHERF also began competing aggressively for managed care business during the 1990s, some of which were "full-risk" contracts under which the hospital contracts to take care of all HMO member health care needs for a percentage of that member's HMO policy premium. Competition with other hospital networks bid down the prices paid, and inexperience with full-risk management caused expenses to rise, resulting in substantial losses. Yet in the short run these contracts brought in additional cash (as HMO premiums were paid) that could be used for more acquisitions, and only in the long run, as services were paid for, did the losses appear on the balance sheet.

By 1996, AHERF was beginning to suffer on a number of fronts. Economies of scale from owning multiple facilities were not coming to fruition quickly enough, since it takes time to consolidate operations. Bidding wars for physician practices resulted in lower returns. Bidding wars for HMO contracts resulted in lower reimbursement rates. To hide poor financial performance, AHERF executives transferred funds from one division to another to make each appear profitable at the time of the division's audit. Some of these transfers included restricted funds that are intended for use at one institution only for a specific purpose; such transfers are illegal. Lack of diligence by both AHERF's Board of Directors and auditors left these transfers hidden. Like Enron, this financial shell game eventually came unraveled. In 1997, AHERF became the largest not-for-profit bankruptcy in U.S. history, and its CEO, Sherif Abdlehak, was eventually sent to jail.

Hospital debt was subsequently viewed in the bond market as being much riskier, so all hospitals had to pay higher interest to compensate for the actions of this rogue entrepreneur.[14] Simple yet powerful economic forces put AHERF in jeopardy. AHERF leadership, through deliberate acts of top executives and passive acceptance by the Board of Directors, compounded the failure.

*This section researched and prepared by Prof. Patrick M. Bernet, Florida Atlantic University.

In this environment with tax-exempt debt, willing investors, and cost reimbursement, it is not surprising that hospitals went on a borrowing spree, loading up with more than $10 billion in debt by 1980. However, any business that takes on lots of debt is more likely to come under financial pressure. Despite being organized as nonprofit organizations, hospitals were no exception. With millions of dollars of interest payments to make each year, hospital managers had to become more and more bottom-line oriented. As the threat of bankruptcy became more real, the social welfare and community benefit orientation that had prevailed since the turn of the century increasingly gave way to a business orientation.

Hospital borrowing rose so rapidly that it had to lose steam eventually. Too many new beds were added, and debt loads became insupportable. Also, pressures on the Medicare budget led to tighter and tighter reimbursement. In 1985, the first bond defaults began to occur. Investors quickly revised their expectations and treated hospital debt as risky, and hence required a higher rate of interest. Municipalities were less and less pleased about the loss of property and income taxes, and calls were made to limit the use of tax-exempt revenue bonds such as those issued by hospital financing authorities. Access to capital became more difficult. Old and decrepit facilities could not tap the bond market and were acquired by for-profit hospital chains that could use the stock market to quickly raise equity, refurbish the physical plant, and make money. Many towns were willing to sell their hospitals for nothing, even provide special subsidies and tax breaks, rather than let them go bankrupt and disappear. The environment also had changed so that more hospitals felt it necessary to become part of a system covering all types of care over a broad geographic area. To do so, strong hospitals wanted to merge with or buy weaker ones and to buy nursing homes, home health agencies, physician practices, and medical office buildings. In most cases, it was not legal to use tax-exempt debt to do so, nor could the hospitals borrow the hundreds of millions of dollars necessary in the corporate (taxable) market.

The stand-alone community hospital was a good structure for creating a social contract.[15] Business leaders, citizens of the town, and the poor all participated in a visible symbol of community responsibility that was governed by a local board of directors. The move toward larger and more integrated health care systems has shown that this structure is inflexible and increasingly outmoded. People no longer identify primarily with a community or look to voluntary action to provide health care, and the solo hospital has no way to move capital from where the funds are (in wealthy suburbs) to where the needs are (in distressed urban and rural areas, in providing assistance to elderly people with disabilities). Creating a chain of hospitals is one way to regionalize and rationalize the allocation of capital. Recently there has been a spurt of acquisitions and conversions of hospitals to for-profit status, although it is still unclear how far this trend will go and to what extent the government, as the primary payer for hospital care, will let it go. What has become clear is that private equity markets have far outstripped private philanthropy as a source of capital for meeting the demands for new health care services and new health care facility construction in the twenty-first century.

12.6   HMO OWNERSHIP AND CAPITAL MARKETS: SUCCESS AND FAILURE

Business Risks for an HMO

An HMO, especially a closed-panel group practice HMO, is a hybrid combining insurance (financial intermediary) with operations (hospitals, physicians, etc.). The major risks to the individual patient, random variation in illness, are diversified away. A group of 10,000 people has reasonably predictable health care costs, and a group of 100,000 has negligible variation in average costs due to the random variation among the individuals who make up the group. The more relevant patient risks to an HMO are related to marketing: selection and volume. An HMO attracting a larger proportion of seriously ill people will suffer financially from adverse selection as much as any other insurer.[16] An even more serious marketing risk is the inability to attract a sufficient number of clients. To break even, a certain volume must be attained to cover fixed costs, and growth is a primary determinant of cash flow and profitability. In this regard, HMOs are similar to most other businesses. Indeed, the primary risks an investor must evaluate in considering HMO profitability are standard business risks: obtaining clients ("lives" or number of persons); pricing (capitation rate); expenses (e.g., wage rates, per diem hospital costs, cost of referrals); productivity (how much labor and capital it takes to run the HMO); and financial leverage (debt obligations relative to reserves).[17] The "core competency" of an HMO is the ability to keep the growth rate of medical costs below the rate of growth in premiums while maintaining or increasing patient satisfaction.

Kaiser Health Plan: The Evolution of an HMO

Kaiser Health Plan, with more than 9.8 million members, is the largest HMO in the United States and one of the largest medical delivery systems in the world. Its origins lie in the efforts of a young surgeon, Sydney R. Garfield, to find a place to practice when he completed residency at Los Angeles County Hospital in 1933.[18] The disastrous economy of the depression made it impossible to open up a new solo fee-for-service practice in Los Angeles as he wished to do, so Dr. Garfield reluctantly began looking for a salaried job to tide him over until times improved. The Metropolitan Water District was building an aqueduct from the Colorado River to Los Angeles and was looking for a physician to staff a small clinic to treat construction workers in the desert. Garfield thought the salary they offered, $125 a month, was too little for someone as well trained as himself. With the support of a local doctor as partner, he decided to open his own hospital at Desert Center. The construction companies were very anxious to have a doctor for their workers and agreed to help Garfield and send all their industrial medicine cases insured under the new workers' compensation plan to his facility. Garfield opened a top-notch hospital, complete with modern operating facilities and air conditioning, an unheard of luxury for industrial workers at that time.

The injured workers and the construction companies loved the facility, but two financial problems quickly arose. The workers' compensation insurance companies thought Garfield treated the workers too well, and they argued over many of the bills submitted. Garfield also treated the men for nonindustrial illnesses, but few could afford to pay private practice fees for extended hospital stays or major surgery, even though Garfield felt obligated to treat them. Garfield threatened to close the hospital unless he could obtain a steady source of funding. The foundations of a major innovation in health care financing were laid when an executive of the major workers' compensation insurance companies suggested that they prepay Garfield by giving him one-eighth of the worker's compensation insurance premium, which amounted to $1.50 per month for each of the 5,000 construction workers on the project, and for workers to voluntarily prepay an additional $1.50 per month to cover all nonindustrial accidents and illnesses.[19] Garfield's experiment in prepaid HMO medicine was very successful. He added two more hospitals; at the end of five years, as construction slowed and the hospitals began to close, Garfield had made a net profit of more than $250,000 (equivalent to $4 million after adjustment for inflation to 2010).

Although Garfield intended to take his profits and set up a private practice in Los Angeles, he was lured north to open another prepaid workers' clinic by one of the aqueduct contractors, Henry J. Kaiser, who had just made a deal to complete the Grand Coulee Dam in Oregon. Kaiser was impressed by the efficiency and high quality of Garfield's operation in the desert and felt that establishing a similar facility would help him attract workers to another remote construction site. At Grand Coulee, SR Garfield & Associates provided 24-hour medical coverage to 15,000 workers and family members in a modernized and, once again, air-conditioned hospital with a group of five physicians and six nurses. Garfield himself, however, remained in Los Angeles undergoing more medical training and looking after business interests, flying to Grand Coulee and working in the clinic only once every six weeks. It was as a manager that Garfield made the health plan successful, while his status as a physician gave him a special connection with the professionals who worked under his direction. He was, in the words of one of the physicians who worked for him, "a genius at keeping salaries and expenses down."

With Grand Coulee nearing completion and Garfield ordered up for service in the Army Medical Corps during World War II, it appeared that his days as an entrepreneur were over. However, Kaiser had just been given a new contract to construct 60 freighters at a hastily organized shipyard in Richmond, near San Francisco, and he wanted Garfield to provide the medical care for his wartime crew. Within a year, Garfield built a hospital and was caring for 90,000 workers. His commitment to staying at the forefront of medical practice is evidenced by the establishment of a research program and a new journal, the *Permanente* (Kaiser) *Foundation Medical Bulletin*, in 1943. By 1944, Garfield had a hundred doctors working for him to care for more than 200,000 workers and dependents. Although his first recruits were outstanding doctors from Stanford University, the University of Southern California, and other leading medical schools who wished to join a prepaid group practice, others were hired only because they were unfit for military service and needed a job. From them, Garfield learned an important management lesson, which he later stated as, "No matter how the principles of our plan are meant, if you don't have the physician group who have it in their hearts and who believe in prepaid practice, it won't work," emphasizing that it is the culture and the people even more than the financial contracts that define a successful HMO.[20]

As fast as the war had created a need for the Kaiser medical plan, the end of the war took it away. The only clinic not to suffer a major enrollment decline was the one at the new Kaiser steel mill in Fontana, in the desert outside Los Angeles. The Alameda County and San Francisco medical societies, tolerant during the war emergency, grew openly hostile. Kaiser doctors were denied medical society membership, and hence could not join hospital medical staffs or participate in many forms of professional advancement. Yet Garfield, Kaiser, and many of their closest associates, including health economist Avram Yedidia, decided that the appropriate course of action was to regroup and expand their visionary health plan rather than shut it down. In the immediate postwar period, enrollment stabilized at fewer than 20,000. By 1948, it had rebounded to 60,000, with much of the growth coming from marketing to unions and firms whose employees would join as a group.

Yet the pressures of fluctuating enrollment, requirements for capital, and a need for clearer lines of authority made the entrepreneurial organization, with Sydney Garfield alone in charge of all the Kaiser health facilities, untenable. The new structure had three entities: a charitable corporation for the hospitals, a nonprofit foundation for the health plan, and a private for-profit partnership for the physician group. Garfield was paid $257,000 for his interest in the hospitals, and subsequently gave up his interest in the partnership, so that by 1949 he was just an employee, albeit a very important one. By 1952, enrollment reached 250,000, but the organizational difficulties were not over, and financial disputes between the health plan and the physician groups had become serious. In 1955, Garfield resigned his post as executive director, and a new profit-sharing plan for the physician group was drafted.

The medical group was to be paid on a capitation basis, have a pension plan, and get half of all revenues in excess of the funds needed for expenses, capital replacement, and reserves for distribution as bonuses. This financial agreement between Kaiser Health Plan and the Permanente Medical Group has continued essentially unchanged for the past 50 years.

In 1962, enrollment exceeded 1 million subscribers and dependents, 2.5 million in 1972, and 10 million in 2000. Kaiser health plans have maintained an enviable record of growth over 40 years, more than doubling in most decades. Although Kaiser remains strongest in its initial market areas around San Francisco, Los Angeles, and Portland, it has expanded to Hawaii, Colorado, Connecticut, North Carolina, and Washington, D.C. Yet even as the forces of managed care began to revolutionize the U.S. health care system, Kaiser, the exemplar of prepaid organized medical practice, had begun to falter.[21] The Kaiser plan established in Hartford, Connecticut, was unable to grow past 30,000 members after ten years, below break-even size. To penetrate the competitive Washington, D.C., and North Carolina markets, Kaiser departed from its traditional closed-staff model and set up open IPA HMOs contracting with already-established local physicians. Despite—or because of—these changes, Kaiser in 1994 suffered its first enrollment decline in 50 years. A once-dominant and innovative organization had drifted, giving up its core competency as it imitated the newer IPA HMOs that could grow rapidly by just signing contracts. After losing hundreds of millions of dollars, Kaiser finally regrouped and recovered in the year 2000. When the federal HMO Act was passed in 1973, Kaiser accounted for more than 2 million of the 3 million total HMO enrollees in the United States, a market share of 70 percent. By 2002, although it was still the largest, Kaiser's 10 million enrollees represented less than a 10 percent market share.

The Kaiser Health Plan operated as a nonprofit foundation; thus, there were no stockholders or individual owners who stood to gain by expanding into new markets. To some extent, it might seem as though the physicians were shareholders, but in one important way they clearly were not owners. When each new region got started, it took capital from the existing Kaiser foundation. However, once the region was up and running, no "returns" were paid back. The physicians who had given up some current income to enable the new offshoot to grow gained nothing. Thus, it is not surprising that Kaiser plans grew robustly where they were already established (since that medical group stood to benefit) but had difficulty obtaining the resources to move into new areas. Garfield built Kaiser single-handedly, but after 1949, he held no legal ownership interest, and in 1955 he was forced out. Garfield was apparently willing to do it for the glory, but the fact is that someone of his talent and training would surely have ended up a wealthier man if he had stuck with his original plan to open a fee-for-service surgical practice in Los Angeles. The incomplete and complex ownership structure was not able to protect his interest, nor was it able to maximize the potential of the Kaiser Health Plan.

GHA: A Consumer Co-op Gets Bought Out by a Franchise Chain

The history of another of the first HMOs makes a similar point regarding ownership. Group Health Association (GHA) of Washington, D.C., was founded in 1937 as a consumer's co-operative to provide physician services to its members, who were largely federal employees. The physicians were employees, not partners. The American Medical Association and the D.C. medical society sought to put GHA out of business, and GHA's victorious antitrust suit, which was affirmed by the U.S. Supreme Court in 1943, was considered crucial to the survival and growth of all HMOs, including Kaiser. Yet ten years later, GHA still had fewer than 20,000 members. The cooperative structure legally made every subscriber an owner. Some existing members were ambivalent about letting large unions join, since it would change the dynamics of control. A basic management function, marketing, was the subject of great ideological debates rather than concerted action. GHA did become more solidly established after becoming an option in the Federal Employees Health Benefits Program, reaching 50,000 members in 1962 and 100,000 in 1975. An attempt by the physicians to set up a medical group partnership similar to that at Kaiser met with resistance from GHA members and their elected board. As a chronicle of GHA observes, the physicians "failed to comprehend GHA's special environment, in which the members instinctively reacted against the notion of a profit motive."[22] Unable to form a corporate medical group, GHA's physicians formed a union in 1977 and went on strike in April 1978. GHA continued to suffer financial reversals and labor disagreements. The nurses and physical therapists went on strike in 1982, and the physicians struck again in 1986. GHA weathered the storm but continued to struggle. Enrollment reached 150,000 in 1986 and 200,000 in 1992. In 1994, unable to persevere in an increasingly competitive market, GHA was acquired by Humana. Thus, an organization that had begun as a consumer cooperative became part of a for-profit chain, one of whose founders had honed his business skills developing the Colonel Sanders Kentucky Fried Chicken franchise.

The rapid expansion of HMOs from 10 million enrollees in 1980 to 100 million in 2005 occurred mostly within the corporate for-profit structure. Many HMOs that started as nonprofits switched to for-profit to take better advantage of their market opportunities. Why have for-profit firms been more successful, and why didn't they emerge earlier? Sydney Garfield dreamed of "one organized integrality" that encompassed all of medicine as a business, including hospitals, laboratories, physicians, financing, and marketing under one roof. He was able to maintain unified control by force of personality during Kaiser's formative years, but lost control when confronted by these vital questions: Who can borrow enough money to build a hospital? How are wages to be set once profits start rolling in? How can one physician single-handedly manage a group of doctors too large for all of them to be personal friends? The common answer to all of these questions lay in the "corporatization" of health care organizations.[23]

12.7 CORPORATE ADVANTAGE

In a corporation, control is more clearly defined. The board of directors has the power to appoint senior management, which, in turn, has the power to hire and fire employees, purchase assets, and borrow money. The stockholders have a clear right to the profits. However, being numerous and diffuse, these stockholders usually have little control over the management of operations. The corporate structure is able to delegate authority and establish accountability reasonably well. Opponents of for-profit health care might argue that nonprofit organizations can be very well managed. In fact, nonprofit and for-profit hospitals both have boards of directors and suites full of administrators who seem to look and act similarly in most ways. The difference is the nonprofit organization's lack of direct ownership. No one in a nonprofit organization has the incentive, or the power, to take a big risk in the hope of achieving a large capital gain. Furthermore, the lack of unified control makes it hard for any one person to make rapid and risky decisions on behalf of the whole organization in times of turbulent change and emerging opportunity.

A nonprofit structure with diffuse ownership may actually be an advantage when leadership requires achieving a consensus among a large number of stakeholder groups. Such a situation was characteristic for most community hospitals from 1950 to 1980. Yet when profits and survival depend on hard bargaining, innovation and quick commitments to capture opportunities that expand and disappear in a moment, the diffuse voluntary structure is overwhelmed. It is simply harder for an entrepreneur to work in a nonprofit structure or to take the organization he or she has built and sell it for a large capital gain.

U.S. Healthcare: A Profitable Growth Company

U.S. Healthcare, founded by Leonard Abramson in 1975, is a good example of the new for-profit HMO firms that came to dominate the market. Abramson was from a South Philadelphia family of modest means and had driven a taxi to put himself through pharmacy school. After working as a detailer calling on physicians for a pharmaceutical firm (see Chapter 11), six years in retail pharmacy, and participation in equipment leasing and other health care businesses, Abramson was astounded by the freedom of doctors and hospitals to raise prices whenever they wanted. "It was a blank check," he said in a 1985 interview.[24] Abramson was much taken with the promise of HMOs to bring business methods to health care and knew a number of physicians who shared his enthusiasm. Taking advantage of the government loans made available by the HMO Act of 1973, the Health Maintenance Organization of Pennsylvania was incorporated as a nonprofit prepaid health plan in January 1975, obtained a state HMO license in 1976, and was designated as a federally qualified HMO in 1977.[25] Operations started in April 1977 by taking over the assets of an existing prepaid health plan, Family Medical Care. HMO/PA began enrolling members and grew rapidly. In 1981, U.S. Healthcare went private, using venture capital from Warburg, Pincus and Company, paying back a $2.5 million loan to the federal government. Its initial public offering of stock came in 1983, as did its expansion into New Jersey.

The Philadelphia market of the 1980s was old-style traditional medicine: lots of specialists, lots of hospital beds, and fee-for-service indemnity insurance. With changing medical trends and the advent of Medicare's prospective payment by DRG (see Chapter 8), it was becoming clear that there was a surplus of hospitals in the area and that even good specialists were having some trouble attracting all the patients they wanted. There was room for an entrepreneur who could cut premiums by contracting in advance for surgery and beds at a discount. Abramson was a sharp negotiator. It often seemed that he came into a bargaining session knowing more about a hospital's operations and finances than its administrators. Discounts of 20 percent, 30 percent, or more were often won. Abramson made information a weapon in the fight for market share and low prices, and honed it to a fine edge in repeated competitive encounters.

Not everyone was enamored of U.S. Healthcare's tactics. Some hospitals were terrified that they would lose so much revenue that they might go out of business, and the Philadelphia Blue Cross plan was furious that an upstart was trying to invade its market by cutting prices.[26] The acrimony spilled over into name calling, then full-page attack advertisements in the newspapers, and finally a series of lawsuits charging libel and unfair trading on both sides (most of which were settled or won by U.S. Healthcare, although bad feelings between the two companies continued to run high). By 1985 U.S. Healthcare, with more than 500,000 enrollees, was the sixth-largest HMO in the nation, and probably the most profitable. Its medical loss ratio was only 75 percent, whereas the average was closer to 80 percent, and Kaiser was above 95 percent.[27] The formula of aggressive contracting, meticulous claims review, and conscientious client service made the company successful and financially sound, although with less than a 20 percent market share it was far from dominant and was not universally loved.

Abramson was not content to let the company rest on its laurels and pile up profits. He made a strategic decision to emphasize quality. Whereas most primary care physician incentive payments in the original HMO/PA reimbursement plan were cost controls dependent on reductions in the quantity of referrals and other services used, the Quality Care

Compensation System (QCCS) for primary physicians, inaugurated in 1987, based 40 percent of practice bonuses on quality and consumer satisfaction measures. The 1992 QCCS revision raised the bar further, making 82 percent of incentives reliant on medical chart review, availability of evening hours, retention of existing patients, ability to attract new members, and ratings on questionnaires mailed to patients, with only 18 percent related to reductions in utilization.[28] For hospitals, the CapTainer™ payment system introduced in 1992 paid a quality- and diagnosis-adjusted per diem rate. Quality incentive plans were introduced for obstetrician/gynecologists in 1994 and for other referral specialists in 1996.[29] However, the most important part of the new strategy was the development of a new corporate subsidiary in 1990, USQA, devoted solely to quality measurement. USQA created databanks based on millions of patient records, consumer surveys, pathology reports, and laboratory tests. The physician-information scientists working at USQA published significant studies on the cost-effectiveness of laparascopic cholecystectomy, asthma treatment, influenza immunization, and autologous bone marrow transplantation for treatment of breast cancer. It used $2 million to fund a fellowship in Managed Care and Quality Assessment at Jefferson Medical College. In 1993, U.S. Healthcare was the first HMO to release the full 1992 Health Employer Data and Information Set (HEDIS) report and, in 1994, the first to provide members with a detailed report card on each participating physician.[30] U.S. Healthcare had clearly gone far beyond compliance and had established a leading presence in the quality assurance and health care information field.[31]

Growth continued to climb, reaching 1 million members in 1989 and 2 million members in 1995. In the face of such rising demand, Abramson's announcement that he would cut premiums in order to build market share came as quite a surprise.[32] Publicly traded HMO stocks fell by as much as 16 percent the following day. Yet the strategy of favoring long-term growth over short-term profitability was sound, and share prices soon recovered. U.S. Healthcare ended the year trading at $46\frac{1}{2}$, with a total market capitalization of $7.1 billion. In April 1996, Aetna Life & Casualty declared that it would acquire Abramson's company, paying more than $8 billion.[33] The information and quality assurance systems of USQA would now be deployed to serve 14 million members, reaching roughly one out of every twelve people with health insurance in the United States.

Why did Abramson decide to sell if U.S. Healthcare was such a successful company? Although any analysis of internal motivations and assessments is largely speculative, some plausible reasons do appear upon reflection. Although U.S. Healthcare had created start-ups and/or joint ventures in Florida, Illinois, Delaware, and Maryland, as well as ten other states and even in Europe, by 1996 it was becoming more difficult to maintain the 10 to 20 percent annual growth it had enjoyed. Every major market now had an established HMO, often several, and the indemnity insurers such as Blue Cross, CIGNA, and New York Life had developed their own HMO plans; therefore, signing up each additional employer group was a struggle. Merger with Aetna meant that 11 million (mostly indemnity) members could be transferred over rather than fought for. Tremendous economies of scale in the use of USQA's software and statistical profiles could be immediately obtained. In 1992, heady with success, the management of U.S. Healthcare envisioned that USQA would attract other HMOs as clients and that soon it would be spun off as a separate company, perhaps growing larger than its parent. Later, it became clear that such a strategy was not viable. Monitoring quality and developing information systems is intimately intertwined with the core business of an HMO, so much so that most HMOs would never allow a competitor to participate in that task or to access such sensitive data. Hence, USQA technology could only be used in-house or sold only in regions (such as England) where U.S. Healthcare could never be a competitive threat.

In the end, it may have been Abramson himself who was the most compelling reason for selling the company. U.S. Healthcare never developed a faceless corporate style—it was always Leonard Abramson's company, where he personally made most of the important decisions. Although he had groomed several of his children for leadership roles and brought in a number of senior executives, there was no clear successor in sight.[34] The genius and prime mover of the company was now 63. He sold the company—at the peak, for $8 billion.

Even though U.S. Healthcare was bought by Aetna, the smaller company, U.S. Healthcare, was supposed to colonize the larger old-line insurer from within, with its executives taking leading roles and spreading the managed care and quality measurement techniques to transform the older indemnity insurer. How well did the deal work? It vaulted Abramson into the role of leading philanthropist, and threw Aetna/U.S. Healthcare into a tailspin. Most of the U.S. Healthcare executives targeted to lead the combined firm drifted away or were let go. An Aetna insurance executive took the reins, tightened controls, cut payments—and drove the hospitals and physicians into revolt. The market had changed, and providers were no longer willing to do anything and make sacrifices to get an HMO contract. Providers threatened to pull out—and Aetna had to pull back. Finally, a new CEO, a doctor from academia with almost no insurance experience, was brought in to restore confidence and rebuild relationships. Marginal lines of business were cut or sold. Aetna/U.S. Healthcare kept losing money, and after five years its total market capitalization had fallen below $6 billion—less than it had paid for U.S. Healthcare.

Aetna is no longer the largest health insurer in the United States. It reformed operations and turned the company around to become profitable—by 2005 its share price had increased 600 percent. However, the Aetna of today is not the ultimate managed care company envisioned in the waning years of the last millennium, but simply a strong, solid health insurance company servicing clients and earning a good return. Aetna suffered because it overpaid for U.S. Healthcare's assets. Those in control lacked business acumen, despite the expertise of their staff and financial consultants. This chapter reviewed a number of financial concepts and techniques, serving as a mere introduction to the intricacies of legal structure, corporate finance, risk, and the time value of money. Yet perhaps even these simple lessons can be a caution to help you avoid making big mistakes with billions of dollars.

SUGGESTIONS FOR FURTHER READING

CFO Magazine, http://www.cfo.com
Fitch Ratings, *Rating Process for Nonprofit Healthcare Credits*, http://www.fitchratings.com/
Louis C. Gapenski, *Healthcare Finance: An Introduction to Accounting and Financial Management* (Chicago: Health Administration Press, 2004).
Healthcare Financial Management Association. http://www.hfma.org.
Moody's U.S. Municipal Bond Rating Scale, http://www.moodys.com/
Kristin R. Reiter, John R. C. Wheeler, and Dean G. Smith, "Liquidity Constraints on Hospital Investment When Credit Markets are Tight," *Journal of Health Care Finance* 35, no. 1(2008): 24–33.
J. B. Sivers, "The Role of Capital Markets in Restructuring Health Care," *Journal of Health Politics, Policy and Law* 26, no.5 (2001): 1019–1030.
Standard & Poors, *Understanding Capital Markets*, http://www2.standardandpoors.com

SUMMARY

1.   Every organization must have cash inflows that exceed cumulative cash outflows (**no margin, no mission**). This means that start-up funds are required, that regular operations (plus fundraising and/or reserves) must generate a surplus, and that at the close of operations, some entity must be designated as residual claimant (owner) of remaining funds.

2. The value of an asset is the cash flow it generates. Anything that increases earnings, such as a medical degree, can be evaluated in terms of financial rate of return. Considering all present and future costs and benefits, **the internal rate of return (IRR) of a project is the interest rate at which the sum of the present value of all cash flows (NPV) is zero**.

3. Although medical school tuition is expensive, running as much as $40,000 per year, it is still a very good **investment in human capital**. The average medical student will graduate with a debt of about $85,000—but this is less than six months of the average physician's earnings. Overall, taking into account the tuition, years of training, extra hard work, and other factors, going to medical school provides an annual inflation-adjusted return of about 12 percent, three or four times what one could expect if one invested in financial assets rather than education, and about 1.5 to 2 times as much as one gains from most undergraduate and graduate education.

4. Assets with risks that are independent (uncorrelated) can be bundled together into **a diversified portfolio that reduces variability**. Insurance companies are financial intermediaries pooling individual risks, and pharmaceutical companies are diversified corporations with multiple projects and are thus able to maintain profitability in most years. However, if the risks are correlated, then bundling assets together may increase volatility and lead to a system-wide financial crisis.

5. If equity capital is replaced by borrowed funds, that **debt increases financial leverage**, raising returns on equity when outcomes are better than expected but reducing returns when outcomes are worse, and may even bankrupt the company leaving stockholders with nothing under adverse circumstances.

6. The largest sources of **risk in health care are changes in regulation and reimbursement** rather than the changes in interest rates or GDP that are the most important risks for most financial markets.

7. In a sole proprietorship, the owner is responsible for everything and can claim all the profits, but in larger organizations **agency problems arise where there is a separation of ownership from control**. Management may behave in ways that are not in the interest of the stockholders (publicly traded firms) or the community (nonprofits).

8. Although accounting for just 9 percent of operating costs, **access to capital** has been crucial in shaping the growth of hospitals. Philanthropy was first replaced by government construction grants through the **Hill-Burton** Act of 1946, and subsequently by **tax-exempt municipal revenue bonds** in the 1970s. **Equity** financing through the stock market is becoming increasingly important as hospitals try to acquire nursing homes, physician practices, and other hospitals to form integrated health care systems.

9. Most HMOs started as nonprofit organizations. Some were explicitly collectivist and anticapitalist in origin, but have become increasingly businesslike. **Kaiser**, founded just after World War II, is **the largest HMO** with more than 10 million members. However, the lack of a clearly defined ownership structure, limited access to capital, and resistance to capital mobility between regions have been major impediments to further growth. Over time, the more rapid **growth of for-profit firms** has led them to dominate the industry, and now even many nonprofit HMOs have for-profit subsidiaries.

10. Growth and/or downsizing through mergers and acquisitions are inherently more complex for nonprofits. With no market for corporate control there are no forced takeovers; **ownership changes and reorganization among nonprofits is limited mainly to distressed facilities** in financial trouble that need capital to survive.

PROBLEMS

1. {*financial definitions*} What is the value of an asset? What is its NPV? Its IRR?

2. {*annualized returns*} If the rate of return on human capital is 15 percent and the opportunity cost of time for a newly graduated physician is $60,000 per year, how large an incremental increase in annual earnings should the physician expect to obtain from a four-year postgraduate residency?

3. {*NPV, IRR*} If a project requires an initial investment of $25,000 and then is sold for $42,000 after five years, what is its NPV at an interest rate of 6 percent? What is its IRR?

4. {*NPV, IRR*} If Dr. Smith buys a machine for $5,000 and is able to improve the earnings of her practice by $2,000 a year for five years, and then can sell the machine for $600 as scrap, what is the NPV at 15 percent? What is the IRR?

5. {*NPV, IRR*} Dr. Smith opens a lab at a cost of $10,000 that provides revenues of $3,000 in the first year, with revenue growing by 15 percent a year after that. Expenses in each year are equal to 20 percent of revenues. In five years the lab is obsolete and worthless. What is the NPV of the lab at 8 percent? What is its IRR? What would the value be if you kept all the other assumptions the same, but sales in the first year were $2,000? What if instead of growing by 15 percent each year, revenues shrank by 15 percent each year?

6. {*ownership*} Are doctors usually employees, owners, or managers of hospitals?

7. {*ownership*} Who owns most hospitals? Who gets the profit when a nonprofit hospital makes money? Can nonprofit hospitals be bought and sold?

8. {*capital financing*} Are the ways in which hospitals obtain capital different from the ways in which doctors obtain capital? Why?

9. {*rate of return, incidence*} How does a philanthropist who donates funds to a hospital get "returns on capital"? Are these returns measured as a dollar amount, as an annualized percentage rate, or by some other method?

10. {*ownership, nonprofit, capital financing*} Hospitals received special treatment from the government and were able to borrow subsidized capital using tax-exempt municipal revenue bonds. During the 1970s and 1980s, billions of dollars of tax-free capital flowed into nonprofit hospitals. Did this make them more or less like for-profit firms?

11. {*financial reporting*} Which is more important in determining the type of financial reports a hospital must prepare: the type of ownership or the major sources of funding? If capital is attracted from different sources, are different types of financial reports required?

12. {*property rights*} What are the advantages and disadvantages of (a) nonprofit status and (b) publicly traded stock that provides incentives to physicians?

13. {*property rights*} Who owns Kaiser Permanente? Is there stock? Have ownership rights ever been sold?

14. {*property rights*} Why were HMOs formed in the 1930s often collectives attracting physicians with liberal or socialist leanings, whereas today HMOs are most often formed by entrepreneurs with capitalist ideals?

15. {*pricing*} How did Sydney Garfield set the monthly premiums for his first prepaid health plan? How are premiums set for Kaiser today?

16. { *regulation*} Did the HMO Act of 1973 affect competition and capital expenditure in a manner similar to the certificate of need (CON) acts passed during the same period?

ENDNOTES

1. Good general sources of information is *CFO magazine* at www.CFO.com and *HFM magazine* at www. hfma.org.

2. Gary S. Becker, *Human Capital* (Cambridge, Mass: Harvard University Press, 1975).

3. William B. Weeks and Amy E. Wallace, "The More Things Change: Revisiting a Comparison of Educational Costs and Incomes of Physicians and Other Professionals," *Academic Medicine* 77, no. 4 (April 2002): 312–319; see also Sean Nicholson, "Medical Career Choices and Rates of Return," pp. 195–225 in F. A. Sloan and H. Kasper, *Incentives and Choice in Health Care* (Cambridge. Mass.: MIT Press, 2008).

4. The calculation would be $(1.17) \times (1.17) \times (1.17) \times (1.17) \times (1.17) = 2.1924$, which is slightly less than 2.20, so a more precise answer would be 17.0805 percent; it just depends upon how exact you try to make your approximation.

5. Diversification that would help to reduce risk due to macroeconomic shifts in the U.S. economy would be foreign stocks (especially emerging markets), commodities, special purpose arbitrage funds, and other investments relatively uncorrelated with movements in the stock and bond markets. See also Joseph H. Golec and John A. Vernon, "Financial Risk in the Biotechnology Industry," NBER working paper #13604, November 2007.

6. The classic DuPont Equation for Return on Equity is:

$$\text{ROE} = \text{Net Income}/\text{Equity} = (\text{Net})/(\text{Sales}) \times (\text{Sales})/(\text{Assets}) \times (\text{Assets})/(\text{Equity})$$

7. Some beginning corporate finance texts refer to revenue risk and operating leverage together as "business risk" or "enterprise risk" and assume that one knows in advance all cash flows from operations. This allows them to focus solely on how financial leverage affects earnings without having to worry about revenues and expenses. In understanding the finances of health care organizations, that particularly simplification is usually untenable. Most of the action is on the "revenue and expense" side, with pure financial engineering having limited relevance. It was important in the case of the nursing home industry because it is largely for-profit, publicly traded, and asset heavy with simple services and limited technology that doesn't change very rapidly—that is, compared to most of medicine.

8. There are several references to economics in the Oath. The classic translation is W. H. S. Jones, *Hippocrates*, The Loeb Classical Library, Harvard University Press, (1923). A more recent translation is provided by Heinrich von Staden, "in a pure and holy way:" Personal and Professional Conduct in the Hippocratic Oath. *Journal of the History of Medicine and Allied Sciences* 51 (1996): 404–437.

9. "Entrepreneur" is taken from the French, and means one who undertakes a venture, who grabs the chance, who organizes resources and brings an idea to business fruition.

10. Michael C. Jensen and William H. Meckling, "Theory of the Firm: Managerial Behavior, Agency Costs and Ownership Structure," *Journal of Financial Economics* 3 (1976): 305–360.

11. Odin W. Anderson, *Health Services as a Growth Enterprise in the United States since 1875* (Ann Arbor, Mich.: Health Administration Press, 1990).

12. Jonathan Betz Brown, *Health Capital Financing* (Ann Arbor, Michigan: Health Administration Press, 1988), 14–18.

13. Patrick M. Bernet and Thomas E. Getzen, "The Company you keep: Spreading effects of financial fraud on investor trust," *Journal of Health Care Finance* 33; 3 pp. 48–66 (Spring 2007); Cain Brothers, *Strategies in Capital Finance 27* (Summer 1999): 1–26; Lawton Burns and John Cacciamani, "The Fall of the House of AHERF: The Allegheny Bankruptcy," *Health Affairs* 19; 1 pp. 7–42, (January/February 2000).

14. Mary Chris Jaklevic, "Pricier, Less Plentiful," *Modern Healthcare* 30, no. 21 (May 22, 2000): 52–56.

15. Robert Sigmond, "From Charity Care to Community Benefit," *Hospitals & Health Services Administration* (Summer 1994).

16. Charles Wrightson, "Selection Bias and Premium Rate Setting," in *HMO Rate Setting and Financial Strategy* (Ann Arbor, Mich.: Health Administration Press, 1990), 245–292.

17. The term "risk" is used to mean many different things. The technical definition frequently used in finance is "random variation over which managers have no control" and is equated with the *standard deviation* of some statistical series. Most businesspeople use "risk" to mean something such as "all of the things that can happen." In health care, "taking on risk" means accepting capitation—and taking a fixed monthly payment would be seen by most businesses as getting rid of the risk from an uneven flow of FFS payments. A leading health care business consultant said, "What cannot be controlled should not be assumed as risk," (Joseph

Coyne, *Healthcare Financial Management*, August 1994, p. 33). This definition, relying on managerial control over clinical processes, is quite at odds with the definition of risk used by currency and bond traders, who strive to make money contracting strictly for things they cannot control.

18. Much of the information in this section comes from John G. Smillie, M.D., *Can Physicians Manage the Quality and Costs of Health Care: The Story of the Permanente Medical Group* (New York: McGraw-Hill, 1991); and Paul de Kruif, *Kaiser Wakes the Doctors* (New York: Harcourt, Brace & Co., 1943).

19. Prepaid medical group practice had existed in America since at least 1790, when such a plan was used at the Boston Dispensary. The innovative prepayment contract between The City of Los Angeles Department of Water and Power and Drs. Ross and Loos to provide all medical services to 12,000 employees and 25,000 dependents for $2 per month (excluding hospitalization) was a more proximate example that probably influenced Garfield.

20. Quoted on page 55 of John G. Smillie, M.D., *Can Physicians Manage the Quality and Costs of Health Care: The Story of the Permanente Medical Group* (New York, McGraw-Hill, 1991).

21. Louise Kertesz, "Kaiser Retools to Fight for Lost Ground," *Modern Healthcare* (July 17, 1995): 34–40.

22. Edward D. Berkowitz and Wendy Wolff, *Group Health Association: A Portrait of a Health Maintenance Organization* (Philadelphia: Temple University Press, 1988), 144.

23. Paul Starr, *The Social Transformation of American Medicine* (New York: Basic Books, 1982).

24. As quoted in Gilbert Gaul, "U.S. Healthcare's Abramson: Dedicated, Perhaps Ruthless," *The Philadelphia Inquirer*, April 2, 1996, sec. A, p. 5.

25. Much of the information in this case study comes from interviews with Sandra Harmon-Weiss, M.D., Medical Director of U.S. Healthcare, and other executives, "A Brief Overview: U.S. Healthcare" by Hyman R. Kahn, M.D. (mimeo, November 28, 1994), and annual financial reports of U.S. Healthcare.

26. In the words of Pulitzer Prize–winning journalist Gilbert Gaul, "For years, some of the most prestigious hospitals in Philadelphia refused to sign contracts with U.S. Healthcare. Those that did often complained bitterly about the hard-line negotiating style of Abramson and his colleagues, which resulted in lower reimbursement rates for the hospitals." in "U.S. Healthcare's Abramson: Dedicated, Perhaps Ruthless," *The Philadelphia Inquirer*, April 2, 1996, sec. A, page 5.

27. Accounting practices are significantly different in the nonprofit Kaiser plan, so the figures are not entirely comparable. It is, however, generally accepted that of the major HMOs, Kaiser probably has the highest percentage of premiums going to medical costs, whereas U.S. Healthcare had among the lowest.

28. Neil Schlackman, "Evolution of a Quality-Based Compensation Model: The Third Generation," *American Journal of Medical Quality* 8, no. 2 (1993): 103–110.

29. Nicholas Hanchak, Neil Schlackman, and Sandra Harmon-Weiss, *U.S. Healthcare's Quality-Based Compensation Model*, 32 pages (mimeo) (Blue Bell, Pa.: U.S. Healthcare, 1996).

30. Paul Kenkel, "U.S. Healthcare 'Report Cards' Expanded to Primary-Care Docs," *Modern Healthcare* (April 11, 1994).

31. Eleanor H. Kerns, health care analyst for Alex Brown & Sons, a leading investment banking firm, has opined publicly that U.S. Healthcare's information systems were superior to those of competitors: see Marian Uhlman and Andrea Knox, "Aetna, U.S. Healthcare Plan Merger," *The Philadelphia Inquirer* (April 2, 1996): A1, A5.

32. George Anders and Ron Winslow, "HMO Stocks Skid on U.S. Healthcare Announcement," *The Wall Street Journal*, April 20, 1995.

33. Leslie Scism and Steven Lipin, "Aetna Near $8 Billion Deal to Acquire U.S. Healthcare," *The Wall Street Journal*, April 1, 1996, sec. A, p. 3.

34. Gilbert Gaul, "U.S. Healthcare's Abramson: Dedicated, Perhaps Ruthless," *The Philadelphia Inquirer*, April 2, 1996, sec. A, p. 5.

CHAPTER 13

MACROECONOMICS OF MEDICAL CARE

QUESTIONS

1. Does inflation affect health care spending? If so, does it affect health care spending permanently or temporarily?
2. How does a person decide what is the right amount to spend each year on health care?
3. How does a nation decide the right amount to spend on health care?
4. Is community health the same as individual health?
5. Why do general tax revenues pay for so much personal health care? Who will pay if (when?) the Medicare trust fund runs out of money?
6. Which is more important in determining how much to spend on medical care: how sick people are or how much money is available?
7. Do price controls work? If not, why might people think that they do?
8. Do professional licensure, third-party reimbursement, and nonprofit organization make it easier or harder to adjust health care spending to changes in prices?
9. What determines wage levels in the health care industry?
10. Is it easier to adjust to growth or to a recession?

13.1   WHAT IS MACRO?

Macro means large. Macroeconomics deals with large-scale properties and institutions that characterize the system as a whole. Individuals become an economic system only when they start to trade with one another. In doing so, they create a whole that is larger than the sum of its parts, develop a government to set the rules under which trade will occur, and create a special medium, money, for conducting trade.[1] Macroeconomics evaluates gross domestic product (GDP) as a measure of national economic activity, whether growing (expansion) or falling (recession), and the dynamics of the process by which change occurs (investment, trade, unemployment, bankruptcy). Rather than investigating the income of a particular individual or firm, macroeconomics investigates growth and distribution of income. Macroeconomics seeks to determine how many people are rich, how many people are poor, whether the same people always make up the same groups over time, and whether the gap is widening or narrowing toward more economic equality.

Macroeconomic (system) properties

- Growth
- Dynamics
- Distribution

Macro (system) institutions

- Government
- Laws
- Money

The macroeconomics of health is concerned with a parallel set of large-scale system issues concerning (a) spending, employment, and other aspects of medical care as a part of the economy and (b) the biological health status of the population as a whole and its relation to economic changes. Thus, it must address how GDP growth affects the number and income of physicians as well as how GDP growth affects the health (longevity, morbidity) of the population and, consequently, how an increase in longevity affects both spending on medical care and growth in overall GDP.

Health System Properties

Economic	*Biological*
Spending	Longevity
Employment	Fertility
Prices	Productivity

Health (System) Institutions

- Medical professions
- Hospitals and caring organizations
- Financing (insurance and reimbursement) structure

The central issues in the macroeconomics of medical care are growth and distribution: how much, for whom, by whom? Where is more money spent on medical care: Bangladesh or Boston? Why? Who gets the care? Who pays for it? Although these issues are clearly related, they can also usefully be distinguished.

Micro and Macro Perspectives on Spending

The main reason people in Boston spend more on medical care than people in Bangladesh is that they have more money. Medical expenditures depend upon the size of the available budget, as do most other types of spending (housing, food, transportation, entertainment). This simple budgetary dynamic also explains why more is spent on health care in 2010 than in 1910, and more will certainly be spent in 2050 than today (see Figure 13.1). From the graph, it is apparent that the amount spent per person on health care is aligned very closely to the amount of income per person. Income explains a lot of the growth in health spending over time; so much so that once an analyst takes account of income, there is not a lot of variation to be explained by other factors. However, if we ask how much is spent on this particular person in Boston compared to that person in Boston, the answer will be about illness and the need for medical care, not about budgets or per capita income. Even if we

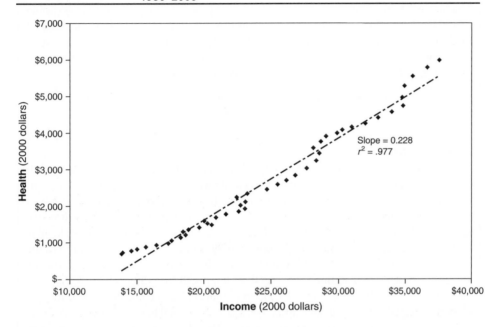

FIGURE 13.1   U.S. Income per Capita and Health Expenditures per Capita, 1950–2005

compare this person in 2010 with the same person in the year 2000, or 2020, most of the answers will be in terms of differences in health, not differences in income.

Why is there such a big difference in the answer when we ask about a particular person rather than the per person national average? Note that the discussion made a subtle shift, from "how much this person spends" to "how much is spent on this person," and therein lies part of the answer. Most medical expenditures in Boston are paid by insurance, rather than by the individual.[2] Budgets matter, for health as for other types of spending, but whose budget? The person? Their employer? The insurance company? The state of Massachusetts or the United States of America? All of these matter. For candy or cars, it is likely to be the personal budget (or maybe the family budget) that matters most, but for health care the most important budget is the national budget. For candy and cars, I have to spend my own money. For medical care, expenditures come from insurance, pooled funds from many people, and assistance from tax subsidies. The constraint that matters is not how much I earn; it is how much everybody else earns and contributes to "our" health insurance.

13.2 THE CONSUMPTION FUNCTION

The relationship between income and spending is known as the **consumption function**. Some people spend less than they earn so that they can save. Some people spend more than they earn, dissaving or going into debt. What is always true is that *consumption + savings = income*.[4] This is an accounting identity, a definition that cannot be changed by obfuscation or by wishing it were not so. A corresponding accounting identity holds across people and nations: for each person who borrows, there must be someone who saves and can lend the borrower money. Unless there are people with savings to lend, people (or nations) that want to spend more than they earn cannot do so. This accounting identity is

INCOME ELASTICITY

The income elasticity of medical care is measured by the percentage increase in spending relative to each percentage increase in income. Suppose that the income elasticity of medical care were 1.6; that would mean that for a 10 percent increase in income, spending on medical care would increase 16 percent. If the income elasticity were 0.2, then a 10 percent rise in income would lead to only a 2 percent rise in spending.

$$Income\ Elasticity = (percent\ change\ in\ expenditure)$$
$$\div (percent\ change\ in\ Income)$$

On average, items have an income elasticity of about 1.0. Such "unit elasticity" has a special constancy: since a 10 percent rise in income leads to a 10 percent rise in expenditures, the share of the total budget spent on that item remains unchanged. If 0.133 of all spending was on an item that had unit income elasticity, then the share spent on that item would remain 0.133 if income rose 10 percent, rose 20 percent, or fell 10 percent. Items whose income elasticity is less than unitary (0.999 or less) will take a smaller and smaller share of total spending as income grows. Food, for example, may be the largest item in the budget of a poor family, and as the family grows richer the amount spent on food increases, but not by as much as income is increasing, and so the share of total spending accounted for by food might fall from 30 percent ($3,000 in a budget of $10,000) to 25 percent ($5,000 in a budget of $20,000). Items with income elasticity greater than 1.0 will take up a larger share of the total budget as income rises. By convention, items with income elasticity greater than 1.0 are termed luxuries, whereas items with income elasticity less than 1 are termed necessities.[3] This does not mean that one group is more or less important, only that the relative rates of expenditure increase as income rises are different. An item may be a necessity at some times or places and a luxury at others; spending on automobiles as a share of total spending, for example, goes up and down for different groups and for different income levels.

The total income elasticity of all things (consumption + savings) necessarily must equal 1.0. If your income goes from $30,000 to $55,000, then the additional $25,000 is either spent or saved. Spending may go up more for some types of goods than others (travel and entertainment maybe rising more than food and newspapers), but overall every additional dollar of income is spent on something or saved. Mathematically, if one takes the budget share of each item (weight) multiplied by the income elasticity of that item, such a weighted sum must exactly add up to 1.0. To account for all possible expenditures, one must of course include savings and debt (and taxes, or count income only after taxes).

most easily obfuscated when dealing in money rather than goods; therefore, it is better to think in terms of a specific item, such as food. If country A wants to consume 80 tons of lettuce but produces only 60, it has to borrow 20 tons from country B. Country B can do so only if it produces more lettuce than it consumes. Country A will usually pay off the debt with oil or wheat or money instead of lettuce, but the mechanics of transfer are clear: total consumption of all people globally = total production (plus amount saved for next year or minus amount taken from storage). For services and perishables that cannot be stored, the relationship simplifies to *total production = consumption + investment*.

A 10 percent increase in income must therefore result in a 10 percent increase in expenditures if all possible uses of income, including savings, are counted. Mathematically, the average income elasticity for all goods (with each good weighted by its share of the total budget) must equal 1.0, unit elasticity (see the box section on "Income Elasticity" or a standard economic text for a discussion of income elasticity). Economists are interested in why one good, such as food, entertainment, or medical care, increases more or less than proportionately as income increases. For many years, economists were perplexed by the following observation: rich individuals tended to save a larger percentage of their incomes than the poor, making the income elasticity of individual savings greater than 1.0 (thus "saving" was categorized as a superior or luxury good). In contrast, rich countries do not save a larger percentage of income than poor countries do; both save about the same fraction of national income. Furthermore, when gross domestic product (GDP) rises over time, there is no tendency for a larger percentage of national income to be saved. The disparity between individual and national income elasticities of consumption and savings posed a major puzzle, one that forced economists to scrutinize and reconsider the relationship between individual and national spending.

The Permanent Income Hypothesis

A major conceptual advance coming from the micro and macro economic analysis of consumption is that of **permanent income**—the hypothesis that the amount consumed is determined by expected average earnings over the long term rather than current earnings today. Thus, a medical student entering a surgical residency buys a new Volvo and a house for a growing family because she is confident that although her current earnings are near $0, they will jump to $40,000 next year and to several hundred thousand dollars per year as soon as her residency is completed. Conversely, a trial lawyer who has just earned $15 million from a case will not spend it all this year. He is aware that such big paydays are rare, and that the next major settlement, *if* it occurs, may take five, ten, or twenty years. Hence, although earnings and consumption are matched in the long run, they can deviate widely in any given period. Nobel Laureate Milton Friedman began his economics career as an assistant in the construction of the first national income and product accounts used to measure GDP, GNP, current account surplus and deficit, and so on.[5] His task was to measure the incomes of doctors, lawyers, and engineers. Measuring the incomes of these people was problematic because their spending did not seem to match their incomes. Employees with steady wages seemed to consume about the same amount each year—but so did these professionals, whose incomes fluctuated widely from year to year. Friedman hypothesized that the spending of doctors, lawyers, fishermen, farmers, and other groups with highly variable earnings was based not on their actual income, but on their expected long-run income.[6] Franco Modigliani examined how people's income and spending varied over their lifetimes, showing that they typically began with a period of borrowing at the start (to buy a home, automobile, furniture and other goods), followed a period of saving in their 50s and 60s, and then dissaving in retirement.[7] Like Friedman, Modigliani found that spending is related to average long-run income rather than the size of the current paycheck. Together, the ideas of Friedman and Modigliani have become known as the life-cycle permanent income hypothesis.

The permanent income hypothesis resolved the empirical inconsistency between micro and macro studies of consumption and savings. It recognized that a disproportionate number of high-income individuals are people who only temporarily earn so much money (such as the malpractice lawyer who just received $15 million, or the 59-year-old house carpenter saving for retirement) and hence would naturally hold some for later periods, whereas a disproportionate number of low-income individuals (such as the surgical resident, the carpenter in winter, and most undergraduate economics and finance students) are only temporarily poor and hence rationally spend more than they currently earn. For countries, however, the budget constraint is binding. Total national consumption is limited by what the country produces each year (except for the limited flexibility allowed by international borrowing and investment) and thus automatically adjusts to match national income.

Shared Income

What is your income? If you are not working and your parents are sending you to school, the more relevant question is: What is your family's income? For the child of the young surgical resident, it is the parents' or grandparents' earnings, not the child's, that matter. The surgeon may also eventually have to support her aged parents. Families tend to share income; therefore, it is usually the resources available to all family members on average, not the amount earned by an individual family member, that determine personal consumption. How extensive is such sharing? Who counts as a member of your family? Do you owe anything to your brother, who moved to Alaska 12 years ago and only contacts you once a year when he sends a Christmas card? Do you owe him more if he loses his leg and his job due to an accident and moves back home? Do you owe anything to a neighbor who lost his job, or a homeless person sleeping on the street? The surgeon may or may not feel that she owes a lot to a neighbor or a homeless person, but will pay taxes that are used to help both of them.

Just as the permanent income hypothesis suggests that long-run expected earnings rather than current measured earnings determine current spending, a similar **shared-income hypothesis** suggests that the average income of a group of people who share determines their consumption, rather than the earnings of each person individually. Most consumption is shared within the family, and some public goods are shared within the community (schools, roads, fire and police protection). Clothes, food, entertainment, and most other private goods are shared within a family, and perhaps within a circle of friends, but not within a larger community. What about medical care? Although care of an individual may seem like a private good, the infrastructure (hospitals, medical education, pharmaceutical companies), clinical standards, and funding of care are arranged collectively. Shared group spending is not just the 45 percent paid by taxes, or the 5 percent paid by charity and community programs. The 35 percent paid by private insurance is regulated by the Employee Retirement Income Security Act of 1974 (ERISA) and state insurance commissioners to meet public policy objectives. Even the remaining 15 percent paid out of pocket by individuals is subject to special treatment in the tax code and thus is affected by collective political decisions. A physician office practice and a for-profit hospital may be private enterprises, but both are subject to regulation and social expectations much greater than those faced by other firms. Thus it could reasonably be said that almost all health spending is subject to collective decisions made on the basis of partially shared perceptions and incomes.

Studies of individuals show that utilization of medical resources is only slightly related to income (elasticities of 0.0–0.4), but studies of nations show that rich nations spend more on health than poor nations (with income elasticities > 1.1). The reason for this disparity is that individuals' ability to consume medical care is based not on their own personal income, but on the average income level of all the people in their family, in their community, in their insurance plan, and in the nation as a whole.

Consider two people employed by a company that provides insurance benefits. Both employees, who are covered by the same insurance plan, a file clerk and the chief financial officer, have the same illness. They do not live in the same type of house, drive the same type of car, or take the same vacations, but they will receive similar hospital care. Even if the clerk does not make much money, most of the hospital bill is already taken care of. It would be foolish for him not to take advantage of his employee benefits when he is sick just to save a few dollars on copayments. Now consider the chief financial officer. There is little more medical care that she can buy, no matter how much she is willing to spend. If she wants to have the new gene therapy or positron scans she has read about, the decision is up to the medical staff, not her. Indeed, every effort is made to keep such medical decisions from being influenced by payment considerations. This is not to say that there are no differences in the treatment of the rich and the poor, but the differences are deliberately kept small by professional ethics within the system. Government provision of care for the poor and tax subsidies to pay for health insurance are parts of that system. The consequences, relatively similar sorts of care for all people with the same illness, are not an accident; they are some of the reasons that these collective policies receive wide public support. Insurance converts personal medical care into a public good, and as a society we have collectively decided that all citizens should have reasonable access to quality medical care.

For public goods, such as clean air, national defense, and control of communicable diseases, society's willingness to pay determines how much will be provided (see Chapter 15). Since everyone is able to consume the same amount of a public good, individual income is irrelevant except for its contribution to the total tax base. For a public good, or within a group insurance plan, the individual's income is not a binding budget constraint. It is possible to spend more curing one sick child than the child could earn in three lifetimes, and the amount of money spent to clean up the air in Los Angeles is hundreds of times greater than the money earned by a Hollywood movie star. It is the resources available to the group as a whole that determines the average level of spending.

The shared-income hypothesis implies that income becomes more important in determining spending as the unit of observation gets larger and becomes similar to the budgetary unit.[8] For individuals, income is relatively unimportant, and income elasticities are near 0. For small areas, such as a census tract, average per capita income is somewhat more important, with income elasticities rising to perhaps 0.4. For counties or states, their budgets are a constraint, but it is still possible for them to obtain money from the federal government. Per capita income is significantly more important as a determinant of health care spending than health status, and elasticities are about 0.9. For the nation as a whole, the budget constraint is binding. No other country is going to reimburse us for our medical bills. Every dollar paid to doctors, nurses, and drug companies must be collected in taxes, insurance premiums, or direct fees. Income thus becomes the dominant determinant of spending at the national level, with elasticities greater than one, usually about 1.3 (see Figure 17.2).

Public and Private Decisions

Economics is a decision science. The implications of shared income are that an economist must consider who is making the decision, a person or a group, and even how that decision gets made and implemented (tradition, majority vote, popular will, law). Most individual and family decisions are private. Corporate employers are "private" in the sense of not being government entities, but insofar as they use rules and incentives to regulate and coordinate the behavior of many people, they are obviously public in nature. As soon as we begin to consider larger and/or less well defined groups of people, the simple utility maximization model is more difficult to implement and less plausible. What is "the" utility of the people living in Flagstaff, or Arizona, or the United States? Should we count immigrants, legal or illegal? How does a group such as "General Motors employees and their dependents" make up its mind about what medical benefits it wants and how much to pay for them. The role of government will be discussed in Chapters 14 and 15, but the ramifications of public decision making go far beyond anything that can be presented in two chapters, and indeed much is still beyond the grasp of economic analysis. Certain economic ideas have proven very helpful in understanding politics and public decisions. The concept of budget constraint is central to this discussion and to an understanding of the determinants of health spending for individuals, for larger groups, and for the nation as a whole.

Budget Constraints: Borders that Matter

The financing of a health care system is a macro system characteristic. For most countries, including the United States, funding is national in scope. Thus, we do not expect to see major differences in health care as we cross the border from Texas into Arizona, or in Mexico as we cross the border from Sonora into Chihuahua. Yet crossing the national border from Arizona into Sonora, or Texas into Chihuahua, reveals a vast disparity in the use of medical resources, costs, and prices.

Disparities in health care of this sort were once found within a single country. At the end of the nineteenth century, New Yorkers living on Park Avenue and those living in the tenements of lower Manhattan occupied different social and medical worlds. To some extent, disparities still exist within a country today—between the suburbs and the inner city, between the mainstream medicine provided to most Americans and the care available to residents of isolated Indian reservations in the United States or the remote Inuit villages in Canada. In Australia, studies have demonstrated that the health and health care of aboriginal populations is much worse than that of the majority white population.[9] In South Africa, studies showed large differences in health spending per capita for blacks and whites under apartheid, which has been greatly reduced but not entirely removed under the new political system. The crucial determinant of the health care available to a group of people is the amount of resources available to that group, often measured by average income per capita. The essential question then becomes: what is a group? Why are Mexican-Americans living in San Diego getting more medical care than their relatives and friends across the border in Tijuana? Why are some Indian tribes not sharing in the wealth of the average American? Defining who is and who is not part of the group determines who does and who does not have access to health care.

13.3   ADJUSTING TO CHANGE: DYNAMICS

If per capita income falls, health care spending must also fall. Yet it is impossible to make this economic adjustment all at once. Usually the country goes into debt during the transitional period. Even for an individual, adjustments to changes in income are not instantaneous. If you were to lose your job today, you would not immediately move into a smaller apartment, drive an older car, or wear less fashionable clothes. In fact, if you lose your job today, you will probably go out and spend a little extra money to keep up your spirits. Next week you will cut back, but not too much, because you probably expect to find another job soon. If you are still out of work six months later, you will find that your clothes, house, and car start getting shabby, and you think about downsizing your lifestyle. Once you do get a new job, it will take years to build your savings back up.

When college students graduate and begin to earn good wages, they find it easy to live and save part of their salary because their lifestyles are still somewhat geared to being a student. Their consumption does not move upward as quickly as their incomes. During this "I can't figure out how to spend it all" period, savings accumulate. Later on, with a fancy lifestyle suitable for a young stockbroker or lawyer, they find it difficult to see how one could have lived on so little money as a student, or even on what they earned three years ago. Consumption is geared to expected income, whether $15,000 or $150,000. The amount of income saved depends not so much on how high the income is, but on transitional (permanent income/life-cycle) factors and the extent to which a person is willing to give up current pleasures for retirement or future consumption.[10] If a young lawyer who has just bought a new Mercedes loses his job, he will discover one of the underlying asymmetric truths of human behavior: it is a lot easier and more fun to adjust spending upward rather than downward.

The dynamics of adjustment for individuals (micro) and for nations (macro) are similar, except that it usually takes longer for macro adjustment, because the system as a whole must change. People who still have their jobs must be convinced that it is necessary to cut back, to reduce the provision of public goods, or to change the tax code. Achieving a consensus to alter organizations and revise institutional structures is extremely time-consuming. The health care system, based on professional ethics, institutional obligations, and shared public values, reliant on a complex set of public and private financing mechanisms, is even more difficult to change than most other sectors of the economy. In the stock market, expectations of the future are traded every day, and prices change by the minute. Commodity sectors, such as farming and metals, are forced to respond quickly due to market discipline. Although the number of houses cannot change rapidly, housing sales are sensitive to macroeconomic conditions. The decision to buy a house is based on an individual's assessment of job prospects. The effective price of a house, the monthly mortgage payment, depends on interest rates, which are both volatile and forward-looking. For these reasons, housing tends to be one of the sectors that leads the economy into or out of a recession. Health care is slow to change, and it lags behind other sectors in adjusting to macroeconomic conditions.

How long does it take for health care to adjust? It takes from one to five years on average, but some parts take even longer. Even if everyone in Congress decided today that we need more health care or less health care, this decision could not be carried out for months, and its full effects would take years to work their way through the system. If a medical school decides to accept more students, it takes at least a year to enroll them, and to build new medical schools takes much longer. Medical students take four years to graduate, and another three or four years to complete a residency and enter practice. Thus, eight years after a decision to expand a medical school has been made, there are still no extra doctors in practice. Something might be done to reduce the rate of retirement, but effectively the quantity of doctors in practice who graduated in a particular year in the past was fixed once they left school. It took until 1985, 20 years after the Health Professions Educational Assistance Act of 1963, before the expansion in physician supply was a real force in the market—and by then Congress had changed its mind. It takes 40 years, until all graduating physicians have retired, before the full effects of such decisions work through the system (see Chapter 7).

Not everything in health care takes as long to adjust as physician supply. The supply of nurses is much more flexible, because typically there are many licensed nurses who are temporarily not working or working part-time; therefore, an increase or decrease in demand quickly translates into a change in the numbers employed. Clerical, maintenance, and other less-specialized labor adjusts even more smoothly and rapidly, because people can move between health services and other sectors of the economy in response to changing conditions. Although we do not have data to look at each segment of the health care sector separately, the National Health Expenditure (NHE) Accounts, the analogue to the National Income and Product Accounts established by the U.S. Department of Commerce to track GDP and the economy as a whole, do categorize health care spending by type (hospitals, physicians, dental care, drugs, nursing homes) and enable us to examine the patterns of adjustment separately for each component.

Hospitals, the largest component of health care expenditure, are quite rigidly institutionalized and dependent upon public or third-party financing. In a study of how rapidly health spending adjusts over time, hospitals took longer than the average 2.7 years.[11] Physician services are somewhat more flexible and adjust a bit more quickly, with a lag of 2.5 years. Spending on drugs, much of which depends on direct consumer decisions and is paid for out of pocket with current income, takes only 1.3 years. Long-term care, a mixture of flexible personal spending and rather inflexible Medicaid spending, adjusts in 2.5 years on average. The component that takes the longest to adjust is construction, at 3.5 years. Capital must be accumulated in advance to fund new construction, and the decision to build depends on long-run future economic considerations, not just revenues and expenses today. The estimated average lag for adjustment of dental spending, 2.5 years, seems longer than one would expect since most dental bills are paid by individuals with limited third-party reimbursement, are a result of personal decisions, and occur in an office setting rather than within the large institutions. However, this estimate is the least reliable statistically, and it may just reflect how hard it is to pinpoint the timing of adjustment in a complex area with many segments and subsegments. Consider hospital expenditures again. Because of the way NHE accounts are kept, construction is listed as a separate component, making it possible to see that construction took longer to adjust than labor. However, some construction (clinics, equipment installation) probably takes less time than others (new buildings), but we cannot tell because they are categorized together. If supplies were listed separately, they would probably be seen to adjust more quickly than labor. The "average lag" is just that: an average. Some parts are moving faster and some slower. It is also an average over time—in some periods the organization may respond more quickly than in others. In particular, it appears that managers are quicker to step up purchasing when the economy expands than they are to cut back when the economy contracts. Everyone hopes that a slowdown is just temporary, and delays firing people or closing clinics. The time required to adjust also depends on the magnitude of the change. The statistical techniques used here can only detect changes in the one-to-ten-year range, but a truly massive revision of the system, such as that which occurred in 1965, may take several decades to complete. Some argue that one reason health spending is so high in the United States is because it is still stuck with a health care system constructed on the lines of the Great Society envisioned during the 1960s, when economic growth was steady and strong. This system is not appropriate to the more constrained conditions and budget deficits prevailing in 2010.

Permanent Income and Adjustment of Health Spending to GDP

Government is based on stable rules that change slowly and only with the consent of citizens. For example, any amendment to Medicare must be approved through the courts, the legislature, and public opinion. What are the consequences of slow adjustment in the health care sector? Importantly, it buffers the economy. During a downturn, Medicare and Medicaid spending usually continue; therefore, health care workers are less likely to lose their jobs than workers in the farming, housing, or financial services sectors (Figure 13.2).[12] Conversely, an increase in employment during an economic recovery is delayed.

The delay in adjustment can have adverse budgetary consequences. Because spending continues to rise in a recession even though government tax revenues fall, a deficit builds up. In theory, such periods of excess spending average out over time with underspending during periods of rapid growth. However, it is easier to obtain agreement to pour money into the health care sector and save jobs during a recession than it is to hold back and save money during good times. In a recession, people hope that normal growth will soon return, and they may bend their spending rules to temporarily soften the impact of macroeconomic disorder. An economic boom feels so good that people may not realize that such high growth

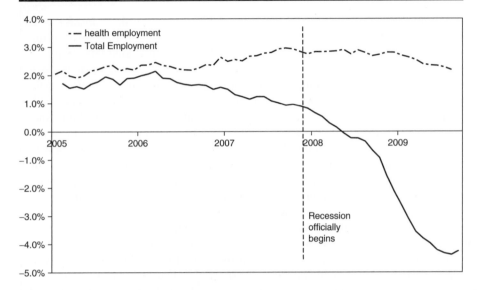

FIGURE 13.2   Annualized Employment Growth Rates, 2005–2009

rates are abnormal, that another recession is bound to come eventually. People may claim that this time around will be different and that we never have to worry about going hungry again, thus we do not need to save money for bad times or give up much to pay off old debts. As a consequence, it is much easier to accumulate deficits than build up surpluses.

Politicians want to get elected. They need results that will affect the economy and the voters in the near term. Extra government spending during a recession meets these needs; extra saving when the economy starts to grow again usually does not. The benefits of a balanced budget—low inflation, steady or falling interest rates, strengthening the dollar in foreign exchange, stability for businesses to invest in productivity improvements, and a modest but sustainable path of optimal growth—are long term. However, none of these benefits can be realized quickly enough to help the politician worried today about the next election. In a pinch, a politician (or a professor) will sacrifice the long-term good that helps others in favor of near-term benefits they can capture for themselves. It is difficult to get politicians to behave in a way that benefits the long-term public interest, because it is difficult to get voters to behave that way. One consequence of this is well known—a U.S. federal debt of ten trillion dollars. Eventually, just like the out-of-work lawyer running up his charge card balances, we will have to bring spending back into line and balance the budget. That is in the long term, though, and right now the elections keep coming up fast.

Adjustment to Inflation

Inflation is defined as a general rise in prices (or equivalently, a fall in the real value of the dollar). With 5 percent inflation, it will take 5 percent more dollars to purchase the same amount of real goods (pounds of butter, acres of land, hours of landscaping, gallons of gasoline, and everything else people buy) each year, and after 15 years of inflation at that rate, it will take more than $2 to buy what $1 used to buy.

The slow adjustment of the health care sector to inflation means that during a period of more rapidly rising prices, spending is less than expected.[14] To see why, we can trace the process of adjusting spending to changing price levels, as illustrated in Table 13.1. Suppose that a hospital spent $100,000 in 2000 and wanted to spend the same amount in real terms

ARE RECESSIONS GOOD FOR YOUR HEALTH?

Just as spending may respond differently to permanent and transitory income, it is possible that the effect of income on health may differ in the long run and the short run. The evidence reviewed in Chapters 16 and 17 makes it clear that long-term trends in health are strongly and positively related to growth in GDP per capita. Since that is well known to be the case, many economists assumed that disruptions in economic growth, recession, and the unemployment that accompanies it would temporarily cause health to worsen. Christopher Ruhm, in a series of careful empirical articles, has shown that exactly the opposite occurs.[13] For every 1 percent increase in unemployment, there was a 0.5 percent *decrease* in mortality rates. The primary reason that recessions appear to be good for health is that peoples' lifestyles improve; they exercise more, eat better, lose weight, and smoke less (however, they also appear to drink more). Motor vehicle fatalities show a large drop, in part because unemployment means less work and less money, so people drive less. Back injuries decline, perhaps because people no longer have to do so much heavy lifting. Diseases that are less affected by lifestyle, such as cancer, do not show much correlation. Contrary to the general trend, suicides increase during recessions, as do some forms of mental illness. This is consistent with the common perception that the fact or threat of unemployment increases stress. Related research shows that over the long run (20 years or more) job loss is strongly related to reduced life expectancy and increased mortality. What is fascinating about these studies is how clearly they illustrate the fallacy of composition. The short-run effects of macroeconomic fluctuations in this case are, for most conditions, exactly the opposite of the long-run effects.

(e.g., full-time equivalents (FTEs) in labor, gallons of fuel, square feet of office space) in each succeeding year. If the expected rate of inflation is 5 percent, 105 percent of 2000 spending will be budgeted for 2001; that is, $105,000. If actual inflation equals the expected 5 percent, the same quantity of all inputs bought in 2000 can be bought with the 2001 budget. If inflation is again expected to be 5 percent in 2002, $110,250 is budgeted for that year. However, suppose that inflation actually turns out to be 12 percent in 2002. The budget does not buy $100,000 worth of goods in constant inflation-adjusted dollars, but only $110,250 ÷ (1.05 + .12) = $94,000. With a 12 percent rise in prices, the budgeted 5 percent wage increase leaves employees worse off, with less purchasing power. The budgeted 5 percent increase in the supply budget is not enough; thus, equipment purchases will have to be cut back. In 2003, inflation is expected to be, and actually is, 5 percent. However, the hospital has to make up for the lost purchasing power resulting from underestimating inflation the previous year. Therefore, the budget for 2003 will be up 12 percent to $123,480. Having

TABLE 13.1   Adjustment to Inflation

	2000	2001	2002	2003
Nominal spending	$100	$105	$110	$123
Price index	100	105	117	123
Real spending	100	100	94	100

Note: Hypothetical example of adjustment to inflation. The hospital tries to spend exactly the same amount ($100 in year 2000 dollars) in each year. In the first year, inflation is 5% and spending increases 5%, so there is no change in real deflated expenditures. In the second year, spending increases by 5% again, but inflation is 12%, so the real spending power declines. In the third year, inflation is 5%, and the hospital catches up by increasing spending 12% (7% to catch up and 5% for current inflation).

caught up, spending will once again be $100,000 in real (year 2000) terms (see last line of Table 13.1).

National health care spending shows this type of lagging adjustment to unexpected changes in the price level for several reasons. First, government and nonprofit organizations such as hospitals usually set a budget at least a year in advance, which limits their flexibility. Second, most wage contracts run for at least one, and usually several, years. A set of inflation adjustments is already built into raises, and any difference between what negotiators expected to happen to prices and what actually happens falls on the workers. If inflation is less than expected, workers are lucky and can buy more. If inflation is worse, they have to tighten their belts. Estimates calculated from Bureau of Labor Statistics (BLS) data indicate that for any 1 percent change in the rate of inflation, only about 0.5 percent shows up in the wages of health workers in the first year, and another 0.3 percent in the following year. It takes three years for wages to fully adjust to a change in inflation. In the long run, all wages do adjust, making inflation neutral, neither raising nor lowering real health care spending. The government can only temporarily trick workers and firms into accepting a dollar that is only worth $0.90. Any government that tries to "save" money by printing lots of currency ends up with chronic inflation, as Argentina and Russia have had. Therefore, most governments aim for price stability and a sound currency. Yet the year-to-year fluctuations caused by temporary inflation adjustment problems may be larger than any real changes in health care spending due to GDP growth or changes in health care policy.

The distorting effects of a surge in inflation are shown in Table 13.2, which traces prices and employment in Canada during the oil price shock of 1973.[15] Inflation, which had previously been averaging 3 to 5 percent, suddenly leapt to 9 percent in 1973, peaked at 14 percent in 1974, and remained high at 10 percent in 1975. However, by this time, the health sector had begun to build in expectations of high inflation. It looks as if spending, measured by the fraction of GDP devoted to health care, fell during 1973 and 1974. However, real resources, as measured by the number of nurses working in the Canadian health system, continued to rise throughout this period.[16] Indeed, employment for nursing rose not only in absolute numbers, but also as a fraction of total employment. In terms of real labor, spending was rising. It only appeared to decline because the nurses were temporarily underpaid, getting raises smaller than the rate of inflation. Their wages had gone up somewhat during 1973 and 1974, but not as rapidly as the prices of the things they bought with those wages. Thus, the nurses' real purchasing power fell, which is why the fraction of GDP spent on health declined. This "decline" was entirely transitory, because the nurses were not willing to make less than everyone else and were able to get their wages revised upward to take into account the increase in inflation during the next contract period. In the long run, whatever was taken away by a delay in adjustment had to be given back. When this was done, in 1975, there appeared to be a jump in the share of GDP spent on health care. Actually, this rapid rise

TABLE 13.2 How Inflation Distorts Reported Health Expenditures

| Canada | Inflation | Employment | | Ratio | Health Share of GDP |
		Nurses	Total		
1972	5.6%	152,005	8,447,000	.0180	7.3
1973	8.9%	159,274	8,860,000	.0180	7.0
1974	14.4%	168,530	9,220,000	.0183	6.9
1975	9.8%	177,182	9,364,000	.0189	7.4

Note: Inflation rates, nurses and total employment, and health spending as a share of GDP show how sudden price increases distort budgetary measurement of the relative size of the health sector.

Source: OECD 1990.

is accounted for by the removal of the earlier distortion—eventually the health care sector had to catch up with the rest of the economy.

Although expected inflation is built into contracts, a surge in overall prices is not immediately matched in the health care sector. Because wages are slow to adjust, workers bear the burden by being made worse off temporarily. Because budgets are slow to adjust, health care organizations must make do with fewer supplies, drugs, buildings, and so forth, or temporarily go into debt. However, in the long run, inflation has no effect on real health care spending. After about three years, health care wages and other contracts have fully taken account of earlier shifts.[17]

Adjustment to GDP: Rates of Change and Time Series Analysis

It is evident from Figure 13.1 that there is a close relationship between per capita income and health care spending per capita in the United States. A similar relationship will be seen across countries when an international comparison is made in Chapter 17 (see Figure 17.2). From the discussion regarding permanent income and the time required for adjustment of large systems, it should be apparent that one would not expect national health spending to respond immediately to any rise or fall in GDP, but rather to adjust over the long term. Indeed, looking at the growth in health expenditures from one year to the next compared to the growth in GDP, it almost seems as if there is no relation at all (Figure 13.3). That is because the year-year-change in GDP is a measure of current income, and the health system is responding to permanent income. Giving some time for adjustment to occur, and measuring not just the change in GDP over a single year but over three years, the relationship between health expenditures and per capita income starts to become more visible (Figure 13.4). Adding a better measure of permanent income stretching over decades would increase the correlation.

Reflection will indicate several reasons why there is so little connection between current income and current health spending. Government accounts for more than 45 percent of

---

FIGURE 13.3   Annual Percentage Rates of Change

FIGURE 13.4   Annual Percentage Rates of Change (lagged moving average)

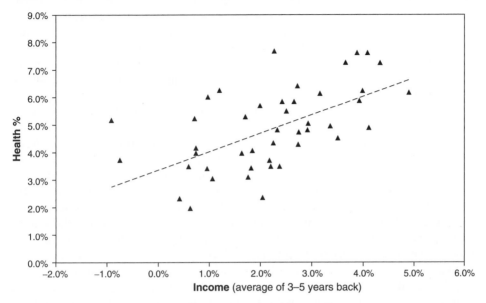

health expenditures, and government budgets must be proposed, debated, and passed well in advance of the current year. For the federal government, all money is committed at least 12 months in advance, if not more. A decision to build a hospital, create a medical school, or provide a new benefit like Medicare Part D involves a commitment to years and years of future spending. As shown in Tables 13.1 and 13.2, and as we will discuss in Section 13.6, wages of health care workers are slow to adjust to changing economic conditions, and thus it can be expected that spending in health care would lag a bit behind most sectors of the economy. The long-run trends in technology and organization are even more important. Decisions that affected spending in 2010 were made last year, the year before, and even decades ago. The enactment of Medicare in 1965, authorizing major increases in federal spending, was not unrelated to the surge of prosperity that the country was experiencing then. When times are bad, the public thinks more about cost controls than about providing new benefits.

13.4   FORECASTING FUTURE HEALTH EXPENDITURES

Using the permanent income hypothesis and the lagging inflation adjustment hypothesis allows economists to create a model to project future national health expenditures.[18] Analysis of the correlation between actual spending, fluctuations in prices, and per capita income indicates that health expenditures are a function of the average percentage rate of growth in real per capita GDP during each of the preceding five years (but not the current year) and over the preceding 25 years. This analysis also indicates that health care expenditures lag by 40 percent of the change in inflation for the current year and 20 percent of the change in inflation for the previous year. This model can be used to project future national health care spending quite well for the next three to five years, and is fairly satisfactory for a 10-year or maybe even a 20-year projection.[19]

The fact that the health care system is slow to adjust is an advantage in forecasting. Next year will usually look a lot like last year, and the trend over the last few years is a pretty good guide to spending, wages, and prices next year. Also, for a one-year forecast it will not make much of a difference if the average growth in health expenditures exceeds the rate of inflation by 2 percent or 3 percent—factors specific to a particular person, group, or disease category are likely to be more important for decisions than general trends. However, that relatively minor difference between inflation plus 2 percent and inflation plus 3 percent would gain importance over time, and after 35 years could amount to a 40 percent difference, more than enough to make up the shortfall in the Medicare trust fund (see Chapters 12 and 18).

A rule of thumb applied by forecasters is that for each year into the future, one needs comparable data going back three years in order to make a good forecast; i.e., to make a five-year forecast, the analyst would want at least 15 years of data. The trustees of the Medicare Trust fund are required to make not just a forecast for next year, or past the next election, but for a sufficiently long period to cover the life of current beneficiaries and taxpayers—70 years. With a "times three" rule of thumb for forecasting, that would mean looking at 210 years of historical data, all the way back to 1800. This emphasizes that long-run planning for the future of Medicare involves not only fluctuations in trend, but also major shifts in the entire medical system (consider how different medicine and paying for care was 200 years ago). Most of today's college students will face their largest medical expenses in retirement, and may be in a nursing home (or making use of a titanium hip replacement to hike the Appalachian Trial) 70 years from now. The possibility of major change in the health care system becomes a near certainty given that kind of time span. The recurring difficulty, of course, is predicting what the future system will be.

13.5 COST CONTROLS: SPENDING GAPS AND THE PUSH TO REGULATE

Analysts have questioned why a cost-control policy that seems so successful in one instance, or so successful among individuals or physicians or hospitals alone, fails to reduce total costs. It is because the consequences of income for spending are established only at the level where the budget constraint is fixed. For some types of health care, this is the individual household; for others, it is the hospital, region, or the insurance plan; but for much of medicine, it is the national budget constraint that is most relevant.

The lagging response of the health care sector to macroeconomic changes creates spending inertia that makes it difficult to balance the budget. In a recession, expenditures continue to climb even as revenues fall. The budgetary gaps created by delays in the adjustment of spending to changing macroeconomic conditions may force governments to put cost controls on health care. Almost every inflationary spike or sharp recession is followed by a new attempt to regulate hospital rates, ration health care, establish price controls, cap revenues, or use another method to stem rising costs. The recession of 1970 pushed President Nixon to impose wage and price controls on the economy and to keep hospital prices under control for an extra period. Afterward it became clear that the U.S. experience from 1971 to 1975 served mostly to confirm the lessons learned from wage and price controls imposed by other governments around the world over the last two millennia. The underlying pressures created by excess monetary growth and the fiscal imprudence of waging a war without raising taxes could not be contained, controls were routinely evaded, and prices shot up as soon as controls ended in April 1974.[20]

After the expiration of the Nixon price controls, health care costs were freed from external economy-wide controls, although they continued to be regulated by cost reimbursement rules (see Chapters 5, 6, and 8). Then in April 1977 President Carter proposed a "voluntary effort" (VE) to constrain costs. Flyers and buttons were printed to promote voluntary efforts to have hospitals reduce prices and to lobby Congress. In November 1979 the Carter bill was soundly defeated by the legislature. This tale of voluntary regulation would normally have been forgotten and relegated to footnotes, yet the story lingered on because claims of effectiveness were uncritically accepted. Three reasons for the persistence of the impression that VE worked are that (1) hospital price increases did moderate in 1978 and 1979, (2) claims of VE's effectiveness were loudly voiced, and (3) Congress cited these claims in debate before Carter's legislation was defeated. It is difficult to understand how flyers and buttons could accomplish what the force of law could not, but the claim appeared plausible until the data were examined more closely. Hospital costs had already begun falling in 1977 before VE. They declined further in 1978 and were below the target when the legislation failed. Even VE believers referred to the American Hospital Association's luck, because the VE coalition did not even convene a meeting until December 1977 and, therefore, had no time to directly affect hospital behavior.

Luck, however, was only one factor in the fortuitous "success" of VE. The main reason that nominal health care expenses were lower than expected was that hospital wages and supply prices, because they lag the CPI, had not yet caught up with the surge of inflation that began in 1977. There was no decline in hospitals' use of real inputs (labor FTEs, supply items), only a delay in price adjustment that made nurses and technicians temporarily cheap relative to the CPI (as in the Canadian example in Table 13.2).

In October 1983, Medicare radically changed its method of paying hospitals from cost reimbursement to a new prospective payment system (PPS) based on the expected cost of each admission, categorized into diagnosis-related groups (DRGs). This new cost control plan did work, in some ways. There was a significant reduction in the rate of increase in Medicare Part A (inpatient) expenses and in hospital expenses generally. However, this was accomplished primarily by hospitals shifting services to outpatient and day surgery categories covered under Medicare Part B. Total health care expenditures per capita continued to rise at historically high rates. In 1985, 16.9 percent of the $407.2 billion spent on health care was paid for by the federal government, and by 1990, the fraction actually increased to 17.7 percent of the $643.4 billion spent that year, even though reduction in the federal deficit was an explicit objective of the Medicare legislation. PPS clearly had a large effect on the health care system. Administrators and doctors panicked, employment was (temporarily) held below trends, and the average length of stay for patients fell sharply. However, there were no long-run reductions in the total cost of health care.[21]

The Balanced Budget Act of 1997 imposing significant cuts on Medicare payments was initially more successful in controlling costs. Yet by 2001 total spending was again rising in line with long run trends (with the exception of home health, which had been specifically targeted for reform in this legislation—see Chapter 10, section 7).

The idea that ESP, VE, and PPS regulations were "effective" in reducing expenditures lingers because a superficial before-and-after comparison in each case showed a decline in spending that the public and legislators could understand and that was quickly reported in the newspapers. People did not recognize that these declines were delayed effects of the adverse macroeconomic conditions that had caused the regulations to be proposed in the first place. Also, the declines in spending in one reimbursement category (Part A) due to regulations look like effective cost controls, until it is realized that these costs were just shifted to another area (Part B). A more human reason for the persistence of this belief is that many analysts and politicians worked thousands of hours to draft and implement these regulations, becoming so personally committed that it was hard for them to accept that so much well-intentioned effort had so little effect over the long run.[22]

FIGURE 13.5   Macroeconomic Shock

Health care expenditures are never too high or too low in an absolute sense; rather, they are out of line with the spending that can be afforded under current economic conditions. A theory of health care cost regulation must start with the realization that shared costs, and governmental expenditures in particular, are always regulated even when no external regulatory agency is in operation. Furthermore, costs can be ratcheted up or down within the existing framework by making administrative procedures tighter or looser, even if no legislation is passed. Regulation is always an integral component of health care system management in a modern nation. It is part of the process, not an external shock. What an economist can evaluate is a *change* in the regulatory regime. To do so, one must first ask why the change took place at a particular time.

Legislatures don't get together to pass cost control measures for health care because the economy is doing well. Macroeconomic crises bring about a call for legislatures to do something, but these crises eventually push spending down, regardless of whether legislatures act. The ability of politicians to dictate spending independent of the rest of the economy is limited, particularly during the next one to four years, which are usually all that remain before the next election. The process of adjustment is shown in Figure 13.5. Incomplete adjustment to inflation and recession is apt to simultaneously exert pressure on legislatures to do something about excessive health care costs and force future spending downward, thus often creating a spurious correlation between the enactment of regulation and the temporary moderation in costs. This does not mean that cost controls have no effect, but rather that much of the decline is due to the underlying process of macroeconomic adjustment rather than an explicit effect of regulation.

Capacity Constraints and Budget Constraints

The slow adjustment of the health care sector is one reason that cost controls are ineffective. The number of doctors and hospitals is essentially fixed for the time span of most political action (one to four years). If twice as many people got sick next year, there would be no major increase in physician supply or the number of hospital beds. If the hospital is full, admitting another patient means discharging someone who the doctors feel is less in need of care. Conversely, maintaining capacity means keeping nurses and technicians available even if there are fewer patients than expected—or treating more patients who are perhaps not quite so severely ill. Capacity in health care tends to be constrained rather than flexible. Although it is possible, even easy, to shift costs from one organization to another or to move a few billion dollars back and forth across budget years, real change in the capital and labor employed takes longer and is much harder to achieve. Only a small fraction of the total cost of hospital care (including drugs and supplies, food, nursing overtime) varies with the number of patients. Therefore any changes in the total expenditures will show up as mostly short-run changes in employee wages, and perhaps some temporary hiring or layoffs (although there is usually considerable reluctance on the part of administrators to adding permanent staff when there is a surge in demand, and an even stronger resistance from unions to cutting staff when demand falls).

13.6   WORKFORCE DYNAMICS: "SPENDING" IS MOSTLY LABOR

What does it mean to control costs? Because health services are mostly labor, costs are primarily a function of the number of people employed in the health care sector and the wages (or professional incomes) that they are paid. Cost control must be employment control. Yet it is easier for politicians to say that they will control costs than to say that they will have people laid off or cut wages, which is one reason that there is so much more rhetoric than action in health care cost control.

The most significant government interventions in the health care labor markets have been (1) cooperating with the medical profession in the formulation of effective licensure laws and making medical schools the restrictive gateway for entry into the profession during 1910–30, (2) extending the medical licensure model to other health professions throughout the remainder of the twentieth century, and (3) enacting the Health Professions Education Act of 1963 to expand health care labor (see Chapter 7).

Every occupation within the health services field has its supply and demand most strongly influenced by the particulars of licensure statutes and relations with the dominant medical profession. Yet what is true of each of the parts is not true of the whole. Most of the growth in health employment comes from adding new occupational categories rather than by expanding numbers within an existing occupation. Therefore, to study how health care labor is related to the economy as a whole, it is necessary to look at aggregate employment in the health sector rather than a single occupational category.

Employment

There are two separate sources of data on U.S. health care employment. The decennial census began recording information on the occupation of respondents in 1850 and thus can be used to create a long series of health-related occupations with 15 observations over the past 150 years (Table 13.3). The Bureau of Labor Statistics (BLS) records employment within industries by Standard Industrial Classification (SIC) codes and has identified health care services (SIC 808) as a category since 1958 (SIC 80806 is the subcategory "hospital employment"), providing annual and monthly observations (Table 13.4). The definition of the two series is quite different. The census data is based on *occupation of the individual;* therefore, a secretary, chemist, or accountant employed at a hospital would not be counted as a health care employee. The BLS data is based on the *SIC code of the employer;* therefore, a nurse, medical technician, or doctor employed at a manufacturing firm would not be counted as a health care employee, but a hospital secretary would.

Employment in health care has grown more than twice as rapidly as total U.S. employment over the past hundred years, 3.4 percent versus 1.5 percent for the period 1900–2000. Consequently, the share of total employment accounted for by health care has increased from 1.2 percent at the turn of the century to 8.1 percent (1 out of every 12 workers) now. Yet the 0.6 percent of total employment accounted for by physicians in 2008 was up only slightly from 0.5 percent in 1900. The health care sector (SIC 808) has enjoyed positive employment growth every year for the past three decades. The average annual growth rate of this sector between 1958 and 2008 was 4.8 percent—more than double the annual average growth of total U.S. employment. During this period, health care sector employment never contracted (see Figure 13.6), in contrast to total employment, which experienced four major contractionary episodes. Total U.S. employment contracted in the 1960s, after the oil price

TABLE 13.3 — U.S. Health Care Employment, 1850–2000

	1850	1860	1870	1880	1890	1900	1910	1920	1930	1940	1950	1960	1970	1980	1990	2000
Population	23,192	31,443	39,818	50,156	62,948	75,995	91,972	105,711	122,775	131,669	150,697	180,671	205,052	227,726	249,973	275,372
Employed Civilians	5,372		12,925	17,392	23,318	29,073	37,371	42,434	48,830	51,742	59,230	67,990	79,802	104,058	123,473	131,720
All Health Occupations	46	61	103	114	170	346	486	634	900	1,020	1,450	2,064	3,277	5,403	7,580	10,103
Fraction	0.8%		0.8%	0.7%	0.7%	1.2%	1.3%	1.5%	1.8%	2.0%	2.4%	3.0%	4.1%	5.2%	6.1%	7.7%
H/pop	1.97	1.93	2.58	2.26	2.70	4.55	5.29	6.00	7.33	7.75	9.62	11.42	15.98	23.73	30.32	36.7
MD/pop	1.76	1.75	1.62	1.71	1.66	1.73	1.66	1.43	1.33	1.33	1.31	1.29	1.45	1.90	2.35	2.8
Aid/MD			0.2	0.2	0.5	1.0	1.4	2.1	3.2	3.7	5.1	6.7	8.7	10.1	10.6	10.9
Physicians	41	55	64	86	105	131	152	151	163	175	198	234	297	433	587	772
Dentists	3	6	8	12	17	30	40	56	71	71	76	83	95	125	156	168
Diagnosticians, NEC							8	22	38	40	53	68	40	54	132	94
Pharmacists	2					46	54	64	84	83	89	93	116	146	182	208
Nurse (practical)			18	15	47	120	166	212	236	200	224	276	267	435	429	679
RN-nurses				1	1	12	51	104	214	284	406	592	762	1,285	1,885	2,290
Att-Hosp/Nurse Aides, Orderlies									41	102	212	409	951	1,378	1,860	1,834
Att-Phy/Health Aid										35	42	73	134	292	249	490
Dent Asst													100	158	216	251
Dent Hygienist													17	47	72	148
Opticians, Lens Grinders						6	4	7	14	12	20	21	31		38	67
Therapists (licensed)							2	7	14	18	25	37	78	224	332	296
Psychologists								11	13		5	12	30	93	192	***
Dieticians									14		23	27	43	67	90	97
Med Technicians									14		78	141	260	508	927	1,057
Managers, Medicine & Health													58	111	234	***

U.S. Health Labor: Annual % Rates of Growth

	1850	1860	1870	1880	1890	1900	1910	1920	1930	1940	1950	1960	1970	1980	1990	2000
Population		3.1%	2.4%	2.3%	2.3%	1.9%	1.9%	1.4%	1.5%	0.7%	1.4%	1.8%	1.3%	1.1%	0.9%	1.0%
Employed Civilians		4%	4.5%	3.0%	3.0%	2.2%	2.5%	1.3%	1.4%	0.6%	1.4%	1.4%	1.6%	2.7%	1.7%	1.9%
All Health Occupations		2.9%	5.4%	1.0%	4.1%	7.4%	3.5%	2.7%	3.6%	1.3%	3.6%	3.6%	4.7%	5.1%	3.4%	2.6%
Physicians		3.1%	1.6%	2.9%	2.0%	2.3%	1.5%	-0.1%	0.7%	0.7%	1.3%	1.7%	2.4%	3.8%	3.1%	3.1%
Dentists		6.7%	3.6%	4.4%	3.6%	5.4%	3.0%	3.5%	2.4%	0.0%	0.6%	1.0%	1.4%	2.8%	2.2%	1.3%
Nurse (practical)						10.0%	3.3%	2.5%	1.1%	-1.6%	1.1%	2.1%	-0.3%	5.0%	-0.1%	4.7%
RN-nurses						28.0%	15.6%	7.5%	7.5%	2.9%	3.6%	3.9%	2.6%	5.4%	3.9%	2.0%
Att-Hosp/Nurse Aides, Orderlies								5.5%	7.1%	9.6%	7.6%	6.8%	8.8%	3.8%	3.0%	2.7%
Att-Phy/Health Aid											1.7%	5.6%	6.3%	8.1%	-1.6%	4.0%
Therapists (licensed)										2.5%	3.3%	4.0%	7.7%	11.2%	4.0%	
Psychologists												9.4%	9.3%	7.5%	3.0%	
Dieticians											3.3%	1.5%	4.9%	4.5%	3.0%	3.8%
Med Technicians												6.0%	6.3%	6.9%	6.2%	
Managers, Medicine & Health														6.7%	7.8%	

Source: U.S. Census and Bureau of Labor Statistics, various publications.

TABLE 13.4	Trends in Employment in the Health Care Sector				
Year	Total U.S. (1000s)	SIC 808 Health Services	SIC 80806 Hospitals	SIC 808 % of Total	SIC 80806 % of 808
1960	54,189	1,548	1,030	2.9%	67%
1970	70,880	3,053	1,863	4.3%	61%
1980	90,406	5,278	2,750	5.8%	52%
1990	109,403	7,814	3,549	7.1%	45%
1991	108,249	8,183	3,655	7.6%	45%
1992	108,601	8,490	3,750	7.8%	44%
1993	110,713	8,756	3,779	7.9%	43%
1994	114,163	8,992	3,763	7.9%	42%
1995	117,191	9,230	3,772	7.9%	41%
1996	119,608	9,478	3,812	7.9%	40%
1997	122,690	9,703	3,860	7.9%	40%
1998	125,865	9,853	3,930	7.8%	40%
1999	128,916	9,977	3,974	7.7%	40%
2000	131,720	10,103	3,989	7.7%	39%
2001	131,922	10,381	4,096	7.9%	39%
2002	130,793	10,673	4,225	8.2%	40%

Source: Bureau of Labor Statistics, *Employment and Earnings*.

shocks of the 1970s, and again at the start of the 1980s and 1990s. Although health sector employment grew more slowly during the mid-1970s and early 1980s, annualized year-on-year growth never fell below 2 percent. Health care employment shows less fluctuation because it adjusts more slowly and gradually to macroeconomic shocks (see Figures 13.2 and 13.6). When total employment is shifted upward or downward 1 percent from trend, health care employment moves by only 0.2 percent after one year, 0.17 percent after two years, and so on (Figure 13.7).[23] The cumulative rise or fall in health care is proportionately larger, about 1.2 percent for each 1 percent shift in total employment, but spread out over the entire decade that follows, so that on average shifts in health employment lag by 2.6 years.

The slow rate of adjustment to government intervention is shown in Figure 13.8, which presents the estimated impact on health care employment resulting from the enactment of

FIGURE 13.6   Annual Percentage Change in Employment

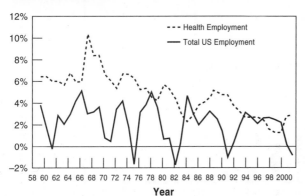

FIGURE 13.7	Health Employment Adjusts Slowly

**Effect of a 1% Increase in Total U.S. Employment on
Health Sector Employment**

FIGURE 13.8	Effect of Medicare on Health Employment in Subsequent Years

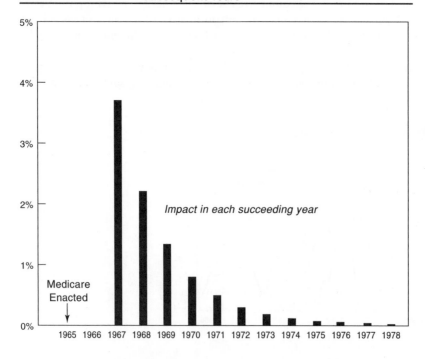

Medicare and Medicaid in 1965. Although this legislation created a fundamental change in reimbursement and flow of money into the system, and was ultimately responsible for a rise of more than 10 percent in the number of health care jobs, it had no visible effect on health employment during 1965 or 1966. Not until 1967 did employment begin to soar, leaping 3.7 percent above trend in that year, 2.4 percent in 1968, 1.2 percent in 1969, 0.6 percent in 1970, and 0.4 percent in 1971 (see Figure 13.7). The average lag between the enactment of Medicare and the creation of an additional job was 3.5 years.

Wages

Health care wage data for the United States are available from the BLS for hospitals from 1968 on, and for all health employment from 1972 on. There were rapid increases in real inflation-adjusted wages of more than 5 percent per year in the late 1960s post-Medicare period. During the 1970s, health care wages were essentially flat, just keeping pace with wages in other industries and with inflation, and growing less than 0.5 percent per year. From 1980 to 2008, while real wages in the rest of the economy were essentially flat (rising by less than 3 percent), average health care wages rose by 27 percent, and the increases for hospital employees and self-employed physicians were even greater. There does not appear to be any consistent correlation between economic growth (GDP) and health care wages, but the 30 years of data available is not enough to be certain of this. Other than the apparent surge

---

THE IRON LAW: MEDICAL COSTS = MEDICAL INCOMES

One person's expenses are another person's income. This economic observation, seemingly obvious, is often overlooked. The circular flow of funds that makes trade possible (Chapter 1) and the structure of the National Income and Product Accounts used to measure GDP and other macroeconomic activity are based on the principle that when a dollar gets paid, it gets paid to someone.

every $100 income = $100 costs

The largest element in health care costs is labor, and it is reasonably clear that the $120 that gets paid for a visit is "expense" on the patient side and "revenue" on the provider side. It is also evident that the salary of nurses, technicians, and administrators must come from patient revenues. What about the payments to suppliers or banks? They too have employees, and for them to pay the rent (and taxes) they must get paid from patient fees (or government subsidies or philanthropy or some other source of revenues). Isn't it possible to improve the efficiency of the health care system so that one can simultaneously reduce the cost of health care and maintain the incomes of doctors and nurses? Nope. The only way an organization can cut its labor bill is to either reduce wages or lay some people off, neither of which is very popular. Increased productivity could make it possible to employ fewer people in medicine, even at higher salary, and thus reduce the total wage bill (and hence reduce the total cost of care). However, for the most part, it is worth remembering that any reductions in the cost of medical care ONLY come through reductions in the incomes of providers, and that making medicine more productive, or getting people to lead healthier lives, only leads to a reduction in the cost of care and health insurance premiums/taxes if the number or salary of health care workers is decreased. Even after technology provided an answer to the Malthusian dilemma (see Chapter 16), economics is able to live up to its name as the "dismal science."

due to Medicare (which occurred before health care wage data was collected) no government policy appears to have significantly altered the health care wage trend. The adjustment of health care wages to changes in the rate of inflation is slow. More than 60 percent of the rise (or fall) in inflation from one year to the next was not incorporated in health care wages until the following year, and 11 percent was still missing after two years, indicating substantial contractual rigidity in health care wages.

Real health expenditures per capita in the United States grew 5 percent a year from 1960 to 2008, outpacing the 2 percent rate of growth in per capita incomes and thus consuming an ever larger share of GDP. The labor portion of this 5 percent annual increase can be decomposed into a 4 percent increase in employment and a 1 percent annual increase in real wages; therefore increased intensity of medical services, more nurses and perfusionists and occupational therapists per patient day, is by far the more important cause of increased spending over this time span. However, since 1980 excessive compensation growth in the health care sector relative to the rest of the economy has accounted for a significant proportion of spending increases. With both wages and employment increasing faster than in other occupations, it may well be that health care professionals are getting more than a fair share of the nation's economic growth, a concern that health economist Uwe Reinhardt of Princeton University has humorously identified as "feasting on healthcare, or the allocation of lifestyles to providers."

Although the power of licensed health professions to control entry and wages is a major cause of delayed adjustment, it is not the only one. The dominance of nonprofit firms and third-party financing are also important factors in creating labor market rigidity. Health care in the United States is currently undergoing significant institutional changes. The pattern of slow and delayed adjustment over the last 40 years indicates that the ultimate outcome of these changes will not be revealed for a considerable period of time (see Chapter 18).

SUGGESTIONS FOR FURTHER READING

CMS, *NHE Projections 2007–2017*, www.cms.hhs.gov/NationalHealthExpendData.

Cynthia Engel, "Health Services Industry: Still a Job Machine?" *Monthly Labor Review* (March 1999): 3–14 (www.bls.gov).

Milton Friedman, *A Theory of the Consumption Function* (Princeton, N.J.: Princeton University Press, 1957) and with Simon Kuznets, *Income from Independent Professional Practice* (New York: National Bureau of Economic Research, 1945).

Thomas E. Getzen, "Aggregation and the Measurement of Health Care Costs," *Health Services Research* 27 (October 2006); and "Health Care Is an Individual Necessity and a National Luxury: Applying Multilevel Decision Models to the Analysis of Health Care Expenditures," *Journal of Health Economics* 19 (2000): 259–270.

Marian Osterweis et al., eds., *The U.S. Health Workforce: Power, Politics, and Policy* (Washington, D.C.: Association of Academic Health Centers, 1996).

SUMMARY

1. Consumption and savings decisions are not based on current income, but on expected **permanent income** over the entire life cycle.

2. Shared financing through government and insurance makes health care into a **quasi-public good**, so that group or national income is the relevant budget constraint, not individual income.

3. The major determinants of total health spending are macroeconomic (inflation, population, and GDP).

4. Professional licensure, nonprofit organization, third-party reimbursement, and other institutional features **make the health care sector slow in adjusting to changes** in macroeconomic conditions.

5. These delays in response create **pressures for regulatory change**.

6. Many of the effects associated with the passage of health care cost control regulations are actually **delayed effects** of inflation and recession.

7. Real **increases in health care spending** are largely **increases in labor**. Much of the growth shows up in the form of new occupations, and some shows up as higher wages and professional incomes.

PROBLEMS

1. {*competition, welfare maximization*} Does the "invisible hand" work in health care markets? Give an example that clearly illustrates the welfare-maximizing effects of self-interested competition and one that calls self-interested competition into question. Is health care more, or less, nonprofit than other types of human productivity and exchange?

2. {*dynamics*} Explain the difference between the comparative statics and dynamics of a market, such as physician services or long-term care.

3. {*transaction costs*} Do all economic exchanges have a monetary price? How would a politician pay the price of changing insurance legislation to cover hospital-sponsored health maintenance organizations (HMOs)? To whom would the price be paid? Do laws regulating exchange make trade more expensive or less expensive?

4. {*dynamics, productivity*} How many nonphysicians are currently employed in the health care sector for each M.D.? Is this ratio more than or less than it was 50 years ago? Does the change in the ratio of physician to nonphysician labor imply that productivity has increased or decreased? Which adjusts more rapidly to changes in demand: ancillary employment or physician supply?

5. {*flow of funds*} Which factor has accounted for more of the increase in the cost of hospital care per patient: increases in the number of physicians, the number of days of care, physician incomes, wages of nonphysician employees, or number of nonphysician employees?

6. {*dynamics*} Do delays in adjustment cause deficits, surpluses, or both?

7. {*elasticity*} If the income elasticity of NHE spending is 1.4 and per capita income increases from \$12,000 to \$15,000, how much will health care spending increase? How much will it increase if income elasticity is 0.9?

8. {*elasticity, aggregation*} Since the amount of income spent on health care for a group is just the sum of the amounts spent on each member, why would the income elasticity be different if the economist measured one person, or groups of 10, or 100, or 1 million? Is individual income elasticity for health care spending larger or smaller than national income elasticity for health care spending? If so, why?

9. {*fallacy of composition*} What determines how much is spent on your health care: how sick you are or how much money you earn? What determines how much is spent on average in the United States: how sick people are or how much money they earn?

10. {*price controls*} Suppose that you read Sunday's newspaper and learn that price controls have been placed limiting the cost of health insurance to $2,500 per employee, significantly below the current average. What effects would you predict to occur?

11. {*inflation*}

    a. Assume that inflation is 4 percent for the years 2000 to 2004, jumps to 14 percent for the years 2005 and 2006, and then falls to 3 percent for 2007 to 2009. Calculate the price index using 2000 as the base year. What is the price in each year of a good whose price changes matched the overall level of inflation and cost $27.42 in 2002?

    b. Suppose that service L's price adjusts with a lag, causing a third of the change in the rate of inflation to show up in L's price in each succeeding year. Calculate the annual percentage rates of price increase for L.

    c. Suppose that good A anticipates future price increases, causing half the change in next year's inflation rate to show up in its price in advance. Calculate the annual rate of price increase for good A.

    d. Which prices in the health care system might show delayed adjustment, lagging behind changes in the general rate of inflation? Which prices might show anticipatory response, changing in advance of the general rate of inflation? (*Hint*: Who sets premiums in advance?) What problems would this pattern of delay/advance present to administrators trying to work within a budget?

12. {*inflation*} Will changes in the rate of inflation affect health care spending? In your answer, distinguish between real and nominal expenditures and between short- and long-run effects.

13. {*dynamics*} Are decisions regarding health care budgets and medical school enrollments based on the past or the future?

14. {*consumption*} What is the permanent income hypothesis? For which type of person would the permanent income hypothesis lead one to expect the greatest error from using tax returns to predict consumption?

    a. Assistant manager at Macy's

    b. Management intern at Macy's

    c. Chief executive officer at Macy's

    d. Retired vice president of Macy's

    e. College student

    f. Medical student

    g. High school teacher

    h. Retired college professor

15. {*dynamics*} Why might it take longer to adjust health care expenditures downward than upward? Frame your answer in terms of the economic incentives facing those who make the decisions.

16. {*equilibrium, segregation*} What determines the level of wages among health care occupations?

17. {*public good*} Why does insurance turn private medical care into a public good?

18. {*price controls, dynamics*} Did health care costs rise less rapidly after President Nixon introduced price controls in 1971? Why or why not?

19. {*dynamics, price controls*} Which forces cause the public to want price controls?

20. {*price controls*} What do you think was the effect of Medicare PPS, which paid a fixed price per DRG after 1983, on the length of hospital stay? What was the effect on the number of outpatient surgeries? On nursing home admissions? On total Medicare hospital expenditures? On total Medicare expenditures for all types of care?

21. {*voting*} If price controls and crazy tax proposals are the economic equivalent of voodoo, why do such proposals continue to gain support? For that matter, why has voodoo continued to be profitable?

22. {*dynamics*} How long is the "long run"? How much difference can the length of the period used for measurement make on the estimates of price and income elasticity?

23. {*productivity*} Is it be possible to raise both employment and wages while still controlling total costs through the development of new technology that increases the productivity of medical care? Why or why not?

ENDNOTES

1. This chapter borrows selectively from a number of authors, including James S. Coleman, *Foundations of Social Theory* (Cambridge, Mass.: Harvard University Press, 1990); Douglass North, *Structure and Change in Economic History* (New York: W. W. Norton, 1981); and Oliver Williamson, Markets and Hierarchies (New York: The Free Press, 1975).

2. Thomas E. Getzen, "Health Care is an Individual Necessity and a National Luxury: Applying Multilevel Decision Models to the Analysis of Health Care Expenditures," *Journal of Health Economics* 19 (2000): 259–270.

3. The economic definitions of "necessity" or "inferior good" and of "superior" or "luxury goods" depend solely on consumer buying behavior, whether income elasticity is less than or greater than 1.0, and not on any judgments regarding the usefulness or importance of the items or how most people think of them. Thus bottled water, new cars, and organic baby food all qualify as luxuries, while hot dogs, cheap costume jewelry, and bus tickets are all termed necessities. This is an example of economists' occasional bad habit of taking a common term and giving it a very narrow meaning within the profession that is at odds with common usage. This twisted professional definition tends to confuse rather than communicate unless a reader has fully interiorized the profession's specific definition (e.g., "luxury" for income elastic, "marginal" for incremental, "rents" for payments for fixed resources).

4. Note that savings may temporarily be negative, as they are for many students who go into debt to support a lifestyle. Yet in the long run, savings aggregated across all people must be positive (or at least zero). It is not possible for everyone everywhere to have more by going into debt. Note also that economists consider savings very different from food, clothing, and other consumer goods because savings determine investment, interest rates, growth, the price level, and many other macroeconomic variables.

5. Milton Friedman and Simon Kuznets, *Income from Independent Professional Practice* (New York: National Bureau of Economic Research, 1945).

6. Milton Friedman, *A Theory of the Consumption Function* (Princeton, N.J.: Princeton University Press, 1957).

7. Franco Modigliani, *The Collected Papers of Franco Modigliani: Vol. 2: The Life-Cycle Hypothesis of Saving* (Cambridge, Mass.: MIT Press, 1980).

8. Thomas E. Getzen, "Aggregation and the Measurement of Health Care Costs," *Health Services Research* 27 (October 2006).

9. David Mayston, "Disadvantaged Populations, Equity, and the Determinants of Health: Lessons from Down Under," in *Health, Health Care and Health Economics: Perspectives on Distribution*, by Morris L. Barer, Thomas E. Getzen, and Greg L. Stoddart, eds. (Chichester, U.K.: John Wiley & Sons, 1998).

10. Take-home advice: if you want to become rich, get in the habit of saving *now*, while you are still in school.

11. Thomas E. Getzen, "Macro Forecasting of National Health Expenditures," *Advances in Health Economics and Health Services Research* 11 (1990): 27–48.

12. William C. Goodman, "Employment in Services Industries Affected by Recessions and Expansions," *Monthly Labor Review* (October 2002): 1–15 (www.bls.gov).

13. Christopher J. Ruhm, "Are Recessions Good For Your Health?" *The Quarterly Journal of Economics* CXV (May 2000): 617–650; "Good Times Make You Sick," *Journal of Health Economics* 22, no. 4 (2003): 637–658; and

"Healthy Living in Hard Times," *Journal of Health Economics* 24, no. 2 (2005): 341–363. Daniel Sullivan and Till von Wachter, "Mortality, Mass-Layoffs, and Career Outcomes: An Analysis Using Administrative Data," NBER working paper #13626, November 2007.

14. Angus Deaton, "Involuntary Savings Through Inflation," *American Economic Review* 67 (1977): 899–910.
15. Although it would be nice to have a more recent example, economists are rather grateful that there has been no need to make rapid adjustments to surging inflation in the last 20 years. However, the increasing federal budget deficit and declining trade balance make the prospect that a future edition of this textbook will have a current example of necessary adjustment to rapid inflation within the U.S. somewhat more likely.
16. The changes in the numbers of RNs are used because the data for all health care workers are, unfortunately, not readily comparable across these years.
17. Sheila Smith et al., "The Next Ten Years of Health Spending: What Does the Future Hold?" *Health Affairs* 17, no. 5 (September 1998): 128–141.
18. Thomas E. Getzen, "Macro Forecasting of National Health Expenditures," *Advances in Health Economics and Health Services Research* 11 (1990): 27–48; see the methodology paper and current projections at www.cms.hhs.gov/NationalHealthExpendData/projected/.
19. Thomas E. Getzen, "Forecasting Health Expenditures: Short, Medium and Long (Long) Term," *Journal of Health Care Finance* 26, no. 3 (Spring 2000): 56–72.
20. Paul Ginsburg, "Impact of the Hospital Stabilization Program on Hospitals," in M. Zubkoff, I. E. Raskin, and R. S. Hanft, eds., *Hospital Cost Containment: Selected Notes for Future Policy* (New York: PRODIST for Milbank Memorial Fund, 1978), 293–323. See also the first and second editions of this textbook, which contained more extended analysis of these historical events.
21. Congressional Budget Office, *Rising Health Care Costs: Causes, Implications and Strategies* (Washington, D.C.: U.S. Government Printing Office, 1991).
22. David Dranove and Kenneth Cone, "Do State Rate Regulations Really Lower Hospital Expenses?" *Journal of Health Economics* 4, no. 2 (1985: 159–165; C. Eby and D. Cohodes, "What Do We Know about Rate Setting?" *Journal of Health Politics, Policy & Law* 10 (1985): 299–327; Michael Morrisey, Douglas Conrad, Steven Shortell, and Karen Cook, "Hospital Rate Review: A Theory and Empirical Review," *Journal of Health Economics* 3, no. 1 (1984): 24–47. Karen Davis, Gerard Anderson, Diane Rowland, and Earl Steinberg, *Health Care Cost Containment* (Baltimore, Md.: Johns Hopkins University Press, 1990).
23. Michael Kendix and Thomas Getzen, "U.S. Health Services Employment: A Time Series Analysis," *Health Economics* 3, no. 3 (1994): 169–181.

CHAPTER 14

THE ROLE OF GOVERNMENT

"To do for the people what needs to be done, but which they cannot, by individual effort, do at all, or do so well, for themselves."

— *Abraham Lincoln*

"In the evolution of economic enterprise, the things which could be produced and sold for a price were taken over by private producers. Those that were not, but which were in the end no less urgent for that reason, remained with the state."

— *John Kenneth Galbraith*

QUESTIONS

1. Is competition better than regulation?
2. Which parts of the health care system are paid for, or controlled, by government? Why?
3. Should I pay taxes to care for the poor?
4. Why is Medicare so much more popular than Medicaid?
5. Does the Food and Drug Administration, or any other agency that regulates health, operate in the interest of the public, in the interest of the people who work there, or for the special-interest lobbies?
6. Is it because health is "priceless" that medical markets are so heavily regulated?
7. Do people vote for what is good for society or what is good for themselves?

14.1 GOVERNMENT HEALTH FINANCING

State, federal, and local government account for almost half of all health spending. However, most "government" health care is actually third-party insurance payment to the highly regulated private health care industry composed of independent physicians, hospitals, nursing homes, and so on. More than 90 percent goes to such providers of personal health care services, and less than 10 percent goes to core government functions such as medical research, infectious disease control, collection of national health statistics, and public health. Government's share of the rapidly growing health care sector tripled from 14 percent in 1929 to 48 percent in 2010. If the tax subsidies for health insurance are included, the government share of total spending exceeds 59 percent. In earlier years, state and local governments were larger sources of funding than the federal government. In 1965, the biggest single category of government spending was state and local hospitals, institutions providing care for both general medical conditions and chronic mental illness. Since then, Medicare and Medicaid have become much larger, and in 2008 they accounted for three-fourths of all government spending on health care.

The bulk of the $1,250,000,000,000 in 2010 government funds came from general tax revenues. Premiums paid by enrollees for supplemental Medicare insurance (set originally to pay a quarter of costs) brought in $37 billion, and the designated Medicare Hospital Insurance tax of 2.9 percent on the wages and self-employment income of all workers brought in another $230 billion. These funding schemes shift the incidence of the tax burden but do not change the total amount. Ultimately, all government spending must come at the expense of private consumption and investment.

Although the U.S. government provides the largest flow of funds into health care services, it has remained relatively passive. Both Medicare and Medicaid are **entitlement** programs, which are open-ended commitments for government to pay the bills incurred by any eligible patient (i.e., age 65 or over or indigent, respectively). Unlike budgeted programs, in which a fixed dollar amount is appropriated each year, there is no limit on the amount that can be spent on Medicaid and Medicare. Explosive growth in expenditures is a major cause of deficits in state and federal budgets and "crowds out" spending on vital public health activities. From 1965 to 2007, the share of federal government health care dollars devoted to public health declined from 4.6 percent to 1.3 percent, and spending for medical research to discover new therapies and diagnostics fell from 26.8 percent to 4.8 percent. The future health of the U.S. population is being compromised to pay for uncontrolled and excessive use of resources (see Figure 14.1 and Table 14.1).

FIGURE 14.1   Sources of Health Financing (% of GDP)

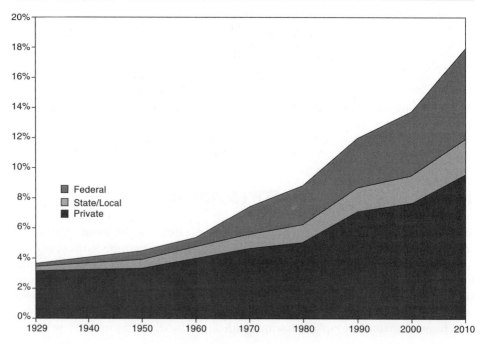

TABLE 14.1	Distribution of Government Funds	
	1965	**2007**
Total (millions)	$ 10,799	$ 1,036,000
Medicare	—	42%
Medicaid*	20%	33%
Veterans/DOD	18%	6%
Worker's compensation	8%	3%
State/local hospitals	22%	2%
Public health	8%	6%
Research	12%	4%
Construction	7%	3%
Other	5%	2%

Source: CMS National Health Accounts.

*Medicaid category includes general assistance (welfare) payments for health care, and in 1965 was composed of a variety of medical care programs for the indigent, as Medicaid was not yet enacted.

14.2   THE ROLES OF GOVERNMENT

Government Is Necessary, Even for Private Exchange

As people go about their daily activities, trying to stay happy and healthy and save a few dollars, they are usually not aware of government. Suppose that you get a headache and go to the drugstore for some aspirin. You are making that choice individually, as a private citizen, and buying from a private company. Yet this simple transaction could not take place unless a government had already done many things to prepare for the welfare of you and the company. To begin with, government provides a medium of exchange (money) and maintains its value. Without money you would have to engage in barter and search for someone who wanted you to cut their lawn, or care for their children, or whatever, in exchange for the aspirin. Not only is the value of money determined by the government, so are the measurements of what you buy. You don't ask for "some" or a scoop of aspirin, but for one hundred 250-milligram tablets. Furthermore, without government policing, you could not be sure whether the white pills were made of aspirin instead of sugar or flour or some noxious chemical. In fact, you depend on your government to keep your local store from selling you anything that could kill you when ingested. Without this form of consumer protection, you would have to spend a lot of time and money making sure that the drugs you bought were safe. All of the government activities that make exchange easy and inexpensive are going on almost without notice.[1]

To make any transaction, you must be able to say, "I own this, and I will give it to you in exchange for that." The most fundamental function of government is to maintain law and order. Unless we can define and enforce rights, including property rights, there is no way for people to cooperate and move beyond the law of the jungle—each person for himself or herself alone. Being killed because somebody wants your house or your cow or your mate is the most basic of threats to your health. Government arose in response to such threats. Families banded together into tribes to protect one another. To do so, they had to agree on how to work together—who would farm and who would fight, who would lead, and when it was OK to disagree with the leader. Douglass North, the 1993 Nobel Laureate in economics, defines the state as "an organization with a comparative advantage in violence, extending over a geographic area whose boundaries are determined by its power to tax constituents."[2] The state monopoly on violence makes it less costly for citizens to defend themselves and their property. Government is there to produce those goods and services that government can provide more efficiently than the market. When we say *efficiently*, we do not mean that government has no waste, or makes no mistakes, only that it does the job on the whole better than private action—or competing governments.

Efficiency of Markets under Conditions of Perfect Competition

The best way to run the economy is usually to let people work, play, and consume what they want without restriction. This interaction of supply and demand in the market leads to an equilibrium at the point where marginal benefits equal marginal costs. The prices that arise direct people to (a) work at the jobs in which their skills provide the most value to society, (b) find the most efficient means of production, (c) limit the consumption of goods that are most scarce, and (d) save and invest for the future. If there were no special problems or difficulties, the entire economy could be coordinated without any central control or direction from the government. The power of market prices to organize production and consumption to maximize welfare is expressed in the two fundamental theorems of welfare economics: under "perfect" conditions, (1) competitive markets will always lead to an efficient allocation of resources for production and consumption and (2) *any* efficient allocation can be obtained through a market system without any central government control by adjusting initial distribution.[3] These theoretical results emerged from a continuing debate among economists and politicians of all persuasions, from conservative to liberal to Marxist, during the early twentieth century. They provide the prime intellectual underpinning for advocating the use of markets rather than government intervention to solve most economic problems.

Economists' most frequent criticism of government intervention is that it distorts prices so that marginal costs and marginal benefits are no longer equated at the margin. In trying to make things better, government gives up some efficiency, and often makes things worse. Governments also inevitably tend to favor certain politically powerful interest groups (e.g., bankers, tobacco producers, the military-industrial complex, sons and daughters of senators), and by helping them, harm the rest of society and reduce the overall efficiency of the economy. Yet recognizing that government action is sometimes wrong or self-serving does not mean that it is not necessary. Conditions are not always perfect, and there are things that only government can do. Carefully examining the conditions of theoretically perfect competition (i.e., many buyers and sellers, all fully informed; costless transactions, with free entry and exit into the market) provides some insight into the roles of government in the real world. **Market failures** necessitating corrective government intervention arise if (a) conditions are such that the market has only one or a few buyers or sellers, (b) access to information is restricted or prohibitively costly to obtain by certain participants, (c) **transaction costs** are so high that many potentially beneficial agreements cannot be negotiated, or (d) the market is closed by constraints of technology, morality, or law. Sometimes the problems with competition are so extreme that they preclude a market from developing at all, making it necessary for government to create one. In the case of **public goods** (Chapter 15), the technology is such that only the government can act as a buyer or seller. Finally, the second theorem of welfare economics states only that the desired outcome "could in principle" be achieved if income were initially distributed in a particular way— which it is not. Therefore, governments must act to bring about a desirable **distribution** of income.

Government in a Mixed Economy

Government has four primary tasks in all economies:

- Maintain law and order
- Provide public goods
- Deal with market failures
- Equitable distribution of goods and services

To achieve these goals, a government may (a) *produce* services, (b) *finance* services that are provided by private contractors, or (c) *regulate* the private market. In practice, programs usually serve several functions and use a combination of methods. The Medicare program, for example, deals with market failure due to adverse selection and redistributes services to the sick elderly. Although functioning primarily as a financing mechanism, Medicare also uses regulation to enforce compliance and participation. In the face of such complexity, a simplified conceptual framework helps organize the analysis and make the fundamental economic forces more evident.

14.3   LAW AND ORDER

National defense and its complex domestic version—law and order—are the most fundamental tasks of governance. Without protection of life and property, society could not exist. A uniform interpretation of the law and a system of taxation must be enforced by the police and the courts. If the law applies to some and not to others, people are split into two different societies, even if they are nominally within the same nation. Coercive powers of taxation and law enforcement are freely given to the state by the citizens—we agree to have the government take our money and punish us if we break the law because we are better off that way. Each of us fighting our own battles is more expensive than all the taxes, parking fines, and so on that we love to complain about. Government is expensive, but anarchy, although it doesn't cost anything, is ruinous.

Getting people to agree that there should be law and order is much easier than reaching agreement on exactly what those laws should be, who pays how much tax, and so on. The philosopher John Rawls, in his book *A Theory of Justice*, suggests a useful way of looking at the problem of reaching a social consensus.[4] Rawls argues that much of the conflict over what is right and wrong is due not to differences in beliefs, but to differences in the positions that people are coming from. Older people want government to provide nursing home insurance, while young families believe that better schools are more important. The rich want taxes to be kept low, while the poor (who hope to benefit from redistribution and government aid) want taxes to be higher. People with AIDS favor a national health insurance system that insures everyone, while healthy workers tend to favor higher take-home pay and insurance premiums based on expected costs. In each case, the supporters tend to be those who can expect to benefit, while the critics tend to be those who stand to lose (through higher taxation, less service, or loss of preference).

Consider the formation of policy on disability. It is expensive to provide home care, prostheses, therapy, and building modifications. Including students with disabilities in regular classrooms (mainstreaming) helps them become integrated into society, but imposes costs on the other students in the diversion of teachers' attention, pacing of lectures, disruption, and so on. If everything that can possibly benefit the disabled students is done, it will cost too much. Yet providing only those benefits that reduce costs (e.g., a prostheses to help someone return to work) is not enough. Whether people focus primarily on the costs or emphasize the benefits depends mainly on whether they are disabled or whether they care deeply about a child, parent, or friend who is. However, even people who are healthy recognize that there is some chance that they might become disabled in the future (e.g., after an automobile accident) and switch their focus. Rawls defines justice as a set of policies people would vote for "behind the veil of ignorance" (i.e., what people would consider an optimal balance of costs and benefits if they did not know whether they were disabled or healthy, farmers or lawyers, or young or old). Formally, Rawls' notion is a lot like insurance, where people willingly contribute enough to cover their expected losses to an insurance plan that spreads the risk. Most health care, disability, and pension financing systems in Europe and Asia are considered "social insurance" operating under principles of fairness and solidarity rather than private actuarial principles (such as rating and payment according to risk category) used in commercial insurance.

Justice is more than an abstract notion; it is necessary for the operation of society. Unless people believe that the system is fair and serves their needs, they will not trust the government, and it becomes prohibitively costly to force them to behave according to the rules. Pervasive cheating will cause the whole system to break down. If members of a group think they are not being treated fairly, the group will lose respect for the law. At the extreme, they will revolt and perhaps set up a separate government that conforms more closely to their ideal of a fair system.

14.4 PUBLIC GOODS AND EXTERNALITIES

A public good is something that everyone consumes collectively. National defense is a public good. So is clean air, the discovery of penicillin, and the publication of national health statistics. Public goods have two distinguishing properties. First, they are *inexhaustible*; therefore, once produced, there is no additional cost for having additional people use them (i.e., the marginal cost of additional users is $0). Second, they are *nonexclusive*; therefore, people cannot be stopped from using a public good once it is there. Private goods are exhaustible and get used up by consumption (a pill, an hour of a doctor's time), whereas public goods (the formula for the pill, the discovery that eating foods rich in vitamin C reduces certain diseases, clean air) do not. If one patient uses a doctor's time, another patient cannot. Yet if one patient uses a formula, clean air, or nutritional advice, the amount available for someone else is not reduced. Private goods are *exclusive*; thus, if one person uses them, another person cannot. This makes it easy to charge consumers for using a private good and to pay the costs of production. Public goods tend to be nonexclusive and indivisible; thus, if anyone gets the benefits, everyone does. Since no one can be prevented from using a public good like clean air, no one has any incentive to pay for it. Selfishly, it makes sense for me to wait for someone else to clean up the air, discover a cure for AIDS, or build the Internet, because whether I contribute or not will make little difference. This is known as the **free-rider** problem. If no one is charged for public goods and no one voluntarily contributes, there is no way to conduct medical research, reduce pollution, or build highways. Therefore, governments are allowed to force everyone to "donate" taxes to pay for public goods.

Many goods are not purely private or purely public, but somewhere in between, and the extent of "publicness" may change with market conditions. For people in an isolated rural area, building and staffing a hospital is mostly a public good. Without the hospital, they have no medical care, but once it is built, anyone who wants to can use the hospital without displacing or reducing anyone else's consumption because there is plenty of excess capacity (i.e., marginal cost of additional patients is near $0). However, if population increases and the hospital becomes full, each additional patient displaces someone else who might have received care, and care becomes more like a private good (and marginal cost rises to approximately equal the average cost per unit). Highways, parks, and movie theaters show similar congestion effects, being almost pure public goods when they are mostly empty and more like private goods once they fill up.

Externalities

The production or consumption of a private good may have social consequences because it affects other people. A firm that produces cars may not pay for the exhaust they emit, an airport may not compensate residents in neighboring houses for the disruption caused by jets taking off at night, a student who cheats may not compensate classmates for the inconvenience caused by new test-taking rules, and a student who comes to class with a cold to take an exam may not compensate classmates for exposing them to illness. Externalities exist whenever a transaction affects an uncompensated party. The term *"public good"* focuses attention on the collective concerns that face all of us: a need for consensus, government control, and a universal tax system. The term *"externalities"* focuses attention on concerns in which the costs and benefits of actions are borne by different people, making private and social costs diverge. Whether considering public goods such as national defense and scientific research, or externalities such as infection control and pollution, we end up with the same issue: how to design appropriate institutions and government rules to align individual incentives with social welfare.

There are positive as well as negative externalities. Governments subsidize schools and colleges because they think that educated people will become better citizens (and able to pay more taxes). A person who fixes up an old house increases the value of all houses in the neighborhood, a cook who washes his hands reduces the risk of spreading infection, and a technological discovery that allows more efficient production by one firm creates external benefits for other firms that copy it. However, that same technology may create negative externalities for some corporations and people, because it puts an obsolete factory out of business and causes workers to lose their jobs. In fact, whether an externality is positive or negative depends on the perspective from which it is viewed. The cook may have thought that he was doing his patrons a favor by washing his hands. The patrons may have thought that being clean is part of his job and that not washing his hands was an unwarranted burden to impose on them. This mirror-image aspect, that an action may be considered either a negative cost reduction or a positive benefit increase, leads to an important insight.

The Coase Theorem: Transaction Costs and Property Rights

If transacting were indeed costless, as is assumed under perfect competition, a factory would pay a fee for the smoke it emits, a cook with dirty hands would pay a fee to customers who became ill, and a student with the flu would not show up for an exam unless he or she was willing to pay each classmate $20 for exposing them to airborne viruses. These externalities would then be internalized by market transactions. If only one or two people are affected by an externality, individual transactions can be used to deal with it. For example, a person who dumps dirt in a neighbor's yard or who breaks a neighbor's window, or a doctor who negligently causes a leg fracture, will pay for it. If many people are affected by an externality, the cost of arranging thousands of individually negotiated transactions becomes prohibitive and **property rights** (who controls what, who must pay whom to use it) become unclear. No market develops to handle externalities at this scale. Therefore, government must act on behalf of many people by creating rules and regulations. It is cheaper to deal with a problem once and for all, despite some inefficiencies, than to make thousands of individual transactions with everyone who might be affected by the problem (e.g., pollution, infection, air traffic control).

Suppose that the socially optimal decision, in which marginal costs equal marginal benefits, is to force factories to reduce the pollution emitted from their smokestacks by 80 percent. The **Coase theorem** asserts that there would be *no difference* in outcome whether the factory has a right to pollute or the people have a right to clean air.[5] As long as all rights are well defined, there are no transacting costs (a big if), and income distribution effects are ignored, the result will be the same. If a factory has the right to pollute, its neighbors will pay the company a fee to install smokestack scrubbers until pollution has been reduced to 20 percent. If the neighbors have a right to clean air, the factory will pay each resident a fee to allow discharge of 20 percent of the smoke and will buy scrubbers to clean up the rest. Either way, the result will be the same: air that is 80 percent cleaner. The ability to make mutually beneficial trades through the market guarantees that whoever values air quality more, whether positively or negatively, will "buy" it from the other party. The Coase theorem is important, not because outcomes would be the same under some hypothetically perfect conditions, but because it shows how transaction costs and assignment of property rights actually affect distribution and efficiency in the real world, and how distortions and difficulties increase to the extent that the characteristics of a good are more public than private.

Politicians: Entrepreneurs Who Try to Get Votes

Markets operate through voluntary exchange, whereas public goods can be provided only through political intervention. You cannot go to the store and buy more clean air, better schools, or safer highways. We depend on politicians to act as entrepreneurs, to propose a plan of action that appeals to us so that we will put them in positions of power. Like all entrepreneurs, politicians expect to be paid for their efforts, extracting "rents" in the form of influence, prestige, perquisites, and salary. To an extent, the political arena can be viewed as a market, with people "spending" votes or influence. However, the correspondence is very imperfect—people are not allowed to buy and sell votes, borrow votes by paying interest, or trade votes by setting up joint-stock corporations. The property rights to votes are much less well defined and enforceable, and thus the transaction costs are very high.

Because it is difficult to make a political bargain, a lot of the effort and money must be wasted. Millions of dollars are used to win support or to keep a wavering supporter in line. Formally, economists talk about the problems of "rent capture." If ordinary entrepreneurs have a good idea, they can trade the idea to a firm for money. For example, inventors, biochemists, and screenwriters avoid the hassles of marketing and production by licensing the rights to their ideas and obtaining royalty payments in return. These profits are called **rents** because once the entrepreneur has the idea, no more work needs to be done to get the money. It is similar to collecting rent on a piece of land. Also, like land, the rent depends entirely on the demand. A good idea (Mickey Mouse, penicillin, mobile phones) is valuable the way land in downtown Tokyo is valuable; bad ideas are like acreage in the Gobi Desert.

Rents and rent seeking are major obstacles to providing an optimal level of investment in public health. Many good ideas (well-child care, genetic counseling for parents, dietary change) offer no simple way for innovators to capture the benefits, and thus there is little incentive to produce them. On the other hand, when large sums of money are available to put good ideas into practice, most of the money is not well spent. The new road primarily benefits a construction company owned by a senator's brother-in-law, the new antismoking campaign is highly visible and impresses voters but doesn't keep children from lighting up, and the new sex education program for teenagers is so dreary that they only use it to make jokes. Even if we know exactly how much to spend on public goods, it is doubtful that all the money will be well spent. Because no single individual has much of an interest, those who are able to capture a piece of the action will distort the program to benefit themselves, and the objective of meeting the needs of the public will be compromised.

14.5 MARKET FAILURE

Monopoly

For public goods, the marginal cost of additional consumption is $0. The production of some private goods has such high fixed costs and low marginal costs that the average cost per unit continually falls as output increases. Such goods (telephone networks, power and water supply) are called **natural monopolies**. Declining average cost means that the largest firm can underbid all the others, and competition will lead to a single firm that dominates the whole market. However, to break even, that firm must charge a price above marginal cost (the high fixed cost overhead means that average cost per unit is always above marginal cost). Since there is no competition, the monopoly firm may push prices up to extract extra profits from consumers, stopping only when the profits are so great that another firm is tempted to enter the market, even at an inefficiently small scale. In a rural area, ambulance transport, hospital services, even a doctor's office, may all be natural monopolies. In addition to the technologically induced natural monopoly, there are monopolies created by political action. For example, a certificate-of-need law may give a hospital an effective monopoly in its local market by barring the construction of new competititors, licensure laws may give a profession monopoly control over supply, quality regulations may give a manufacturer monopoly control over a special medical device, and requirements to hold clinical trials demonstrating safety and efficacy can give a pharmaceutical firm monopoly control over a type of drug.

The desire to maximize profits and the lack of competition leads a monopolist, unlike a firm under perfectly competitive conditions, to charge a price above the average cost per unit, thus generating excess profits known as **monopoly rents**. Monopoly pricing causes the market to be inefficient. With prices above average cost, some consumers choose not to buy even though goods could have been produced and sold for an amount less than their willingness to pay. The amount of consumer welfare forgone is traditionally estimated by the "welfare triangle" (see Chapter 4, Section 5) which, under appropriate conditions, is approximately one-half the difference between the monopoly price and the average cost per unit ($P_{monopoly} - AC$) multiplied by the number of units not purchased due to the excessive price ($Q_{optimum} - Q_{monopoly}$). The magnitude of inefficiency due to monopoly pricing is shown by the shaded welfare triangle in Figure 14.2. Monopoly rents (shown as the lightly shaded rectangle) resulting from high prices are a loss to consumers but are a gain to the seller, and are regarded by most economists as a pure transfer that does not in itself create any loss of market efficiency. However, consumers tend to get upset about being charged extra just because a firm has a monopoly. Also, there is likely to be some fighting between firms for the right to become the monopolist that takes home the rents, and this fighting is a waste of resources that generates inefficiency.

There are four ways for government to deal with the problems created by a natural monopoly:

1. Take over the process and let government become the producer.
2. Subsidize the fixed cost overhead and set a government-controlled price equal to the marginal cost per unit.

FIGURE 14.2   Welfare Loss Due to Monopoly Pricing

3. Set a government-controlled price equal to the average cost, which causes some inefficiency but avoids using taxpayers' money to subsidize a monopoly firm.

4. Do nothing and let the firm set a monopoly price.

Some economists claim that government production is so inefficient that the first option should always be avoided. Options 2 and 3 depend on the government's ability to accurately estimate marginal and average cost, which is always difficult and is inevitably made worse by firms' attempts to overstate costs and hide revenues to make extra profits. However, allowing firms to become monopolies often costs much more than the traditional welfare triangle loss, because firms waste millions of dollars making donations to politicians, hiring lawyers, and competing for (and competing away) the potential monopoly rents. Natural monopoly is a cornerstone of applied welfare economics, but is relatively unimportant in health care. Most medical monopolies arise from government intervention (licensure, regulation, reimbursement rules, patents) designed to ameliorate market failures caused by risk and information difficulties (discussed in Chapter 6) rather than market failures caused by production conditions of declining average costs.

Paternalism

Market efficiency depends on consumers' ability to choose, to correctly balance their demands with prices and available income. Some types of consumers—notably children, the mentally ill, addicts—are considered incapable of making reasonable choices. There is a biological necessity for parents to care for and make decisions on behalf a child, forcing the child to learn by doing many things he or she does not initially want to do (hence the term *paternalism*). Market failure due to mental incapacity is dealt with by having a parent, legal guardian, social service agency, or government bureau make decisions on behalf of those individuals rather than allowing them to do so for themselves. Addicts are prohibited by law from buying drugs they are willing to pay for. To that extent, these people are wards of the state, not fully participating citizens of the country.

Recently there has been a move to provide more freedoms and more rights to people who are mentally ill. "Deinstitutionalization" emptied state mental hospitals as patients were released into the community. In principle, inpatient hospital services were going to be replaced by community services so that former patients could operate at a higher level of functioning and be integrated into the community. The rise of a new generation of homeless people is evidence that things did not work out as planned. Economics, or rather the *failure to consider* the economics of deinstitutionalization, was a contributing factor. The public was more willing to recognize that people with mental illness had rights, and to vote for a change in the law making it difficult to keep people in mental hospitals, than to provide money for the community services needed to take care of them. Once it cost something, voters approached the issue from a different perspective. Unlike a manager or a factory owner, voters are under no obligation to be consistent. Thus, they could vote for their principles on one day and for their pocketbooks on another. Deinstitutionalization created a need for services but not the taxes to pay for these services. Furthermore, the expected transfer of funding from hospitals to community programs did not occur. Employees at state mental hospitals fought to maintain their jobs and their budgets even though most patients were being discharged.

The initial proponents of deinstitutionalization were ordinary citizens who had worked with people with mental disorders and were convinced that most of them could function better and enjoy life more if they lived in the community. Like doctors, they were agents and even advocates for their clients. Yet they were not balancing the interests of all the parties involved. Although living in the community might be beneficial to a patient, it might not be beneficial to the community. Deinstitutionalization has had a large and unrecognized externality that we call the homeless problem.

14.6   REDISTRIBUTION AND CARE OF THE POOR

Every civilized society takes care of its poor. It is generally accepted that no one in the United States should die because he or she cannot afford a necessary operation or medications. However, the poor cannot afford to buy insurance or medical care generally available to most members of society. Not being able to buy is what being "poor" means. Countries that provide health services as a public good just as they provide water and mail delivery services, such as Sweden and the United Kingdom, automatically provide medical care to the poor. In a pluralistic system where individual income affects access to the system, a more explicit mechanism to protect those least able to pay is required. In the United States, Medicaid is the most important program to guarantee that poor people have access to medical care. Originally directed toward impoverished families with dependent children, Medicaid has been broadened to include all people who are medically indigent, and now pays for almost half of all nursing home care, even for the middle-class elderly (see Chapter 10).

Medicaid and Medicare: Dependency or Rights?

Medicaid is fraught with ambiguity and compromise because of an unresolved conflict at its core: Is it charity or a form of social insurance? Is it a program for taking care of people who can't take care of themselves and whose dependency, like that of children, addicts, and the mentally ill, makes them inherently less qualified than other citizens to make decisions? Or is Medicaid the provision of a basic necessity of life, such as safe water and national defense, that poor people can claim as a right of citizenship and, therefore, should not involve giving up any decision-making power?

Some people believe that most or all of the benefits of economic development should belong to society as a whole, and they favor broad government activity to ensure a relatively equal distribution of goods and services. In Sweden, for example, more than half of gross domestic product (GDP) moves through the government sector. Other people believe that individual initiative and luck should determine who gets to consume what and thus want to limit the role of government to referee and provider of last resort. Medical care for the poor is caught between these opposing positions. Some who believe in reducing taxes and the role of government are willing to make an exception for medical care, but expect the indigent (like other dependent beneficiaries) to give up some autonomy and self-respect. Other people who want a more equitable social distribution of all goods and services are willing to settle for a few (medical care, education) rather than none.

In general, rich people will rationally favor a conservative position, since any redistributive government activity is likely to cost them more in taxes than they will receive in benefits. Conversely, the self-interest of poor people rationally favors broad social redistribution. The motivations behind these two positions are in conflict on several levels and it is, therefore, almost impossible to design a practical program that satisfies both at the same time. This tension and its policy implications are well illustrated by comparing Medicare and Medicaid.

Medicare is a universal and popular program to pay on a national basis for the medical care of all the elderly.[6] Medicaid is a much reviled and unpopular part-federal, part-state (local) program that requires each beneficiary to meet a "means test" and covers a complicated patchwork of special programs.[7] Why are these two programs perceived so differently? Medicare is constructed like a public good for all citizens, whereas Medicaid has the punitive elements of a qualified dependency assistance program. To qualify for Medicare, one need only be 65 or older, and it covers everyone, rich or poor, sick or healthy, black or white. Every voter expects to benefit from Medicare and views it as vital to their financial planning for old age. Medicaid is the opposite. Applicants must submit to probing questions and must sometimes misrepresent their economic positions to qualify for benefits. Most voters believe they personally will never benefit from Medicaid, and often feel shame when they help Grandma (and themselves) do so by transferring ownership of her car and her house to their own name so that she can qualify for assistance. Medicaid is not designed to provide satisfaction to its beneficiaries; it forces them to acknowledge dependence and serves as a necessary social backstop so that no one is deprived of minimal (but not comfortable) care.

The expansion of a Medicare-type program (universal access, no means testing, the same care for all) furthers redistributive social and political goals by broadening participation in government activities viewed as helpful and high quality. Replacement with a Medicaid-type program (means tested, differential standards of care by payment class) furthers a narrowed political agenda by making government programs unpopular. Thus, how a public health program is put together affects not just the services people get, but also their future voting behavior and attitude toward government. Each political party fights to get programs that make it easier to say, "I told you so," and that favor the economic interests of its supporters. Attitudes toward public health activities and the design of programs thus depend on political ideology and self-interest as much as any objective evaluation of costs and benefits or morbidity and mortality.

14.7 HOW GOVERNMENT WORKS

Government influence on various parts of the economy ranges from watchful oversight to total control (Table 14.2). Government is least intrusive when it confines its activities to creating a foundation of property rights and contract enforcement within which the market can operate freely. Government is most controlling when it takes over production and replaces

TABLE 14.2	Varieties of Government Action
	Examples
Public production	*Centers for Disease Control and Prevention*
	Veterans Administration hospitals
Public financing	
• **Contract**	*Neighborhood health center*
• **Producer subsidy**	*Vaccine liability insurance*
• **Consumer subsidy**	*Employee health benefits*
• **Entitlement**	*Medicare*
Public regulation	
• **For the market**	*Financial standards for insurance companies*
• **Superseding market**	*Price controls*
Private production	*Self-paid visit to therapist*

private ownership completely. Through regulation and third-party financing, the health care sector has a high degree of government involvement. **Government production** is mostly limited to certain core public health functions, such as setting and monitoring standards, controlling infectious disease, and conducting medical research.[8] Direct contracting with production tailored to government specifications, which occurs in military health insurance, federally qualified neighborhood health centers, immunization programs, and so on, offers extensive, yet not complete, public control since the workers are employed by private firms. With **subsidies**, government can exert influence, but rarely control. For example, tax-exempt municipal bond financing can encourage construction of hospital facilities, but only rarely and indirectly does it affect the type of clinical services offered. **Entitlement financing**, such as Medicare, may leave behavior essentially unconstrained since it is designed to be the equivalent of privately purchased insurance.

A large part of **health regulation** is intended *to make markets more efficient* by providing standard definitions, quality assurance, uniform insurance contracts, and other measures that reduce transactions costs. Other regulations attempt to change the shape of the market *or to supersede the market entirely* and dictate prices and quantities. The regulatory apparatus can be tightened or loosened to allow government to exert more or less control, and can be made compelling without resorting to legal action by combining regulation with financing. Medicare, initially a passive entitlement financing program that provided essentially private funding for the purchase of physician services, now sets prices within a narrow range and may virtually prohibit the use of some medical technology by refusing to pay for it. Direct regulatory control is exercised by government in only a few areas where the threat to public safety is compelling: water and air quality, production and prescribing of pharmaceuticals, and performance of surgery. For the most part, medical care is "regulated" through control over finances rather than laws.

The Voluntary Sector

The public good is sometimes best served neither by a government bureaucracy nor a private firm but by independent "voluntary" organizations. Nonprofit status can free hospitals, social service agencies, professional societies, and other voluntary organizations from the dictates of profit maximization and make it easier for them to pursue the goal of maximizing health. Independence from government often makes voluntary organizations more flexible and creative than the public sector in meeting social needs.[9]

Government as the Citizen's Agent

Government exists, to paraphrase the quote from Abraham Lincoln at the opening of this chapter, to do for the people things that they cannot do for themselves. However, what guarantee is there that a government agency will act as the agent of the people rather than of special interest groups or of the bureaucrats themselves? When information problems cause market failure and thus preclude private action, governments will also have a difficult time collecting information and voters will have a difficult time evaluating the performance of an agency to make sure that it is, in fact, operating in the public interest. Economists examine the performance of government agencies from four perspectives:

1. Maximizing public welfare
2. "Capturing" of regulatory agencies by profit-maximizing firms
3. Maximizing bureaucratic objectives
4. Balancing political interest groups

Public Welfare Maximization The starting point for the economic analysis is to assume that regulation does what it says it does—maximize public welfare. The British Empire, the state of Pennsylvania, and other governments argue as much when they define themselves as a *commonwealth*. However, to define *public welfare*, assumptions about whose preferences count, and how much, must be made. Is everyone equal? Do people who harm themselves through drug use or lack of exercise deserve the same services as people who try to stay healthy? Do people with genetic defects that shorten their lives deserve more, or less, than people without genetic defects? Does a desire for life-saving heart surgery count as much as a desire for face-saving cosmetic surgery? Even if all these issues are resolved, there still may be no way to reach a decision about which government policy is best, as demonstrated in the proof of the famous "Arrow impossibility theorem."[10] The theoretical problems of welfare maximization pale beside the practical problems of public incentives. Unlike a firm, which has an owner, no one has an interest in maximizing the benefits of government. An individual seeks to maximize his or her own welfare. Acts and votes are usually directed by self-interest, even when the cost to others far outweighs the benefits to the individual. Many government programs are characterized by *concentrated benefits* greatly helping a few people and *diffuse costs* spread across many people. For example, lengthening patent restrictions would raise the price of drugs several cents per prescription thus adding millions of dollars to the profits of a few pharmaceutical firms, but would cause just a slight, almost unnoticeable, rise in the medical bills and insurance premiums of millions of consumers.

Regulatory Capture The concentrated interest of the firms most affected by a regulation makes it worthwhile for them to lobby government and try to "capture" the regulatory agency. For example, a hearing on the safety of cardiac pacemakers is sure to be attended by lawyers for the device's manufacturers, but few patients will travel to Washington to testify and will not be paid $400 an hour for doing so. Contributing to political campaigns is an obvious way of attempting to exercise control, but usually is not the most effective way. It is common for firms in regulated industries to appeal directly to bureaucrats, not with money or gifts (which are illegal), but by hiring former regulators and holding informational seminars in Hawaii. It is natural for someone who has worked for years in regulating health to take a job with a company in the same field, but such a **revolving door** is likely to compromise regulatory objectivity. How can a junior analyst in an agency remain clear when asked to make a difficult judgment call if the person on the other side of the table is the well-respected former chairman? Even a bureaucrat who wants to do a good job performing daily tasks can be influenced by the asymmetry between concentrated producer interests and diffuse consumer interests. There are many more patients than producers, yet most complaints to regulators (or complaints to politicians about regulatory decisions) come from producers, because they stand to gain so much from any change in the rules.[11]

Bureaucratic Objectives   Bureaucrats, just like consumers, profit-maximizing owners, union workers, and all other individuals in the economy, prefer not to be harassed. Most people get paid to do tasks that are occasionally unpleasant in order to maximize long-term gains (e.g., impose discipline on second-graders, redo a botched repair job for free, fire an incompetent employee, hold the HMO doctors within budget). The difficulty of evaluating how well a government agency is performing can reduce the competitive pressure to take on unpleasant tasks. This can lead to an agency that is bloated and excessively risk averse. Unlike an owner, who can gain large profits from taking on risk, a bureaucrat will continue to be compensated on a civil service pay scale. Any effort to make changes or take risks could go wrong and cost them their jobs, so they tend to play it safe. If an owner believes that the additional revenues gained are less than the additional cost in wages, then an employee may be let go. A bureaucrat, on the other hand, has almost no incentive to reduce the number of workers. Instead, an increase in employment usually means a larger salary for the director (who now runs a bigger agency) and better working conditions (since the tasks are spread out among more employees, giving them more time to do the job). Unlike a profit-maximizing firm, there is no internal incentive to limit the size of a government agency; therefore, control must be imposed from the outside. Unfortunately, outsiders are, by definition, less familiar with the tasks, workload, and performance of the agency than the employees and managers inside or the industry experts who lobby them. This does not mean that most government agencies are too large, since the fear of "waste" may lead legislators to preemptively cut regulatory budgets. What it does mean is that the difficulty of evaluating performance, which is why this task was taken out of the market and given to government in the first place, also makes it much harder to tell whether the agency is too big or too small or to manage the agency so that the use of employees and other resources is optimized.

Political Interest Group Balance   The actual behavior of government agencies is not determined by the public interest, self-interest of the industry, or of the bureaucrats, but by a complex and shifting balance of all interest groups. Transaction costs shape politics just as they shape markets, and are lower when interests are concentrated or uniform across a large group of people (e.g., all of the elderly tend to favor increased Medicare budgets). However, political deals cannot be negotiated, specified, and enforced by precisely weighing conflicting interests the way the market can so precisely and quickly weigh dollars, making outcomes less predictable. Economists and political scientists devote considerable attention to studying how the process of making decisions affects the decisions made. For example, a majority rule implies that 50 to 49 wins while 49 to 50 loses, thus providing politicians with a great incentive to seek the median (50th percentile) voter rather than maximize the average level of support. Other political structures favor different parts of the voting spectrum. In union representation, for example, seniority is important; thus, the desires of older workers for more health benefits and higher pensions tend to outweigh the desires of younger workers for fewer benefits and higher wages. Several critiques of the health care industry claim that it is dominated by an "iron triangle" of providers, insurance companies, and government agencies, all of whom benefit from higher health care spending rather than difficult, but potentially worthwhile, cost cutting.[12]

Winners and Losers

Although economists try to evaluate how a regulation changes the overall efficiency of the system, most hospital administrators, physicians, and patients are far more concerned with how it affects them personally. Even if a change in Medicare reimbursement is good for the country, a medical equipment vendor will fight it with everything he owns if that regulation would force his business into bankruptcy. Changes in the regulatory structure often have more to do with finding paths that have less resistance than the achievement of noble ends. Many issues have solutions that are nearly the same in terms of overall efficiency but are quite different in terms of who bears the costs or receives the benefits. For example, it may not make a great deal of difference in terms of economic efficiency whether an expanded Medicare drug benefit is paid for through increases in enrollee premiums or an income tax surcharge for the elderly, but the former falls mostly on the poor while the latter falls mostly on the wealthy (who pay more taxes) with predictable consequences in the political support for these alternatives by different groups. Research suggests that when a necessary change in policy involves two mutually exclusive options, the wealthy, even if less numerous and initially less powerful than the poor, may be able to hold out longer and obtain a result more favorable to their interests.[13] A disproportionate share of benefits, from Medicare reimbursement to subsidized medical education, goes to those in the highest income groups, who have the power to make their demands on government effective. Yet, without government intervention, the poor would surely be much worse off.

14.8 PROS AND CONS OF REGULATION AND COMPETITION

Even when markets are suppressed, there is always competition. Physicians try to attract patients with their reputations for quality and with evening office hours. Hospitals try to attract physicians with subsidized office rentals, access to new equipment, and helpful staff. HMOs try to attract enrollees with special benefits, picnics, or free radios. Conversely, even the most open market in health care is highly regulated, with oversight of safety, professional qualifications, and long-term side effects, even when prices are freely set. The issue is not "regulation" or "competition," but what combination and compromises to make (Table 14.3).[14]

Many problems are created by reliance on government intervention. First, regulation itself costs money: agencies must be staffed, salaries must be paid, and information systems must be maintained. Many of these costs have to be paid for with taxes. Other costs, such as for the compilation of mandated reports and time spent in preparing for regulatory inspections, are imposed on private firms, which then pass them on to the public in the form of higher prices. When government takes over production from private firms, it has sometimes been inefficient and inept at customer service. Even if the market is superseded by direct government provision of services, some form of rationing must still take place. Since prices are not used to match demand and supply, the amount distributed often will be too large or too small, and the people served may not be the ones who value the services most highly. Both discrepancies cause deadweight losses of consumer welfare. Government suppression of the price mechanism prevents desirable trades from occurring, and also distorts related markets for inputs and substitute goods.

Government responds well, perhaps too well, to focused interest groups willing to lobby for their positions. Markets are better able to respond to diverse and diffuse consumer groups, and the prices people pay are a superior mechanism for publicly revealing the value of the services they use. Politicians are constrained by public scrutiny to "do no harm," and

TABLE 14.3	Pros and Cons of Regulation and Competition

Limitations of Regulation
- Regulatory agencies are costly to operate.
- Government is sometimes an inefficient producer with inadequate customer service.
- Rationing must still take place, and without prices, deadweight welfare losses are larger.
- Suppression of prices distorts markets in inputs and substitute goods as well.
- Government responds to narrowly focused interest groups, not broad consumer interests.
- Regulators must "do no harm" and avoid losses (except the hidden kind).
- Bureaucracies rigidly impose uniformity, treating everyone according to the same standard.
- All regulation is based on the past as a precedent, not directed toward the future.
- No automatic adjustment is made to changes in supply or demand.
- There are no incentives to be an entrepreneur developing new technologies that anticipate demand.

Limitations of Markets
- Markets are costly to operate and must be policed.
- Entrepreneurs maximize profit, not health or social welfare (which are not paid for).
- Under competition, prices pay for services valued by individuals, not public goods (education, research).
- Health care is not very price sensitive, so it is difficult to control behavior through prices.
- Consumers are willing to pay to avoid using prices to make health care decisions.
- Somebody must still take care of the poor, the chronically ill, and the seriously injured.
- Adverse selection may cause private insurance markets to collapse unless government steps in.
- The ethics of competition do not blend well with the ethics of medicine as a *caring* profession.
- Licensure, insurance, patents, and other erosions of the medical marketplace must be doing more good than harm or they would not be built into the health care system of every country.
- Even the U.S. government must be doing something right, since it has been given increased funding responsibility and control over the medical marketplace.

every dollar spent becomes a "federal case"; therefore, services that are valued by consumers and raise average health levels (e.g., mass immunizations, fluoridation, birth control) may not be available. Government is subject to so much criticism that agencies can become very risk averse. This exacerbates bureaucratic formalism. Government programs designed to deal with the public must impose universal standards and thus are less able to respond to the variation in individual preferences or to make individual exceptions. Legal constraints make bureaucracies rigid and may stifle innovation. A central failing of regulation is its reliance on precedent. There is no flexible equilibration of supply and demand through prices to create automatic adjustments as conditions change, and little scope for entrepreneurs who are willing to make mistakes and go out on a limb to create the next generation of technology.

Markets have their flaws as well. They, too, are costly to operate, requiring salespeople, billing systems, and policing mechanisms. Entrepreneurs are apt to push the newest and most expensive technology because it is the most profitable rather than a more cost-effective substitute that would do more to improve health.[15] Markets reward those who provide what consumers want, not those who provide public goods such as medical research, infection control, and ethical standards of professional education. Furthermore, markets for health do not appear to be very price sensitive, perhaps because of information problems and the potential for death from even small errors; therefore, reliance on prices to motivate behavior seems ill-placed. Even when people can use prices to make decisions about medical care, they seem to want to avoid doing so. For example, the elderly, although well insured with Medicare, overwhelmingly opt to obtain supplemental insurance that reduces the marginal price to zero.

Although advocates of competition emphasize the beneficial effect of creating incentives to win, what about the losers? Who will care for people with mental retardation, an alert but alone and alienated 92-year-old, people with genetic defects, the truly unlucky accident victim? Although markets can enable socially beneficial risk pooling through insurance, adverse selection may be so severe that insurance can become unstable or fail to cover many of those most in need unless government intervenes. Medical *care* is so grounded in a concern for the health of others that any competition sufficiently vicious to really cut costs and close all the unnecessary hospital beds may entail such a fundamental violation of human caring that it is socially unacceptable. One might also ask, "If the erosion of the marketplace due to licensure, insurance, and nonprofit organizations is so terrible, why are these anti-competitive features an integral part of every health care system in the civilized world?"

The approach to health care in the United States is among the most highly privatized and most responsive to individual needs. Yet even in the United States, government is the largest funding source, paying 48 percent of the bills directly, subsidizing much of the remainder through tax relief, and regulating virtually every dollar spent. It is the mixture of competition and market forces, the matching of programs to needs, that must be evaluated, not the pros and cons of one or the other alone.

SUGGESTIONS FOR FURTHER READING

Ronald Coase, "The Problem of Social Cost," *Journal of Law & Economics* 3 (1960): 1–44.

Paul Feldstein, *The Politics of Health Legislation: An Economic Perspective* (Ann Arbor, Mich.: Health Administration Press, 1988).

Theodore Marmor, *The Politics of Medicare* (Chicago: Aldine, 2000).

Douglass North, *Structure and Change in Economic History* (New York: W.W. Norton, 1981).

Joseph Stiglitz, *Economics of the Public Sector* (New York: W. W. Norton, 1986).

Burton Weisbrod, *The Non-Profit Economy* (Cambridge, Mass.: Harvard University Press, 1988).

Charles Wolfe, *Markets or Governments: Choosing Between Imperfect Alternatives* (Cambridge, Mass.: MIT Press, 1994).

SUMMARY

1. **Government accounts for 48 percent of health care spending**. Most government spending pays for private medical services of special populations (the aged, the indigent, veterans). **Only one-tenth pays for core public health** activities such as infectious disease control, research, and monitoring of drugs, food, air, and water.

2. Under certain conditions, a **purely competitive market allocation** of goods and services, where marginal benefits equal marginal costs enforced by the price mechanism, is most efficient.

3. Perfect competition is rare in the real world. There are **market failures** resulting from uncertainty and information problems, transaction costs, **externalities**, and the existence of **public goods**. Government or another paternalistic agency must step in when an individual is incapable of making appropriate market choices due to immaturity, substance abuse, or severe mental illness. Civilized societies **redistribute** goods and services to protect the poor and disabled.

4. Since most benefits of government are public goods available to all without restriction, many people would be **free riders** who avoid paying unless forced to do so through **compulsory taxation**.

5. Government is formed to act as the agent of the citizens to **maximize public welfare**. However, the ability of special interests to exert undue influence may lead to

regulatory capture, where government favors the industry rather than the public. Also, the employees of a government agency may pursue **bureaucratic self-interest**, avoiding risks and controversy, and increasing budgets to obtain higher salaries and more employees to ease workloads. The most realistic model of government action combines all three of these perspectives and a consideration of **transaction costs** in achieving **political interest group balance**.

6. Although people say that they want to do what is best for everyone, **they tend to vote for what is good for themselves.** That is why some government programs, such as Medicaid to care for the poor, are unpopular and grudgingly supported, while Medicare, which most voters believe will benefit them now or in the future, and which incidentally helps keep politically connected doctors and hospitals well off, is very popular.

7. To some extent, **politics is a type of market**, albeit a slow and imperfect one, with legislators trying to get elected by promising the best package of benefits and costs in return for votes. Special-interest legislation benefiting a small group at the expense of the many is most apt to occur when benefits are concentrated on a particular group, making it worthwhile for them to organize and lobby, while the costs are widely dispersed across all of society. **Prices change much faster than laws.** Public goods take longer to adjust because groups and individuals with different interests must agree before any changes can occur.

8. The **voluntary sector**, composed of **nonprofit organizations independent of government** whose objective is to foster the public good, dominates the ownership of hospitals in the United States and the important private disease control and medical research firms.

9. **For the most part, government works with the market**, regulating and financing private activities. Government supersedes the market when it exerts control over prices and quantities and when it prohibits certain kinds of trades. Some critical functions, such as law and order (police and courts) and national defense (military), are produced directly by government employees. The important question is not whether government or markets are "better," but how to **balance and blend regulation and competition** to optimize social welfare and meet necessary constraints. To do this, a consensus about what constitutes **a just society** is needed.

PROBLEMS

1. {*flow of funds*} What fraction of total health expenditures in the United States is paid for by government? Which government programs are the largest? Were the same, or similar, programs at the top of the list for government funding in 1900?

2. {*market failure*} Which aspects of the economic organization of U.S. medical care result from market failure?

3. {*distribution*} In several marches on Washington, demonstrators have carried signs saying, "No Justice, No Peace." Explain what this slogan means, and how it relates to the level of funding for Medicaid.

4. {*incidence*} Why is more dental care paid for privately whereas more hospital care is paid for publicly?

5. {*welfare*} Which results in lower prices: competition or regulation?

6. {*incidence*} Why is Medicare more popular than Medicaid?

7. {*public goods*} Does the demand for public health increase or decrease as the size of a city increases?

8. {*rents*} How are rents different from other input payments? Which of the following are rents?

   a. Royalties from a biotechnology patent

   b. Lease payments for use of a laboratory

   c. Payments to research participants who are observed while sleeping

   d. Surgical fees

   e. A bonus paid to a research assistant who finishes an experiment ahead of schedule

   f. A bonus paid to a Nobel Laureate for switching to another university

9. {*transaction costs*} What is the Coase theorem? What does it imply about the extent of immunization among herds of cattle? What does it imply about the levels of immunization among schoolchildren in a classroom?

10. {*regulatory capture*} Explain how the Food and Drug Administration might be subject to regulatory capture. Who would favor, and who would be opposed to, regulations that limited regulatory capture?

11. {*regulatory capture*} Name several medical professional/trade organizations that have made large donations to political campaigns. Did they get their money's worth?

12. {*incidence*} Who benefits and who loses from deinstitutionalization of people who are mentally ill? Which factors thwarted the original plans for transfer of funding to community treatment facilities?

13. {*flow of funds*} Which of the following are funded as entitlements?

    a. Medicare

    b. Medicaid

    c. Medical research

    d. Public health statistics

14. {*voting*} Who counts for more in political calculus:

    a. The sick or the well?

    b. The old or the young?

    c. The rich or the poor?

15. {*incidence*} Medical savings accounts (discussed in Section 5.2) tend to favor which groups of people?

16. {*dynamics*} Why does it often take longer for a government program to change in response to shifts in external conditions than it takes a private company? Is this good or bad?

17. {*dynamics*} Which is harder to close: a public hospital or a private clinic? Why? Which is more likely to take advantage of information asymmetry to cheat patients?

ENDNOTES

1. Oliver Williamson, *Markets and Hierarchies* (New York: Free Press, 1975).
2. Douglass C. North, *Structure and Change in Economic History* (New York: Norton, 1981), p. 21.
3. Joseph E. Stiglitz, *Economies of the Public Sector* (New York: W.W. Norton, 1986), p. 77.

4. John Rawls, *A Theory of Justice* (Cambridge, Mass.: Harvard University Press, 1971).

5. Ronald H. Coase, "The Problem of Social Cost," *Journal of Law & Economics* 3 (1960): 1–44.

6. Marilyn Moon, *Medicare Now and In the Future* (Washington, D.C.: The Urban Institute, 1993); Mark V. Pauly and William L. Kissick, eds., *Lessons from the First Twenty Years of Medicare: Research Implications for Public and Private Sector Policy* (Philadelphia: University of Pennsylvania Press, 1988). Theodore Marmor, *The Politics of Medicare* (Chicago: Aldine, 2000); Jonathan Oberlander, *The Political Life of Medicare* (Chicago: University of Chicago Press, 2003).

7. SCHIP (the State Children's Health Insurance Program) discussed in Chapter 5 is the sort of "exception that proves the rule." Expansion of coverage to include children is so hard to resist politically that conservatives have pushed to limit funding just to those children who are poor—lest there be another popular universal health insurance entitlement program on the books. However, for an intriguing contrary view of the relative political merits of Medicare and Medicaid, see Lawrence D. Brown and Michael S. Sparer, "Poor Program's Progress: The Unanticipated Politics of Medicaid Policy," *Health Affairs* 22, no. 1 (January 2003): 31–44.

8. A significant exception is the Department of Defense/Veterans Administration health care system. Although national defense is a pure public good, the fact that VA/DOD health is an adjunct to defense does not necessarily make it public, and indeed large parts of the VA/DOD health care are now being privatized through subcontracting.

9. Burton Weisbrod, *The Non-Profit Economy* (Cambridge, Mass.: Harvard University Press, 1988).

10. Peter J. Hammond, "Social Choice: The Science of the Impossible," in George R. Feiwel, *Arrow and the Foundations of the Theory of Economic Policy* (New York: New York University Press, 1987), pp. 116–134.

11. Michael Romano, "Money and Politics: AMA's Lobbying Tab Surges in Second Half of 2000," *Modern Healthcare* (November 12, 2001), p. 14.

12. Lawrence R. Jacobs, "The Politics of America's Supply State: Health Reform and Technology," *Health Affairs* 14, no. 2 (Summer 1995): 143–157. See also Lawrence D. Brown, "Who Shall Pay? Politics, Money and Health Care Reform," *Health Affairs* 13, no. 2 (Spring 1994): 175–184, and "Commissions, Clubs and Consensus: Reform in Florida," *Health Affairs* 12, no. 2 (Summer 1993): 7–26.

13. Alberto Alesina and Allan Drazen, "Why Are Stabilizations Delayed?" *American Economic Review* 81, no. 5 (1991): 1170–1188.

14. Charles Wolfe Jr., *Markets or Governments: Choosing Between Imperfect Alternatives* (Cambridge, Mass.: MIT Press, 1994).

15. Eleena de Lisser, "Ready or Not, Firms Rush to Sell the Public on Laser Eye Surgery," *The Wall Street Journal* (August 24, 1995): A1, A8.

CHAPTER 15

PUBLIC GOODS AND PUBLIC HEALTH

QUESTIONS

1. Should treatment of syphilis be part of the public health system or private medical care? What about psoriasis? Psychosis? Scoliosis?

2. Why not charge people full price for vaccinations?

3. Why are new surgical techniques developed with public funds whereas pharmaceutical research and development is conducted privately by for-profit firms?

4. Who paid for Pasteur to discover bacteria?

5. Why pay for cost-benefit analysis to decide which public programs are worthwhile instead of using prices to let the market decide?

6. Do the preferences of smokers, patients who are mentally ill, or unborn children count when assessing the efficiency of the public health system?

7. Is medical care for homeless and terminally ill AIDS patients a public good or a waste of money?

8. Are "free goods" like air or the theory of relativity public goods? Are they costly?

15.1 CHARACTERISTICS OF PUBLIC GOODS

It is not possible to charge for some goods because no one can be excluded from using them (e.g., clean air), and there are other goods no one wants to charge for because there is no cost to accommodate additional users (e.g., a news release reporting the discovery that eating oranges cures scurvy). How easy and how desirable it is to use market pricing to ration goods or to exclude people from using a service determines whether it is part of public health or private health care. The two dimensions of "publicness," the ability to enforce exclusion with prices and the marginal cost of accommodating additional users, are illustrated in Figure 15.1. A knee brace is costly to produce and easy to charge for. Therefore, it is a pure private good. Arthroscopic surgery for knees falls between being a private good and a public good. Although the surgery has a relatively constant average cost per unit, the development of surgical techniques and instruments is more like a public good. Once knowledge is obtained, it can be used over and over again. It is relatively easy to charge for the surgery, but a bit difficult to charge for the years of development work. Polio vaccine is more of a public good. Once discovered, the cost of production per dose, although constant, is almost negligible. Although it would be relatively easy to charge users for vaccination, it

FIGURE 15.1   Dimensions of Publicness

would not be economically desirable to do so, since the benefits of freeing the population of disease are externalities that benefit everyone, not just the user. The monitoring of infectious disease by the Centers for Disease Control and Prevention (CDC) to discover epidemics is a pure public good. If the agency is successful, there are fewer epidemics, and there is no way to charge individuals for preventing a mass tragedy that does not happen. Also, once the CDC's *Morbidity and Mortality Weekly Report* is printed, there is essentially no additional cost for having more physicians use CDC data to protect their patients.

Publicness can vary with local conditions. A congested suburban hospital can readily charge for services, whereas a quiet rural hospital that is three-quarters empty most of the time cannot. Most of the benefits the community derives from the rural hospital come from the hospital just being there in case of an emergency (option demand) rather than from use of services. There also are goods that are publicly provided, even though some amount could be sold privately. Motor vehicle inspections are required, and thus do not depend on owners' willingness to pay, because there is a compelling public interest in having a car's brakes and emission control system work properly to protect other people. A social calculation of costs and benefits must supersede market pricing.

Privatizing Public Goods

Prescription drugs are an interesting case of a public good being privatized. Once a discovery is made and validated through clinical trials, the actual costs of production are nearly zero. However, unlike vaccine, which benefits the public by inhibiting communicable disease, most of the benefits from a prescription drug accrue to the user. Patent law gives the firm a monopoly on the drug for 17 years so that it can charge users for the sunk costs of discovery and testing.[1] Geographic enclosure also privatizes public goods.

Thus, residents of a resort community will pay privately for maintaining the cleanliness of a lake and have private agreements to limit noise and pollution. Externalities arise primarily because the costs and benefits are borne by different people so that one or the other is external to the market transaction. Patent laws, enclosed communities, and membership clubs are examples of internalizing effects so that government intervention is less necessary.

Social Costs Depend on the Number of People

The extent of externalities depends on the magnitude of the costs and the number of people involved. For example, very strict sterilization procedures are followed for spacecraft because of the possibility that extraterrestrial bacteria could threaten the health of the entire world. Airplane accidents are scrutinized by government safety inspectors more carefully than automobile accidents, and nuclear power plant failures are even more closely scrutinized. The larger the number of people who could be hurt, the more thorough the investigation.

Garbage disposal is an example of how the treatment of public goods changes with the number of people involved.[2] In prehistoric times, people did whatever they pleased with their garbage and no one worried about a waste disposal system. The same is true today in isolated rural areas where people toss the garbage out in the woods or bury or burn it. Keeping one's own house tidy and the neighbors happy is sufficient incentive to maintain a social optimum, and no government rules are needed. However, as people move closer together, creating a town, the divergence between private and social costs widens. Dumping trash in fields or in the yards of strangers rapidly creates a problem. Therefore, rules are formulated designating when and where garbage can be dumped. As the town becomes larger, public spending becomes necessary to handle all the garbage produced. Land is purchased and set aside to serve as a dump. As the town becomes a city, it is not enough just to have a dump; the city must actively collect all the trash and carry it to the dump. Taxes are imposed and trucks come around to collect garbage at people's houses. In this way the private costs of conforming to the social optimum are minimized. Garbage collection is a public activity that requires collective financing through taxes, but the actual work can be done by a private firm, and often is.

Insurance Makes Any Good More Public

Whenever a service is financed through third-party insurance rather than directly by individual purchasers, the service becomes more of a public good. When individuals purchase a good, one person may choose high quality, another low; one wants the color to be blue while the other wants it green; and so on. Within a risk-pooling group, they all become the same. Whether the person being treated is a vice-president of marketing or an assistant janitor, the hospital gets paid the same amount. It is possible for insurance companies to provide extensive coverage for plastic surgery and 200 days of mental health coverage, but everyone in the benefit plan must get it. The differentiation between individuals by payment is eliminated. The quality of services covered by the insurance package is a public good. There is no gain to the janitor for seeking out a cheap hospital, since even if the company does obtain some savings, it won't make insurance any cheaper to the janitor personally. Thus, once medical care is financed on a group basis, any change in quality or standards of service affects everyone and requires collective action.

15.2   INFORMATION

Research on new drugs, new surgical techniques, and new methods of diagnostic imaging is popular and receives billions of dollars in public funding. However, it is the collection of statistics over many years and from millions of patients that makes it possible to determine how medical discoveries work in practice. Statistics and scientific discoveries are both forms of information and are almost pure public goods.[3] Once statistics have been tabulated or a discovery has been made, there are no additional costs incurred as more and more people use them (zero cost). Once discoveries are known, there is no way to stop anyone from using them, regardless of whether or not they have paid for them (zero charges). The discovery of bacteria by Louis Pasteur began a revolution in the treatment of disease. It also saved the wool industry from the plague of anthrax, which had been decimating sheep (Pasteur's original research project); the wine and beer industries, which were having trouble with fermentation irregularities; and the dairy industry, whose unpasteurized products caused diarrhea and many fatalities among infants.[4] Much of Pasteur's work was supported by government grants, just as medical research is today. No single person or firm could obtain enough benefits to justify spending the money required to fund such a large research and development project. It was a collective enterprise. However, there were still many free riders. Although the costs were paid mostly by France and, to a lesser extent, by some industrialists in Belgium and Germany, people in the United States, Africa, China, and the rest of the world benefited. To the extent that those who benefit do not contribute, there is underinvestment in the development of knowledge.

Information is created not only through new discoveries, but also through the compilation and organization of existing data. A landmark breakthrough in the history of medicine and public health was the printing of *Observations on the Bills of Mortality*, by John Graunt, in 1662.[5] Graunt studied death records in the city of London and tabulated the number of people dying each year and their causes of death, thus creating the first modern work in the science of epidemiology. With the causes of death plainly laid out, the years of plague and the probable effects (or lack of effects) of government attempts to improve the health of citizens could be seen.

Measurement and statistics do not come into being just because it is a good thing to have them; they must serve an economic purpose. The census that recorded Mary and Joseph at the birth of Jesus of Nazareth was mandated to enable Caesar to collect taxes. Deaths historically have been recorded to establish inheritance, not to study the effects of medical treatment. The provision of universal public benefits, such as Social Security, made it possible for the United States to easily enforce the requirement that all deaths be recorded. The fact that collecting information is costly explains why there are more statistics on health care expenditures (which must be recorded on each transaction to pay employees, bill insurance companies, and so on) than on medical diagnosis or treatment effectiveness. The U.S. Centers for Medicare and Medicaid Services (CMS) (which has power because it controls the funds) is setting standards for a "uniform bill" that will be submitted electronically by all hospitals and doctors and thus provide an integrated database for comparing the costs and effects of all types of medical care. Potentially, this will not only reduce the administrative costs of running the system, it will also make it possible for researchers to tap into an online database with hundreds of millions of patient years of experience and, therefore, rapidly determine which treatments, types of hospitals, drugs, and so on are most cost-effective.

The National Institutes of Health (NIH) has overall responsibility for medical research in the United States, and the National Center for Health Statistics (NCHS) is responsible for data collection and distribution. NCHS's oldest and most important publication is its *Vital Statistics Reports* on births and deaths. NCHS also conducts surveys on health and nutrition status, insurance coverage, and the characteristics of patients treated in doctors' offices, and compiles statistics on patients discharged from hospitals using billing records. All this information is made available in "public use data tapes" and in free publications (which can be obtained from the library or the Web for your term paper) because it is a public good produced with public money. Those running the agency want to maximize the value of this "free" good so that they can argue for more funding from Congress—and, not incidentally, benefit all of us.

Rational Consumer Ignorance

Why does the government have a better information base for making decisions than most citizens? Because the government paid for it. From safety standards for seatbelts to the efficacy of vitamin supplements, millions of dollars have been spent to determine the best possible answers. Massively wasteful duplication would result if each consumer collected such information individually. If consumers banded together to share the costs of gathering information, such banding would constitute a form of government. Consumers are rationally ignorant of many health and safety issues because it is more efficient to have the government collect information once than for each of us to do it separately. Rational consumer ignorance is sensible free riding. Even for a private good, such as a bottle of vitamins, it is cheaper to perform quality control once in a government laboratory than to do it over and over again in each individual's home.

Consumers remain rationally ignorant by delegating their decision-making powers to the government because it is more efficient for them to do so—they are being smart by staying stupid! Thus, the Food and Drug Administration (FDA) tests the safety of food and drugs, the Environmental Protection Agency (EPA) conducts studies on the effects of pollution, and the Department of Transportation (DOT) monitors the safety of highways and motor vehicles.

Milk or Bread: Which Is More Public?

Whether goods should fall in the public or private arena depends on the characteristics of the goods and the way they are produced and transacted. In general, if something is produced collectively so that one person's consumption cannot easily be separated from another's, more government intervention is called for. If the relevant characteristics are readily observable by consumers at the time of purchase, more reliance on private markets is appropriate. Consider two products that are consumed by almost everyone: milk and bread. Milk was subjected to government regulations more than a hundred years ago, and public milk-dispensing stations were set up in New York and other cities.[6] It is now illegal in most states to sell milk that has not been inspected and processed according to government standards. Bread, although under routine surveillance as a food, is largely unregulated. Why this difference in treatment?

Bread may be mixed in batches, but each loaf is baked separately, and the baking process kills most germs. When bread gets old after sitting on the shelf too long, it becomes stale and hard, and green and white furry spots start growing on it. These signs of deterioration are readily visible to consumers. Milk from many dairies is mixed together when it is being processed for sale; thus, contamination at any one dairy potentially threatens thousands of consumers. Contamination is most likely to occur during the milking process and can best be prevented by keeping the cows clean, keeping the equipment sterilized, and sweeping the manure out of the barn. On-site inspection is the best way to cheaply enforce cleanliness and can be performed at moderate cost by government agents, but it would be prohibitively costly for consumers to visit all the dairies their milk comes from each week and check the floors. Bacteria are killed during the processing of milk, but how is a consumer to know that the "pasteurized" label on the carton is to be believed? When the crucial quality-control step can be monitored efficiently only during processing and compliance is not easily discernable at the point of sale, government oversight and labeling are called for. Most of the dangerous bacteria that people can get from milk, particularly salmonella, do not make milk curdle or smell bad and thus are hard to detect. Milk is an ideal culture medium for many bacteria, making milk distribution, in effect, a perfect way to spread disease. Contamination from one farm cannot be determined later because milk from all the farms is mixed together. The bacteria rapidly grow to infect all the milk and are delivered invisibly, with much of the product going to the most vulnerable segment of the population, children.

Many factors make milk more suitable for government regulation, but the crucial issue is which information consumers can easily obtain at the point of sale. Bad bread is visible to consumers; bad milk is not. The information necessary to protect the safety of the public is available at low cost if regulations are enforced *during production*, a process that would be prohibitively costly for consumers to carry out on their own. The asymmetry of information costs makes milk quality a public good, whereas the quality of bread is largely private.

Given the benefits of good information for both science and political management, it seems that often there is too little of it around. Problems frequently have to reach the crisis stage before the necessary information is collected, and decisions regarding thousands of lives or billions of dollars are made without adequate study. The difficulty lies in the conflict between individual and collective incentives. A lot of data may be useful in solving a public problem, but it is in the interest of no particular person to collect that data unless that person can benefit from it. Even if the person can benefit, he or she will not be able to devote enough resources to the problem because their personal benefits are much less than the total benefits to society as a whole. To see more clearly why free-riding leads to persistent underproduction, it is necessary to consider the theory of pure public goods in more detail.[7]

15.3   THE THEORY OF PURE PUBLIC GOODS

Information is a public good, but it can be provided privately as well as publicly. For example, people may purchase cable television by paying for each channel or show, or they may tap into a broadcast, which is a public good paid for through taxes, donations, advertising, or other collective means. To more meaningfully address the question, "How much of a public good should society produce?" we will consider a society made up of three people, Ann, Bob, and Carl, who can either purchase TV from the cable company at $5 per channel or contribute through taxes to have the signal broadcast to everyone at a collective cost of $10 per channel. The private demand and supply for TV channels for Ann, Bob, and Carl is shown in Figure 15.2a. The total private market demand for this three-person market is obtained by adding horizontally the quantity demanded by each person at any given price, as shown in Figure 15.2b. For example, at a price of $10, Ann would purchase one channel, Bob would purchase three channels, and Carl would not purchase any channels; therefore, total market demand at $10 would be $1 + 3 + 0 = 4$. Similarly, at a price of $5 per channel, market demand would be $2 + 5 + 0 = 7$, and at a price of $1 per channel, it would be $3 + 7 + 4 = 14$.

| FIGURE 15.2 | Public and Private Demand Curves |

(a) Private individual demand and supply curves

(b) Private market demand and supply for all three people

(c) Public goods quasi-demand curve and supply for all three people

The market equilibrium with a perfectly elastic (flat horizontal line) supply curve at a price of $5 per channel is for seven channels to be sold, two to Ann, five to Bob, and none to Carl.

The demand for a public good is different. If the government provides one public channel paid for with taxes, everyone gets to watch it. The value of that public good is the value of the service to each member of society added together. In this example, the marginal value of the first channel is $10 to Ann, $15 to Bob, and $4 to Carl, for a total social value of $29. Similarly, the second channel has a marginal value of $5 + $12.50 + $3 = $20.50, the third $0 + $10 + $2 = $12, and the sixth $0 + $2.50 + $0 = $2.50. Whereas the quantities are added horizontally in Figure 15.2b to find total market demand at a specified price for a private consumption market, the values are added vertically at a specified quantity to find total social value for a public good, as in Figure 15.2c.[8]

Public Versus Private Demand Curves

Social Demand Curve for Public Goods: for each quantity Q,

$$\text{Value}_{\text{total}} = V_A + V_B + V_C$$

Market Demand Curve for Private Goods: for each price P,

$$\text{Quantity}_{\text{total}} = Q_A + Q_B + Q_C$$

The cost of broadcasting a channel to everyone is $10, twice as much as the price of providing it on cable to just one person. It is beneficial for society to produce more of the public good as long as the marginal cost is less than the additional value; therefore, the social optimum is reached at the intersection of the public good marginal cost "supply" curve and the public good quasi-demand curve. In this example, three channels would be supplied at a total cost of $30, because the marginal cost of a fourth channel ($10) exceeds the value to the members of society ($0 + $7.50 + 1 = $8.50).

Public Goods Make Most People Better Off, but Few Happy

In the private market, with channels selling for $5 each, Ann paid $10 for two and Bob paid $25 for five. Who will pay the $30 to broadcast three public channels? Suppose that a tax of $10 is collected from each person. Ann is indifferent to public versus private provision. Although giving up some flexibility, by participating in society she gets one additional channel for the same amount as she was previously paying. Carl is mad and wants to start a taxpayer's revolt. He paid nothing before and now must pay $10 for stations he barely wants. The consumer's surplus ($4 + $3 + $2 = $9) he obtains from getting three TV channels "for free" is worth less to him than the new taxes he has to pay. Carl has an incentive to understate his demand to get the government to provide less. He might say, "I hate the stuff and, as you can tell, don't watch it. If it has to be there, don't make me pay for it." If Carl could force the government to back down from the social optimum and provide just one channel, he would be better off, although both Bob and Ann would be worse off.

Bob loves TV and gets a large consumer's surplus. The value of three stations to him ($15 + $12.50 + $10 = $37.50) far exceeds the new $10 tax. But he is not happy, either. He complains that he used to get five channels and now that the government has taken over, he only gets three! Bob wants five public TV channels. Although these two extra channels would cost $20, he would only get taxed to cover a third of the cost, or $6.67. To a certain extent, Bob would be a partial free rider. He would push for more TV channels than he would be willing to buy in a private market. Even though Bob and Ann are unhappy, they are both better off. Carl is only slightly ($1) worse off. The group as a whole is clearly better off using public provision, but each individual has a reason to complain and try to get a different deal.

For public goods, cost-benefit analysis must replace market pricing as a mechanism for resource allocation and rationing. Voting and administrative procedures are used to make public decisions. In a private market, people who value services more highly pay more to get them. Since a social optimum depends on values, why doesn't government tax people depending on how much they want the services? Besides being unfair (imagine saying to someone, "Since your broken leg forces you to stay at home, we want to double your public

TV taxes"), it cannot readily be done because there is no way to tell how much someone values a public good. In a private market, the act of purchasing demonstrates people's willingness to pay and reveals how much they value the good. With public goods, however, there is no purchase. In our example, both Bob and Carl watch all three public TV stations, but Bob values them more. Suppose we sent a questionnaire asking how much each person likes TV as a basis for adjusting individuals' tax rates. Why should Bob reveal how much he likes TV and then pay more? His paying more will not increase the number of stations. Conversely, Carl will say, "I don't care one bit, nothing, nada, zilch," because he wants to pay $0 and still be able to watch all three channels. This is why Figure 15.2c is only a *quasi*-demand curve. It does not show the choices people make in a market, only what we estimate they should do to optimize social value.

To get the government to provide more "free" services, Bob and people like him have an incentive to overstate their demands because most of the cost will be borne by the rest of the public. Since public goods are provided at no charge, there is no way to use market behavior to gauge demand. Everyone's self-interests might lead them to lie on the questionnaire to get more services. The sensible thing for Bob and every other interest group to do is to act as a rational free rider: always tell their elected officials that they want more and the tax collector that they want less. There is no simple way to get everybody to agree on the social optimum once we consider not only the benefits and who will get them, but also the costs and who will pay them. The social value function is only a quasi-demand curve, because the voluntary actions of individuals will never allow society to reach the optimum and will only lead to name-calling, avoidance, and unstable coalitions (also known as "politics").

The provision of a public good poses two problems: how much of it to provide and how to pay for it. Neither is solvable through individual action. For example, a swimming pool is a semi-public good after it is built; it does not cost very much to allow one more person to use it, yet people can be easily excluded. The pool could be paid for collectively through taxes so that each person would pay the same amount or according to income. It is also possible to pay for the pool with user fees. This way the people who value swimming the most, and go to the pool often, will pay more. However, neither method will get to the social optimum. If we depend entirely on taxes, taxpayers will not be willing to build as many pools as the social demand curve indicates. If user fees are imposed, some swimmers (such as the poor 10-year old who wants to train for the Olympics) will be denied entrance even though the marginal cost of using the pool is $0. The actual method chosen to fund a service depends on the transaction costs particular to that case (pools, yes; clean air, no; TV used to be no and now yes, sort-of). How purely public is the good? Can users be easily charged for use? Can we tell what aggregate demand will be? Are people able and willing to acknowledge their demand up front and promise to pay or vote for the proposed program? (schools, maybe; venereal disease clinics, maybe not). Is a dedicated revenue source available? (Examples would be recurrent proposals to put a tax on hospital bills to fund indigent care and the near-universality of room and airport taxes to extract money from tourists). Is anyone likely to sue?

Purchasing of public goods is problematic even if the money can be raised. Since no particular person has a comprehensive interest in making sure that all the goods contracted for are delivered or that the quality is adequate, a supplier may extract some of the social benefits by providing poor service or inferior goods. Even if we all want a good army, or hospital, or national weather service, none of us individually is willing to spend our time making sure that those who are paid to provide these public goods are actually doing their jobs and doing them efficiently. The free-rider problem goes beyond payment; it makes the enforcement of public contracts more difficult.

15.4 INFECTIOUS DISEASE EXTERNALITIES

One way of looking at the publicness of a good is to ask how much one person's action affects the welfare of other people. As discussed earlier, a mistake by the bread baker will have only a limited effect on consumers, whereas a failure in sanitary procedures at the dairy could cause illness or even death among thousands. Economists observe that milk has more externalities than bread. Infectious disease is a classic example of externalities and the basis for many public health laws. The author's first job was as a sexually transmitted diseases (STD) investigator for the city of New York. Why were tax dollars used to pay civil servants to find out who was infected and who they had sex with, and to bring these people to the clinic for penicillin shots? Didn't people who were infected already have sufficient incentive to come in for treatment? No. Infection creates externalities. The one who is infected bears the personal costs of disease and treatment, but does not bear the cost imposed on society by increasing everyone else's risk of infection. The divergence between private and social costs means that people are not sufficiently motivated to seek treatment. Consider what would happen if you discovered that you are infected. Whether you get treated this week or next week may not make much difference to you, but it may significantly affect the risk you impose on others.

Sexual transmission of diseases heightens the divergences between private and social costs of infection because stigmatization makes information harder to come by. The desire for privacy increases transaction costs. With the flu, everyone knows when you are sick. With syphilis or gonorrhea, the symptoms are usually unobservable, even by your sexual partner. Whereas coughing is a costless signal of flu infection, you must be told that you have been exposed to an STD. This is difficult for most people because it marks them as infected and involves the admission that they have been having sexual relations with others. Although it is beneficial to society as a whole that all your sexual partners be notified that you are infected, it is often costly to you personally—it may cost you some friends, a marriage, or a job. The U.S. Public Health Service (PHS) developed a rule of anonymity to minimize the costs of acting in the interests of society. When sexual contacts are notified to come in for treatment, they are not told who has given their name. One client showed up with his wife and three girlfriends (yes, all at once, in the same room) and demanded to know who had been infected. Although it may have been in his interest to know, violating confidentiality would make it more difficult for the PHS to get people to divulge sensitive information.

Day care centers are a useful and familiar example of infection externalities. Parents with a child who is slightly sick, or who might be coming down with a cold, face a difficult choice. If they stay home with the child, they miss a day of work; if they send the child to day care, other children will be exposed. The first cost is borne personally, but the costs of other children getting sick is a social cost borne by the other parents. Therefore, many busy parents faced with deadlines at work make a decision that is in their own best interests and drop the slightly sick child off at day care. Day care workers hate this and have developed a rule that if a child does get sick at day care, the parents must come immediately and take the child home or they will be fined and/or barred from the facility. The day care facility is deliberately trying to increase the costs of bringing in a sick child to force parents to act in accordance with the collective good, to take account of social costs.

Epidemics

Sudden upsurges in disease have had profound effects on the course of human civilization: the black death of the Middle Ages; the Biblical plagues that afflicted the people of Egypt;

tuberculosis, syphilis, a pandemic (worldwide epidemic) flu outbreak in 1918 that killed hundreds of thousands of young people; and most recently, AIDS.[9] The externality imposed by contagion was recognized long before germs were identified as a cause of disease. Quarantine was among the earliest forms of public health action. In primitive societies, those who were visibly ill were sometimes banished from the tribe. As early as 1400 A.D., ships from ports where plague had been reported were kept out in the harbor for months to see whether any of the sailors would die. Only after sufficient time had passed for the authorities to convince themselves that the ship was not carrying disease was it allowed to unload. The public interest in disease reduction conflicted with the private interests of ship owners. Most of the costs of an epidemic (i.e., deaths) would fall on the population of the city, while the benefits of continuing to trade accrued to the merchants. The plot of the famous play *An Enemy of the People*, by Henrik Ibsen, centers on the disastrous consequences of ignoring the long-run risks of disease to pursue short-run profits.[10]

Leprosy may have been the first communicable disease brought under control by public health measures. Now known as Hansen's disease, after the scientist who discovered the causative agent, leprosy is a slow-growing bacterium that destroys the neural sheath and hence sensation. The infection itself is often less damaging than its side effects. People with leprosy cannot feel pain in the affected area; therefore, they may scratch an itch until they gouge their flesh away, or get burned without even knowing it, and so on. The bacterium is hard to transmit from person to person; thus, infection usually requires intimate contact over an extended period of time. People with leprosy were isolated from the rest of the population to halt the spread of the disease. Although the United States still had leper colonies until 1953, effective treatment with antibiotics has now removed the threat of contagion.

In the twelfth century, there were more than 200 hospitals for the confinement of lepers in France alone. Leprosy almost disappeared from medieval Europe, and permanent quarantine in hospitals appears to have played a significant role in reducing the incidence of disease. But consider the cost. Leprosy is a progressive disease. Without treatment, the person sent to a hospital was put away for life, without visitors. The church would hold a funeral for the leper, the family would mourn, and all the person's property would be passed on through inheritance, just as if that person had died. The signs and symptoms of leprosy (a scaly rash) are common to a variety of ordinary, nonserious disorders (psoriasis, scabies, skin allergy), making diagnosis difficult. Therefore many people without leprosy must also have been permanently confined in such hospitals (where presumably they caught leprosy after awhile anyway). The uncertainty of diagnosis and the severe consequences probably made people very reluctant to visit the doctor for a rash or to share information with neighbors. Claims of leprosy were more apt to be made against people who were not welcome within society (gypsies, Jews), and a disgruntled family member or impatient heir might assert that the wealthy grandfather had leprosy purely out of self-interest. Permanent quarantine probably did help protect the community, but at the cost of making a person with leprosy, or who was suspected of having leprosy, a nonperson. Only when epidemics caused high rates of mortality did the interests of the community (disease prevention) outweigh the interests of the individual (property, freedom).

HIV/AIDS

HIV/AIDS also illustrates economic issues in disease control and public policy.[11] When first diagnosed in the early 1980s, the costs of treatment were very high. The first official estimate, made in 1987, was $147,000 per patient. Subsequent estimates became lower over time. One reason for declining costs was economies of scale. As more cases were treated, unit costs went down. There was specialization of labor as dedicated AIDS units were established, and also movement down the learning curve as infectious disease specialists became better at managing the opportunistic illnesses that affect immuno-compromised people. There was a growing recognition that medical care served an important humanitarian purpose. A crash program of medical research brought about major advances in an incredibly short time span—less than a decade. However, the new protease inhibitor combination treatments that successfully reduced symptoms and increased a patient's ability to function did not cure the infection, they only suppressed it. Thus the extension of life implied increasing the number of years of expensive medical therapy.

HIV/AIDS also increased insurance market failure, due to adverse selection. The association between frequency, type, and number of sexual partners and HIV/AIDS means that the individual may possess private information about risk not available to an insurance company. People who are HIV-positive know they will need considerable medical care in the near future; therefore, insurance companies offering individual policies covering HIV/AIDS would be swamped by purchasers from this 100 percent risk group. The inevitability of illness makes it almost impossible for someone who is HIV-positive to change jobs and switch insurance plans if there is any exclusion of pre-existing conditions. The appearance of a fatal disease at an early age disrupts many economic relationships. A bank might wonder why an 83-year old man wants to borrow $250,000 and be unwilling to lend without security since he no longer has a job, but be quite happy to lend this amount to an employed 33-year-old man to buy a house. However, if the young man is HIV-positive, he might actually want the money to pay his medical bills and the living expenses of his partner, and may figure that there is little the bank can do to collect on the debt when he dies. Therefore, the bank is inadvertently thrust into the role of supplying life insurance to people at high risk. Developing the social mechanisms to deal with the consequences of the AIDS epidemic on economic contracts will take awhile, and it is hoped that a cure will be available long before financial institutions have to make a full adjustment.

The Sanitary Revolution: A Moral Campaign for Public Health

The public health reforms that reduced the threat of cholera, diphtheria, typhoid, and other communicable diseases were part of the nineteenth century social revolution that imposed Victorian middle-class values on society as a whole.[12] Posters that attacked working conditions in the coal mines did not stress that workers had to eat stooped over while standing in pools of water that collected human waste, but instead the fact that women working underground were stripped to the waist because of the heat. Mandating that children under the age of 12 work no more than 10 hours a day seemed an act of kindness, not an attempt to prevent premature disability. Above all else, Victorians hated dirt, and so the social reformers wanted cleanliness and light—which happened to be effective in reducing the spread of infectious disease, although there was no way to know that given the science of the time. A belief in what was morally right, not scientific evidence, underlay the English sanitary revolution.

Not all attempts to remove dirt and immorality proved to be healthful. Sending women to maternity hospitals instead of having a midwife attend birth at home caused the spread of puerperal (childbirth) fever and a rapid increase in maternal mortality. The replacement of breast-feeding with sterile bottles deprived middle-class infants of maternal immunities. Diseases of poverty, such as pellagra, were so consistently blamed on lack of cleanliness and insects that the mounting evidence of dietary deficiency was ignored. The sanitary revolution did much to clean up the environmental mess created as industrial urbanization brought masses of people together in cities, but science was decidedly secondary to morality and ideology. The net result was beneficial overall, but quite unbalanced. These historical lessons are worth remembering as we attempt to evaluate the hazards of environmental carcinogens and other public health issues today.

Formation of the U.S. Public Health Service

The U.S. Public Health Service had it origins in the merchant seamen's hospital founded in 1798.[13] The rationale for government involvement was threefold. First, seamen were engaged in international trade and ships frequently carried diseases between countries, so the government had an interest in making sure that the seamen were willing to report any illnesses. Second, medical care was mostly provided at home by one's family, but sailors spent years abroad on ships and rarely had families to depend on. Ordinary laborers without kin who became sick or disabled were the responsibility of local communities, but sailors were travelers who might have been born in Boston or Chicago or Kankakee or anywhere, and thus could not rely on any town to support them in their time of need. Third, international trade was vital to the economic growth of the nation. Unless the national government was willing to take care of people who became ill or disabled, few would have been willing to leave home and become sailors.

Public health activity was much more limited in the United States than in England during the nineteenth century. American cities were not as old, or as crowded. There were fewer innovations in the United States, but European social programs and sanitary reforms were quickly adopted. Massachusetts set up the first state board of health following the Shattuck report in 1850. By 1900 the New York City health department had become an active center with special support programs for immigrants and free sterile milk distribution for mothers and children. The Pure Food and Drug Act was passed in 1906, and in 1920 the Shepard-Towner Act provided the first national government-sponsored medical care for mothers and dependent children. Other milestones in U.S. public health include the formation in 1952 of the National Institutes of Health, now by far the largest public health agency, to conduct medical research; the 1965 passage of amendments XVIII and XIX to the Social Security Act, which established Medicare and Medicaid; and the 1970 acts creating the Environmental Protection Agency (EPA) and the Occupational Safety and Health Administration (OSHA).

15.5 SEX, DRUGS, AND WAR: PUBLIC HEALTH IN ACTION

Government uses police powers to enforce health and safety regulations. It acts as the agent of all citizens to perform collectively beneficial activities more efficiently than individuals could on their own. Rules made by the people and for the people are not an intrusion on liberty, but a way of making the people more free by maintaining order. Government is not there to enforce public health standards because people are too ignorant to know what is in their own best interests. Instead, government exists so that citizens can remain rationally ignorant and devote their time to sports, making money, and art rather than checking the temperature at the pasteurization facility each hour. However, government does sometimes intercede directly against the will of the individual, overruling his or her own desires. Such paternalism is based not on ignorance, but on a determination that the individual is incompetent; thus, it is reserved for people who are assumed to be unable to make decisions on their own: children, addicts, the mentally ill and retarded.

Sexual behavior reveals some of the underlying value judgments that are at the heart of any paternalistic decision to override individual decision-making authority. For centuries, children's sexual behavior fell under the control of parents because inheritance was a major form of economic exchange. Thus, the rules regarding whom to have sex with for the aristocracy (who had inheritable land) were much different from the rules for the peasantry. Aristocrats, who were not allowed to have sex with the 17-year-old sons and daughters of neighboring lords, could have sex with their serfs because any children born from such a union had no property rights.

Sexual preferences are value laden, with active debates over homosexual marriage and the acceptability of gays and lesbians serving in the military and holding public office. The American Psychiatric Association until 1974 listed homosexuality as a disease and, although difficult to imagine today on a college campus with prominent gay organizations, young men and women then were treated for having the illness of "abnormal" desires. The labeling of behavior as illness is not limited to homosexuality. Activities such as eating pork, piercing lips and noses, circumcision, lying down to sleep with the dead, taking hallucinogenic drugs, speaking in tongues, and mortification of the flesh are viewed as normal or exemplary in some cultures and as clear signs of illness in others. The line between using power to make someone "do something for your own good" and dictatorial thought control is not always easily drawn, and it is rarely more contentious than when it touches on the continuation of society through procreation. In one society, it may be routine for a young person to be taken to a prostitute or religious center for sexual initiation, whereas in another such behavior would be seen as cruel or immoral.

Advocates for people with mental illness and mental retardation are willing to push for the fullest participation in "normal" activities, but are often placed in a quandary regarding the desire of the mentally disabled to have children, especially when the disability is genetically related. Can that person understand the consequences? Is it fair to the unborn child? Even if the child has no genetic abnormalities, is it fair to the child to be raised by parents whose capacity is severely constrained, making it likely that the child will be raised in a foster home? Externalities forcefully raise the question: Who counts, and do some count more than others?

Who Counts as a Citizen? Abortion and Other Dilemmas

Nowhere is the conflict over whose views are to count more apparent than in decisions regarding abortion. American society has been unable to achieve a clear resolution, and we will not attempt to do so here. What we can do is see how abortion poses a dilemma that affects many other problems in public health, and thus we will use it to clarify the nature of a general issue: Who is to be counted as a citizen, and do everyone's views count equally?

In the marketplace of third-century Rome, there was a law stating that no citizen could be sold a fish that was more than three days old (which, given the lack of refrigeration, seems plenty).[14] What happened to fish more than three days old? They were sold to noncitizens. Although this kind of blatantly discriminatory behavior seems inconceivable to us today, most countries follow similar policies. Pharmaceuticals that are not approved for use in the United States are routinely sold overseas, and for years many drugs whose shelf lives had expired were disposed of profitably this way. The most forceful statement regarding who is not a citizen, and what the country is willing to do to protect and enrich those who are its citizens, is war.

Even more difficult questions are posed by pregnancy. The right of a mother, as the one most proximately involved, to make decisions regarding her pregnancy seems reasonable, but it does elevate her rights over those of others. Could this position, if accepted logically, be used to claim that someone else is even more proximate (a grandparent for example, especially if the mother is incapacitated by substance abuse or illness)? This position is also directly in conflict with what pro-life activists describe as the right to life of the unborn child—*if* such an entity can be said to be a citizen. In general, societies seem to accede that mothers have special rights over their infants, and this extends with even greater force to before their birth. Yet this interest is not absolute. Similarly, it is accepted that a fetus does not have the same standing as a child. Consider how differently a court would treat a pregnant woman who took heroin because she was anxious and upset and a mother who gave the drug to her baby to keep the baby quiet. There is no social resolution to these issues other than in crafting some new set of rules and in agreeing to live, however uneasily, within them. It is possible that for many years two or more sets of rules will be in effect for different groups of people who can only agree not to talk about the issue or to fight in the courts rather than in the streets.

Ultimately the question of who counts as a citizen, and how much, is a moral one, but it is heavily conditioned by economic considerations, and transactions costs in particular. Experience has shown that it is virtually impossible to stop women who desperately want an abortion from having one. Making the practice illegal leads to many unsafe operations that cause infertility, disability, and death. Furthermore, any woman who can afford an airplane ticket to a country where abortions are legal can choose that option; thus, the practical effect may be to limit access for those who are young and poor and perhaps less able to care for a child. Indeed, the cost-benefit argument (that abortion is much cheaper than years of social services) may have sufficient appeal to some people that their moral positions are influenced by it. How strongly we support another person's right to self determination depends in part on our own self-interest.

Addiction

Addiction, which is sometimes treated as a mental illness, also reveals the tensions surrounding overrule of the individual by the state. Economists do not really understand addiction, but then, doctors don't either.[15] Many foods and substances are habit-forming, and many people have bad habits without engaging in self-destructive addictive behavior. Yet legally, a rather sharp distinction must be made between substances that are legal (e.g., candy, coffee, cigarettes, alcohol) and those that are not (e.g., steroids, marijuana, cocaine, heroin). The distinction is sometimes as much social and historical as it is biological. Heavy alcohol use is probably more likely to impair judgment and lead to injury than marijuana, and heroin taken regularly over years has fewer adverse physical effects than cigarettes. Yet alcohol has been a part of human culture for thousands of years and thus is not only well accepted, it is also subject to some social controls. Cigarettes are a relatively recent innovation. Only in the last 50 years have large numbers of people been able to afford to smoke many cigarettes daily. They are also a rather mild addiction and are cheaply available. Heroin, on the other hand, is such a powerful drug that addicts will do almost anything to get it, and illegality raises the price so high that it becomes necessary for many to steal to stay high. It is the externalities (stealing, dirty needles) rather than use that makes heroin so harmful to society. Cigarettes may be bad for your health, but they provide income to farmers, bring us sporting events, elect senators and representatives, and contribute mightily to the profits of large multinational firms. In trying to understand how morality is shaped by economics, it is useful to point out that the British Empire started a war with China to enforce its "right" to cross the border and sell opium to Chinese workers, a practice the Emperor wanted to prevent.

There is no way to fully separate the moral issues from the economic ones. Who is or is not a person, and how much their wishes are to be respected, is ultimately more than an economic decision, but it is always conditioned by economic factors. Government usually acts as a collective agent to carry out the wishes of (most) people, not as an omniscient ruler dictating standards of good behavior. Borderline cases can never be solved to everyone's satisfaction, and there will always be conflict over the appropriate boundaries of action for criminal and social justice.

War and Public Health

A common wall poster during the 1960s read, "War is not healthy for children or other living things." Activity dedicated to killing seems obviously inimical to public health, and indeed, the American Public Health Association has passed several resolutions condemning war. Yet many advances in public health have been associated with war: Florence Nightingale's reform of field hospitals during the Crimean War led to modern nursing, malaria was eradicated during the Spanish-American War, and the campaign against venereal disease and the development of rapid psychotherapy occurred during World Wars I and II. The number of times that medical breakthroughs occurred during or because of a war raises the question: How (un)healthy is war?

As economic historian Douglass North points out, competition between states forces them to meet the needs of the people.[16] A government with no rivals does not need to develop new technologies. When kings or countries are vying for people's loyalty, it is in their interest to build hospitals, clean up the water supply, and perform all the other public health activities that are costly but also yield net benefits to society. North points out that we cannot understand the development of laws and political organization unless we recognize that rulers put their own interests first. War has a positive long-term effect on medical science because it heightens the interest of rulers in the health of the population—sick civilians make lousy soldiers.

In every war throughout history, at least until the twentieth century, many more soldiers died from diseases than from wounds inflicted on the battlefield. Armies of 20,000 or more would gather and camp in open fields with no toilets or running water. Contamination of food and drink were a more likely cause of death than enemy attack. Even in battle, it was often infection rather than bullets that killed, because lack of sanitation made minor wounds fatal. Conscripts were often drawn from isolated villages and so had never been exposed to common diseases. The result was uniformed disaster. Armies that spent any long period together were decimated by disease. Rulers' incentives for finding ways to keep large numbers of people living in close proximity without illness and epidemics were much greater in war than in peacetime.

When the United States entered World War I, the first thing it did was to call up an army of young, healthy men. To the chagrin of leaders at that time, one out of every four volunteers was medically unfit for service. They had tuberculosis, or syphilis, or vision so poor that they could not shoot straight. Prior to this time, it had been assumed that Americans were much healthier than their European counterparts who lived in crowded conditions with less food. The 1917 mobilization was the first time the nation collected information on the health of its citizens on a large scale, and the results were appalling. After the war, campaigns for the control of disease and malnutrition were promoted based on the data collected at induction centers.

The war also radically changed the practice of medicine. What had been a local trade practiced without a license was transformed in the military. Standards to determine how diseases should be treated and which doctors should be in charge were established. Physicians who had never seen modern medicine were educated by three years of practice in an organized setting, with antiseptic surgery under anesthesia saving thousands of lives. New occupations were developed to assist the harried field surgeons, and the organization of medicine was decisively changed from solo individual practice to cooperative expertise centered in the hospital. Although most people were skeptical of medical science at the turn of the century, the stories and living examples of what medicine could do were spread as the injured soldiers returned home throughout America.

War changes the calculus of individual costs and benefits. As the collective interest looms larger, massive investments in new knowledge and infrastructure are made. The attempt to place as many men as possible on the front lines leads to the rapid acquisition of knowledge on nutrition, surgery, psychology, and infectious disease. Without ignoring the shameful horror of death and destruction that wars impose on humankind, the fact that they have been a powerful force in advancing public health must be recognized.

SUGGESTIONS FOR FURTHER READING

American Journal of Public Health and *Public Health Reports*, published monthly.
Senator William R. Frist, M.D., "Public Health and National Security: The Critical Role of Increased Federal Support," *Health Affairs* 21, no. 6 (November 2002): 117–130.
Institute of Medicine, *Public Health in Crisis* (Washington, D.C.: National Academy Press, 1990).
John R. Lumpkin and Margaret S. Richards, "Transforming the Public Health Information Infrastructure," *Health Affairs* 21, no. 6 (November 2002): 45–56.
George Rosen, *A History of Public Health* (New York: MD Publications, 1958).
Paul Samuelson, "A Diagrammatic Exposition of a Theory of Public Expenditure," *Review of Economics and Statistics* (November 1955).
U.S. Centers for Disease Control and Prevention (http://www.cdc.gov/).

SUMMARY

1. A **pure public good** is something that is **consumed collectively** by all. It is indivisible so that **no one can be excluded** (zero charges), and one person's consumption has no effect on another's **(zero marginal costs)**. Examples are clean air, statistics, and the discovery of penicillin.

2. Many goods are both public and private. The degree of **publicness** of a good increases with **the number of people**, the use of **insurance**, and the **transactions, information, and measurement costs**.

3. Although decisions about private goods can be made through the market, the **indivisibility** of public goods **means that governments must make these decisions through voting**, political compromises, or cost-benefit analysis. Invariably, this means that there is a **moral or social justice** dimension as well as an economic one.

4. **Externalities** are said to exist when the actions of one person affect another (e.g., smoking, disposing of garbage). Infectious disease externalities have shaped public health, from the foundation of the U.S. Public Health Service as the homeless seaman's hospital to the pasteurization of milk. The increased risk of infecting others is a cost the individual does not bear, and government intervention is required to achieve (or get closer to) an optimum level of prevention.

5. To improve public health, it is necessary to determine exactly **who the public is**; whether some people or **some preferences count more than others**. Conflict over who is and is not worthwhile and able to make decisions lies at the heart of some of the most contentious public health issues: abortion, substance abuse, and care of people with mental illness.

6. People's **attitudes toward a particular public good** are always affected by their **private interests**. Universal access to high-quality medical care and redistribution of goods and services *may* be important public goods. Whether you think so depends a lot on whether you are poor or identify with those who are.

7.   **Competition** between governments over the provision of public goods may be just as important as competition between people or firms in creating economic efficiency, particularly in **forcing beneficial change over time**.

PROBLEMS

1.   {*property rights, public goods*} Why is most drug research paid for by companies, whereas most medical research is paid for by the government?

2.   {*public goods*} Explain which item in the following pairs is more "public" and why:

   a.   AIDS or lung cancer

   b.   Milk or bread

   c.   Saturday morning cartoons or a Sunday night late show

   d.   Stroke or lung cancer

3.   {*externalities*} Why not charge people full price for vaccinations?

4.   {*welfare*} Which type of good is apt to have a larger consumers' surplus: a public good or a private good? Why?

5.   {*property rights, scale*} Why have wars often given rise to improvements in medical technology?

6.   {*property rights*} Caring for the poor costs money, much more than they are able to pay directly or in taxes. Why would different government jurisdictions compete to provide medical care for the poor?

7.   {*incidence, voting*} Many goods are desired by some people and not by others. Since diversity of tastes is universal, why does it create more problems for public goods than for private goods?

8.   {*aggregation*} Draw the demand and supply curves for (**a**) a public good and (**b**) a private good for two people, Adam and Barbara, and (**c**) the market demand for a two-person (Adam + Barbara) market.

9.   {*exclusivity, marginal cost*} Some forms of health care are public because the marginal cost of serving additional people is zero. Other types of health care are public, even though marginal costs are positive, because it is impossible to exclude beneficiaries who do not pay. Some forms of care meet both criteria—zero marginal costs and a lack of exclusivity. Give examples of all three categories (recognizing that no real goods or services are perfectly public or fall entirely in one category or another).

10.   {*welfare*} Why pay economists to conduct a cost-benefit analysis for a new medical technology if the market will show its value to consumers?

11.   {*public goods*} Which has more externalities: cigars or chewing tobacco? Guns or knives? Laptop computers or portable telephones?

12.   {*externalities*} What are the externalities of heroin addiction?

ENDNOTES

1.   After 17 years, other firms can manufacture the drug in generic form if they meet certain standards and obtain approval from the FDA. See Chapter 11 and also Sam Peltzman, *The Regulation of Pharmaceutical Innovation: the 1962 Amendments* (Washington, D.C.: American Enterprise Institute, 1974).

2.   Elizabeth Fee and Steven Corey, *Garbage: The History and Politics of Trash in New York* (New York: New York Public Library, 1994).

3. Donald A. Dunn and Aristides C. Fronistas, "Economic Models of Information Services Markets," in Robert Goldberg and Harold Lorin, eds., *The Economics of Information Processes* (New York: Wiley, 1982), Vol. 1: 141–162; Michael R. Rubin, *Information Economics and Policy in the United States* (Littleton, Colo.: Libraries Unlimited, 1983).

4. Bruno Latour, *The Pasteurization of France* (Cambridge, Mass: Harvard University Press, 1988).

5. John Graunt, *Natural and Political Observations on the Bills of Mortality* (London: John Martyn, Printer to the Royal Society, 1662); see Charles Creighton, *A History of Epidemics in Britain*, 2nd ed. (New York: Barnes & Noble, 1965), p. 532.

6. George Rosen, *A History of Public Health* (New York: MD Publications, 1958), pp. 354–360.

7. The classic paper setting out these results is Paul A. Samuelson, "A Diagrammatic Exposition of a Theory of Public Expenditure," *Review of Economics and Statistics*, November 1955.

8. Note how difficult pricing is in the real world of broadcasting. The network stations are in effect "priced" by making the consumer watch advertisements, whereas "PBS public broadcasting" uses a mixture of taxes and voluntary donations. Such pricing problems, and the blandness of much government programming, may also explain why cable and satellite TV are doing so well in newly developing countries.

9. David Rosner, ed., *Hives of Sickness: Public Health and Epidemics in New York City* (New Brunswick, N.J.: Rutgers University Press, 1995).

10. Henrik Ibsen, *An Enemy of the People* (1882) in *Henrik Ibsen, The Complete Major Prose Plays*, translated by Rolf Fjelde (New York: Farrar, Strauss, Giroux, 1978), pp. 277–388.

11. Paul Farnham, "The Economic Cost of HIV/AIDS," in J.M. Pogodzinski, ed., *Readings in Public Policy* (Cambridge, Mass.: Blackwell, 1995). Recently there have been a number of press reports that a new type of treatment using protease inhibitors may be effective against the HIV virus, but only under such strict treatment regimens and at such great cost that a new set of economic issues is raised.

12. George Rosen, *A History of Public Health* (New York: MD Publications, 1958).

13. Fitzhugh Mullan, *Plagues and Politics: The Story of the United States Public Health Service* (Basic Books: New York, 1989); Odin Anderson, *Health Services as a Growth Enterprise in the U.S. Since 1875* (Ann Arbor, Mich.: Health Administration Press, 1990).

14. George Rosen, *A History of Public Health* (New York: MD Publications, 1958).

15. The attempt to explain why people do things to their bodies that are clearly not in their own best interests and hence seem to contradict the assumption of rationality has led to a spate of research by economists on "rational addiction." Although these models have been well received within economics, they have had limited effect on the substance abuse and psychiatric community. See Donald S. Kenkel, Robert R. Reed III, and Ping Wang, "Rational Addiction, Peer Externalities and Long Run Effects of Public Policy," NBER working paper w9249 (October 2002); or Jonathan Gruber and Botond Koszegi, "Is Addiction 'Rational?' Theory and Evidence," NBER working paper w7507 (January 2000), (www.nber.org).

16. Douglass North, *Structure and Change in Economic History* (New York: Norton, 1981).

CHAPTER 16

HISTORY, DEMOGRAPHY, AND THE GROWTH OF MODERN MEDICINE

QUESTIONS

1. Does economic growth cause population growth?
2. Is medical care the main reason life expectancy is increasing?
3. Must a society be wealthy to invest in medical care?
4. Do economic failures cause plagues and other mortality?
5. Was Malthus right? Will populations continue to expand until food supplies are exhausted?
6. Why do families have fewer children today?
7. Does medical technology create economic growth or does economic growth create new medical technology?

16.1 ECONOMIC GROWTH HAS DETERMINED THE SHAPE OF HEALTH CARE

In order for a modern health care system to develop and be supported economically, four conditions must exist:

- Effective medical technology
- A sufficiently low risk of death that improving health is worthwhile
- Ample wealth to pay for advanced medical treatment
- Financial organization through insurance and government programs to pool funds from many people

Although medical care has been provided for as long as human society has existed, these four conditions have been met only within the past hundred years, and only in developed countries. Most of Africa and parts of Asia and Latin America are still characterized by high mortality, subsistence farming, and a lack of social and financial organization so that the risks of dying are high and heavily influenced by the amount of income available.[1] Economic

373

development creates the foundation for modern medicine. As large numbers of people live longer and have more wealth, they become more willing to pay for medical care. They pool funds to finance care through insurance (Chapters 4 and 5) and to support medical research so that collectively they can obtain the technological wonders that none of them could afford individually (Chapters 14 and 15).

Food was the primary limitation on the number of people in a population and their health until perhaps 200 years ago. Only after the Industrial revolution did medical technology become important. Yet close study indicates that changes in economic organization, from simple tribes to complex multinational corporations and global markets, have done as much to increase human health and welfare as have advances in medical technology.[2]

16.2 BIRTH RATES, DEATH RATES, AND POPULATION GROWTH

Population growth is determined by the number of births minus the number of deaths (ignoring immigration, which just transfers people between different parts of the world). Stated in percentage terms:

Natural Rate of Population Increase = Birth Rate − Death Rate

If the birth rate is 4.2 percent and the death rate is 3.9 percent, the rate of increase is 4.2 percent −3.9 percent = 0.3 percent per year. As a first order of approximation, the death rate ≈1/(life expectancy), thus a life expectancy of 25 years implies that 1/25, or 4 percent, of the population will die each year.[3] Birth and death rates fluctuated wildly through most of history, but were forced quite close to each other on average because of the uneasy equilibrium between population and food supply. If the birth rate was high for a while, there would be too many mouths to feed in the winter and starvation became more likely. If food was scarce for many years, people delayed marriage, thus reducing the birth rate. On the other hand, years of bumper crops meant people were more likely to survive and reproduce.

It is important to recognize the numerical effects of **compounding**: how small differences in rates turn into large differences in size over time. If births and deaths are both 4 percent per year, the population is stable, neither growing nor shrinking. If there is a slight increase in births, to 4.1 percent a year, the natural rate of increase becomes 0.1 percent and population will double in 700 years, as it did through much of the Agricultural Age. If the birth rate rises further to 4.2 percent (i.e., a 0.2 percent net increase), the population will be four times larger in 700 years. A growth rate of 1.0 percent a year means the population will double every 70 years—a total population growth of 106,000 percent in a 700-year time span.[4]

16.3 THE STONE AGE

Time span: 5 million to 10,000 B.C.	**Economy:** Subsistence hunter-gatherer
Total population: Beginning to 4 million	**Distribution of income:** Roughly equal
Growth rate (doubles): .0007% (100,000 years)	**Medical care:** Shaman/witch doctor
Life expectancy: 28 years	**Medical $:** Not applicable

The **Stone Age** began with the emergence of the first hominids in Africa about 5 million years ago. People lived in small bands as hunter-gatherers, with a simple family/tribal social structure and little physical or intellectual capital to improve productivity. Population was limited by the amount of food in the immediate area. Life expectancy was less than 30 years, and more than half the children did not live long enough to start families, although some elders lived into their forties or fifties.[5] For millennia upon millennia, the rate of population growth was so slow as to be almost unnoticeable. It took about 100,000 years for global population to double, an annual growth rate of 0.0007 percent. At the end of the prehistoric Stone Age around 10,000 B.C. there were about 4 million people in the world, mostly in Asia, Africa, and the Near East, with only a few in the Americas. For Stone Age hunter-gatherers, everyone lived pretty much equally at a subsistence level. Violent death and starvation in the winter were constant threats, but during the good times, life was relatively easy. Studies of remaining hunter-gatherer tribes that rely on Stone Age "technology" in the Amazon, Philippine jungles, and Africa indicate that only three to six hours per day is required to obtain food and repair simple shelters and tools, with much of the rest of the time taken up by other pursuits. Exchange between groups was rare, so there were no organized trading systems.

Population growth during the Stone Age occurred primarily by expansion into new territory. As a tribe got too large for the local area, some family groups split off and occupied new land. Evolution and new technology (i.e., bows and arrows, flint knives) meant better exploitation of the existing food supply, not increased productivity. *Homo sapiens* displaced *homo erectus* because the former was more efficient at hunting and killing, gathering and storing food, and building shelter. This increased efficiency did not increase the productivity of the land, and in some cases even reduced it as large game species (mammoths, sloths) were exterminated. Each additional person required more land, and the ultimate size of the population was limited by the area under settlement. By the end of the Stone Age, those limits had already been reached in some fully populated areas. The rising population pressure in long-settled lands overfilled with people may have contributed to the development of animal husbandry and plant cultivation to feed the excess population, initiating the Agricultural Age.

16.4   THE AGRICULTURAL AGE

Time span: 10,000 B.C. to 1800 A.D.	**Economy:** Farming and harvesting
Total population: 4 million to 400 million	**Distribution of income:** Top-heavy, unequal
Growth rate (doubles): .046% (1,500 years)	**Medical care:** Empirical
Life expectancy: 24 years	**Medical $:** Perhaps 1%

Population growth accelerated with the development of agriculture, but only slowly at first. Agriculture appears to have originated around 10,000 B.C.–7000 B.C. in the river valleys of the Tigris, the Euphrates, and the Nile, and subsequently developed independently in China and the Peruvian highlands. People began to settle permanently in one place. Irrigation canals were dug and roads were built. The same acreage could support more permanent farmers than roaming hunter-gatherers. The productivity increases that made agriculture a stable way of life depended on countless and often incremental innovations occurring at different times and places. Furthermore, the geographic diffusion of ideas was slow, only about one kilometer a year. As late as 4000 B.C., global population was still growing at a rate of only about 0.01 percent a year (doubling in 7,000 years). Agriculture meant greater reliance on just one or a few crops so there was less diversity in foodstuffs and nutrients, reducing health. Cultivation of a single food also exposed the population of a village to catastrophic declines as drought or infestation caused crop failure. Thus, although the population grew larger, life expectancy sometimes declined.

Investment and Trade

Farming takes investment. Seed must be saved, fields plowed, and animal pens erected. A hunter might have worked at making a sharper spear or better root gatherer, but the increase in output was small compared with the gains obtained from farm improvements (building an irrigation ditch, selecting superior seed, inventing the harrow or plow). In the **Agricultural Age**, many farm investments, such as building a road or a large corral, were collective, benefiting the entire village. The returns on investment became larger when more people were involved. There is a synergy (economy of scale) in bringing people together. Whereas each person could know something about farming, a hundred could compare experiences and draw on the best ideas. Each person could make tools, but collectively, in a village of a hundred, the few people who were best at it could spend more time making tools for others and get food in return. Specialization, trade, and division of labor arose. Towns and cities were built. Trade between regions became a regular part of economic activity.

For trade and investment to occur, societies must develop property rights. To have farms, people needed to be able to stay on their land and improve it from year to year. They had to own a portion of the extra grain that was stored for times of famine or traded for tools, salt, and other necessary items. Stored grain had to be defended against the marauding bandits who showed up at harvest time. Once an agricultural society formed an army, it quickly discovered that force was useful for things other than defense. Neighboring tribes were displaced from their more productive lands or conquered and made into slaves. Leaders who successfully rallied the troops in battle gained power and, through a hierarchy of princes and priests, effectively controlled most of the wealth of society. Yet the development of governance was more than a military necessity. To grow, agricultural societies needed rulers who could accumulate and manage the excess output necessary for collective investments in irrigation, laws, and war making.

Civilization, War, and Government

With the advent of the first great civilization—the Sumerians—population began to increase rapidly. Population growth rates increased to .07 percent per year (doubling in 1,000 years), about a hundred times the hunter-gatherer growth rate. Although the Sumerian empire soon fell, the Pharoic theocracy established along the banks of the Nile in Egypt endured for centuries. Between 1000 B.C. and 1 A.D., many other large and vigorous civilizations developed. The classical Greeks rose to unprecedented heights, and Alexander conquered the world before being displaced by the Romans. In China, the Han dynasty unified 50 million people, and in the Americas the great Inca and Olmec/Maya/Aztec civilizations began. By 1 A.D., empires spanned continents and trade routes stretched for thousands of miles. World population exceeded 200 million and was growing about 0.12 percent per year (doubling every 600 years).

As cities grew, the population split into two classes: peasants who worked the land and continued to live at subsistence level and rulers who controlled all the wealth. Whereas hunter-gatherers were all at the same level, working three to six hours a day to obtain subsistence plus a little extra, farmers had to work much harder, eight to twelve hours a day, to obtain the same amount of food. Why, then, did anyone become a farmer? People became farmers probably out of necessity rather than choice. When a climatic change caused a succession of bad years, or a stronger band of tribes pushed people out of favored territory, they were forced to try to get more out of what was at hand: husbanding animals rather than just hunting them, planting roots and grain rather than just picking them wild, and so on.

Many peasants were "recruited" as they were captured and placed under the domination of a warlord. Once the shift from hunting to farming occurred, farming acquired a momentum of its own and the trend became irreversible. There were too many people in the valley to go back to the old ways, and the kings did not want to give up the wealth they obtained by ruling others. Even if doubling the population of the city did not make the average person better off, it made the king and the court twice as well off.

Prosperity depended on the willingness of people to support (or at least tacitly cooperate with) the existing system and to work toward improving it. Although the king might coerce peasants into paying taxes, he had to deliver order and a stable standard of living in return or face rebellion. The taxes collected had to be directed toward appropriate public works and services to maintain progress. The rapid growth in population could only be sustained by new forms of social organization, by creating the cultural, political, and economic institutions that make up civilization. Having enough wealth left over to indulge idle priests and philosophers as they researched mathematics, astronomy, chemistry, physics, and medicine also fostered the conditions for technological advance. This process of economic development was mutually reinforcing, because growth required more government and investment and made it possible to free up resources to support them.

The Decline of Civilizations Leads to Population Declines

The amazing growth of classical civilizations was followed by almost equally sensational declines when social order decayed. There were more people in ancient Greece at its apex in 440 B.C. than at any time during the next 2,000 years, and it was not until 1850 A.D. that the population again exceeded 3 million. As the Roman Empire shrank, the total population of Europe fell from 44 million in 200 A.D. to 22 million in 600 A.D. By 1000 A.D., European population had only partly recovered, to 30 million. Similar though less severe declines occurred in China and Africa. A recent example is found in the traumatic transition of the Soviet Union as communism disintegrated in 1990. The sharp drop in economic output, widespread moral and social disorder, and precipitous decline in life expectancy was catastrophic.

IMPLOSION OF THE SOVIET ECONOMY CAUSES DRAMATIC DECLINES IN LIFE EXPECTANCY

Life expectancy in Russia in 1989 was 64.2 years for males and 74.4 years for females, slightly higher than it had been 30 years previously.[6] The reconstruction (perestroika) of the Union of Soviet Socialist Republics (USSR) under Mikhail Gorbachev brought hope, and then disaster. The Soviet economy crumbled, the USSR fragmented, and quality of life declined. For some people on fixed incomes, hyperinflation took food prices beyond their reach, causing malnutrition. More important, the loss of jobs and hope meant despair. In such a grim situation, deaths from alcohol poisoning and accidents soared. By 1994, life expectancy had fallen 6.6 years for males (to 57.6 years) and 3.3 years for females (to 71.1 years), a decline that is virtually unprecedented in modern industrial countries. Fertility dropped below replacement level and total population declined. In 1992, births exceeded deaths by 184,000. By 1993, there were 800,000 more deaths than births.[7] For every live birth, there were 2.2 abortions. Only now are the true dimensions of this contemporary social and demographic catastrophe being measured.

The Plague

As European populations began to recover robustly toward the end of the Middle Ages (500–1500 A.D.), they were hit by a new and rampantly destructive force, the plague. Bubonic plague, or black death, swept through Europe in 1347–1352 and repeatedly thereafter, wiping out a quarter of the population.[8] Half the citizens of Genoa and Naples died as a result of the plague of 1656.[9] Although bouts of plague continued to appear until 1700, changes in immunity, social structure, the plague bacillus itself, or a combination of these, reduced the impact over time, and population growth resumed after 1500 A.D. The peoples of the New World were not as fortunate. After contact with the Spanish conquistadors, plagues of measles and smallpox spread rapidly, with devastating effects. The native population of Aztecs dropped from 17 million in 1532 to 2 million in 1580, and fell to just 1 million by 1608. It was not just disease, but also the collapse of social order that caused the permanent decline in numbers. Much of the repopulation of the Americas after 1600 came from the growth of immigrant populations from Europe and Africa.

Food Supply Determines Population

From 1500 to 1750 the European and world populations grew at an average annual rate of 0.25 percent (doubling in 300 years). Food supply was the fundamental constraint on growth since the great majority of people lived at a subsistence level. A study of the Italian district of Siena for the period 1550–1715 shows that increases in prices for grain were associated with malnutrition and death.[10] Each time the cost of food rose, the meager salaries of the residents were stretched thinner and mortality climbed. The cycle is self-correcting and self-reinforcing. As people die, there are fewer mouths to feed; therefore, demand falls and prices fall. When food is abundant and prices are low, peasants are more able to marry and have children, the number of mouths to feed rises, demand increases, prices jump, and the cycle starts over again.

As the Agricultural Age drew to a close and the transition to an urbanized industrial society began, scarcity of food continued to be a major issue. Salaried workers were little better off than peasants, because it took 80 percent of their salaries to get enough to eat. For example, in 1790 France was a highly developed country with perhaps the greatest cultural and political influence in the Western world, yet most of its citizens were impoverished and undernourished. The average 30-year-old Frenchman of 1790 had to live on 2,250 calories per day, was just 5 feet 3 inches tall, and weighed only 110 pounds.[11] The bottom 10 percent of society had so little to eat that they were usually ill, and most people below the twentieth percentile did not get enough food to meet the caloric energy demands of regular work. Even relatively well-off people at the eightieth percentile were sufficiently stunted and wasted (height and weight below current U.S. standards) that they were at substantially higher risk of chronic health conditions and premature mortality.

The Rise of Economics

The intellectual ferment of the Renaissance (1350–1650 A.D.) and Enlightenment (1650–1800 A.D.) brought advances in government, science, and commerce (although major changes in medicine did not occur until 1900). In 1662, John Graunt published his *Natural and Political Observations on the Bills of Mortality* in London, a work now recognized as the beginning of the science of epidemiology. In 1671, Sir William Petty made the first estimate of national wealth (gross domestic product [GDP]) in his essay *Political Arithmetik* (economic statistics). As people moved from rural estates, where they had been cared for (and/or owned) by a feudal lord, into cities where they worked at jobs for wages, the economic organization of society evolved from one based on tradition to one based on money. Only after exchange became standardized through the use of money could regularities be observed and statistical analysis be performed.

The development of accounting and statistics marked the emergence of a new "information technology" that revolutionized trade. Financial markets in London and other cities traded government bonds and shares in joint stock companies, shifting tons of gold with the stroke of a pen. Factories were built, and thousands of people changed occupations and even nationalities to better their standard of living. Capital investment and labor mobility of this magnitude had been impossible during the Middle Ages because the necessary economic structure was not available or was too rudimentary. Corporations, rental contracts, taxes, ownership, and other property rights had to be refined before trade between individuals, firms, and governments could be conducted on a large scale. *The Wealth of Nations*, Adam Smith's insightful analysis published in 1776, is recognized as the start of modern economics.[12] Yet Thomas Malthus's *Essay on the Principle of Population* (1798) often has been more influential, clearly presenting the consensus of thinkers at the end of the agricultural age and responsible for labeling economics "the dismal science."

The Malthusian Hypothesis

Malthus's hypothesis was that any increase in productivity could provide only a temporary boost to the standard of living.[13] Over time, increases in the number of people to be fed would use up all the productivity increase; therefore, on average, people would be no better off than before—still living at a subsistence level. The **Malthusian hypothesis** is based on two key assumptions: that (1) *food supply* is a primary constraint on population growth and (2) any increase in the number of people would inevitably lead to more crowding or to farming of less desirable land, so that the *declining marginal productivity* of labor (and hence, wages) would bring down the standard of living.

Ireland became a natural experiment for testing the Malthusian hypothesis. The importation of a new crop, potatoes, led to a tremendous increase in yields per acre. Using the new crop, the acreage that could support only one family in 1700 could be split up and support three families by 1800. Potato farming was so much more efficient than other types of agriculture that the peasants ate little else, consuming up to 10 pounds per day. The population of this small and already fully settled island grew 50 percent in the half century before Malthus wrote, and by another 50 percent over the next 30 years. Farms were divided into smaller and smaller parcels, and the Irish people, with a diet consisting almost entirely of potatoes, lived no better than before—there were just more of them. Then came the fungus blight that damaged the potato harvest of 1845 and destroyed the crop of 1846 entirely: 1.5 million people died and another 1.5 million people emigrated, mostly to America. Those who were left tightened their belts and stopped having children (the women born before the blight who remained in Ireland were four times as likely to remain unmarried as those who emigrated to America).[14] Out of a population of 8 million in 1840, there were only 4.5 million left by 1900, and by 1950, only 2.8 million.

The assumptions in the Malthusian hypothesis had been valid through the thousands of years that spanned the Agricultural Age and continued to apply in countries that remained essentially rural, such as Ireland. The law of diminishing returns, as elaborated by Malthus, was a major intellectual contribution to economics. However, it applies only if the technology of production stays similar in essential ways (as agriculture had up until then). In England, Germany, France, and the United States, the intellectual revolution that stirred Malthus to write his treatise led others to create a technological and commercial revolution so profound

---

ECONOMIC MODELING

Malthusian Hypothesis: An increase in productivity will not make most people better off in the long run.

- The total population is held in check by the food supply.

- An external change (new land or new technology) increases food production. As (Total Food / Total Population) rises, the average welfare increases.

- More food per person allows people to have more children (or for more of the children born to get enough to eat to live to maturity).

- Increasing population means more workers per acre of land.

- More workers per acre of land means that the additional output per person (marginal product) will be lower (*"the law of diminishing returns"*).

- Adding in a declining marginal product per person will make the average fall.

- The population stabilizes with a larger number of people living at the same average "subsistence" level of welfare (food per person) as before the new land or new technology was discovered.

The Malthusian hypothesis is presented here in step-by-step detail to provide an example of what economists mean by "modeling" a process. The crucial insight (economic concept) articulated for the first time by Malthus is step 5—what is now generally known as the *law of diminishing returns*. This insight is what makes Malthus famous as a founder of economic thought.

---

that productivity increases were continuous, and output grew much more rapidly than any natural increase in the number of people.[15] A continuous excess of food and other goods became available for all to enjoy.

16.5   THE INDUSTRIAL AGE

Time span: 1800 to 1950 A.D.   **Economy:** Manufacturing
Total population: 0.4 billion to 1.6 billion   **Distribution of income:** Mixed
Growth rate (doubles): .65% (108 years)   **Medical care:** Empirical
Life expectancy: 35–65 years   **Medical $:** 2% to 4%

Life was difficult at the start of the Industrial Revolution and often got worse for those who moved into cities to work in factories. Crowded slums and harsh working conditions caused disease. Whereas diets on a farm could be supplemented by gardens and occasional hunting, in the cities food was monotonous and lacking in vitamins. As the countryside became enclosed (put under ownership of a lord rather than held in common) and people moved into cities, illness increased. Life expectancy in England, about 38 years in 1600 A.D., declined throughout the next hundred years and did not regain earlier levels until about 1850.[16] Yet as the Industrial Revolution took hold, productivity increases caused the average person's standard of living to improve. There was a sharp rise in the rate of population growth to 0.43 percent for 1750–1800, almost twice the rate of the preceding three centuries, rising to 0.53 percent for 1800–1900, 0.88 percent per year for 1900–1950, and surging to 1.8 percent after 1950. World population quadrupled from about 750 million to 2.5 billion. Overall life expectancy rose by more in these 200 years than it had in the previous 2,000, going from 27 to 40 years. The rise was even more remarkable in the most developed countries, such as Sweden, where life expectancy rose from 37 years in 1750 to 71.3 years in 1950.

Why Malthus Was Wrong

There are two reasons Malthus's gloomy predictions went wrong. First, technological advance, rather than being a one-shot improvement, became a continuous process. Output expanded at an exponential rate as one invention led to another. In the Agricultural Age, the primary productive inputs were land and labor. The total supply of land is fixed, and any increase in the supply of labor meant more mouths to feed. In the **Industrial Age**, capital equipment, skilled labor, and knowledge became more important than land and unskilled agricultural labor. By 1950, a single farmer, sitting in an air-conditioned cab operating a combine harvesting genetically engineered wheat, could feed more people per 100 acres than a dozen farmers could in 1750. Although the rate of productivity increase during the Agricultural Age averaged about 1 percent a year, in the Industrial Age it rapidly tripled and sometimes exceeded 5 percent a year. A second reason that Malthus's immiserating population growth failed to occur was that as death rates declined, birth rates also declined. With fewer children dying, parents chose to have fewer babies, and invested more in the education, medical care, and nutrition of each one. Cumulatively, these individual decisions brought about a social revolution. They also changed the character of labor (more education, more skills, fewer new entrants) and accelerated technological advance, leading to higher wages and a rising standard of living.

Why did Ireland suffer a Malthusian catastrophe and lose two-thirds of its population while most other European nations experienced surging growth during the Industrial Revolution? Ireland was not a self-governing nation, but a colony exploited by absentee landlords from England. Profits from Irish estates were not invested in Ireland but used to build factories in England or sent overseas through joint stock companies. Irish farmers did not own their land but were tenants working the fields for the benefit of the landlord. As crop yields went up, rents were raised, keeping workers in subsistence conditions typical of the Agricultural Age. With no claim on the profits, the tenant farmer had no incentive to raise crop yields and had little ability to save and improve the lot of the family in the next generation. The only way for Irish farmers to capture any of the economic surplus created by increased agricultural productivity was to have more children, and so they did. Irish citizens wishing to leave the farm and build a better life in the city had to leave their country and go to New York. The lack of property rights for citizens and restrictive colonial economic organization were significant factors in keeping Ireland from joining the ranks of industrialized countries during the nineteenth century.

Malthus's predictions were never as dismal or as wrong as his critics claimed. He hoped that by clearly laying out the logical conclusions of agricultural demographics, he would encourage people to delay marriage and have fewer children. Birthrates did, in fact, decline, but for other reasons. Women gained more opportunities and spent less time on child rearing. More children survived, so fewer births were needed to make sure that one or two children in a family lived to maturity. Dependence on children in old age was replaced by reliance on savings. Children went from being a form of supplemental income (as productive family farmworkers) to a form of consumption (bringing joy but costing money). All these changes either raised the price of or reduced the demand for children. Average total fertility per mature female in England fell from 5.3 births in 1750, to 4.6 in 1850, to 1.96 in 1900 (below the replacement rate of 2.0; therefore, national population actually would have decreased over time if not for foreign immigration).

Demographic Transition

The process of economic development is linked to a dramatic change in national population known as "demographic transition." When societies are in the agricultural stage, many children die before reaching adulthood. High rates of mortality (4 to 5 percent) are matched by high rates of fertility (also 4 to 5 percent), so the total number of people is stable or just slowly increasing. This equilibrium between births and deaths changes radically during the process of economic development. With greater material well-being, mortality rates decline toward 1 to 2 percent. Since birth rates are still high, the rate of population growth (births–deaths) is very rapid, 2 to 4 percent a year, enough to double the population in each generation (every 15 to 40 years). Such explosive growth does not continue indefinitely. Although constantly increasing economic output should not necessarily cause birth rates to fall, it is observed that birth rates do in fact fall in virtually every developed country. As children cease to be productive farm assets and become a costly form of family consumption, families decide to concentrate more care and investment on fewer children.[17] This decline in fertility does not require the use of modern birth control techniques. Delayed marriage, extended breast feeding, infanticide, and other methods have been used to restrict population to desired levels in many countries without recourse to contraceptives. As economic development continues, low mortality (1–2 percent) is eventually matched by low fertility (1–2 percent) so that the total population is again stable or slowly growing, and the process of demographic transition is complete (see Figure 16.1).

Population growth spurts during the Agricultural Age occurred when settlement of new territories caused an increase in births, whereas population growth during demographic transition is caused by a decline in deaths. These two demographic patterns have different long-run consequences on the average level of individual wealth. When new territories

| FIGURE 16.1 | Demographic Transition |

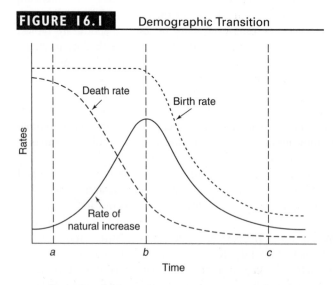

a = Beginning of the transition
b = Greatest difference between birth and death rates
c = End of the transition

are settled, the pioneers have much more land per person than in the country they came from and thus initially enjoy a much greater marginal productivity of labor and greater wealth. This advantage is eroded over time as more and more people are born in the new territories. Eventually, the new territories are just as crowded as the old country, the marginal productivity of labor is pushed back down to the subsistence level, and the total population, although larger, is not much better off. In contrast, the economic advances that mark demographic transition, rather than fading over time, are reinforced with each succeeding generation. Healthier adults can work longer and harder and thus accumulate more surplus for investment, while a smaller number of children means that each one receives more in the way of education, nutrition, and inheritance. These gains lead to even lower mortality, even fewer children, and so on. Each generation is better off and material advantage is concentrated among fewer offspring until transition is complete. By then, the share of family income required to buy food has fallen from 80 percent to 20 percent. Getting enough to eat is no longer a significant factor in demographic change or labor productivity.

Demographic Change, Income Distribution, and the Rise of the Middle Classes

In a hunter-gatherer society, there are no wealthy people. The tribe as a whole is living at the subsistence level with only a little accumulated wealth in the form of weapons or religious objects. One or two bad years can spell disaster. An agricultural society, in contrast, is hierarchical and often has considerable wealth, almost all of it concentrated at the top. Most of the agricultural population consists of rural peasants. As agricultural civilizations develop, the number of traders, soldiers, craftspeople, merchants, and other members of the bourgeois who live as free "citizens" in (mostly small) cities increases, but they are always a minority. The king's authority is absolute, and almost all of the wealth stays under his control.

To industrialize, the bulk of the population has to move into cities. People who leave the land are no longer under the control of the lord, and they enter into wage labor contracts with factories. As businesses and bureaucracies replace the feudal manor as a means of organizing production, the fruits of economic development are spread more widely. Although the wages of industrial workers are near the subsistence level at first, real earnings rise rapidly for two reasons. First, the decline in the number of births during demographic transition means fewer new workers entering the market; thus, the supply of labor grows less rapidly than demand, putting upward pressure on wages. Second, the labor market becomes specialized. Initially, the threat of starvation drove unskilled workers off the farm to take subsistence wages in the city. However, the later movement of skilled mechanics, clerks, and managers to the city was driven by the premium wages required to attract these workers. These well-paid workers and shopkeepers could afford some luxuries. They could also save for retirement, and in so doing, contribute to the pool of capital funds for investment and entrepreneurial ventures.

Although feudal blacksmiths took pride in their art, most of the benefits went to the lord. Master mechanics in the industrial era had a much greater incentive to improve their skills because they were paid directly and captured more value from increases in quality and productivity. They were apt to take the risk of innovating and start new businesses because they might become rich. Even when their ventures failed they could get other jobs and keep their families from starving.[18]

In the city-states and empires of the Agricultural Age, lords and kings exercised centralized bureaucratic power to raise taxes, build roads, and support armies. Building factories and inventing new technologies in the industrial era required decentralized entrepreneurs who acted as managers on their own behalf rather than on behalf of the king. Working

FIGURE 16.2		Distribution of Income at Different Stages of Development		
Upper classes		$$$$$	$$	$$$$$$$$
Middle class	$	$$	$$$$$$$	$$$$$$$$$$
Lower classes	$$$$$	$	$$$	$$$$$$$
	Hunter-Gatherer	Agricultural	Industrial	Informational

independently or in small groups, entrepreneurs convinced investors to put up capital and attracted skilled labor with high wages. By the end of the Industrial Age, even people of modest means could go to school, start a business, and save for retirement. A startling change in the distribution of income and wealth had occurred—the bulk of the money was held by the large and growing middle class of laborers, tradespeople, and small-business owners. In 1750 the market for art, education, travel, housing, and almost everything except food was concentrated in the upper 2 percent of families who were truly wealthy. By 1950, the market for such goods in the United States, England, Germany, and other developed countries was dominated by the middle class. The wealthy bought luxury in a few shops, while the millions shopped in department stores (see Figure 16.2).[19]

The hierarchies that dominated the Agricultural Age were broken up by tremendous increases in economic mobility and a general improvement in wages. The crowd at the bottom was replaced by a bulging middle class of people who actively participated in a monetary economy. This shift in social and economic structure, rather than the discovery of new technology per se, was the driving force that powered growth of the industrial revolution. Many countries today remain poor and rural, struggling to make the demographic and economic transition to development. It is not because they lack technology (which can be found in many textbooks, ordered from catalogs, or shared in commercial joint ventures), but because they lack the property rights, social order, and administrative structure to create a context in which technology can be applied productively.[20] The deficit that allows starvation to remain a threat to people's health is not a lack of knowledge, machinery, or money for investment, but a lack of organization.

16.6 THE INFORMATION AGE

Time span: 1950 to future
Total population: 1.6 billion to 20 billion?
Growth rate (doubles): 1.88% (40 years) but slowing
Life expectancy: 70+ years

Economy: Services
Distribution of income: Not yet clear
Medical care: Scientific

Medical $: 6% to 16%+

The advent of a post-industrial **Information Age** is marked by the ubiquitous appearance of the television and the computer. The economy is global, linked by communications networks where massive amounts of capital flow between countries with a few keystrokes. Labor is concentrated in services rather than agriculture or manufacturing. Information specialists, the dominant workers, spend their entire childhood and many years of adulthood in school investing in skills. Such training can be prevalent only in a population with long life expectancies and few children per family. In this era, most people are healthy and wealthy enough that personal income affects longevity and fertility primarily through lifestyle choices, rather than lack of food or shelter. What was rare throughout history, the ability to retire with independent means and sufficient fitness to travel the world after age 65, has become not just attainable, but an ordinary reality for most people in postindustrial economies.

U.S. life expectancy was about 35 years in 1750, 49 years in 1900, and rose to 68 years by 1950 and 78 years in 2008. Although people will continue to live longer, incremental years of life expectancy are added at a slower rate as infectious diseases and childhood maladies are removed as major causes of death. More important from a demographic point of view is that almost all the gains in longevity after 1950 occurred for mature adults who had already completed their families. Each generation may live longer, but will not have more babies. Additional increases in life expectancy will not increase the number of children and thus will have little effect on the long-run total size of the population.

During the demographic transition of the Industrial Age and its final phase, the 1950s baby boom, rapid population increase created expansive economic growth as more houses, roads, and factories were built. However, expansion due to demographic transition is a one-time occurrence. After transition, population returns to a steady state of slow or zero growth, typically a small natural decrease offset by immigration of people from less-developed countries seeking higher wages. It is important to recognize that the "normal" conditions of industrializing countries from 1770 to 1970 were actually abnormal periods of spectacular but transitory growth. In comparison, the 1 to 2 percent growth rates of recent decades can seem inadequate, particularly since most of the added value comes in the less visible form of service improvement and information content (HD television, the internet, cheap mobile phones and travel), rather than in the number of countable goods (cars, houses, tons of corn) that are most readily measured in GDP accounts.

Much of the world is still undeveloped, caught somewhere between an agricultural society and the modern information era. A world map shaded to show which nations today still have economies dominated by agriculture is almost identical to a world map showing which nations have the most premature mortality under age 30.[21] Such nations have the potential for fantastic growth as they industrialize (e.g., Korea, Singapore, Indonesia) but also for tragic population explosions without economic advancement, leading to starvation and social ruin (e.g., Somalia, Rwanda). In a developing country, such as Indonesia, the average age of the population is about 17, longevity is less than 70 years, many people still work on farms, and a sizable fraction still live at the subsistence level. Such countries have a tremendous "population momentum." Even if every family immediately limited fertility to the replacement level of 2.2 births, the total population would still double in size because so many young women have already been born. In the United States, as in most developed countries, the natural population growth is already zero to negative; thus, the increase in population is due to immigration from less developed countries. If current trends continue, almost every country in the world will be developed within a hundred years (by 2100) and have a steady or shrinking population.[22] Total world population will stabilize somewhere between 10 to 20 billion, Mexico City will be much larger than Los Angeles, and food supply will be a trivial health problem compared to pollution and congestion (see Table 16.1).

16.7 INCOME AND HEALTH

The connection between poverty and poor health was noted long ago. The connection is described in ancient Greek and Chinese commentaries, and detailed empirical studies were conducted in London and Paris in the nineteenth century.[23] As economic historians carefully review the data, it becomes clear that although economic growth may have been the major

TABLE 16.1   Timeline: Economic History, Population Growth, and Medical Care

	Stone Age	Agricultural Age				Industrial Age			Information Age	
	5 million–10,000 B.C.	4000 B.C.	1 A.D.	1200 A.D.	1800 A.D.	1900	1950	1975	2000	????
World population	Beginnings to 4 million	8	250	400 million	950	1.6 billion	2.5 billion	4 billion	6 billion	Stops @ 20 billion
Rate of growth	*.0007%*	*.01%*	*.09%*	*.04%*	*.14%*	*.52%*	*.88%*	*1.88%*	*.20%*	*(Slowing)*
(years to double)	*(100,000)*	*(7,000)*	*(800)*	*Varies*	*(500)*	*(130)*	*(80)*	*(40)*	*(Slowing)*	
Life expectancy	28 years		24 years			40 years			80 years	
Organization	Family/tribe		Fief/city/empire			National states			Global village?	
Information	Oral		Written			Statistics			Electronic	
Economy	Hunter-Gatherer		Farming & harvesting			Manufacturing			Services	
Incomes	Subsistence		Rich rulers/subsistence serfs			Wages			Wages & entitlements	
Equivalent $ per capita	$200		$300			$300 rising to $5,000			$35,000 (developed countries)	
% Spent on food	All		Almost all—90%			80% falling to 30%			12%	
Income distribution	Roughly equal		Highly unequal			Mixed			Not yet clear	
Type of medicine	Witch doctor/shaman		Healer priest			Empiricist		Scientifically trained physicians		
Medical spending	—		? maybe 1%			2% rising to 4%		6%	10%	?

TABLE 16.2	Mortality Ratios by Social Class 1931–1981				
Class	**1931**	**1951**	**1961**	**1971**	**1981**
I Professionals	90	86	76	77	66
II Managerial	94	92	81	81	76
III Skilled manual	97	101	100	104	103
IV Semi-skilled	102	104	103	114	116
V Unskilled	111	118	143	137	166

Source: The Black Report (note 25). Standardized Mortality Ratios, Men 15-64, England and Wales, age-adjusted: 100 = average mortality rate for that year.

contributor in lengthening life expectancy, its effects were neither uniform across groups nor steady over time. Average health appears to have declined significantly in the United States during the early decades of the nineteenth century despite rising per capita incomes; therefore, life expectancy was probably not much greater in 1900 than it was in 1800.[24] Most commentators assume that extreme poverty has the most deleterious effects and that the relationship between income and health is nonlinear, with gains in life expectancy becoming smaller as one moves up the income scale (see Figure 17.4). However, the famous "Black Report" on civil service employees in the United Kingdom established that, even among high-income people, mortality was lower for those at the very top. In addition, the report established that although the absolute effect got smaller over time as general life expectancy increased, the relative importance of rank did not disappear and perhaps even widened between 1930 and 1981 (Table 16.2).[25] This finding is often viewed as indicating that health insurance alone cannot remove the effects of poverty on health because this period includes the formation of the National Health Service in the United Kingdom, which provides essentially free medical care for all citizens. Studies of U.S. populations show a similar gradient, with smaller but still significant income effects even at very high income levels.[26]

The relationship between income and health is strong, but the nature of that relationship is far from clear. Getting sick makes people earn less, thus observing that "sicker people are poorer on average" does not establish whether the lack of income led to poor health, or bad health led to less income.[27] It seems as if income may affect health more than vice versa for young people, but not for older people, for whom bad health is more likely to be responsible for a loss of income. The Social Security "notch" (some people receive higher retirement incomes because they were born a week earlier than others) provided a natural experiment—which showed that just giving people bigger checks did not make them live longer.[28] It is not income per se that makes people healthy, but all the things associated with higher income: more education, better nutrition, social connections, family stability, and so on. For children, it appears that the things that tend to go along with income (better environment, better education, better educated mothers) may be more important than money per se.

16.8   REDUCING UNCERTAINTY: THE VALUE OF LIFE AND ECONOMIC SECURITY

Economic development not only meant that most people had more; it also meant that the risks of losing it all were vastly reduced. For the first time, it was possible and reasonable for ordinary people to plan for the future—to decide how many children to have, whether or not to go to school or start a business, and to save for retirement. The improvements in health and income brought about by economic development had a powerful and paradoxical effect: the more secure the future became, the more afraid workers became of losing that security.

The Value of Risk Reduction

Even if medical care is responsible for only a small incremental improvement in health, the value of that increment is increasing as workers become healthier and wealthier. Consider how the value of reducing the risk of dying in the next 10 years by 1 percent changes as workers gain greater life expectancy. If the average person has a 50–50 chance of dying in 10 years, it is not worth much to change the probability to 51–49. Yet if a healthy person has only a 1 percent chance of dying, eliminating this risk, or just cutting it in half, is worth a lot.[29] The value of risk reduction also depends on the level of income. In a subsistence economy where workers get paid only enough to buy food and rudimentary housing, they cannot afford to give up much of what they earn to buy medical care, even if such care would help them avoid future illness and death. On the other hand, a skilled industrial worker earning $40,000 a year can probably afford to pay $300 a month for health insurance and another $100 for vitamin supplements and a health-club membership. A rock star or corporate CEO earning $5 million a year can afford to spend hundreds of thousands of dollars just to keep looking young.

By reviewing a number of studies conducted during the twentieth century, Dora Costa and Matthew Kahn constructed a consistent set of estimates of the value of life (reducing mortality risk) for workers. Valuation increased by thirty-fold, from $427,000 to $12,000,000 in inflation adjusted dollars, during the last 100 years (Table 16.3).[30] The value of life tends to increase more than proportionately as income rises, since life itself is necessary to enjoy the benefits of having goods. Costa and Kahn estimated that the income elasticity of the value of life is about 1.6 (i.e., a 160 percent increase in value for every 100 percent increase in income), indicating that life itself is a "luxury good" in economists' terms (see Section 13.2).

It is not just the increase in the length of life expectancy that is valuable; a reduction in the variance is also important. Most people would rather be faced with a life that might vary from 73 to 83 years in length than a life that is equally long on average but varied from 53 to 103. Knowing approximately when one will die could alleviate substantial existential anxiety, and would be incredibly helpful for pension and estate planning. A recent study

TABLE 16.3	Changes in the Estimated Value of Life, 1900–2000
Year	**Value of Life (2002 dollars)**
1900	$427,000
1920	895,000
1940	1,377,000
1950	2,426,000
1960	2,884,000
1970	5,176,000
1980	7,393,000
2000	12,053,000

Source: Dora L. Costa and Matthew E. Kahn (note 29).

estimated that for the current U.S. population with a life expectancy of 78 (s.d. ±15) years, a reduction in that standard deviation by two years (i.e., to ±13 years) is worth almost as much as a one-year increase in average life expectancy.[31]

Social Security and Health Insurance

Whereas the poor agricultural masses may have been happy to get a chance to stay alive and perhaps get ahead, the industrial middle-class expected progress. If their lives did not constantly improve, or if something went wrong, they expected their employers or the government to do something to correct the problem. Originally, coal miners went underground to work to get higher wages. They began to demand safe working conditions, compensation for accidents and disability, and retirement plans. As early as 1700, a few English industrialists offered health insurance to their workers. Such employee benefits made the workers loyal to these firms and willing to work harder. The risks of disability and sickness were no longer borne by the workers individually, but by the firm. This sharing of risk reduced the uncertainty and variability of wages to workers (Chapters 4 and 5).

Industrialization and the change to wage labor shifted the distribution of political power. Workers' revolts spread across Europe during the nineteenth century, stretching from Paris in 1789 to Russia in 1917. Economic, legal, and health security were fundamental demands of what became known as "socialism." In 1883, to forestall further labor unrest, Chancellor Bismarck created the first national social security system in Germany, providing pensions to workers over age 65, sick leave, and health insurance.[32] In the United States, private insurance provided by employers became the dominant mode of health care financing in the 1950s. These plans have been supplemented by the government Medicaid program for the poor and Medicare for the elderly. Today 89 percent of all health care spending and 97 percent of hospital costs are paid for through third-party financing mechanisms. In 1850, medical care was still largely a personal transaction. Workers paid, or did not pay, for what they thought they could afford, rather like they bought clothes, food, or heating oil. Whereas in less-developed countries, medicine must still rely primarily on personal purchases for financing, pooled financing through government and private insurers has dominated the economic organization of medical care in developed countries since 1960. Now the shape of the health care system is determined by negotiations over benefit packages and government appropriations, not consumers' personal purchasing decisions.

16.9 THE RISE OF MODERN MEDICINE

Medicine is as old as humankind. One of the earliest-known written documents, the "Code of Hammurabi," contains references to medical price controls and malpractice in the laws of this Assyrian kingdom circa 2200 B.C. The Hippocratic Oath, written about 1 B.C. and still quoted in medical writings today, put forth the principle that physicians should "first, do no harm." This was good advice, because for thousands of years physicians could do little to cure illness or reduce the risk of death. Despite the vast amount written about medicine, and the great store of practical knowledge transmitted orally in many cultures, this knowledge was largely unsystematic and did not create therapies that made a significant impact on the health of most people.[33] Medical theory, such as it was, usually consisted of a strange mixture of mysticism; serious looks and kind words; some sound advice about eating, sleeping, and getting fresh air; and a few favorite remedies, some of which might sometimes be useful. Hospitals were places where sick or disabled people were housed, and little was expected in the way of treatment. Physicians were counselors who could make someone feel better and preside over the deaths they prognosticated, but could do little to change the course of illness. Many were also priests, and the distinction between morality and medicine was often unclear. Plagues were more likely to be blamed on infidelity or blasphemy than on unseen organisms in the blood.

Preconditions for Change

This chapter began with a list of four preconditions for the development of modern medical care: effective technology, sufficient wealth, low risk of death, and insurance financing. These factors are not independent of each other, but mutually reinforcing. Increasing wealth meant more food, which reduced the risk of dying. Increased longevity also meant greater productivity and hence even more wealth. As trade developed, financial markets increased in complexity and insurance contracts were needed to better manage capital. Broad participation in pooled financing could only occur when most workers were relatively healthy and well-off. The development of medical technology was the result of an interactive process, requiring advances in biology, chemistry, physics, statistics, and data management. Gaining knowledge and reducing the uncertainty caused by illness takes both science and economics. It is now quite possible that the most commonly used medical instrument is the computer.

The Growth of Medical Science and Technology

The change from mysticism and fear to scientific investigation was the defining characteristic of the Enlightenment. Some milestones include the demonstration of proteins in urine by Paracelsus in 1500, the discovery of the microscope and "little worms" (bacteria and protozoans) by Athanasius Kircher in 1569, William Harvey's discovery of the circulation of blood in 1619, and Anton von Leewenhoek's microscopic description of red blood cells in 1668. The growing accumulation of knowledge presaged a form of medical practice that eventually would be able to provide effective treatment against disease. The crucial link, however, was organizational rather than technical—more a matter of changing the way knowledge was collected, used, and transmitted than any particular scientific breakthrough or discovery. The formation of "clinics" in the great hospitals of Paris around 1750 is particularly noteworthy.[34] These clinics were organized by what would now be called specialties: one for the eye, another for the hand, another for mental illness, and so on. Instead of trying to create a holistic theory that covered all aspects of health, the clinics broke medical problems into component parts. A single doctor would become an expert in diseases of the hand, or the eye, and so on, and then train others. The clinic provided the working classes with access to trained physicians whom they otherwise could not afford. The physician was provided with a large group of compliant patients all suffering similar illness so that he could experiment with new therapies, teach students, and perfect his techniques. Practicing on the masses of poor workers allowed him to charge higher fees to wealthy patients and to collect tuition from students eager to learn the latest advances. The creation of clinics was a success because they provided a social exchange mechanism that yielded gains to both parties.

Organizational innovation was complemented by an intellectual innovation—statistics. Clinic doctors began to count how many people were treated and how many got well. Numerical comparisons of outcomes began to replace doctors' personal assessments. Instead of evaluating quality of care by the reputation and experience of the physicians who vouched for it, now clinical experiments and statistical observation were used. The impact of this new approach to medical science is well illustrated by Edward Jenner's discovery of vaccination for smallpox in 1798. The act of making a healthy person sick (inoculating them with cowpox) to prevent possible future illness is a form of therapy that can only be defended statistically. No single patient feels better or gets cured because of what the doctor does.

Scientific advances accumulated rapidly throughout the latter part of the nineteenth century; Pasteur, Semmelweiss, and Koch determined that bacteria cause anthrax, childbirth fever, tuberculosis, and other infectious diseases; Eijkman discovered vitamins; and Roentgen discovered X-rays. Whereas France was preeminent in the eighteenth century, Germany was arguably the world leader in medical technology by the end of the nineteenth century when Chancellor Bismarck provided the landmark social insurance legislation. American physicians tried to improve the quality of practice in the United States with the Flexner Report of 1910, promoting the "Johns Hopkins model" (actually the German model, but Americans needed a local champion to make it more acceptable). By the end of the 1930s, a license and modern scientific education were required to enter the practice of medicine, and most doctors treated their difficult cases in the hospital using a range of technical devices and nursing support (Chapter 7).

Information systems and access to capital gave hospitals economies of scale and made them necessary adjuncts to medical practice. As modern surgical techniques using anesthesia and antiseptics turned what were formerly warehouses for the sick into technologically sophisticated treatment facilities, written medical records became the locus for storage and communication of test results, diagnostic information, and treatment documentation that linked all the trained medical practitioners together. Florence Nightingale, through her work in military hospitals during the Crimean War and subsequent books, is most often credited with developing the hospital as an organization. Her patients may have seen nurses as "angels of mercy," but she saw them as soldiers gathering intelligence and carrying out orders as part of a grand campaign against disease. As technology became more advanced and specialized, it cost more—too much for individual physicians to purchase on their own. In 1816, Laennec invented the stethoscope to investigate the body, and every doctor bought one. In 1885, Roentgen's X-ray machines peered inside the body, but the equipment was so large and so expensive that most doctors had to join the staff of a hospital to use one. The computed axial tomography (CAT) scan developed in 1973 costs millions of dollars, depends on software that few radiologists understand, and can transmit images through the Internet to be digitally enhanced and read by a specialist thousands of miles away in another country.

Although medicine has been actively practiced since ancient times, only fragmentary technological advances were made until the end of the industrial era. In the eighteenth and nineteenth centuries, scientific discoveries came more and more rapidly, yet there was still little improvement in treatment outcomes. **Only after 1900 did effective medicine start** to become widely available, 150 years after the productive expansion that marked the beginning of the Industrial Age. Between 1900 and 1950, a virtual revolution took place, and medicine became one of society's most valued occupations.

Medical progress resulted more from planned effort and massive public investment than serendipitous discovery or any preordained march of ideas: Florence Nightingale's scientific hospital was supported by kings who wished to cut the cost of putting soldiers into battle; Pasteur's discovery of bacteria was made under contract to the French wine and beer industry; and Walter Reed worked to conquer yellow fever so that construction of the Panama Canal could be completed in tropical jungles. Rising incomes, falling mortality, and commercial organization were more than just contributing factors; they were the central forces driving the demand that created medical technology.

Although all four conditions needed for the development of modern medicine (technology, wealth, low mortality, organized financing) operate concurrently and reinforce each other, medical technology is more a result of the process than a cause. Society's accumulation of the necessary prerequisites for modern medicine began with the rise in wealth brought about by trade and technology, which quickly led to a decline in mortality and subsequently to a decline in the birth rate. The application of science and industrial technology to medicine not only took time, it also took money and an independent profession dedicated to continuous improvement. Both organized medicine, with its schools and professional associations, and organized financing, with insurance risk pooling and government funding, were necessary to carry out that research and pay for years of trial and error as treatments were perfected. The development of integrated health care systems and decentralized contracting will bring medicine to the final stages of the industrial revolution's productivity enhancements, and will evolve in new directions to meet the challenges of the information age.[35]

Did Better Medical Care Increase Life Expectancy?

It seems obvious that providing more and better medical care improves life expectancy, but it is actually quite difficult to show conclusively that this is the case. Given the strong relationship between mortality and income, questions have arisen regarding the relative importance of medical care by itself. After all, the catastrophic decline in Russian life expectancy in 1989–1994 was not caused by any loss of medical technology or reduction in the number of hospitals. More and better medical care is usually associated with higher incomes and better public health, making the independent effect of medicine harder to disentangle.

It is clear that life expectancy has risen steadily over the last 150 years. The causes are not so clear or so steady, making it likely that the truth is complex, with different factors being more or less important at different times and places. Nutrition, housing, and other income-related factors were probably most important during the eighteenth and early nineteenth centuries. With the subsequent advance of science and the "Sanitary Revolution," public health became a major factor, and one study estimates that one-half of the gains in life expectancy during this period can be attributed to improvements in water supply alone.[36]

Prior to 1910, it is unlikely that medical care had much effect on life expectancy because it was so ineffective. In a famous study, Samuel Preston showed that around the turn of the century the mortality rate of the children of doctors was no different than that of factory workers.[37] Medical care became increasing efficacious during the twentieth century as the extensive availability of inexpensive fresh food, clean water, and advanced waste meant that the major gains from income (nutrition) and public health had already been made (i.e., the law of diminishing returns was setting in with regard to these factors).[38] Since 1960, much of the +7 year gain in life expectancy has been due to reduced cardiac mortality, with about two-thirds of that attributable to better medical care and one-third attributable to lifestyle changes (primarily decreased smoking).[39]

The gains from medical *science* are much larger than the gains from *care* because advances in knowledge improve nutrition and public health as well as medical therapy. Indeed, these boundaries can become blurred when vitamin deficiency diseases are treated by dietary supplements, fluoride in the water reduces dental caries, and infectious disease get made less threatening with vaccination. What was once advanced treatment can become routine (treating ulcers with Zantac bought at Walmart, taking an aspirin every day to reduce heart attacks and strokes). In the future, a healthy lifestyle might replace prescription medication with genetically engineered personal foods. The importance of knowledge as the underlying driver of increased life expectancy is demonstrated by the mortality trends in Africa during the 1970s and 1980s. There, despite disastrous decades in which dysfunctional governments and economies led to declining per capita income and closed many medical clinics, life expectancy continued to rise (however, note also that the plague of the 1990s, HIV/AIDS, caused heavy losses that are only now being reversed).

SUGGESTIONS FOR FURTHER READING

David M. Cutler, *Your Money or Your Life.* (Oxford, UK: Oxford University Press, 2004).

David Cutler, Angus Deaton, and Adriana Lleras-Muney, "The Determinants of Mortality," *Journal of Economic Perspectives* 20, no. 3 (2006): 97–120.

Angus Deaton, "Health, Inequality and Economic Development," *Journal of Economic Literature*, 41 (2003): 113–158.

Robert G. Evans, Morris Barer, and Theodore Marmor, *Why Are Some People Healthy and Others Not? The Determinants of Health of Populations* (New York: Aldine De Gruyter, 1994).

Robert W. Fogel, "Economic Growth, Population Theory and Physiology: The Bearing of Long-Term Processes on the Marking of Economic Policy," *American Economic Review* 84, no. 3 (1994): 369–395.

Robert W. Fogel, *The Escape From Hunger and Premature Death, 1700–2100.* Cambridge, UK: Cambridge University Press, 2004.

Massimo Livi-Bacci, *A Concise History of World Population* (Cambridge, Mass.: Blackwell, 1992).

Angus Maddison, *The World Economy: A Millennial Perspective* (Paris and Washington, D.C.: Organization for Economic Cooperation and Development (OECD), 2001).

Douglass C. North, *Structure and Change in Economic History* (New York: Norton, 1981).

Mancur Olson, Jr., "Big Bills Left on the Sidewalk: Why Some Nations are Rich, and Others Poor," *Journal of Economic Perspectives* 10, no. 2 (1996): 3–24.

Roy Porter, *The Greatest Benefit of Mankind* (New York: Harper-Collins, 1998).

James P. Smith, "Healthy Bodies and Thick Wallets: The Dual Relation Between Health and Economic Status," *Journal of Economic Perspectives* 13, no. 2 (Spring 1999): 145–166.

Rodrigo R. Soares, "Mortality Reductions, Educational Attainment and Fertility Choice," *American Economics Review*, 95, no. 3 (June 2005): 580–602.

SUMMARY

1. Four conditions must be met for modern medicine to develop:

   a. The risk of dying must be low enough (i.e., **life expectancy** long enough) that spending money to improve health is worthwhile.

   b. People must have **sufficient income** to pay for medical care.

   c. There must be a way to pool funds and **organize financing** for large numbers of people through insurance or government programs.

   d. **Medical technology** must be effective enough at improving health to be worth paying for.

2. **Life expectancy** averaged about 28 years from 10,000 B.C. to 1 A.D., and populations grew slowly, taking 100,000 years to double. From 1 A.D. to 1750, life expectancy averaged 22 to 28 years, and population doubled every 1,000 years. From 1750 to 1900, life expectancy averaged 30 to 45 years, and population doubled every 200 years. Today, life expectancy in the United States is more than 70 years, and the number of births is almost identical to the number of deaths, making the total population stable. In less-developed countries, life expectancy is still less than 50 years, and population growth is still very rapid, doubling every 30 years.

3. **Demographic transition** involves the movement of the population into cities, a rise in output per capita, a decline in mortality rates followed by a decline in birth rates, concluding with the stable and well-off populations characteristic of developed countries.

4. Development has always had some adverse effects (crowding, pollution); however, improvements in nutrition, security, and technology make the overall effect of economic development positive.

5. The dismal hypothesis of **Thomas Malthus** was that any increase in productivity would bring an uncontrolled increase in population, eventually making people worse off as the number of mouths to feed expanded faster than the food supply. Although Malthus's analysis provided insight into forces that had previously governed population growth, he did not foresee the rapid and continuous rise in productivity due to the industrial revolution, nor did he understand how the newly emerging middle-class families would choose to have fewer children so that they could invest more in their care and education.

6. In the hunter-gatherer economy of the prehistoric Stone Age, no one had much more than basic necessities. In the Agricultural Age, most people lived at a subsistence level, but the rulers controlled vast wealth and made major investments. In the Industrial Age, workers' wages rose rapidly above the subsistence level, economic organization became more complex, and most income was held by a large **middle class**.

7. A 1 percent reduction in mortality is worth more to people with a 70-year life expectancy than to people with a life expectancy of only 25 years. With good salaries and savings, people can afford to pay more to protect their health than could their grandparents, who barely earned enough to eat.

8. The **reduction in uncertainty** brought about by lower mortality and better jobs made it possible for ordinary people to plan for the future. Having a taste of freedom from fear and loss, they wanted more. In time, the demand for insurance and social security became universal.

9. The development of **medical technology** came after the industrial revolution was already well advanced. Improvements in the productivity of medicine (the ability to actually heal and extend life expectancy) began about 150 years after technological change had begun to raise industrial productivity. Although scientific advances are to some extent accidental, **the rate of technological change in medicine is largely determined by the economic resources** devoted to making new discoveries and applying them in practice.

10. The **economic organization** of medical care is rapidly evolving. From prehistoric times until 1900, most care was given by doctors practicing alone as independent practitioners. By 1950, the hospital and an organized medical staff funded through third-party payment were common. By 2030, most care probably will be provided by integrated health care systems with thousands of employees. **The most important medical advances are being brought about by improvements in information technology,** not pills and scalpels.

11. The astounding improvements in health that have more than **doubled life expectancy** over the last 200 years are attributable first to **better nutrition due to rising GDP**, second to improvements in **public health**, particularly water supply and sanitation, and third to better **medical technology**, especially for reducing cardiac mortality, the leading cause of death, over the last 50 years.

PROBLEMS

1. {*life expectancy*} What is the current average life expectancy? What was life expectancy 100 years ago? One thousand years ago? Ten thousand years ago? Is life expectancy likely to increase more rapidly or less rapidly during the next 100 years?

2. {*population growth*} How rapidly is the population growing in the United States? Is population growing more rapidly or less rapidly elsewhere in the world? Was it growing more rapidly or less rapidly 100 years ago? One thousand years ago?

3. {*population growth, dynamics*} What were the causes of the baby boom? How long did it last? How long will it affect the U.S. economy? Which part of the health care system was (is, will be) most affected?

4. {*population growth*} If the birth rate is 5 percent and the death rate is 3.5 percent, what is the rate of population increase? The death rate is consistent with a life expectancy of approximately how many years? The birth rate is consistent with approximately what family size? (*Hint:* Family size = number of children per year times number of fertile female years.)

5. {*population growth*} How long will it take population to double if it is growing 1 percent a year? If it is growing 0.1 percent a year?

6. {*distribution*} Is the distribution of income per capita more equal or less equal now than in the past? Is the distribution of life expectancy more equal or less equal now than in the past?

7. (*life expectancy*} Which has been more influential in raising life expectancy: economic growth or the development of medical technology? What evidence would support your answer? What evidence would contradict your answer? What evidence would support either answer?

8. {*population growth*} What is the Malthusian hypothesis? How did Malthus link population growth to declining marginal productivity?

9. {*population growth*} What are the most common reasons for population declines in the world today? Give examples.

10. {*family dynamics*} Will a family with higher income have more or fewer children? Which other economic factors affect choice of family size?

11. {*demographic transition*} Why do birth rates fall during demographic transition? How can population growth be accelerating if birth rates are declining?

12. {*demographic transition*} Why might death rates rise at the end of demographic transition? Can you give an example of a country where death rates might be rising now for this reason? Would such a situation imply more or less growth in per capita income? Why?

13. {*flow of funds*} Why is the development of a middle class a precondition for the development of medical insurance? Why is insurance necessary for the development of a modern, high-technology medical care system?

14. {*risk*} Does an increase in uncertainty, especially life-threatening uncertainties such as famine and plague, make medical care more or less valuable?

15. {*dynamics*} Did the productivity of medical technology start to increase before or after improvements in the productivity of industrial technology? Why? What determines the rate of technological change in medicine?

16.   {*productivity*} Assume that you are writing a science-fiction book that takes place in the year 2050. Which would be more devastating to the health of the world: loss of the drugs that cure HIV/AIDS or loss of computers?

17.   {*statistics, productivity*} In which field was the application of statistics necessary to improve productivity: industry, agriculture, or medical care?

18.   {*productivity*} Which has grown more rapidly: the productivity of farmers or the productivity of doctors?

19.   {*health production*} If the cities were the growing centers of economic opportunity, why did many of the people that moved to the city during the industrial revolution experience shorter average life spans than those who remained in the country?

20.   {*industrial organization, dynamics*} Was it economic organization, social organization, political organization, medical organization, or technology that led to the creation of a national medical insurance plan in Germany in 1883?

21.   {*distribution*} Does health insurance make income distribution more equal or less equal? Who is favored by such redistribution? Would a national health plan such as that proposed by President Clinton in 1994 be more redistributive or less redistributive than the current mixed public/private health insurance system in the United States? Which groups were most likely to benefit from the Clinton plan? Which groups of people would have been most likely to gain or lose from President Bush's proposals to privatize Medicare?

22.   {*distribution*} What is the difference between income and wealth? Which has grown more rapidly in the United States?

23.   {*social insurance*} What is the difference between "social security" and "insurance"?

24.   {*pricing, productivity, risk*} To whom will a drug that provides a 1 percent increase in 10-year survival be most valuable? List factors that might expand or reduce the impact of a 1 percent survival effect of on the market value of the drug.

ENDNOTES

1.   *Mortality* is the death rate—the number of deaths per 100 (or 1,000 or 100,000) persons alive at the beginning of the period. *Morbidity* is the incidence of illness or ill health—the number of cases per 100 (or 1,000 or 100,000) persons. Although clearly related to mortality, morbidity should also be clearly distinguished from mortality rates. While it is possible to obtain mortality rates from a variety of sources throughout history and so to create a reliable record, morbidity rates were available only under special circumstances (i.e., epidemics, aboard ships or in school or prison populations) until the advent of routine health surveys in the twentieth century, and are still lacking in many low-income countries with less comprehensive government statistical capabilities.

2.   Douglass C. North, *Structure and Change in Economic History* (New York: Norton, 1981).

3.   Note that this relationship, death rate = 1/(life expectancy), is a stock/flow equation analogous to the relationship between interest rates and the value of an annuity, interest = coupon/(price of bond), presented in finance texts, and is also rather similar to the stock/flow relationship between medical graduates and physician supply discussed in Section 7.3.

4.   A rule of thumb for compounding is known as the "rule of seventy-two." If you divide 72 by the interest rate, it gives the approximate length of time required to double your money. For very small rates of increase, such as those discussed here, a better approximation is to use 70 rather than 72. Thus $70 \div 2 = 35$ years to double at 2 percent per year, $70 \div 0.35 = 200$ years to double at 0.35 percent, and $70 \div 0.1 = 700$ years to double at a 0.1 percent rate of growth. This rule is quite accurate for rates less than 5 percent, and can be computed by hand or with a simple calculator until you have time to check the result with a spreadsheet.

5.   For a large empirical study of conditions in the Americas, see Richard H. Steckel and Jerome C. Rose, eds., *The Backbone of History: Health and Nutrition in the Western Hemisphere* (Cambridge, UK: Cambridge

University Press, 2002). An earlier assessment is found in Mark Nathan Cohen and George J. Amelagos, eds., *Paleopathology at the Origins of Agriculture* (New York: Academic Press, 1984), and a general overview in Mark Nathan Cohen, *Health and the Rise of Civilization* (New Haven: Yale University Press, 1989). It must be recognized that "life expectancy" varied widely (plus or minus 10 years or more, even for groups living within a few miles of each other during the same time period). Hence any comparisons of relative health are only rough indicators subject to many caveats and assumptions. The demographic data in this chapter are drawn largely from the books and articles by Deaton, Fogel, and Livi-Bacci listed among the Suggestions for Further Reading, as well as Wrigley and Schofield (note 16), McKeown (note 32), and McEvedy and Jones (note 9).

6. Theodore Tulchinsky and Elena Varavikova, "Addressing the Epidemiologic Transition in the Former Soviet Union," *American Journal of Public Health* 86, no. 3 (1996): 313–320; Vladimir Shkolnikov, Martina McKee, and David Leon, "Changes in Life Expectancy in Russia in the Mid-1990s," *The Lancet* 357 (March 24, 2001): 917–921; Elizabeth Brainerd and David M. Cutler, "Autopsy of an Empire: Understanding Mortality in Russia and the Former Soviet Union," NBER working paper 10868, October 2004.

7. Barrie Cassileth, Vasily Vlassov, and Christopher Chapman, "Health Care, Medical Practice, and Medical Ethics in Russia Today," *Journal of the American Medical Association* 273, no. 20 (1995): 1569–1573.

8. Johannes Nohl, "The Black Death: A Chronicle of the Plague, Compiled from Contemporary Sources" (London: Unwin Books, 1971); Philip Ziegler, *The Black Death* (New York: John Day Company, 1969).

9. Massimo Livi-Bacci, *A Concise History of World Population* (Cambridge Mass.: Blackwell, 1992), pp. 47, 106; Colin McEvedy and Richard Jones, *Atlas of World Population History* (Middlesex: Penguin, 1978), p. 25.

10. Massimo Livi-Bacci, *Population and Nutrition* (Cambridge: Cambridge University Press, 1991).

11. Robert Fogel, "Economic Growth, Population Theory and Physiology: The Bearing of Long-Term Processes on the Making of Economic Policy," *American Economic Review* 84, no. 3 (1994): 369–395.

12. Maurice Brown, *Adam Smith's Economics: Its Place in the Development of Economic Thought* (London: Croon Helm, 1988); E. G. West, *Adam Smith and Modern Economics: From Market Behavior to Social Choice*, (Aldershot, Hants, England: Edward Elgar Publishing, 1990).

13. Thomas Robert Malthus, *An Essay on the Principle of Population*, 1803, new edition by Patricia James for the Royal Economic Society (Cambridge: Cambridge University Press, 1992).

14. Livi-Bacci (1992), p. 65.

15. Gary D. Hansen and Edward C. Prescott, "Malthus to Solow," *American Economic Review* 92, no. 4 (September 2002): 1205–1217.

16. E. A. Wrigley and R. S. Schofield, *The Population History of England, 1541–1871: A Reconstruction* (Cambridge, Mass.: Harvard University Press, 1981).

17. Gary Becker, *A Treatise on the Family* (Cambridge, Mass.: Harvard University Press, 1981).

18. A surprisingly large number of successful entrepreneurs and inventors go bankrupt several times before and after they strike it rich. Such risk taking is not feasible if two bad years in a row means starvation.

19. Note that the rise of the middle class economy applies only within the small subset of developed countries. For most of the world's population, sharp divisions between rich and poor continued to be the rule. Francois Bourguignon and Christian Morrisson, "Inequality Among World Citizens: 1820–1992," *American Economic Review* 92, no. 4 (September 2002): 727–744.

20. Mancur Olson, Jr. "Big Bills Left on the Sidewalk: Why Some Nations are Rich, and Others Poor," *Journal of Economic Perspectives* 10, no. 2 (1996): 3–24.

21. The World Bank, *World Development Report 1993: Investing in Health* (Oxford, UK: Oxford University Press for the World Bank, 1993), p. 237.

22. United Nations, *World Population Prospects*, New York: United Nations (1989); The World Bank, *World Development Report 1986* (Oxford, UK: Oxford University Press, 1986); Livi-Bacci, op.cit. (1992): 199–208.

23. Angus Deaton, "Policy Implications of the Health and Wealth Gradient," *Health Affairs* 21, no. 2 (March 2002): 13–30.

24. Clayne L. Pope, "The Changing View of the Standard-of-Living Question in the United States," *American Economic Review* 83, no. 2 (May 1993): 331–336.

25. "The Black Report," reprinted in *Class and Health*, Richard G. Wilkinson (London: Tavistock, 1986). See also G.D. Smith, Mel Bartley, and David Blane, "The Black Report on Socioeconomic Inequalities in Health 10 Years On." *British Medical Journal* 301 (August 18, 1990): 373–377.

26. E. Rogot et al., *A Mortality Study of 1.3 Million Persons by Demographic, Social and Economic Factors: 1979–1985 Follow-Up* (Bethesda, Md.: National Institutes of Health, 1992); P. McDonough et al., "Income Dynamics and Adult Mortality in the United States, 1972 through 1989," *American Journal of Public Health* 87, no. 9 (September 1997): 1476–1483; Angus Deaton, "Health, Inequality and Economic Development," working paper, Center for Health and Wellbeing, Princeton University, Princeton, N.J. (May 2001), (www.wws.princeton.edu/~chw/).

27. James P. Smith, "Healthy Bodies and Thick Wallets: The Dual Relation Between Health and Economic Status," *Journal of Economic Perspectives* 13, no. 2 (Spring 1999): 145–166.

28. Stephen E. Snyder and Wiliam N. Evans, "The Impact of Income on Mortality: Evidence from the Social Security Notch," NBER working paper 9197 (September 2002).

29. The value of risk reduction is also high at the other extreme, where a person faces near certain death. If you knew that otherwise you would die, you might well be willing to give up half of your money for just a 1 percent chance of continuing to live. See also Gary Becker, Kevin Murphy and Tomas Philipson, "The Value of Life Near its End and Terminal Care," NBER working paper 1333 (August 2007).

30. Dora L. Costa and Matthew E. Kahn, "Changes in the Value of Life, 1940–1980," *Journal of Risk and Uncertainty* 29, no. 2 (September 2004): 149–80; and "The Rising Price of Non-Market Goods," paper presented at the American Economic Association Annual Meetings, Washington, D.C., January 4, 2003.

31. Ryan D. Edwards, "The Cost of Uncertain Life Span," NBER working paper 14093 (June 2008). The risk of dying between ages 18 and 38 is currently about .02 (2 percent). Eliminating that risk of "unfortunate young death" would increase life expectancy by a bit over one year. If we were get rid of the risk of dying from 18 through 38 by accepting that we could live no older than 90 or by doubling the risk of dying between 75 and 80, such a trade-off would leave average life expectancy unchanged, but most of us would consider ourselves much better off.

32. Isidore S. Falk, *Security Against Sickness* (New York: Doubleday, 1936); Jesse George Crownheart, *Sickness Insurance in Europe* (Madison, Wisc: Democrat Printing Company, 1938).

33. Thomas McKeown, *The Modern Rise of Population* (London: Edward Arnold, 1976).

34. Michel Foucault, *The Birth of the Clinic* (New York: Pantheon Books, 1973).

35. Institute of Medicine, *Crossing the Quality Chasm* (Washington, D.C.: National Academy Press, July 2001), http://newton.nap.edu/catalog/10027.html#toc.

36. David M. Cutler and Grant Miller, "The Role of Public Health Improvements in Health Advances: The Twentieth-Century United States." *Demography*, 42, no. 1 (2005): 1–22.

37. Samuel H. Preston, *Fatal Years: Child Mortality in Late 19th Century America* (Princeton, N.J.: Princeton University Press, 1991).

38. David Cutler, Angus Deaton, and Adriana Lleras-Muney, "The Determinants of Mortality," *Journal of Economic Perspectives* 20, no. 3 (2006): 97–120.

39. David M. Cutler, *Your Money or Your Life* (Oxford, UK: Oxford University Press, 2004); Robert Hall and Charles Jones, "The Value of Life and the Rise in Health Care Spending," *Quarterly Journal of Economics* 122, no. 1 (2007): 39–72; David M. Cutler, Allison Rose, and Sandeep Vijan, "The Value of Medical Spending in the U.S. 1960–2000," *New England Journal of Medicine* 355 (August 31, 2006): 920–927.

CHAPTER 17

INTERNATIONAL COMPARISONS OF HEALTH AND HEALTH EXPENDITURES

QUESTIONS

1. Which country is the healthiest?
2. Which country has the best medical care system?
3. Which country has the largest health care market?
4. Is health care trade more or less international than other goods and services?
5. Is there more trade between countries in goods, services, people, or ideas?
6. Are the differences among countries larger in terms of doctor supply, hospital technology, or per capita spending?
7. Is it high income or high medical expenditures that makes wealthy countries more healthy?
8. Does the distribution of income within a country determine the distribution of health?

17.1 WIDE DIFFERENCES AMONG NATIONS

There were more than 6 billion people in the world in 2006, distributed across some 200 countries. Health care expenditures for these 6 billion people totaled $3.8 trillion that year.[1] The 303 million people living in the United States represented 5 percent of the worldwide total, but U.S. health care expenditures, $2.1 trillion, accounted for more than 40 percent of total spending (see Table 17.1). Although China was the world's largest country, with 1.3 billion people, it accounted for only $0.1 trillion in health care spending. Health expenditures per person in the United States were 12 times the worldwide average in 2006, two and a half times as much as the $2,690 per person spent in Japan, and 70 times the per person average of $90 (approximately $342 in international purchasing power parity (PPP) exchange rates) in China (Table 17.1).[2] The extra $1,900 billion purchased a lot more hospitals, physicians, drugs, and technologically sophisticated equipment for U.S. citizens. But how

TABLE 17.1   Comparison of Health and Expenditures across Nations, 2006

	Population (millions)	Growth % rate	Life expectancy	% age 60+	Mortality Under 5	Mortality (15–59)	GNP (per capita)	GNP (ppp)	Health % of GNP	Expenditures (per capita)	Expenditures (PPP)	% Govt	% Private	Out of pocket	Prepaid plans
World	6,581	1.3	67.0	10.0	.071	.191	$ 7,708	$10,223	5.8	$ 681	$ 579	.56	.44	.23	.18
Sudan	38	2.2	60.0	6.0	.089	.296	$ 1,109	$ 1,780	3.8	$ 38	$ 61	.38	.62	.59	.00
Kenya	37	2.6	53.0	4.0	.121	.416	$ 406	$ 1,470	4.6	$ 29	$ 105	.48	.52	.41	.04
Pakistan	161	1.8	63.0	6.0	.097	.206	$ 756	$ 2,410	2.0	$ 16	$ 51	.16	.84	.82	.00
India	1,152	1.5	63.0	8.0	.076	.241	$ 880	$ 2,460	4.9	$ 39	$ 109	.20	.80	.76	.01
China	1,328	0.6	73.0	11.0	.024	.116	$ 1,226	$ 4,660	4.5	$ 90	$ 342	.42	.58	.54	.04
Turkey	74	1.3	73.0	8.0	.026	.123	$ 5,294	$ 8,410	5.6	$ 406	$ 645	.72	.29	.20	.04
Mexico	105	1.2	74.0	9.0	.036	.122	$ 7,930	$11,990	6.2	$ 500	$ 756	.29	.71	.67	.04
Poland	38	(0.1)	75.0	17.0	.007	.145	$ 8,707	$14,250	6.2	$ 556	$ 910	.70	.30	.26	.01
U.K.	61	0.4	79.0	22.0	.006	.080	$40,624	$33,650	8.4	$3,361	$2,784	.87	.13	.12	.01
Canada	33	0.9	81.0	18.0	.006	.072	$38,651	$36,280	10.0	$3,912	$3,672	.70	.30	.15	.13
Japan	128	-	83.0	27.0	.004	.067	$35,139	$32,840	7.9	$2,690	$2,514	.82	.18	.15	.03
Germany	83	-	80.0	25.0	.005	.081	$36,029	$32,680	10.4	$3,669	$3,328	.77	.23	.13	.09
U.S.	303	1.0	78.0	17.0	.008	.109	$44,070	$44,070	15.3	$6,714	$6,714	.46	.54	.13	.36

Source: World Health Statistics Report 2008.

many additional years of life, how much reduction in morbidity and mortality, did all these extra medical inputs yield? Could the United States have done as well or become even more healthy while spending less? Many factors other than hospitals and doctors are responsible for differences in health among China, the United States, and other countries, but an extra $1,900 billion is a significant amount to spend on health care.

Any assessment of health economy across the world must take into account the tremendous diversity in population, economic growth, and health status. Mozambique, Tanzania, and Ethiopia are among the world's poorest countries. These predominantly rural countries depend on subsistence agriculture and have limited government, little accumulation of savings or investment, per capita incomes of less than $600, and rapidly expanding populations facing repeated threats from starvation. One out of ten children die before age five, and life expectancy is less than 60 years. At the other extreme are Sweden and Switzerland, whose urbane citizens enjoy incomes of more than $40,000, where most deaths occur after age 75, and where average life expectancy exceeds 80 years. Development economists categorize countries as low, middle, or high income. More than half the world's population still lives in low-income, rural agricultural countries. Most countries in Africa are toward the bottom of the distribution. The two undeveloped giants, China and India, have 1.328 and 1.152 billion people, respectively. China's recent rapid development could, if maintained, transform the economy within 20 years. Middle-income countries ($2,500 to $10,000 per capita income), in which 1.5 billion people live, include many Latin American countries; most of the formerly socialist countries of the former Soviet Union and Eastern Europe; South Africa, Saudi Arabia, and other oil-rich states of the Middle East; and Asian countries with emerging economies such as Korea. High-income countries ($10,000+ per capita income), in which 850 million people live, include Western European countries and the United States, Canada, Japan, Australia, and New Zealand.

A nation's health resources generally increase with income, while the extent of illness and need for medical care is reduced. The high-income countries had 2.5 doctors and 8.3 hospital beds per 1,000 people in 2006.[3] The average life expectancy was 78 years, with more than half of all deaths occurring after that age. The perinatal mortality rate was 9 per 1,000 births, and the rate of tuberculosis (TB) infection was 0.2 per 1,000. In contrast, the low-income countries of sub-Saharan Africa could afford to spend only $12 per person on health care and had just 0.1 doctors and 1.4 hospital beds per 1,000 people. Life expectancy averaged 50 years, the perinatal mortality rate was 68 per 1,000 births, half of all deaths occurred in children under age six, and the TB infection rate was 2.20 per 1,000.

Size of the Market

From the perspective of the marketing department of a profit-maximizing health care firm, the importance of a country is determined not by the number of people, illnesses treated, or unmet needs, but by the number of dollars spent there. In these terms, the United States is by far the largest market in the world, with a 40+ percent share. In contrast, the world's most populous country, China, has only a 2 percent share, and the second most populous, India, has only a 1 percent share. In dollar terms, China's market is roughly the same size as the state of Ohio. All of the very-low-income countries together, 2.5 billion people, account for less than 2 percent of the world's health care spending (about one-third as much as the state of California) (Figure 17.1).

The disparity in health resources is not as great as the disparity in health spending because wages are lower in low-income countries; therefore, 75 percent less health care spending usually translates into a somewhat less severe reduction in the number of doctors or nurses.[4] Still, the gap between high-income and low-income countries is substantial

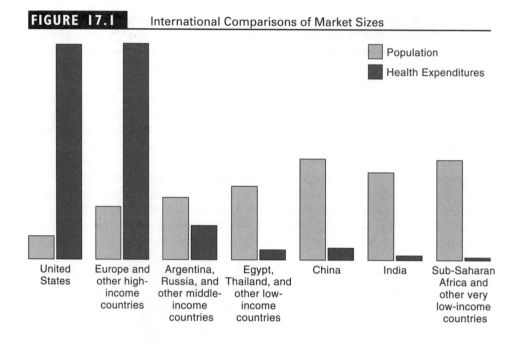

FIGURE 17.1 International Comparisons of Market Sizes

(Table 17.1). Some goods, such as pharmaceuticals, are traded internationally, and their prices are somewhat consistent across countries; thus, any decline in spending causes an equivalent decline in usage. Such internationally traded items take a much larger portion of health care budgets in low-income countries (25 to 50 percent) than in high-income countries (5 to 15 percent). There are vast disparities between rich and poor. Haves and have-nots face such different choices that they almost seem like inhabitants of different planets or different centuries. What is common and readily accessible to most citizens of high-income countries are the favored privileges of a few government officials, industrialists, and celebrities in low-income countries. Medical care as practiced in the developed world is but a dream as distant as Hollywood for most of the world's population.

17.2 MICRO VERSUS MACRO ALLOCATION: HEALTH AS A NATIONAL LUXURY GOOD

Economists call entertainment, travel, and other expenditures "luxury goods," not as a judgment regarding the necessity or importance of such items, but because they observe that the percentage of income spent on these goods increases as income increases. Items for which a 10 percent increase in income leads to a greater than 10 percent increase in spending (i.e., income elasticity > 1.0) are labeled luxury goods, regardless of their use (see Section 13.2). Differences in relative wages between countries may complicate dollar comparisons, but a country that spends 12 percent of its gross domestic product (GDP) on health care is using more of its resources for medical care than a country spending 8 percent.[5]

Nations spend more money on health care because they have more money to spend, not because they have greater medical needs. This conclusion is not very surprising when considering whether Bangladesh (GDP $500 per capita) will spend more or less than Belgium (GDP $45,000 per capita) on health (Figure 17.2). Yet the finding that health care spending

FIGURE 17.2 Per Capita Health Expenditures Related to Income

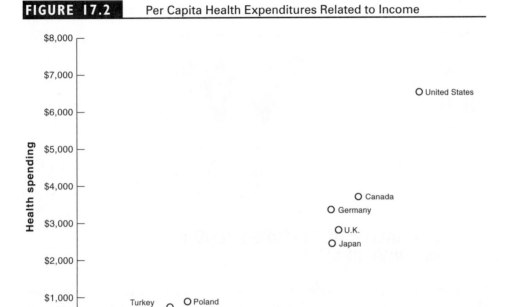

Source: World Health Statistics Report, 2008.

is unrelated or inverse to medical needs contradicts most personal experience—individuals spend more on health care if they become sick. Decisions on how much will be spent by or for a particular individual (micro) are significantly different from, and based on different factors than, national decisions made collectively through the political process about how much of the budget or GDP should be spent on health (macro) (see Chapter 13). Health expenditures come mostly from pooled funds raised through taxes and employee benefit plans. Given that pooled set of funds, decisions will be made about how to spend these funds on a covered individual based on personal medical need. Insurance and government financing are ways to make sure that people's ability to pay does not limit the care they receive when they need it. Yet collectively, the ability of all to pay, their aggregate prior contributions in taxes and insurance premiums, puts an absolute limit on how much can be spent in total on all the individuals treated. As the focus shifts from micro to macro allocation, the significant determinant of spending shifts from "medical need" to "available income" (Figure 17.3). For example, most countries spend two to five times as much on elderly people as they do on young and middle-aged people. However, this does not mean that if a country's population is older it will spend more on health care (take it to the limit and suppose everyone were old and retired—who, then, would be working to pay for the extra nursing homes, hip replacements, and heart medications?).[6] As shown in Table 17.1, England has an older population than the United States and health statistics that are roughly equivalent on many measures (life expectancy 79 years versus 78 years, infant mortality 0.6 percent versus 0.8 percent), but England spends significantly less on health care on average ($3,361 versus $6,714), partly because per capita income is lower ($40,226 versus $44,070).[7]

| FIGURE 17.3 | Micro and Macro Determinants of Health Spending |

Micro ←——————————————————————————→ **Macro**

Health status
Individual differences in medical spending are determined mostly by differences in health status, i.e., whether or not the person is sick.

GDP per capita
National differences in spending per person are largely determined by differences in income.

17.3 CAUSALITY: DOES MORE SPENDING IMPROVE HEALTH?

Wealthier countries are healthier, and they spend more on medical care. Can one then conclude that more spending buys better health? Not necessarily. Many factors associated with higher incomes, such as education, nutrition, and sanitation, are also known to improve health (see Chapter 16). Furthermore, life expectancy has increased greatly in many poor countries over the past 20 years, even when the availability of doctors and GDP per capita declined. A full assessment of all the influences on health status and relative contribution of each factor is not possible, but a rough appraisal of the relative importance of *economic growth*, advances in *public health and medical research*, and the *use of medical care services* can be made. However, it must be recognized that all these influences interact with and modify one another. With no knowledge of what to do, money is worthless, and medical knowledge alone is useless in the face of extreme poverty, which leads to death from starvation. Any specific estimate of how much each factor contributes to health is to some extent artificial and is also limited to what can readily be observed (i.e., differences noticeable within the range covered by statistics, such as those presented in Table 17.1). Perusal of data from many countries indicates that only large differences, increases of ten-fold or hundred-fold, consistently affect health outcomes. Income differences on the order of 50 percent or 100 percent are not reliably associated with increases or decreases in life expectancy and appear to be within a range of indifference or minor variation or measurement error. Hence, they should either be treated with caution or ignored. It is the big picture that matters in this appraisal of relative importance.

Figure 17.4 illustrates that there is a relationship between per capita income and average life expectancy, and that the relationship has changed over time. A plausible interpretation is that movements along the curve reflect the combined effects of more income and more medical care, while the shifting of the curve reflects the universal effect of increased knowledge, which is a public good. Between 1960 and 1990, life expectancy in Africa increased by about 10 years, from 43 to 52, despite the lack of improvement in living standards or incomes. Another piece of evidence for the effect of knowledge on health is provided by studies of childhood mortality in the United States around 1900.[8] In that era, children of well-to-do physicians were just as likely to die before age five as children of poor laborers living in tenements, since both the wealthy and the poor used the same ineffectual health practices. As the importance of infection and nutrition were revealed, physicians' families were able to take advantage of their better education and resources so that child mortality declined much more rapidly in this group than among low-income laborers. In poor countries today, sanitation, basic nutrition supplements for infants, and control of preventable

FIGURE 17.4   Life Expectancy and Income per Capita

disease are still of primary importance. In these situations, studies have indicated that maternal education and literacy is often more important than income in preventing childhood
disease and death.

Separate assessment of the effects of living standards and utilization of medical care
is difficult because both generally rise or fall together. Japan, for example, has achieved a
phenomenal 25-year increase in life expectancy since World War II, but there is no easy way
to determine how much is due to the rapid economic growth and how much is due to the
deployment of modern medical care. The achievement of relatively high life expectancies
in some low- or middle-income countries with relatively low use of sophisticated medical
treatments (72 years in Malaysia, 75 years in the Czech Republic, 76 years in Costa Rica)
suggests that the incremental effect of medical care alone is probably modest. Analysis across
many countries reveals that the absolute level of income may not be as important in many
cases as **income distribution**.[9] It is not surprising that where there is greater equality of
income, the average level of health is higher. The relationship between income and health is
nonlinear. A 20 percent drop means much less at the middle or top of the distribution than
it does toward the bottom. High rates of illness are a function not of poverty but of extreme
deprivation. The greater the degree of inequality, the more likely it is that some families will
be so lacking in food and amenities that deaths from infantile diarrhea, tuberculosis, and
other preventable or treatable illnesses will occur.

17.4 LOW-INCOME COUNTRIES

Low-income countries face health care problems that are very different from those of wealthy,
industrialized countries. The populations of low-income countries are rural, with many

children, and a heavy burden of infectious disease and stunting (abnormally low height and/or small body size) due to occasional malnutrition. However, government officials living in the capital have incomes, tastes, and health care needs much more like those of developed countries. This can lead to a major misallocation of resources, such as building a modern research hospital in the capital providing excellent tertiary care, while much of the country lacks access to a doctor or a nurse and children remain unvaccinated so that preventable disease epidemics remain common. It is not unusual for as much as half the entire health budget of a low-income country to be spent in the capital city, with a large part going to equip and staff the leading hospital (in contrast, the Johns Hopkins University Hospital takes about 0.6 percent of the U.S. health care budget). Convincing local medical leaders to change the allocation of resources to a more appropriate emphasis on low-technology primary care is difficult, since they do not wish to give up their expensive research hospital, which might bring the doctors and government officials prestige and international fame. The world may admire a European doctor trained at a leading university who spends years alone treating cases in an isolated river village, but a local physician who spends his days treating diarrhea and wound infections without any chance to practice in a modern surgical facility is simply considered to have minimal skills of little importance to outsiders. Incentives are not aligned with the health needs of the majority of citizens. Both ruling politicians and leaders of the medical profession will naturally tend to favor maintaining a state-of-the-art facility with modern technology and capability for research, even when doing so drains funds from the village clinics and nursing care that can do more to reduce infant mortality and raise life expectancy. Even in very-low-income countries, medical schools train many specialists who want to perform technologically advanced procedures rather than primary care generalists able to treat most common illnesses.

Studies by the World Bank have found that the status of women is a major determinant of health in low-income countries. Access to knowledge is one factor. In countries where most women are illiterate and uneducated, there is no way for them to know about sterilization of water, proper nutrition, or care of childhood infections. Women are also more likely than men to make family health a priority. In subsistence economies where women have some control over spending (because of tradition or because they have a job with wages), a larger fraction of the household budget gets spent on food and less on alcohol and tobacco.

Starvation remains a problem in many of the lowest-income countries. In Nigeria, 43 percent of children aged two to six are stunted (their height is low for their age), 32 percent in Kenya, and 65 percent in India, compared with 22 percent in Mexico, 4 percent in Japan, and 2 percent in the United Kingdom and United States.[10] This situation occurs not because food supply is insufficient, but because the supply is maldistributed. Organizational disarray, lack of transport, disruptions due to war and political upheaval, and poorly functioning markets mean that food does not get to where it is needed most. No simple solution presents itself, since the defects in economic organization that cause mismanagement of food are the same as those responsible for a lack of economic development in the first place. National governments that maintain order, handle their budgets and money supply prudently, and support market-oriented policies are able to grow out of the low-income category.

Sudan

Sudan* is a low-income, highly indebted poor country on the northeastern coast of sub-Saharan Africa. Sudan's population of 38 million people is spread out over 2.5 million

*This section on Sudan was contributed by Muneef Abdelbagi Babiker, Assistant Professor, Department of Economics, University of Khartoum.

square kilometers and is growing rapidly at a rate of 2.2 percent a year despite desperate poverty. Per capita income is estimated at about $1,100 for 2006. As has been the case in most African countries, the public health system was the main provider of health care services, employing physicians, nurses, pharmacists, and paramedical and other support staff on a salary scale comparable to the public service salary scale. Physicians and facilities were overconcentrated in urban areas, although indicators point to the rural areas as being the most in need. Taxation was historically the primary source of funding, with all premises and equipment owned and maintained by the government.

Although historically services were offered free of charge at the time of use, economic retrenchments and severe natural and human-made disasters, including floods, droughts, and armed conflict in the southern part of the country, have caused serious dislocations in the national health system. The promise of free health services for all citizens became increasingly hollow as inadequate budgets left buildings, equipment, and professional time of salaried health personnel seriously underutilized. Economic waste was further aggravated by purchases of capital equipment, building materials, and medical staff training using scarce foreign exchange. Spending on social services in general and on health in particular was low and declined during the 1980s and 1990s. In times of financial stringency, the obligations to pay salaries and rent and to pay for maintenance and replenishment of assets frequently used by physicians (e.g., cars, stethoscopes) are given priority, making the impact of reduced spending on services even more severe than the financial figures alone indicate.

The adverse economic situation since the 1980s has had a great impact on health services, health status, and funding. The private sector in medical care witnessed a qualitative and quantitative expansion. Traditionally the private sector was restricted to after-hours consultations by government-employed doctors during their free time in the evening. However, more doctors have converted to full private practice, and private inpatient hospitals are being built. A World Health Organization (WHO) consultant estimated that the central government spent $2.50 per person on health care in 2002, about 0.65 percent of GDP.[11] Most total health spending, 62 percent, comes from fees paid by private households, 17 percent from the compulsory National Health Insurance Scheme, 19 percent from ministry of health and other central government ministries, and 2 percent from international organizations (mainly WHO and United Nations Children's Fund (UNICEF)). Other sources of financing for health services include small company-based health insurance schemes, humanitarian national and international nongovernmental organizations, and private expenditures on traditional healers. According to a 2003 World Bank report, Sudan, both in absolute and relative terms—at perhaps US$4 per capita and under or around 1 percent of GDP—government health spending in Sudan ranks among the lowest in the world. This relatively low level of public health spending is supplemented by household out-of-pocket spending and health insurance spending. According to World Bank, "... it is estimated that total out-of-pocket expenditures are as large or larger than total government health spending (that is, 1 percent or more of GDP). In addition, the national health insurance scheme similarly spends around 1 percent of GDP, so that total health expenditures in Northern Sudan are likely in the range of 4 or 5 percent of GDP, or US$ 15 to 20 per capita. This level would be consistent with the lower range of total spending in countries in Sub-Saharan Africa." Because most of the public and private health facilities and personnel are concentrated in urban areas, the actual coverage by health services is expected to be very low. By law the health insurance scheme is supposed to cover all employees of public and private enterprises that employ at least 10 people, but currently this plan covers only 6 percent of the population.

People who can afford to use the current fee-based health services system more tend to benefit most. Reliance on private funds has increased inequity. With less public funding, many individuals wait until their illness reaches a serious stage before contacting the health services system. There is less spending on routine care and prevention and more on catastrophic events. The trend toward privatization has even encroached on public health services. In Khartoum, the upkeep of a number of previously unattended, filthy, and deserted public lavatories attached to mosques, market areas, bus stops, and other public areas have been contracted to private individuals or institutions. The average annual rents for a lavatory unit are 615,000 Sudanese dinars (approximately $2,460). The contractors can charge a small fee ranging between 10 and 20 dinars (4–8 cents) for every episode of use. Although no formal study has been conducted to evaluate this privatization experiment, a limited survey revealed that contractors and users were satisfied. This, along with the fact that these arrangements have been functioning since 1995 and that more units are being constructed, indicates success.

Health Care in Kenya

The economy of Kenya is dominated by agriculture. Its most significant exports are coffee, tea, cotton, and minerals. Kenya's 24 million people had a per capita income of about $340 in 1990. By 2006 population had surged to 37 million but income had increased only slightly, to $406 per person per year (about $1 per day). Income is much more difficult to measure or define in a traditional agricultural economy; therefore, any figure should be considered approximate. The population is growing very rapidly (2.6 percent per year), with almost half under the age of 15. Enrollment of children in primary school is 88 percent, and more than half of all adults are literate. About a quarter of the population lives in cities. The single-party KANU government, in power since 1963, is relatively stable for such a poor country. Life expectancy at 53 years is above average for sub-Saharan Africa. However, half of all deaths occur in children under the age of 15, and adults are about three times as likely to die in any given year as they are in the United States.

The health system is split almost equally between the public and private sector (see Table 17.2). The Ministry of Health runs 80 hospitals, 41 district health centers in the

TABLE 17.2	Health Expenditures in Kenya, 1990	
	$ Millions	**Percentage**
Government		
Ministry of health	204	42%
Municipalities	27	6%
Other government	6	1%
Private Sources		
Voluntary agencies	6	1%
Religious missions	28	6%
Corporate clinics	2	*
Household spending		
Hospitals	45	9%
Physicians & healers	36	7%
Drugs	114	24%
Other	16	3%
Total	484	Approximately $20 per person

Source: The World Bank Development Report 1993, and Bloom et al., Expenditure and Financing of the Health Sector in Kenya (Nairobi: Ministry of Health) 1986.

provinces, 178 rural health centers, and about 1,200 subcenters and dispensaries. District medical officers are physicians, usually assisted by one or more nurses and a hospital secretary (administrator).[12] Below the district level, most facilities are operated by paraprofessionals, and at the dispensary level, by community workers or untrained auxiliaries. Despite a stated emphasis on primary care and rural development, more than 35 percent of the entire national budget is spent on the showcase Kenya National Hospital in Nairobi. Some government agencies, such as the Ministry of Transport and the Coffee Board, run health services for their workers, as do the dozen or so corporations with more than 500 employees.

Religious missions are a very important part of the health care system, running 40 hospitals, 84 health centers, and 173 clinics. Although the origins and management of these facilities are religious, 60 percent of their funding comes from patient fees, about 25 percent from government subsidy, and only 15 percent from donations. Thus, they are considered part of the private sector. Overall, about 22 percent of Kenyan health expenditures are derived from foreign aid.

The government actively encourages private sector health care. Private hospitals, supported entirely by fees, are viewed as being of higher quality and are growing rapidly. The government runs a National Hospital Insurance Fund for high-income workers through a mandatory 2-percent wage tax (there is no employer contribution) designed to reimburse people for stays in private and religious hospitals or private rooms of public hospitals. However, this plan covers only 12 percent of the population. The effectiveness of the plan may be further limited by its low payout rate: only 60 percent of the hospital insurance premiums collected were used to pay claims or administrative expenses, allowing 40 percent to be held by the central government.

Most physicians (70 percent) work full time in private practice. The 30 percent who work for the government or missions also engage in private practice after clinic hours. There are, perhaps, 2,000 physicians actively in practice in Kenya, almost half of them in Nairobi (although it has only 7 percent of the nation's population). In contrast, there are about 19,000 traditional healers and herbalists practicing in Kenya, most of them in the countryside. A physician earns roughly 30 times as much as a traditional healer. A small fraction of the population, the 2 or 3 percent who belong to upper-income families living in the major cities, accounts for more than half of all private expenditures for medical care. About one-third comes from the 10 percent who are middle-income city dwellers. The poor who have flocked to the cities account for less than 2 percent of private spending, and the bulk of the population still living in rural areas (about 75 percent) accounts for just 17 percent of private expenditures. The flow of medical resources clearly follows the flow of funds. The disparity between members of the elite who live in the capital and the vast rural population that subsists by farming is clearly visible in morbidity and mortality statistics, and remains the largest problem facing health care in Kenya.

17.5 MIDDLE-INCOME COUNTRIES

Turkey, Mexico, Thailand, and South Korea are examples of countries that are in the midst of development. Subsistence agriculture and poverty are still the norm in the remote rural regions, but the bulk of the population has moved into cities and works for wages. The shift from rural agricultural labor to urban wage labor presents a major organizational problem: how to develop a comprehensive health insurance system able to fund a higher level of health care. Rapid economic growth allows some countries to expand government services; thus, a predominantly public system is created. In other countries, such as Korea, a strong tradition of industrial paternalism leads to private insurance based on employment benefits. Some countries began with a public system and switched to reliance on the private sector, while others are moving in the opposite direction. In almost every middle-income developing country the health insurance system is in transition. Even when coverage is universal by law, the reality is that access to medical care is very uneven. The urban ghettos and impoverished rural villages frequently lack sanitation. Restrictions and incompleteness in the health insurance system may prevent poor citizens from using medical facilities even when these facilities are accessible geographically. Thus, the disadvantaged populations are disproportionately represented in morbidity and mortality statistics. At the same time, expanding incomes have brought the lifestyle illnesses of the wealthy countries, such as heart disease and lung cancer, to prominence. The growth markets for cigarettes in the twenty-first century are China, India, and Asia, not Europe and North America. Finally, the middle-income countries are still likely to misallocate resources, emulating the advanced health care systems of high-income nations: large research hospitals in the cities matched by a lack of village clinics in the countryside and the training of too many specialists and not enough primary care physicians or public health experts.

The Health Care System of Mexico

With a 2005 per capita GDP of $6,820, an average life expectancy of 73 years for males and 78 years for females, and a young population (30 percent younger than age 15) of 106 million that is growing rapidly (1 percent per year), Mexico* is similar to many other countries with transitional economies. The bulk of the people have moved off the farms into cities to find industrial and service jobs, but agriculture and export of raw commodities still make up a substantial part of the economy, and illiteracy is still a problem in rural areas. The government is politically stable, with a new party coming to power in 2000, shifting away from 80 years of single-party rule to a more open, multi-party democracy.

The government enacted a comprehensive social security system (IMSS, in 1943) relatively early for a transitional economy, but it only covered industrial workers and their dependents.[13] A nationwide network of IMSS health centers, polyclinics, and hospitals was built. The Ministry of Health and IMSS-Solidaridad provide services for around 40 million uninsured Mexicans, mainly the rural and urban poor. In 1960, a plan for government employees, ISSSTE, was established, and a modern and technologically sophisticated network of hospitals and clinics was built with generous funding to accommodate this favored group of employees. ISSSTE, IMSS, and the medical services for the armed forces and employees of the national oil company (PEMEX) provided the top tier of health insurance and covered about half the population (see Table 17.3).

TABLE 17.3	Health Insurance Coverage in Mexico
Mexican Institute of Social Security (IMSS)	39%
Institute for Governmental Workers (ISSSTE)	8%
Other federal agency health plans	2%
Secretariat of Health & Welfare (SSA)	21%
Marginal families program	13%
Private medical care	5%
Unprotected population	12%

Source: Milton Roemer, *National Health Systems of the World*
(New York: Oxford University Press, 1991).

*This section was revised by Julio Frenk, M.D., Ph.D., Minister of Health, and Octavio Gomez, M.D.

The organization of services in Mexico is rigidly segregated, and quality is considerably heterogeneous. The Ministry of Health, IMSS, and ISSSTE provide primary, secondary, and tertiary services, with specialty services concentrated in the three largest cities: Mexico City, Guadalajara, and Monterrey. The private market provides services both at the bottom of the income distribution (where SSA is inadequate) and at the top (where wealthier people can buy state-of-the-art medical care), with the middle occupied by three separate tiers of public care. The private sector consists of providers working in hospitals, clinics, offices, and folk medicine units on a for-profit basis. In theory, this component should provide services for around 10 percent of the population. However, according to recent surveys, around 25 percent of the people enrolled in social security agencies report a private provider as their usual source of ambulatory care. In the same vein, around 40 percent of the uninsured population report a private practitioner as their usual source of primary care.

Most physicians in Mexico work in salaried positions for ISSSTE, IMSS, or SSA and also have a private practice as well. Yet even though Mexico has considerably fewer physicians per 100,000 population than in the United States (about one-fourth as many), there is a large pool of unemployed or underemployed physicians (more than 30 percent of all physicians) who cannot find a government job or attract enough private patients to make a living from medicine.

The present administration promoted a major legislative reform establishing a system of social protection in health, which was approved by a large majority of the Mexican Congress in 2003. This system is reorganizing and increasing public funding by a full percentage point of GDP over seven years in order to provide universal health insurance, including the 50 million Mexicans, most of them poor, who had been excluded until now from formal social insurance plans because they are self-employed, are out of the labor market, or work in the informal sector of the economy.

The increased funding is spearheading a major effort to realign incentives throughout the health system. Poor families can now enroll in a new scheme called "Popular Health Insurance," which is the basis for allocating federal funds to states. The old model of "bureaucratic budgeting," which subsidized providers without regard to performance, is being replaced by "democratic budgeting," whereby money follows people through a demand-side subsidy. Capitated payments and freedom of choice assure an optimal balance between quality and efficiency.

To achieve this aim, the macro-level financial reform is being complemented by a micro-level management reform, which is strengthening delivery capacity through a series of specific interventions, such as long-term planning of new facilities, technology assessment, efficient schemes for drug supply, human resource development including managerial training, outcome-oriented information systems, facility accreditation, provider certification, quality assurance, and performance benchmarking at both the state and the provider levels.

Poland

Poland* has 38 million people, with an average per capita income of $8,200 in 2005 and a life expectancy of 69 years for males and 78 years for females. There are about 22 doctors, 49 nurses, and 50 hospital beds per 10,000 people. Total expenses for health care in Poland were about $540 per capita (6.6 percent of GDP) in 2002.[14] The main sources of financing are public sickness funds (Kasy Chorych), but private resources have recently grown to contribute almost 40 percent. Since 1999, social insurance funds have accounted for 80 percent

*This section was contributed by Katarzyna Tymowska, Director of Postgraduate Study in Health Economics, Warsaw University.

of public resources. Insurance is mandatory for all workers. The amount of the premium (7.5 percent of wages) is established by Parliament as a part of personal income tax. Employers do not finance the premiums, but withhold the amount from wages and submit them for collection by a nationwide public agency. The government pays premiums for about 35 percent of the citizens (farmers, the unemployed, people collecting social security payments). Administrative information systems have many weak points; thus, these estimates must be used with caution. Payments between sickness funds are equalized to account for differences in participants' income and ages. The sickness funds practice cost control by establishing rates and limiting the number of services. However, administrative inefficiencies and the difficulty of enforcing agreements mean that budget limits are frequently broken. Hospital services accounted for approximately 50 percent of the total expenditures of public funds in 2002. Cost shifting also takes place. Teaching hospitals receive financial resources for research from a special quasi-budget fund and from pharmaceutical company grants. Part of these resources covers expenses for patients' treatment. Thanks to the extra funding, the quality of care rises, which attracts good physicians and more patients. Due to the lack of standards, these specialized hospitals also admit patients with minor health problems.

Pharmaceuticals account for one-third of total health expenditures in Poland. The percentage is high not only because drug consumption is high, but also because of the relatively low cost of medical staff. Half of households' private expenditures for health are for buying pharmaceuticals. Drug expenses, both public and private, have increased considerably during recent years. Among the causes are the elimination of the state monopoly in the drug market, intensive marketing by pharmaceutical companies, and the strong belief of many Poles in the efficacy of expensive drugs produced by foreign companies. Hospital managers have responded to the squeeze caused by rising drug expenditures and limited budgets by introducing standardized pharmacological procedures and prescription books and requiring approvals by the head of a hospital unit to order expensive drugs.

In Poland, copayment for services is unimportant. Because patients incur few charges, services are overused (moral hazard). However, there exists a culturally conditioned custom of giving gifts to facilitate access to services or obtain greater kindness from hospital employees. Such informal gratuities constituted 36 percent of private out-of-pocket health spending in a recent study.

Private resources are of increasing importance in Poland. Earnings are going up, educational levels are rising, and social expectations regarding easy access to health care (and to higher quality care) are escalating. Medical services have become consumption goods, which has encouraged development of private medical companies. Unlike in the times of communist rule, one no longer needs administrative permits to establish a firm. These companies, often operating with foreign capital, react quickly to a growing demand for medical services. Some have signed contracts with public payers, while others are planning to take part in the competition offering medical services to the insured. Dissatisfaction with the low quality of public sector medical services has been a major cause of increasing demand for the private companies. Large employers are able to buy services in advance, especially ambulatory care, using prepayments (called "subscriptions"). This is not the same as the workers' health plans, but has similar benefits: tax advantages for employers and employees and "golden cuffs" to keep valued workers. Another factor favoring this development is the partial transfer of treatment costs so that the private sector does not bear full financial responsibility. High-risk patients are directed to specialized diagnostic centers and hospitals financed with public money. In Poland, private facilities act as a kind of "gate" through which patients can get into a facility maintained by public resources more easily.

The present system of contracts creates a special inducement for cost shifting through the use of capitation payments to primary care physicians. Primary physicians receive a fixed amount of funds to pay for their work, for the work of nurses and record-keepers, and for basic diagnostics (physicians are not allowed to own pharmacies but can own diagnostic centers). In some regions, capitation fees also cover specialized health care and diagnostic services. A primary care physician, especially one with an individual practice, prefers to send a patient to a specialist. The primary care physician keeps the capitation payment, the specialist takes over the patient's treatment, and public insurance pays a fee-for-service amount to the specialist.

Both primary and specialist physicians have reason to transfer diagnostic expenses to hospitals, especially when ambulatory diagnostics are underdeveloped or require a long waiting list. Patients, who eagerly accept hospital referrals, contribute to this situation. Despite attempts to limit the number of admissions, the number of hospitalized patients has increased greatly, as has the amount of hospital diagnostic testing. The contracts signed by ambulatory care physicians as well as those signed by hospitals create hidden incentives for cost shifting.

These comprehensive capitated payment plans, resembling managed care in the United States, have caused many conflicts between primary and specialist physicians. Primary care physicians created their own network of service providers, paying for the specialists' work and supervising them. This supervision, a type of utilization review, has brought many complaints from specialists. Very soon all capitation fees will cover primary medical care and an extended range of diagnostics. Some primary care physicians, having funds for a wide range of services, have been motivated to limit the number of referrals. These restrictions are seen as threats to the quality of care, particularly given the lack of standards and of treatment monitoring. Strong protests and lobbying by specialists have resulted in a number of changes, but it is unlikely that the problems of cost shifting and quality deterioration will go away soon.

17.6   HIGH-INCOME COUNTRIES

Among high-income countries, there is considerable variation in the use of medical care inputs (doctors per 1,000 population ranging from 1.4 to 4.3; hospital beds per 1,000 ranging from 3.9 to 16.1), organization of services, reliance on taxpayer financing, and total cost (from $450 to $4,500 per capita), but remarkably little variation in health outcomes. Life expectancy in the 22 high-income countries is between 76 and 81 years and infant mortality is between four and eight per 1,000 births. Much greater variation in health statistics exists between regions within any one of these countries than across all 22 of them. Given the small differences in average health outcomes, it is difficult to say that one country's system is better or worse than another's. What is clear is that many health problems are concentrated in specific, underserved populations, usually ethnic minorities or areas of extreme poverty.[15] Although tremendous resources are available for advanced experimental treatment, electronic scanning for diagnosis, and long-term rehabilitation, there is still a lack of primary care resources ensuring that every child is immunized, that all pregnant women receive adequate prenatal care and nutrition, and that every person has a primary physician to contact when in need of advice or care. In many ways, high-income countries face the same problems of maldistribution and misallocation in the delivery of medical care as low-income countries, but at a different level (see Figure 17.5).

Japan

Life expectancy in Japan* is the highest in the world: 78 years for men and 85 years for women. However, the level of health care spending is only half that of the United States,

---

*This section was contributed by Etsuji Okamoto, M.D., M.P.H., National Institute of Public Health, Saitama, Japan.

FIGURE 17.5   Health Expenditures and Life Expectancy across Countries

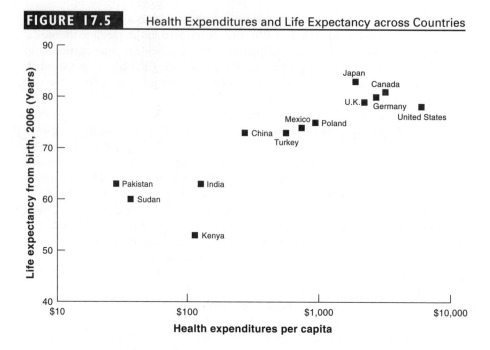

about $3,500 per person, 7.3 percent of GDP in 2006. Although the technology used in the Japanese health care system is similar to that used in the United States, the organization and flow of funds and, hence, the quantity and intensity of use, are considerably different.[16] In Japan, all citizens are covered by some form of insurance and are able to choose any physician or hospital they wish, with no bills other than modest copayments per visit or per day.

Physicians are clearly split into two groups. Generalist physicians are private solo practitioners providing primary and secondary care as small businesses, earning a substantial portion of their income from mark-ups on pharmaceuticals and laboratory tests. Specialist physicians work in hospitals on salary and generally earn much less. Unlike in the United States, a patient undergoing surgery at a hospital in Japan receives a single bill that includes both room and board and the surgery fee. Surgeons are employees of hospitals and are not allowed to charge patients independently. Some argue that this combined bill may be one reason that giving gifts to the doctor is a customary practice in Japan. Private practitioners cannot attend to hospitalized patients, and hospital physicians are not allowed to have a private practice on the side.

Hospitals are also split into two groups. Large public and university hospitals contain medical schools and research facilities, but may also have large outpatient departments providing primary care. Small facilities owned by private practitioners provide less sophisticated treatments and simple therapeutics. For-profit, investor-owned hospitals are prohibited in Japan. Controls over utilization are not stringent. There is no preauthorization for surgery, no requirement for a second opinion, and no statistical profiling or concurrent review as under managed care in the United States. With no limits imposed, length of stay tends to be very long, 30.4 days for general acute hospitals and 377 days for psychiatric hospitals.

Universal health insurance coverage is obtained through myriad funding bodies, all regulated by the Ministry of Health, Labor, and Welfare (MHLW) (see Figure 17.6). Society-managed health insurance (SMHI) covers the employees of the large corporations. Corporations with a minimum of 700 employees may opt to establish their own health insurance societies as distinct legal entities whose assets are shielded from liabilities of the parent

FIGURE 17.6 Flow of Funds in the Japanese Health Care System

corporation. Approximately 1,800 such SMHI societies exist, and virtually all corporations known worldwide, such as Sony and Toyota, have them. SMHI premiums are 6 to 9 percent of salary, split equally between the employer and the employee. Large-company employees tend to have the best salaries, with young workers (typical retirement age is 60) in good health, making these societies financially viable without subsidy. Coverage for civil servants and their dependents under the Mutual Aid Associations (MAA) is rather similar to the SMHI. Small- and medium-sized corporations (less than 700 employees) are covered by the Japan Health Insurance Association (JHIA). The JHAI premiums, 8.5 percent of salary, are not sufficient to cover costs, and subsidies are provided through the MHLW, amounting to about 14 percent of funding. The JHAI was formerly part of the government-managed health insurance but was privatized in October 2008. The self-employed, the unemployed, retirees, and all others are insured by municipal governments (municipal National Health Insurance (NHI) program) using a combination of individual sliding scale premiums and substantial government subsidy (about 50 percent). There is a substantial inequality in the enrollment of the elderly among fragmented insurance systems: since most employed workers retire at about the age of 60 and migrate to municipal NHI programs, municipal NHI will inevitably enroll a higher proportion of the elderly population and hence higher burden of health care cost. To balance this inequality, a financial redistribution system called the Elderly Health System has been in place since 1982. In April 2008, the EHS was abolished and a new independent insurance system called "the Health Care System for the Old (HCSO)" was established. The HCSO is operated by quasi-governmental organizations established in each of 47 prefectures and financed by government subsidies (50 percent), premiums withheld from retirement pensions (10 percent), and compulsory financial supports from all health insurers (40 percent). Hence, although the Japanese health care finance system superficially resembles a large number of independent insurance pools, the extent of transfers and cross-subsidies means that these plans are linked through the MHLW into a form of social insurance that equalizes medical purchasing power across all people.

In contrast to the fragmentation among insurance plans, reimbursement to providers is standardized, with little concern for differences in the type of facility, severity of illness, or geographic variance. The fee schedule and drug prices are set by the government every two years after negotiation with the Japan Medical Association and insurance plans (see Table 17.4). These fees are administratively negotiated provider payments, not "prices," and are adjusted in response to political agreements, not changes in demand. The fee schedule implemented in 2002 introduced a 30 percent cut for hospitals whose surgical cases do not reach specified minimum numbers in each category, giving an obvious incentive to concentrate surgery into a smaller number of hospitals. With the exception of government

TABLE 17.4	Medical Fee Schedule in Japan
1. Acute nasopharyngitis, visit outpatient clinics twice, direct dispensing	
Initial consultation fee	2,700
Follow-up visit	740
Medication	1,580
Total	5,020
(Patient copayment)	1,510
2. Acute appendicitis, emergency surgery and hospital stay 7 days	
Initial consultation fee	2,500
Hospital charge (7 days)	116,270
Laboratory	31,690
X-ray	18,760
Medication	1,510
IV	14,950
Bandages, etc.	3,520
Surgery (appendectomy)	64,200
Anesthesia	10,680
Total	264,080
(Patient copayment)	63,600

Charges for typical cases, in yen ($1 = 125 yen).
Source: MHLW fee schedule revision, March 2002.

subsidies for public and university hospitals, *all payments from insurers are made according to a single uniform fee schedule*, which dictates what will be paid for each of thousands of different services and procedures. Even though there are many different insurance plans on paper, they are all forced into uniformity by the fee schedule. No balance billing is allowed (i.e., the provider gets the specified insurance payment and copayments only). No extra charges to the patient or family are allowed, although the practice of giving gifts to the doctor, a form of tipping, is not infrequent. Fees are set so low for most complex surgical and diagnostic procedures that only public university hospitals, which receive government subsidies, can afford to provide them.

Since all reimbursement is regulated by the uniform fee schedule, it is possible for the government to exert rather rigid control over total expenditures, even in the absence of a global budget. The administrative operation of the fee schedule system can reverse the dynamics of a market (where the services most in demand have higher prices, which in turn, brings forth a larger supply). In Japan, if a procedure becomes popular, its fees are often cut to discourage provision. A notable effect of this shift in remuneration is that there are two-thirds fewer surgical operations in Japan than in the United States.

Japan's complex and bureaucratic health care system has remained viable because of strong price regulation, constant economic growth, and a relatively young population. The Japanese system is a way of reaching equilibrium through consensus, which is vastly different from the sprawling mixture of regulated and competitive markets in the United States.[17] However, many of the conditions that previously favored Japan are now being reversed: the economy is stagnant and weakened by a long slump, the population is rapidly aging, and calls for deregulation are increasingly popular. How Japan copes with these daunting challenges will be one of the great social experiments in health economics.

The Health System in Germany

The health care system in Germany* has its roots in legislation initiated by Chancellor Bismarck in 1883 that made enrolment in pay-as-you-go sickness funds mandatory for certain groups of workers nationwide. This system of statutory social insurance, financed by payroll taxes, has since been greatly expanded to include more and more groups of workers and now covers more than 90 percent of Germany's population. The remaining 9 percent have chosen private insurance. The objectives of the **social insurance** system are equality in access to medical care and a progressive distribution of the financial burden. Social insurance contributions are made through sickness funds (Krankenkassen) and set at a specified percentage (usually around 15 percent) of gross wages, half of which is deducted in the form of a payroll tax and half of which is paid by the insured to the sickness fund of her choice.

Since the reunification of East Germany and West Germany in 1990, the share of GDP devoted to health has risen to more than 10 percent, widely considered a cost crisis. The government eventually responded in January 2009 by superimposing a new national health fund (Gesundheitsfonds) that distributes all revenue from the 15.5 percent payroll tax on the insured's gross wages among the 200 autonomous sickness funds that remain at the core of the statutory system. **Enrollees in the statutory system still make a personal choice for one of the sickness funds,** with family dependents without significant income of their own, such as homemaking spouses and underage children, covered free of extra charges.

Introduction of the health fund was part of a much broader reform effort that was implemented through the 2007 "Gesetz zur Stärkung des Wettbewerbs in der gesetzlichen

*This section was contributed by Dr. Michael Stolpe, Institute of World Economics, University of Kiel.

Krankenversicherung" (GKV-WSG) and intended to foster competition within the health system and help to contain costs. Ninety-five percent of each sickness fund's expenditure must be covered by the flow of money from the health fund, a flat monthly base payment of €185.64 per insured, and an **adjustment that depends on the insured's categorization into one of 152 risk groups,** including 40 age- and sex-categories, 6 earnings capacity categories, and 106 morbidity categories, which in turn are based on 80 well-defined chronic conditions, such as HIV/AIDS, diabetes, and schizophrenia, and in some cases differentiate the severity of the condition. For example, the adjustment for an insured male between the ages of 85 and 89 is plus €1.28, for dementia €86.87, and for hypertension €38.48, so that the total adjustment where all three conditions are met amounts to plus €312.27. For younger people, the age adjustments are negative; in the case of a female between the ages of 13 and 17 it is minus €117.45 as long as she does not suffer from a chronic condition. This morbidity-based risk adjustment scheme, nicknamed Morbi-RSA in German, is meant to eliminate the incentives for positive risk selection that Germany's sickness funds had under the previous rudimentary risk equalization system that was based merely on the insured's age and sex. Under that plan, cream skimming, by providing inconvenient service for the chronically ill and by offering attractive extra services for the young and healthy, was a successful strategy. Free aerobics classes and health food cooking courses proved particularly popular.

Although sickness funds still use more than 90 percent of their budget for a long list of legally mandated medical services with little scope for product differentiation, the new law gives them much greater leeway to offer extra services, incentive plans for enrollees and elements of managed care in relation to care providers. For example, all sickness funds are now required to offer at least two different elective contracts, one of which must offer reduced patient copayments in exchange for a binding agreement to see a registered primary physician, who will act as a gatekeeper, before consulting any specialist or a hospital (Hausarztmodell). In addition, sickness funds are allowed to offer contracts with retrospective bonus payments to the insured in exchange for pre-agreed deductibles. At the other end of the spectrum, sickness funds are allowed to offer supplementary insurance that may cover direct consultations with a specialist practitioner or expensive drugs not covered by the standard contract in exchange for a supplementary premium. Sickness funds can also design their own disease management programs for the chronically ill and make special deals with preferred providers, such as hospitals, rehabilitation clinics, pharmacies, and medical practitioner networks, that did not exist before.

All sickness funds whose expenditures exceed the income received from the health fund must charge a supplementary premium directly to their enrollees. However, the supplementary premium may not exceed one percent of the insured's income, or €8 per month in the absence of means testing. The insureds have the right to switch to another sickness fund in order to avoid paying the supplementary premium. For the first time, sickness funds are allowed to go bankrupt, in which case the insureds are protected because they are automatically transferred to some other sickness fund.

The Morbi-RSA has been criticized for introducing incentives to manipulate the coding of medical diagnoses with the aim to obtain more money from the central health fund. Some sickness funds reportedly pay doctors around €10 per case to provide "more detailed" diagnoses in the hope that more detail could justify claiming a chronic condition or a higher level of severity in one of the 80 predefined conditions that trigger the morbidity-based supplementary payments to the sickness fund. Diabetes mellitus, for example, would trigger an annual supplementary payment per insured patient of €794 if diagnosed without any or with unspecified complications, but €1,825 if diagnosed with ophthalmologic manifestations, €2,022 with acute complications, €2,161 with neurological or peripheral circulatory manifestations, and even €2,887 with renal manifestations. Diagnoses follow the money, say the critics, raising the suspicion that sickness funds will want to reward rather expensive treatments and introduce innovative disease management programs that attract patients in financially attractive Morbi-RSA categories, at the expense of patients suffering diseases that are less profitable from the sickness funds' perspective. Doctors would have an incentive to collude, since treating more severe conditions is often more generously remunerated under the statutory system's new payment scheme for physicians' services. Hence, if the Morbi-RSA sets some of its morbidity adjustment payments too high, it could trigger the opposite of cream skimming: a hunt for the sickest.

Private health insurance is confined to the self-employed, civil servants, and the relatively small number of workers making more than approximately €48,600 per year who are allowed to opt out of the statutory system. Since 2009, the law requires every German to have full health insurance coverage, eliminating the approximately 200,000 who were previously uninsured in Germany. Anybody caught at a doctor's office or in a hospital without insurance may be fined and required to pay up to five years' worth of health insurance premiums. Private insurers assess premiums on the basis of the age, sex, and individual health risks of an applicant, who usually must answer a long health-related questionnaire and often undergo a medical examination. After signing a contract, an insurer cannot unilaterally change its terms in response to changing health risks of the individual; the insurance promise is for the rest of the insured's life, and premiums are allowed to rise only by the same percentage as the general rise in medical care prices. In a similar vein, people opting for private insurance cannot revert to the statutory social insurance plan, but must remain with private insurance for the rest of their lives. For those who can no longer bear the premiums for an existing health insurance contract, the new law requires all private insurers to offer a basic contract (Basistarif) that covers the same set of services covered in the statutory system. Because all people not in the statutory system must purchase private health insurance, the Basistarif is regulated to charge no more than the maximum wage-based premium in the statutory system, about €570 per month, regardless of individual health risks. Another regulated contract with similar conditions is offered for pensioners.

The fee for medical services that private insurers reimburse can be three times higher than the official prices listed in the Federal Health Minister's list; therefore, doctors prefer to treat patients with private insurance. To lure them, waiting times in the physician's office tend to be shorter and treatment is sometimes more generous than for the socially insured. Many private health insurance plans provide strong financial incentives to refrain from seeing a doctor for small, self-limiting health problems. If an insured makes no claims during a given year, many plans refund up to half of the annual premium payments. Because income is positively correlated with health status, the privately insured tend to be healthier and utilize medical services less frequently than the enrollees of statutory sickness funds. To foster consumer choice and competition, insurers are allowed to offer, in addition to regular full-coverage plans, a type of supplemental insurance, mainly used to upgrade the level of hospital amenities or dental care, to enrollees of any sickness fund.

There is still a relatively **strict separation of ambulatory care from hospital care in Germany**, but cooperation and competition between the two sectors is increasing. For example, hospitals are getting involved in outpatient care for chronically sick patients, such as cancer and AIDS patients, living at home. Moreover, the elderly have the right to rehabilitation services after an injury or disease that might otherwise prevent them from returning to their homes. Only one-third of doctors in the ambulatory sector are general practitioners, whereas two-thirds are specialists with their own private practices. Independent specialists often invest heavily in diagnostic and surgical technology, sometimes setting up their own clinics to rival the services offered by small hospitals. This high degree of medical specialization in ambulatory care has long been encouraged by Germany's system of **fee-for-service** payments. New technology creates more and more billable events, and patients are free to take themselves to any office-based physician but not to a hospital.

Remuneration for the individual physician treating statutory patients is a combination of fee-for-service and prospective health-status related payments. However, many ambulatory care practitioners still rely on collective contracts, such as the Hausarztvertrag with individual sickness funds, which are negotiated by regional physician associations, called "Kassenärztliche Vereinigungen," on their behalf. These associations also continue to allocate the funds to individual practitioners according to the official euro prices listed in the Federal Health Minister's list. Office-based physicians retain the opportunity to generate income from private patients.

German **hospitals** employ their own salaried physicians, and physicians in private practice do not have admitting privileges. However, chief physicians of German hospital departments have strong incentives to increase the amount and quality of care, since they are allowed to treat private patients and thereby supplement their personal income in proportion to the number of beds filled with patients with statutory insurance. Hospital reimbursement is generally according to a prospective payment (diagnostically related group, DRG) system that was implemented gradually between 2003 and 2005, accompanied by the obligation to publish regular quality audits. Most municipalities, especially in rural parts of Eastern Germany, have since seen their local public hospitals move into deficit. Also, because the municipalities find it difficult to make the investments that would move hospitals back into profit—for example, by improving quality and increasing specialization on a set of profitable hospital services—more and more hospitals have been put up for sale. This has created a profitable investment opportunity for the fast-growing private-sector hospital chains, especially those that can raise funds on the stock market. Private-sector hospital chains seem to be in a better position to make a profit under DRG because they can invest, restructure, and capture economies of scale from specialization and coordination among the different units in the chain. Some analysts predict that up to 40 percent of German hospital beds may be in private hands by 2015, compared to less than 15 percent in 2009. There is still a significant oversupply of hospital beds per capita, which has long encouraged the export of stationary care to foreign patients (mainly from Scandinavia and the United Kingdom, where rationing of hospital services has created long waiting lists for certain procedures).

In the **pharmaceutical sector** a *reference price* (set by the government) system limits drug spending. Sickness funds are required to reimburse retailers for part of the cost of any prescription drug that contains the chemical entity ordered by a medical practitioner for the insured; fixed reference prices are used for drugs with similar properties. The net effect on prices is unclear because drug competition almost collapsed as generic prices were brought into line with reference prices. Patient copayments are set at 10 percent of the price of the drug up to a maximum of €10 per refill. Some particularly low-priced drugs are dispensed without patient copayment. Sickness funds are free to negotiate volume and other rebates for branded prescription drugs directly with drug suppliers and to restrict reimbursement to one brand in each therapeutic category. This may be coupled with lower patient copayments or with a copayment waiver.

To further strengthen sickness funds' bargaining power vis-à-vis the pharmaceutical industry and prevent them from incurring steep cost increases for new drugs that may have only marginal improvements on the benefit side, comparative cost-effectiveness research has been given a much larger role than in the past. The mandate of the Cologne-based Institut für Qualität und Wirtschaftlichkeit im Gesundheitswesen (**IQWIG**) that since 2004 oversees and undertakes this type of research has been extended so that it assesses not only the benefits of new drugs, but also their costs. This enlarged mandate is likely to set an example for the handling of other issues in technology adoption and economic evaluations of technologies and services in the future.

At present, informed observers generally agree that many restrictions on sickness funds' ability to become efficient negotiators and buyers still exist. Changing this would further undermine the corporatist cartel of ambulatory physicians and meet fierce resistance from this well-organized and powerful political lobby. Instead of further reform, the government may therefore choose to accommodate future hikes in health expenditures by tax increases. Making it easier to infuse general tax money into the health care system on a temporary or permanent basis was actually said to be one of the motives behind setting up the new health fund in the first place.[18] Yet increased government funding would clearly move the German health system away from Bismarck's design of financially autonomous sickness funds.

The Expensive Exception: The United States

In 1970, Denmark spent 7.9 percent of GDP on health care, while the United States spent just 7.0 percent. Since then, expenses have grown in every country, but they have soared far out of line in the United States. There has been a degree of convergence across the developed nations so that most spend between 8 percent and 12 percent of GDP on health care (Denmark spent $4,828 or 9.5 percent of GDP in 2006), with the notable exception of the United States, which spent 15 percent in 2006 and continued to rise to 17 percent in 2010. No other country spends as much on health care as the United States, yet the United States has still not been able to achieve the universal coverage that is standard in other developed countries, and life expectancy in the United States lags behind that of comparable countries. Although considered to be the most "privatized" of major health systems, U.S. government spending on medical care exceeds that of every other country except Luxembourg and Norway. The United States does not have more doctors or hospitals per capita than other developed countries. It ranks 22nd out of 23 countries in number of patient bed days per 1,000 population (only Greece is lower), 9th out of 14 in number of physician visits per person, and 12th out of 18 in number of prescriptions.[19] More important, the results of this very expensive care are hardly exceptional. Life expectancy at 78 years is lower than that of Canada (81), England (79), France (81), Germany (80), Sweden (81), Australia (82), or Japan (83). American medicine does appear to be more dynamic and technology intensive, with more rapid introduction of new drugs, more tests, more complex surgical procedures, and more sophisticated diagnostic equipment. Health care in America also provides an extraordinarily wide range of insurance plans and contracts, whereas other countries may have only single national health insurance plan or a limited number of alternatives (although almost countries offer free choice of physician). Although Americans express a desire for high-tech medicine with lots of choices and multiple insurance plans, they do not seem happy with what they get. Overall performance on a number of clinical and patient access measures is average or below average, and U.S. respondents' confidence and satisfaction with health care ranks in the bottom third in the Gallup World Poll.[20]

How were Japan and Europe able to keep health care costs so much lower than the United States while maintaining equal or better health outcomes and patient satisfaction? Many attempts to control costs in the United States have been motivated at the individual level, using deductibles and copayments to moderate demand, yet the use of pooled financing that protects patients from risks also insulates them from costs. Consumer choice does not lead to lower expenditures when consumers are spending someone else's money. European countries have operated largely on the supply side, constraining the provider system rather than individual demand. The number of health care workers and their wages has been limited and is often subject to nationwide bargaining and controls. Purchasing of expensive new diagnostic and therapeutic technology has been restricted.[21] Open-ended entitlements that reimburse patients for all bills have been avoided in favor of contracts for large groups of patients on a per capita or fixed-budget basis. In analyzing the evolution of payment systems, it has been argued that the flaws of bureaucratic governmental control (lack of innovation and consumer responsiveness) and the flaws of insurance markets (lack of cost control and gaps in coverage) are leading toward a convergence of public and private in a blended contractual model—what is known in the United States as managed care (Chapter 5).[22] Government will be responsible for setting the rules and the overall limits on the amount to be spent and ensuring that everyone receives coverage, while market competition will be used to maintain the quality and amenity of services and provide local control.[23]

Whatever explains the lower cost and better statistics for health systems in other countries, it is clear that health care in the United States does not consistently provide more care or yield better results, and although very dynamic and high tech, it is also financially fragmented, managerially disorganized, and lacking in modern information technology. The public and patients express significant dissatisfaction with the current system, and expenditures are seriously out of line with what is spent in comparable systems.

17.7   INTERNATIONAL TRADE IN HEALTH CARE

Health care is among the world's largest industries, accounting for 10 percent of gross world product but only a tiny fraction of world trade. Products (drugs, equipment) are much more likely to be bought and sold across national boundaries than services. Although in principle there is no reason why an X-ray performed in Seoul cannot be read in San Francisco, licensure and other regulations currently make such international service flows difficult. Trade in services is usually limited to a small amount of border crossing—for example, when a Canadian citizen disgruntled with a long wait for elective surgery crosses into the United States or an uninsured Hispanic worker from Texas crosses to Mexico for cheaper hospital and physician care.[24] The part of the health care system most subject to international movement—trade in people and skills—does not appear in the world economic accounts.

People and Ideas

In stark contrast to the lack of international trade in medical services is the substantial movement of medical personnel and ideas across national boundaries. Most specialists in developing countries receive some of their training in Europe or the United States, bringing home skills of immense value. The extraordinary increase in life expectancy that has swept over the world is perhaps one of the greatest benefits of international trade, made no less significant by the fact that, as public goods, information and scientific discoveries cannot be owned or charged for by a particular firm or country. What is somewhat surprising is the extent of trade in the reverse direction—doctors and nurses who come to work in the United States from low-income countries. At its peak, in 1978, more than half of all medical residents who were in training (and providing care) in urban teaching hospitals were foreign medical graduates. In the less remunerative and attractive specialties, such as psychiatry, this is still the case today. More than 12 percent of all U.S. physicians are immigrant doctors. Similarly, a large number of licensed nurses were educated overseas. There are more Filipino nurses practicing in the United States and Canada than in the Philippines. This anomalous flow of highly trained labor from less-developed to more-developed countries has much to do with the economics of restrictions on labor supply and with the incentive structure created by the size of the market. Limits on the numbers of physicians and nurses imposed through the U.S. educational system mean that there is room for those who have received training overseas and are willing to work for less. Also, truly outstanding neurosurgeons are able to earn more in the United States than in Mexico, and they may be tempted to go where their skills command the highest reward—just as Latin baseball players and movie stars do. There is also a niche at the bottom of the market that attracts foreign labor. Caring for the elderly in nursing homes is so demanding and underpaid that it is difficult to find competent staff willing to work for the minimum wage. These positions are attractive to immigrants who are able to obtain steady employment and benefits in jobs that require a lot in the way of patience, endurance, and strength but not in language or education. The lack of dollar-denominated trade obscures the extent to which medicine and health care became globalized in the twentieth century.

Services

Health care is sharply demarcated at national boundaries. The U.S. Medicare program does not pay for operations in Mexico, nor will it cover Canadians who come to the United States. Therefore, the border-crossing trade in services that does occur is usually paid for privately. Private investment in the small fee-for-service or insured hospitals and clinics that exist alongside national health facilities in the United Kingdom, Sweden, and elsewhere is often international. The largest hospital in Singapore used to be owned by an American firm, National Medical Enterprises. Yet the true test of international trade in medical care looms in the proposals for full integration of service markets within the European Union. A Belgian patient might prefer heart surgery in one of the major Parisian hospitals, or a Swiss factory worker might decide to seek psychiatric care in Germany. Conversely, a German hospital would find it cheaper to obtain nurses or doctors from Greece and pay travel expenses rather than hire them locally. To date, every country has jealously guarded its health care system, and such freedom of choice is available only to a few employees of international companies.

Equipment

Medical equipment is less amenable to international trade because it cannot simply be packed in a box and shipped. Skilled technicians are required to maintain and use these sophisticated devices, and the ongoing labor costs are much larger than the manufacturing cost. Once a new technology is developed, it will usually be produced and supported by a local firm or the local branch of a global firm within a few years.

Pharmaceuticals

The pharmaceutical trade is one of the world's truly global businesses (see Chapter 11). Drugs made in England or France cross pharmacy counters in the United States as readily as drugs made in Des Moines, and research is as likely to be conducted in Genoa or Geneva as it is in Georgia. Companies such as Rhone-Poulenc Rorer and Astra-Merck cross international boundaries and link major markets. Protectionist legislation still gives local firms an advantage, but it is common for more than 25 percent of a large pharmaceutical company's sales to occur outside the country where it is headquartered, and some, such as Ciba-Geigy, are mostly international. There are three major markets: Japan, the United States, and the European Union. The ability of Japanese doctors to profit from prescribing gave them the highest rate of prescription drug use in the world. Thus with only half as many consumers, the Japanese market was larger than the U.S. market in 1990 ($51 billion versus $48 billion). However, the decade-long recession in Japan has caused a relative decline even though the percentage of health expenditures spent on drugs there still exceeds that in the United States (16.8 percent versus 10.4 percent). The European Union accounted for about $40 billion, and all of the developing low- and middle-income countries accounted for $44 billion.[25] Only the major market countries have the research infrastructure and a protected domestic market of sufficient size to cover the massive fixed costs of discovering and testing new drugs. Canada presents an interesting case. Because the nation lacked significant pharmaceutical development capacity, it decided to free ride on the technology produced by the rest of the world. Canada refused to recognize the property rights created by patents and mandated that foreign companies license their drugs for manufacture or use in Canada in return for set royalty payments. This way the Canadians could obtain the benefits of research but not pay the cost. Vigorous protests eventually led to this system being overturned, and now Canada recognizes international patent protection, as do other industrialized countries. However, free riding is still the rule for many developing countries, either through mandatory licensing or simple failure to enforce patents, which allows local companies to make copycat versions of brand-name drugs. Clinical tests constitute a sizable portion of drug companies' costs and provide an interesting opportunity for international trade. By carrying out trials in a foreign country, a firm may be able to significantly reduce the cost per patient of developing a drug and may face lower liability from adverse reactions the experimental drug might produce.

Although the future growth and evolution of the global pharmaceutical industry is inherently uncertain, past trends do allow for some reasonable speculation. The United States has come to dominate the world pharmaceutical market to an increasing degree since 1950, but is unlikely to continue to do so for the next 50 years. Previously the pharmaceutical industry had been centered in France, then Germany, and then England before moving to the United States. In each case, development of the pharmaceutical industry was preceded by growth in manufacturing, science, and industrial research. As global production moved toward America after World War II, so did the pharmaceutical companies—albeit with a lag. Europe and Japan retained strong pharmaceutical manufacturing centers long after their overall share of the global economy had begun to decline. Following the growth of the American economy and the extraordinarily generous reimbursements provided by an expensive open-ended health care system, a majority of the pharmaceutical industry had migrated to the United States by 2010. Just as the industry migrated from France and Germany as their economic power waned, it is likely to move on from the United States to the growing economic powerhouses of the twenty-first century—India and China.

A recent study showed how regulation of pharmaceutical prices in the EU (one of the factors contributing to a lower cost of care) reduced profits of pharmaceutical companies in those countries, thus creating an incentive to move headquarters and R&D facilities into the United States.[26] EU citizens enjoyed lower pharmaceutical prices but lost some high-paying R&D jobs. The European share of pharmaceutical research dollars went from 24 percent above that of the United States ($4.8 billion versus $3.9 billion) in 1986 to 14 percent below ($26.8 billion versus $30.6 billion) in 2004. That is, the European pharmaceutical industry has continued to grow, but more expansive reimbursement overseas shifted a sizable part of that growth to the United States. The authors estimate that price regulation made European drugs 40 percent less expensive, but shifted about 1,680 jobs from the EU to the United States. The tradeoff between paying more for drugs and loss of jobs is inherently problematic. However, long-run growth in a dynamic global industry such as pharmaceuticals will inevitably tend to trail along the path of economic development in search of bigger markets and higher returns.

SUGGESTIONS FOR FURTHER READING

Rupa Chandra, "Trade in Health Services," *Bulletin of the World Health Organization* 80, no. 2 (2002): 158–163, www.who.org

David M. Cutler, "Equality, Efficiency and Market Fundamentals: The Dynamics of International Medical Care Reform," *Journal of Economic Literature* 40 (September 2002): 881–906.

"The Danish Health System," special issue of *Health Policy* 59, no. 2 (January 2002).

Bruce J. Fried and Laura M. Gaydos, eds., *World Health Systems* (Chicago: AUPHA Press, 2002).

Alan Garber and Jonathan Skinner, "Is American Health Care Uniquely Inefficient?" NBER working paper 14257, August 2008.

Philip Musgrove, Riadh Zeramdini, and Guy Carrin, "Basic Patterns in National Health Expenditure," *Bulletin of the World Health Organization* 80, no. 2 (2002): 134–1146, www.who.org

Wynand P. M. M. van de Ven and Frederik T. Schut, "Universal Mandatory Health Insurance in the Netherlands: A Model for the United States?" *Health Affairs* 27, no. 3 (2008): 771–781.

World Health Organization, *World Health Statistics 2008*, http://www.who.int/whosis/whostat/2008/en/index.html

SUMMARY

1. There is **a tremendous disparity in health** between rich and poor nations. The poor countries of sub-Saharan Africa have very little health care and low life expectancies. Many people there die before the age of five. The wealthier countries of Europe, North America, and Japan have more health resources to be applied to much less need. People in these countries have a longer life expectancy, with most deaths occurring after age 70.

2. Average **spending on health care is determined primarily by national income** per capita, not the health needs of individuals. Increased per capita income is also a major factor explaining increased life expectancy.

3. More health expenditures usually mean more health professionals and more use of technology, not more visits to physicians or days in the hospital. It is the **intensity of service, rather than quantity**, that increases as spending is increased.

4. **The United States is the world's largest health care market**, accounting for 40 percent of all health expenditures, even though it has only 5 percent of the world's population. U.S. health expenditures per person are 10 times the worldwide average and 100 times the average per person in India. With more than 15 percent of the world's population, India accounts for less than 1 percent of the global health care market.

5. Significantly **higher medical expenditures do not** appear to have made U.S. citizens significantly healthier. U.S. life expectancy ranks about in the middle of developed high-income countries.

6. The curve depicting the relationship between national income per capita and life expectancy has shifted upward over time. This illustrates the productive impact of **new knowledge** as well as the **transmission of that knowledge across national boundaries**.

7. The **distribution of income** across people and social groups, as well as the average, is important in explaining differences in health and life expectancy.

8. **Lack of organization, maldistribution, and political instability** are perhaps even more important than low income in causing poor health among many low-income countries. Even in middle- and high-income countries, many of the worst health problems result from the uneven distribution of health care and an inability to effectively target care to those most in need.

9. Most countries assert that their health care systems emphasize **primary care**, but their **funding favors specialty training and tertiary hospital care**.

10. **Cost control** in Europe, constraining supply and putting limits on the system as a whole, appears to have been more effective than in the United States. Japan's inexpensive health care system is much less technology-intensive than that of the United States, using only a third as much surgery but more drugs.

11. There is very little **international trade** in health care services. Global trade in health care is dominated by pharmaceuticals. However, the invisible trade in knowledge and health professionals has the largest effect on national health care systems.

PROBLEMS

1. {*flow of funds*} How many people are there in the world today? What fraction of them live in high-income developed economies? What fraction of total health expenditures is accounted for by high-income countries?

2. {*flow of funds*} How much is spent per person on health care in China? How much is spent per person on health care in the United States? In the United Kingdom? What are the primary factors accounting for these differences?

3. {*market size*} What is the largest global health care market?

4. {*correlation vs. causality*} Is more spending on health care associated with more health?

5. {*incidence*} As an officer of the World Health Organization with a budgetary allocation of $100 million, which programs would you fund if you wanted to make the greatest impact on health, measured as the increase in life expectancy multiplied by the number of people affected?

6. {*nominal vs. real*} Mexico spends less than a tenth as much per person on health care as the United States. Does it have more than or less than a tenth as many hospital beds? Physicians? Is the real amount of health care provided overestimated or underestimated by dollar comparisons? Why?

7. {*international trade*} Which types of health care labor are most likely to be traded between countries? Why?

8. {*international trade*} Which types of health care goods are most likely to be traded between countries? Are there more or fewer barriers to trade in health care than in other sectors?

9. {*trade*} Which aspects of medical care are most international? Which are the most parochial?

ENDNOTES

1. World Health Organization, *World Health Report 2002*, http://www.who.int/whr/2002/en.
2. In converting local expenditures and income into U.S. dollars, two methods are used. The value in local currency can be converted using the foreign exchange rate (the rate at which dollars are traded for local currency in the market) or it can be converted in terms of "purchasing power parity" (PPP), the amount required to purchase an equivalent amount of goods and services. In India, GNP per capita was $880 measured in terms of foreign exchange, but $2,460 in terms of the value of goods. This is largely because the cost of food, transportation, etc. is much lower than the price of such goods in the United States, converted at the currency market exchange rate (i.e., whereas 100 rupees = $2.07 U.S. dollars, that amount cannot buy a good meal in the U.S., but would be sufficient to purchase more than three good meals in India).

3. The World Bank, *World Development Report 1993: Investing in Health* (New York: Oxford University Press for the World Bank, 1993). This report provides comparative data on a number of health issues not available elsewhere, and thus is used here despite the age of the data (mostly from 1990). Making comparisons requires not only that the data exist, but also that the data be made comparable in terms of definitions, time periods, etc., a tremendous task for 191 countries.

4. Victor Fuchs, "The Health Sector's Share of the Gross National Product," *Science* (2 February 1990), 534–38.

5. Mark Pauly, "When Does Curbing Health Costs Really Help the Economy?" *Health Affairs*, 14, no. 2 (1995): 68–82.

6. Thomas Getzen, "Population Aging and the Growth of Health Expenditures," *Journal of Gerontology*, 47, no. 3 (1992): S98–104.

7. Thomas E. Getzen, "An Income-Weighted International Average for Comparative Analysis of Health Expenditures," *International Journal of Health Planning and Management* 6 (1991): 3–22.

8. Samuel H. Preston, *Fatal Years: Child Mortality in Late Nineteenth-Century America* (Princeton, N.J.: Princeton University Press, 1991).

9. G. B. Rodgers, "Income and Inequality as Determinants of Mortality: An International Cross-Section Analysis," *Population Studies*, 33, no. 2 (1979): 343–351; also The World Bank, *Population Change and Economic Development* (New York: Oxford University Press, 1985).

10. The World Bank, *World Development Report 1993: Investing in Health* (New York: Oxford University Press for the World Bank, 1993).

11. Zineeldine Alidrissi, *Summary Report of the Establishment of the Sudan Health Economics Unit*, planning section, Sudan Federal Ministry of Health, November 7, 2002.

12. Milton I. Roemer, *National Health Systems of the World* (New York: Oxford University Press, 1991), which includes information reproduced from G. M. Bloom, M. Segal, and C. Thube, *Expenditure and Financing of the Health Sector in Kenya* (Nairobi: Ministry of Health, 1986). The World Bank Statistics, used for most of the tables in this chapter, estimate national health spending in Kenya at $375 million for 1990, of which 63 percent came from the public sector. Roemer argues that private sector spending is much less visible and usually underreported since no regular statistics are kept. Bloom et al., through extensive surveys and several alternate methods, estimate that private sector spending actually slightly exceeded public sector spending, 51 percent to 49 percent, in 1986. Table 17.2 takes the World Bank estimate of public spending of $237 million, derived from government budget reports, as correct. Private sector spending is then estimated to be 51 percent of the total, or $247 million, following Bloom et al. The percentages of total spending within each category in Bloom et al. for the year 1986 are then applied to the $484 million total to create breakdowns by category. The net effect of the adjustment for underreported private expenditures is to raise the estimate of per capita health expenditures in Kenya from $16 per person to $20 per person.

13. Milton Roemer, *National Health Systems of the World* (New York: Oxford University Press, 1991), pp. 345–51.

14. Katarzyna Tymowska, "Health Care Transformation in Poland," *Health Policy* 56 (2001): 85–98.

15. WHO Regional Office, *European Health Report 2002*, http://www.euro.who.int/europeanhealthreport.

16. Some of the information presented here came from Kozo Tatara and Etsuji Okamoto, *Health Systems in Transition: Japan*, (Copenhagen: World Health Organization, 2009).

17. Can you imagine a group of U.S. executives or lawyers suspecting they have heart failure being willing to wait patiently for hours in a public clinic to be served alongside the unemployed, or accepting a situation in which two out of three who currently would be receiving a bypass graft or new pacemaker are sent home with pills instead? Then, when adversity strikes, can you further imagine that they would not sue? The sources of such a disparity go beyond language, currency, and government. Although cultural studies lie a bit beyond the scope of this book, it is clear that culture profoundly affects the health systems of the two countries just by looking at the differences in physician salaries, relative differences in the uses of drugs versus invasive therapy, and ownership of facilities and equipment.

18. For an introduction to this debate, see Banafsheh Siadat and Michael Stolpe (2005), "Reforming Health Care Finance: What Can Germany Learn from Other Countries?" Kiel Economic Policy Paper 5, Institut fuer Weltwirtschaft an der Universitaet Kiel 2005, http://www.ifw-kiel.de/pub/kepp/2005/kepp05.pdf.

19. *OECD Health Systems: Facts and Trends 1960–1991* (Paris: OECD, 1993).

20. Cathy Schoen et al., "Toward Higher Performance Health Systems: Adults' Health Care Experiences in Seven Countries, 2007," *Health Affairs* 26, no. 6 (October 31, 2007), w717–w734; Angus Deaton, "Income, Aging, Health and Wellbeing Around the World: Evidence from the Gallup World Poll," NBER working paper 13317, August 2007.

21. Dale A. Rublee, "Medical Technology in Canada, Germany and the United States: An Update," *Health Affairs*, 13, no. 4 (1994): 113–117.

22. Wynand P. M. M. van de Ven and Frederik T. Schut, "Universal Mandatory Health Insurance in the Netherlands: A Model for the United States?" *Health Affairs* 27, no. 3 (2008): 771–781; Jeremy Hurst,

The Reform of Health Care: A Comparative Analysis of Seven OECD Countries (Paris: OECD, 1992), pp. 140–151. See also Alan Maynard and Karen Bloor, "Introducing a Market to the United Kingdom's National Health Service," *New England Journal of Medicine* 334 (1996): 604–608.

23. The fact that so many health policy experts in so many countries all agree on the essential elements of what the future of health care organization and financing will and should be is probably reassuring, although such a consensus has not always guaranteed either insight or good results in the past.

24. Theo Francis, "Medical Tourism Is Still Small," *Wall Street Journal*, 6 May 2008, p. D2.

25. The World Bank, *World Development Report 1993: Investing in Health* (New York: Oxford University Press for the World Bank, 1993), p. 145; *OECD Health Data 2002* (Paris: OECD, 2002), www.oecd.org.

26. Joseph H. Golec and John A. Vernon, "European Pharmaceutical Price Regulation, Firm Profitability, and R&D Spending," NBER working paper 12676, November 2006; Eddy van Doorslaer et al., "Equity in the Delivery of Health Care in Europe and the U.S.," *Journal of Health Economics* 19, no. 5 (2000): 553–583.

CHAPTER 18

VALUE FOR MONEY IN THE FUTURE OF HEALTH CARE

QUESTIONS

1. What, how, and for whom is medical care provided?
2. Is Medicare likely to go broke, or continue to grow?
3. Will investors put more money into biotechnology or nursing homes?
4. How will economists affect the allocation of health care? Of health care incomes?
5. Are people willing to spend more and get less health?
6. Why is it so hard to reach a consensus if everyone knows what the problem is?

18.1 FORCING THE QUESTION: WHO GETS HEALTHY AND WHO GETS PAID?

The most important contribution economists can make to the operation of the health care system is to be relentless in pointing out that every choice involves a trade-off—that certain difficult questions regarding who gets what, and who must give up what, are inevitable and must be faced even when politicians, the public, and patients would rather avoid them. In the words of Paul Samuelson, "Every economy must answer a triad of questions: *what, how,* and *for whom.*"[1] In the case of cancer, for example, one could ask what symptoms or diagnoses are to be treated, should this treatment be inpatient or outpatient, by generalists or specialists, and who is to receive first priority for treatment (those who are most ill, most likely to recover, best insured, or those who plan ahead and show up first). Although these questions can be asked independently, the answer to one influences all the others: "for whom" affects "what" and "how," and vice versa. Any answer also determines who pays, who gets paid, and how much; that is, it determines the distribution of income as well as the distribution of health care.

It is the job of economists to give advice, not patient care. They estimate, evaluate, and elucidate the decisions to be made; they do not make the decisions or carry them out. The analysis of decision making can be divided into three levels:

WHAT ARE THE QUESTIONS?

WHO IS GOING TO DECIDE?

WHAT ARE THE ANSWERS?

For most economists, it is necessary to work backward, starting with the data collection required to make comparisons among different treatments (i.e., cost-benefit analysis), then consider how different systems for making medical care decisions can affect efficiency (e.g., physician practices versus hospital IT systems, patients or regulatory authorities), and only then approach the top level—framing the questions (What is fair? Public or private financing? Are new discoveries more important than caring for the elderly?). Tracing the flow of money over the last 17 chapters reveals that although data can be used for clarification, the questions are fundamentally *economic*: they are about choices and thus have to do with values as well as numbers. Are some lives worth more than others? How much should a surgeon be paid for a one-hour operation if it saves a life? If it fails to save a life? Which product of the health care system is more important: social justice or cancer mortality?

The pragmatic and detailed collection of data for comparing the costs and outcomes of different drugs, different surgical procedures, and different treatment settings has grown

---

BEHAVIORAL ECONOMICS: RATIONAL CHOICE WITH A NUDGE

Modern ("neoclassical") economics has been based on the logical structure of "rational choice theory," which assumes that each person acts in a way that maximizes her or his own well-being ("utility"). It was always recognized that some behavior did not meet this standard of perfection, yet most economists assumed that deviations were random, due to lack of experience or foresight, or were eventually brought into alignment with utility maximization over time. Two psychiatrists, Daniel Kahneman and Amos Tversky, demonstrated clearly that there were common and quite predictable deviations, "consistently irrational" choices.[2] The new "behavioral" economics has provided several interdisciplinary findings of great importance to health economics. Having more choices, which economists used to assume always makes consumers better off, frequently leaves people less satisfied and more likely to make poor choices, or none ("I just couldn't pick one—there were too many to choose from"). The Medicare supplemental market actually became more competitive and more satisfactory to many elderly participants once the options were limited to 10 well-defined choices. Paying people to attend smoking cessation or exercise classes gets much more participation than providing "equivalent" rewards in the form of tax breaks. Although economists used to assume that people would always make a deal, any deal, that made them better off, a series of experiments have shown that people will often not participate if they think the deal is unfair (i.e., two people split a reward with one getting $2 and the other $998), and will sometimes use their own money to "punish" unfairness even though such acts of conscience do not benefit them directly. Although cost-benefit analyses often assume that "having" something and not losing it is worth the same as "getting" it, this turns out rarely to be the case. A person may only be willing to pay $2,000 to partially reverse a hearing loss caused by a birth defect, but want to sue for $500,000 if an accident causes the same loss.

These insights provide a more nuanced understanding of how incentives affect behavior and are beginning to be used in a number of practical ways to improve health policy (for example, automatically enrolling new employees in health insurance and then giving them options, rather than making them sign up and choose a plan; a cash bonus of $500 for new mothers that get all of their baby's shots on time instead of a deduction on income taxes). Behavioral economics does not so much contradict the traditional rational choice model as supplement it, and provide methods to improve efficiency in the real world.

rapidly over the last decade. Doing such work requires a tremendous amount of clinical knowledge and an understanding of basic economic principles: equilibrium at the margin, production functions, comparative advantage, opportunity cost, and so on. Increasingly, such work is being carried out by clinicians who have training in economic concepts, while economists concentrate on developing theory and new measurement techniques.

Upon this mass of detailed data collection and analysis rests the second layer of issues regarding how to design a better health care system. At this level, the question is not whether radiation is better than chemotherapy, but whether capitation or fee-for-service leads to better decisions or whether group practice is more efficient than solo practice. The focus shifts from the particular decision being made to the issue of who is making the decision—physicians, patients, or payers (see the box section on "Behavioral Economics").

As economists trace how the flow of money follows the path of decision making, the assumptions embedded in the current medical care system become more evident. Analysis at the third level becomes reflective. What does "better" mean? According to which value system? Better for whom? Is it fair? Analysis transcends the current system as it is by asking: "What are the questions?" Reaching beyond the veil of money and grasping the concept that every dollar spent on health care is a dollar earned by a health care provider helps clarify how the distribution of income and health are connected, and suggests fruitful directions for assessing the health implications of changes in economic organization.

18.2   SPENDING MONEY OR PRODUCING HEALTH?

The distribution of health is unequal. This has a profound impact on economic well-being. Some people work productively for years and die contentedly with wealth and happiness in old age, while others struggle for a few months or decades in agony as they are relentlessly drawn down into premature mortality. The question is not whether the distribution of health is fair, or whether it determines or is determined by income, but whether and how it can be changed. More narrowly, one might ask how, and how much, change can be brought about by spending more on medical care? What is that change worth? The marginal productivity of medical care spending declines as more is spent. Increasing spending from $7,000 to $8,000 per person increases average life expectancy, but not by as much as increasing spending from $2,000 to $3,000, which, in turn, does not have as large an effect as going from $0 to $1,000. As more and more money is spent, fewer and fewer gains are achieved in life expectancy as the "flat of the curve" is reached, where marginal productivity, although still positive, is barely above zero.

Reaching a consensus on how much to spend becomes more complicated when there are two or more types of people who are to receive care. Suppose that one group is relatively healthy and would maintain a high level of health even if no money were spent on them, while another group begins at a disadvantage and even with maximal effort would still remain less healthy. If the same amount is spent per person on each group, the total and marginal impact of medical care will be very low in the healthy group, which seems wasteful, while the sicker group would still be forced to do without a lot of potentially beneficial care. To jointly maximize the average healthiness of all people for a given health care budget, it would be necessary to equalize the marginal productivity of medical care (increase in health per additional dollar spent) across both groups, spending much more per person on the sicker people. Such an allocation of medical care resources might seem both fair and efficient, but it also might not. Suppose that the healthy group consisted of employed people who paid insurance premiums, whereas the sicker group were heroin and cocaine users living on the streets. Most voters would not be willing to cut funding for those who take care of themselves and go to work every day in order to provide more funding to people who stick needles in their arms. Further complications are posed by groups such as infants born with genetic defects or severely wounded policemen who are likely to die even with the best medical care. Should they be denied treatment on the grounds that it would not do them much good anyway? Questions such as these evoke strong emotional reactions because they touch on deeply held beliefs and assumptions about humanity and the allocation of health.

The distinction between "medical decisions" and the "determinants of health" is important. Stating that the goal of medical care is to *maximize health* may appear both accurate and appropriate. However, some reflection and reading the last 17 chapters shows how inaccurate and irrelevant such a measure often is. If taken literally, maximizing health would mean that most hospitals in the United States would close so that more food, clothes, books, and medicine could be provided to Afghanistan, Indonesia, Mozambique, and other undeveloped countries. It would also force most surgeons to give up their operating rooms in favor of sewage treatment plants, and force psychiatrists to give up the provision of therapy and the prescription of psychoactive drugs in favor of immunization campaigns and early childhood education. To assert that the goal of medical care is to maximize health for all is not only inaccurate, but profoundly misleading. It confuses a measure of social welfare with the incentives of the groups that make up society to maximize their own welfare. Doctors, nurses, hospital supply company executives, National Basketball Association players, healthy industrial workers, college students, and other definable groups have multiple objectives, including the health of their families and their own incomes, many of which are more important to them than the advancement of global health averages.

It is relatively easy to understand why most Americans do not want all of their hospitals to close, and why most of the doctors who work in them are not eager to practice in Mozambique, even if they are certain that the number of additional life years produced would be higher. It is less obvious why Americans keep spending more and more on medical care if technological advances are making medicine more productive and efficient. Given that the baseline life expectancy at birth, even in the absence of medical care, is much higher now than it was a century ago, each year of life expectancy added becomes more difficult and more expensive to obtain; therefore, marginal productivity (gain in life expectancy per additional dollar spent) is much lower today than it was 50 or 100 years ago. If society were actually optimizing by choosing the point at which the value of health matched the price of health, and the value of health were the same as before, then less money would be spent as technology improved (due to diminishing marginal productivity).[3] Instead, we now spend more per person, implying that the incremental increase in health per additional dollar is even smaller. Extrapolating from the comparisons with Japan, Germany, and England in Chapter 17, it appears that it would be possible to cut spending by a third or more with only a minor decrease in health, leaving average life expectancy in the United States almost unchanged at 78 years.[4] The declining marginal productivity of health care is offset, to some extent, by the increasing aggregate wealth of society, which raises the dollar value of each additional year of health gained (see Table 16.3). The increased medical buying power of specific groups of people who are likely to be high utilizers of care (the elderly, children with disabilities) is perhaps more important as a factor in augmenting demand. Yet even so, the vastness of the increase in medical expenditure cannot be explained purely in terms of productivity and relative prices.

18.3   DYNAMIC EFFICIENCY

A major difficulty for health economics is that the question of "how to improve efficiency" is usually less relevant to reform than the question of "how to make a deal." Deals are tough to make because any significant change in the allocation of resources is going to hurt somebody, and thus generate resistance.[5] Groups that will be harmed are not sure that their concerns are adequately weighed or the harm done to them is balanced off fairly by benefits gained from other programs and policies. Assurances of fair treatment are harder to believe the more distant in time and uncertain the compensating benefits are. Thus, although a group of elderly people may possibly be willing to accept less technologically advanced treatment for a reduction in their premiums and out-of-pocket costs, they might not be willing to make such a sacrifice in order to fund research that will only bring results 20 or 30 years from now. Although this reluctance may be short-sighted, it is perfectly reasonable.

THE VALUE OF MEDICAL PROGRESS

Is the development of new medical technology worth the cost? Should we have spent so much money trying to improve health? William Nordhaus concluded that the growth in longevity in the United States during the twentieth century was worth almost as much as all of the growth in GDP (market goods and services) in the economy.[6] However, a substantial portion of that increase in longevity was due to better housing, nutrition, heating, transportation, and other nonmedical factors. David Cutler and Mark McClellan examined technological advances in five conditions: heart attack, low birth weight, breast cancer, depression, and cataracts. Table 18.1 summarizes their findings. For heart attacks, the cost of treatment increased from $12,083 in 1984 to $21,714 in 1998 (inflation adjusted), a real increase of $9,631 per case.[7] Life expectancy increased from just under five years to a bit over six, a gain of more than a year. If society values an extra year of life at $10,000 or more, it appears that the gains in health are worth more than the cost. (Usual assumptions for the value of a year of life are in the range of $75,000 to $375,000 per additional year.) Conversely, treatment of breast and most other cancers has become substantially more expensive but has not provided sizable increases in life expectancy. Overall assessment depends on the mix of treatments and individuals considered. On balance, averaged across all types of people and all kinds of treatments (the good, the mediocre, and the truly awful), investment in medical technology appears to have provided substantial net benefits to society, although it is also evident that some kinds of treatment still in use are not worth the costs.

TABLE 18.1   Costs and Gains of Medical Technology

Condition	Period	Incremental Cost	Gains from Treatment
Heart attack	1984 to 1998	$9,631	One more year of life
Low birth weight	1950 to 1990	$40,000	Twelve years of life
Depression	1991 to 1996	(decreased)	Better quality of life
Cataracts	1969 to 1998	($0 or decrease)	Better quality of life
Breast cancer	1985 to 1996	$20,000	Two months of life

Source: Cutler and McClellan (2001).

The problems of allocation are often formalized by economists in terms of technical productivity (maximizing the output from any given set of resource inputs), cost minimization (choosing the least expensive set of inputs), and current economic efficiency (balancing marginal costs and marginal benefits) (see "Efficiency" in Section 2.8 and the section "The Value of Medical Progress" above). More sophisticated analyses may also consider how systems are structured to deal with transactions costs and public goods. In medicine, the most important allocation may be that between current consumption and future productivity. The difference between adequate and outstanding current practice is far smaller than the gap between what was possible 20 years ago and what is expected within the next decade (e.g., gene therapy, real-time imaging, robotic laser surgery, in vitro diagnoses). The challenge is to structure a health care system for *dynamic efficiency*, creating technological and organizational change to improve health and productivity. Some current allocative efficiency must be sacrificed for scientists to spend time tinkering to make new discoveries and to give managers the slack to come up with ideas for new products and service delivery systems. A purely cost-minimizing organization is not creative enough to be economically efficient in the long run.

18.4   DISTRIBUTION, DISTRIBUTION, DISTRIBUTION

When asked which three factors are most important in determining value, real estate appraisers reply, "location, location, and location." In a similar vein, health economists asked to determine the value of the money spent on health care might say "allocation, allocation, and allocation," focusing repeatedly on distributional issues: the distribution of resources, the distribution of health, the distribution of medical care, and the distribution of provider incomes. Although a high value is often placed on the quality of nursing care, the skill of the physician, or the use of new medical technology, none of these matters much if the care is provided to the wrong person or at the wrong time. Health economists are asked to assess economic efficiency—how well the health care system has used the resources available to achieve its stated (and unstated) goals. The following short list contains a few of the questions that must be answered in this regard:

- Which diseases should be treated?
- More research or more primary care?
- Which people should be treated?
- How much care should be given?
- Who will pay?
- If the money is to come from taxes, who should be taxed most—those who benefit most or those who can most afford to pay?
- Should more money be spent on prevention or cure?
- How much should healers be paid?
- Should treatment be given by specialists or primary care providers?
- How should the power to make decisions be allocated?

Allocation is the subject of economics. Why, then, haven't economists been more successful in reforming health care? First, it must be recognized that the study of health economics has indeed improved efficiency to some degree. It has made the system better, although it is still far from perfect. Cost-benefit analysis has led to a reduction in the over-investment in hospitals, to the support and improvement of immunization programs, and to the more rapid and objective evaluation of new drugs. Assessment of incentives and risk bearing has led to the creation of new types of insurance and to the refinement of managed care contracting. The application of microeconomics to decisions regarding individual allocation has only limited potential, however, because the most crucial issues in health are likely to involve personal values, public goods, macro allocation, contentious questions of how the costs and benefits are to be distributed between different groups of producers and consumers, and the political dynamics of change.

18.5   PATH DEPENDENCE AND THE POSSIBILITIES FOR REFORM

Path dependence is the term social scientists use to describe the fact that the current system is not only a function of current conditions, but also of the path taken to get here. Whereas the external demographic, economic, and technological forces matter, so do the organizations, institutions, and culture that have developed over the years, and also the habits and rules they have accumulated. What "path dependence" means for health care is that any reforms likely to actually take place will grow out of the existing system—perhaps removing some flaws and adding some innovative elements, but not creating anew from scratch.[8] The "new" will be a pragmatic extension of the old. Rather than a pure and idealized structure, a reformed U.S. health care system will make compromises with history and the give-and-take of American politics.

How Did We Get Here?

Two signature institutional characteristics of the U.S. health care system, professional licensure and voluntary community hospitals, gelled and formalized during the 1920s and 1930s. Medical care was just becoming scientific and therapeutically relevant (although most of our science was still borrowed from Europe). Costs were low at $30 per person per year (about $385 in 2010 dollars), and amounted to less than 4 percent of GDP. From 1935 to 1955 the prestige of medicine grew tremendously, although costs remained modest. Advances such as antibiotics and artificial kidneys were announced with awe as "medical miracles," and medical care got much of the credit for increases in life expectancy that were as much due to better nutrition, sanitation, and other public health measures as to therapeutic improvements (see Section 16.9). The major institutions of insurance and technology-driven academic medicine coalesced in the 1950s and 1960s (Medicare, Medicaid, NIH, Health Professions Educational Assistance). Flooding the system with money after 1965 created a new technocracy, with medical specialties growing as if on steroids. The fusty gentlemen's club of the 1920s with its quaint rules and traditions that excluded minorities and women from the profession was pushed aside in favor of selection by merit and scientific knowledge. Medical care grew rapidly, but GDP was also growing rapidly. With the help of employer-based health plans, most Americans could afford to pay for all of the new medical care available with little problem, since it still added up to less than 6 percent of GDP.

The story of medicine in the twentieth century would seem to be one of triumphant success if we were to stop there, but tensions inherent in the system created in 1965 began to appear soon afterward and have worsened over time. Too many specialists meant not enough individual attention from a family doctor. Costs kept rising even as some of the medical "miracles" began to lose their shine. Hospital bills became a major cause of personal bankruptcy. Health insurance from an employer became harder to obtain, and kept requiring more copays and more paperwork, while the inability to cover 47 million uninsured nagged at the nation's conscience. Faith in technical progress and trust in the profession sagged. By 2008 it was common to see newspaper articles labeling the health care system as "broken," and the Congressional Budget Office had already fingered rising health care costs as "unsustainable" and the major cause of future budget deficits.[9]

The United States still has the path-dependent remnants of a medical profession based on the reality of the 1920s, an insurance system based on the employee benefits of the 1950s and 1960s, and academic medical centers built on the expansive funding of the 1970s. The organizations built on those foundations were great back then but are now in need of a makeover. Yet change in the health care system is slow and inertial, with a delayed and drawn-out response to changes in the economic, social, scientific, and political environment.

What Did Medicine Miss?

Most of the economy has gone through substantial change since 1970, becoming leaner and more flexible to deal with inflation, foreign competition, and aggressive investors that moved capital and labor around to achieve greater efficiency. Not medicine. IBM was a giant of the 1960s that has been supplanted by a succession of firms over the decades: Intel, Microsoft, Google. Sears and A&P dominated retailing, and no one had heard of Wal-Mart, much less Amazon. In retrospect, it can be difficult to appreciate how painful and harsh this process, termed "creative destruction" by Joseph Schumpeter in his classic 1942 economic text, *Capitalism, Socialism and Democracy*, was to those who lost jobs and had to find new careers. It is not fun to compete in the economy, just necessary. Losing hurts, and you do not always get to start again from the same place. In medicine, entrenched practices, revered traditions, and a rising flow of funds kept the profession from undergoing many of the changes in management, financing, workflow, and information processing that gradually revolutionized most of the rest of the economy. Long after bar codes and online ordering had become common elsewhere, medical professionals still shuffled paper records.[10] Medicare "Part A" and "Part B" enshrines a distinction between inpatient and ambulatory care from the 1960s that has become increasingly irrelevant and whose continuation makes it difficult to bundle prices meaningfully. Whatever else the emerging medical system accomplishes, it must bring **teamwork** and modern **information technology** to the practice of medicine. Inadequate management structure and IT means that administrative costs are higher, and the ability to track results lower, in the U.S. health system than in most other developed countries.[11]

What Went Wrong? Notable Failures and Unresolved Dilemmas

The United States has been recognized throughout the twentieth century as the technological leader in medicine, with more Nobel Laureates than any other country—but also as having developed a health care system that is overly expensive, does not deliver particularly good health (mortality and morbidity are average or below that for other developed countries), and leaves many citizens without insurance or lacking access to quality care. It has become increasingly apparent that the most critical problem is a continual increase in costs without commensurate improvement in health outcomes. Paying a lot might be worthwhile if people felt they were getting a lot out of the system, but they do not. Surveys show dissatisfaction with medical care as a whole, and a pervasive sense that professional and business relationships have deteriorated.[12] For many Americans, it seems that health insurance premiums are becoming unaffordable, that hospitals and doctors do not "care" as personally for patients as they used to, that medical advances are increasingly of a "me-too" variety that provide only incremental gains—in short, that health care is not as good as it used to be (see the section "How Rising Costs Created a Distributional Crisis").

HOW RISING COSTS CREATED A DISTRIBUTIONAL CRISIS

In 1950, the average income per person in the United States was $1,929 and the amount spent on health care averaged $83 per year. Even without insurance, such expenses were manageable. For those whose incomes were below average, or perhaps had a bad year so that their expenses were 3× (three times) as much, or even 10×, it was still often possible to find a way to cover the costs by relying on friends or family. By 2007 income per capita had risen to $45,681, but the cost of medical care had risen even more rapidly, to $7,421. Paying 1/20th of your salary for health insurance in 1950 did not seem unfair, but trying to put aside two months of paychecks just for health insurance could make it hard to cover rent, food, and taxes. Trying to handle a bad year in 2010 (or a chronic health condition) that made your expenses 3× the average would be more than difficult, and a real health crisis—pretty much anything that required hospitalization for more than one night—would cost more than 10× (i.e., $80,000) and probably leave you bankrupt.

Distributional problems are made more severe by the skewness of incomes. The "average" of $46,000 per person per year is pulled upward by a few very high incomes: lawyers, professional athletes, CEOs, investment bankers, and so on. The median, or what many would consider the "average family" income, is much less than the mean (mathematical average). In 2007, the mean family income was $84,300, but the median family had about half that much: $47,300 (the disparity in wealth, or savings, is even greater).[13] Since that family often had several adults and one or more children to pay for, "average" health insurance coverage cost $12,680. Those fortunate enough to have good health insurance from an employer paid only about one-quarter of that ($3,380), but others were in trouble and very likely to fall into the pinched camp of those who were "employed but uninsured," for whom any significant illness meant financial catastrophe.

Paying for health insurance, or even covering most bills out of pocket, was not an unreasonable expectation for most families in 1950. Today, just the copays and coinsurance on a good employer-provided health plan take more than the 5 percent of income workers had to pay out for everything back then. It is not reasonable to expect that someone making minimum wage, or even three or four times that much (i.e., about the median family income of $47,300) can afford $8,000 or $12,000 or $24,000 or more just for medical coverage.[14] When health care costs were a problem only for a small segment of the lower middle-class or near-poor without good jobs in the 1950s, they could be ignored by most people. Today, when affordable health care is a problem for half or perhaps even three-quarters of all working families, the public and the politicians are forced to take notice.

Given the broad agreement that rising costs and falling satisfaction are the main problems in health care, it is a bit surprising that there is no consensus regarding what to do. Instead, health policy is faced with a series of contentious questions and enduring conflicts. Should funding be public or private? Do hospitals and doctors need more regulation or more competition? Are new drugs priced too high, or too low? How can we cover the uninsured? These conflicts can be traced to fundamental *unresolved dilemmas of dynamics and distribution*. Path dependence means following an American path, as determined by American culture and history—the frontier society that embraced liberty and innovation to become the capitalist leader of the free world and dominant economy of the year 2000. Sometimes this means aggressive free-market competition so that entrepreneurs can advance the process of creative destruction by which new technologies and new companies wipe out the old.

However, path dependence also means that entrenched interests (professional monopolies, pharmaceutical firms, political parties) will fight to maintain profits by deflecting or stifling competition. Everyone admires competition and growth in theory, yet no one wants their job to be the one that is replaced by computerization or low-cost foreign labor. The conflict between open entrepreneurialism and closed protection of existing organizations creates sharp tensions.

Failures in health policy are best illustrated by looking at the extremes: an unregulated market of "consumer-driven health care" with purely private ownership at one end, and totally regulated "universal health care" organized and financed collectively by the government at the other. Plans emphasizing personal responsibility for medical costs (MSAs, HSAs, and other "consumer directed health plans" described in Section 5.2) were crafted during the 1990s in imitation of the "defined contribution" 401K, individually owned retirement plans that were increasingly being used to replace company-provided defined-benefit retirement plans. MSAs shifted risk and responsibility onto the individual, rather than relying on broad government or employer financing pools that covered thousands or millions of people. Originally a niche within the self-employed individual health insurance market, high-deductible MSAs were held by advocates of an "ownership society" to be a superior alternative to existing employer-provided health insurance because they would give patients "more skin in the game" (i.e., a larger financial stake in each episode of care) and hence be able to use consumer choice to control health care costs (and incidentally relieve employers and government from doing so, just as the 401k had shifted responsibility for retirement from the employer to the individual). Employees, however, did not embrace consumer-directed plans with much enthusiasm. The niche expanded but remained a niche rather than a mainstream alternative.

People whose 401k's got clobbered in 2008 and 2009 had even less enthusiasm for picking up another such financial vehicle in an MSA or HSA. The idea that the individual employee should take personal risk for retirement and health care rather than relying on large scale risk pooling through employers or government fell quickly out of favor. Some advocates still push to replace most existing health insurance with MSA-type plans, but the limited ability to attract more than a narrow segment of the market and a fear of financial crisis make it doubtful that any broad move to privatize most risks will become politically acceptable within the next few years. Even before the political reversals brought about by the 2008 election, legislation to privatize social security was unable to pass Congress. Privatizing Medicare is a nonstarter. Other factors that make regulation seem more appealing than purely market-driven for-profit solutions are the series of convictions and fines levied against private hospital chains (AMI, HealthSouth, National Medical Enterprises, Columbia-HCA, Tenet) and health insurance companies (Oxford Health Plans, United Health, Ingenix) for market abuse violations, as well as the accumulating evidence that private Medicare Advantage plans, rather than saving money, actually cost more than regular Medicare.[15]

The other extreme is represented by "universal health care," financed by government and uniformly available to everyone without charge. Many doctors feel that medical care should be allocated to those who need it most, not those who can afford to pay the most. They point to wasteful advertising of expensive new drugs (which have high profit margins) and elaborate surgical interventions yielding only slight improvements, while proven low-cost remedies (aspirin, vaccinations) are not promoted among the populations most at risk. Yet universal health care for the United States, despite persistent legislative efforts by advocates, has consistently failed to gather majority support at any time since it was first proposed in 1918. A minority has always been strongly in favor, but the majority of the public has refused to accept a purely public health care system. This political failure has been influenced by doctors, who are often entrepreneurs in solo (or small group) practice fiercely protective of their independence and autonomy, and also by the public's generally negative perceptions of the post office, public housing, drivers' licensing bureaus, and other government-run enterprises. The American electorate tends to value independence and personal liberties more, and trust government less, than do most Europeans, Asians, or citizens in the rest of the world. Rarely do people in the United States willingly allow government control over their daily lives, or make it illegal to spend money on some service because it is not worthwhile.[16] "Managed care" generated a huge backlash in part because it crimped doctors' incomes, but more because it was perceived as an interference with "freedom of practice," restricting what patients could obtain from their private doctors. Distributional issues create tensions and trade-offs between the sick and the well, the old versus the new, urban versus rural, as well as the rich and the poor. Even when it is agreed that everyone should have health care, it is hard to reach consensus on who is going to pay for it, and how much each person should get.

18.6   THE PATH FORWARD: STEP BY STEP

Every country that has extended health insurance to the entire population and achieved some degree of success in controlling costs built upon existing blocks of partial financing, filling in the cracks over time. The first national health insurance program in Germany in 1883 covered only miners and industrial workers (Chapter 4). Australia, France, Canada, and Japan similarly started with partial coverage of a limited group of workers. Later new plans (or expansions of existing ones) extended coverage to dependents, farmers, the elderly, the self-employed, and so on. The English NHS is perhaps a bit different in that virtually all of the hospitals had already been taken over by the government during the war, and most doctors and nurses had been in the military, so the step to a government-run system with doctors and nurses as public employees was just a small shuffle that rationalized an existing situation when the NHS began operations in 1948. Those who favor a government-run national health service for the United States must face the facts that the situation in 2010 is far different from that in postwar England, and that legislation sponsoring universal health coverage has been repeatedly rejected by the U.S. Congress.

Private employer-based health insurance, along with voluntary hospitals and insurance plans (Blue Cross and Blue Shield), became entrenched as pillars of health financing in the United States during the twentieth century. The social insurance program that was tried and accepted in the United States is Medicare, which has become immensely popular and has strong political support. These forms of health financing may be supplemented or modified but are unlikely to suddenly disappear. Medicare was originally crafted in imitation of existing private medical insurance plans with UCR and indemnity reimbursement based on charges. As Medicare moved from a secondary role to become the biggest player in the health insurance market, it went from being guided by the private market to creating its own system of terminology and administered prices (DRGs, RBRVS, etc.) that are now guidelines leading the rest of the market.

What Might Work?

Although each polar extreme is loved by its partisan advocates, neither government-provided health care (NHS) nor pure private ownership (HSAs) is probable in the United States right now. What health care reforms could plausibly be implemented by 2012? One incremental step that builds on existing solutions is to **extend Medicare**, making it possible for individuals in their 50s or 60s to buy into this program when they cannot obtain health insurance at work.[17] Another extension of Medicare is to make greater use of its various administered pricing systems as standards for private health insurance contracts. It is also likely that Medicare will push forward trial programs that bundle payments together (e.g., a single payment for heart transplant rather than separate payments for hospitals, surgeons, drugs, etc.) and finally carry through on the competitive contracting experiments that would, for example, let providers bid to provide all of the medical equipment rentals (e.g., oxygen tanks, wheelchairs) in a region on the basis of price. The 2009 financial crisis made the public more willing to rely on government-regulated competition and less trusting of pure free-market control with voluntary policing of prices and contracts by private companies.

Employer-provided private health insurance plans are likely to continue to provide coverage to the largest number of Americans (even though government has paid more in total dollars since 1968, and is projected to cover more than 50 percent of all medical costs by 2018). The Federal Employees Health Benefits Plan (FEHBP) discussed in Chapter 5 has been suggested as a potential model for extending coverage. When politicians say "the same health insurance that members of Congress get," it is the FEHBP that they are talking about. The basic structure is as follows: in each area different insurance companies and HMOs put forth plans, each of which must meet certain standards of coverage. Employees can choose any plan that is offered, but the amount of premium paid by the government is limited to the amount charged by the lowest-price acceptable standard plan in the area. Thus the employee pays the full costs of any additional services or benefits (or inefficiencies). The need to attract enrollees in an open market provides incentives for insurers to keep premiums down and service levels up. Since the FEHBP has been operating successfully across the country with openly competing insurers covering millions of enrollees for more than 50 years, it is well tested and generally accepted. Allowing the rest of the country to buy health insurance through the same FEHBP plan would require expansion but not any radical new structure. However, it would require finding a means or formula for how the base financing (i.e., cost of the lowest cost local health insurance) would be obtained (e.g., individuals pay up to 10 percent of personal income, with the remainder paid by government or employer).

The real challenge is not just to provide coverage, but to reform the health care system so that it performs better and costs less. Creation of a **"Federal Health Board"** that would evaluate health technologies to determine which ones did and did not meet standards for full or partial coverage by health insurance has been discussed.[18] The examples of NICE (National Institute for Clinical Effectiveness) in England and IQWIG in Germany have been pointed to in this regard. In addition to establishing standards for medical effectiveness, the style of practice needs to be shifted to emphasize primary care. The concept of a **"medical home,"** or, in its more expensive version, **"concierge practice,"** is increasingly discussed. In both models, a primary source of care, be it a neighborhood health center or a patient's internist, is responsible for providing regular care, maintaining communication, encouraging compliance and lifestyle changes—and is paid a reasonable amount for doing so.[19]

Legislation establishing a "Federal Health Board" and promoting "medical homes" is almost inevitable given the amount of high-profile discussion these ideas have already generated. The important long-run issue is, will they be used? Will they be strong enough to reform a $3 trillion system, or just another ineffectual committee that advises and reports? In principle, Medicare officials could go ahead now and regulate payment so that only effective therapies are reimbursed using existing rule-making powers and technical advisory panels. So far, Medicare officials have usually backed away from such direct regulation. It is not the legislation that creates change, but the change in organizations and institutions that creates a new "path." As long as Americans believe that access to the latest medical technology is more important than the financial insecurity of uncontrolled costs escalation, as long as it is accepted that American health care is obviously superior to that practiced in other countries where greater life expectancy and patient satisfaction are provided at less cost, then little will change. Until doctors and other medical professionals are willing to shift from autonomous cottage practices to modern management and information technology, very little systematic change can occur.

18.7   THE SHAPE OF HEALTH CARE SPENDING TO COME

It is never possible to predict the future with certainty, but a review of historical trends (Chapter 16) and the simple fact that spending is eventually constrained by the availability of funds make it likely that the long-run trend of health care spending will take on the "S-shape" that characterizes most growth curves. After a long period of unsteady growth with little cumulative increase, a tipping point or sudden acceleration pushes growth exponentially upward. Ever more steeply inclined growth meets inherent constraints that begin to bend the curve back (inflexion point) toward moderation and eventual stability. For medical expenditures, the long period of vacillating slow growth extends back before the founding of the United States. Health care accounted for perhaps 1 to 3 percent of total consumption for hundreds of years. During the period 1929–1955, U.S. spending grew at an annual rate of less than GDP + 0.9 percent, and amounted to less than a 5 percent share of total consumption. From 1955 through 1993, the average rate of growth exceeded GDP + 3 percent, and health care accounted for more than 13 percent of total GDP. Since then, the rate of growth has slowed and averaged about GDP + 1.3 percent. Exactly when or at what level health expenditures will finally stabilize is far from clear. Excessive growth is likely to continue at least for a decade, and perhaps beyond 2025. However, it is likely that the average rate of long-run growth will begin to level out in the range of GDP + 0 to 1 percent sometime before 2050 (see Figure 18.1).

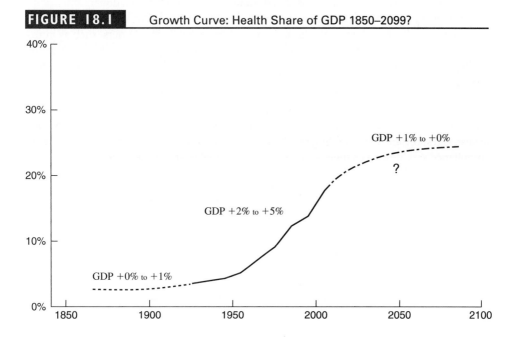

FIGURE 18.1   Growth Curve: Health Share of GDP 1850–2099?

18.8 THE LONG RUN: 2050 AND BEYOND

What can be said about the future of health and medical care over the next 50 years? Table 18.2 lists some expected trends. It is relatively certain that there will be continued increases in longevity, greater technological capability to treat disease, and continuous increases in expenditure. Although there will be more spending overall, the sources and uses of funding will change rather markedly, and it is probable that at some point the annual rate of increase will moderate. An older and healthier population implies more long-term care, with greater emphasis on caring and rehabilitation. Thus, the fraction of medical spending accounted for by acute illnesses of the employed tax-paying population will fall. The tension between public and private financing is likely to remain unresolved, with payers operating under a mixture of market incentives and regulatory structures to provide a middle ground. Treatment and production will become less and less important relative to the provision of caring and information management. Organization and teamwork will be more important as solo practice continues to fade. Quality control will rely on outcomes more than the initial qualifications and resource use by specialists and clinical technicians, with integrated assessment of processes in real time rather than examination of each part or profession separately. Some of these changes will be the disruptive consequences of medical and organizational entrepreneurship, but most will be slow, inertial, and incremental. The net effect of all these changes will on balance be beneficial, yet most are apt to be painful and resisted by some constituency.

The best prototypes for studying health economics in the twenty-first century are probably biotechnology and hospice. Physicians will become technical team leaders operating within a corporate organization, rather than independent medical practitioners. Cost shifting in the form of marked-up prices and open-ended reimbursement will continue to wither and be replaced by new forms, such as mandated benefits pools. The use of economic information and cost accounting for comparative decision making will continue to increase. Greater knowledge about actual costs and the actual effectiveness of clinical practice will provide greater clarity in the questions raised about the trade-off between dollars and health. Some fields (dietary modification, parts of mental health and disability care) are being spun off and are less likely to be counted as an integral part of medicine. Others, such as information systems and genetic engineering, are becoming more integrated and will blur the traditional boundaries between what is medicine and what is information or environmental modification.

TABLE 18.2　　　Future Trends

- Greater longevity, better health
- More long-term and chronic care, less acute illness
- More spending overall, but a smaller fraction spent on the working population
- Less ability to shift costs by overcharging for treatment
- A middle ground between public and private control
- More assessment of cost and outcomes
- Declining trust in organized professions
- Physicians lead teams within organizations, less autonomy and independence
- Successful organizations based on information (e.g., biotechnology) and caring (e.g., hospice)
- Special characteristics previously found mostly in medical care become more typical of many service organizations in a post-industrial economy

The special institutional features that set medicine and health apart from the rest of the economy may become less distinctively special over the coming years. In part, this is because medicine is becoming more organized and more corporate, more subject to a bottom-line assessment of costs and benefits. Yet the extent to which medicine is becoming like the rest of the economy may be of less importance than the extent to which the rest of the economy is becoming like medicine, where information, service, and public goods matter more than manufactured commodities. Previously, health economists have taken models from the study of industrial production and applied them to health and medical care. Ideas may increasingly flow in the other direction as the issues of special interest to health economists—uncertainty, agency, trust, service delivery, and quality—become central to the economy as a whole in a postindustrial era. Models developed for the study of medical care may in the future be applied to banking, entertainment, automation, fashion, and other industries, leading to applications and discoveries as spectacular as genomic sequencing and heart transplants.

SUGGESTIONS FOR FURTHER READING

David M. Cutler and Mark McClellan, "Is Technological Change in Medicine Worth It?" *Health Affairs* 20, no. 5 (September 2001): 11–29.

Victor Fuchs, "Economics, Values and Health Care Reform," *American Economic Review* 86, no. 1 (1996): 1–24.

Atul Gawande, "Getting There from Here: How Should Obama Reform Health Care?" *The New Yorker*, (January 26, 2009), pp. 26–33.

Institute of Medicine, *Crossing the Quality Chasm*, July 2001, http://www.newton.nap.edu/catalog/1027.html

Ian Morrison, *Health Care in the New Millennium* (San Francisco: Jossey-Bass, 2000).

Jonathan Skinner and Douglas Staiger, "Technology Diffusion and Productivity Growth in Health Care." NBER working paper 14865, April 2009.

SUMMARY

1. A primary role of health economists is to **force the public and politicians to consider the trade-offs** implicit in every health and medical care decision. Who gets helped? Who gets hurt? Who makes money?

2. Health economics can be viewed as answering questions in levels of ascending generality. At the base are the questions, **Which treatments are better?** and **How much do they cost?** At an intermediate level, **Who is going to have the power to make decisions?** Finally, **Which questions should be asked** to shape and judge the health care system?

3. The purpose of the health care system is to **satisfy the interests of the groups that participate** in it. Maximizing health is but one of many objectives. The average health of the population often may matter much less than *who*, in particular, gets healthy.

4. The increase in health and life expectancy that can be obtained from any given set of medical resources depends largely on the **allocation** of treatment to those most likely to benefit. Often, this is not the group that is most able or willing to pay.

5. Rising costs have created a distributional crisis as the **affordability** of health insurance, which used to affect only a few, has now become a problem that affects most working families.

6. Major **difficulties in economic appraisal** of health care policies arise because the most important issues frequently involve **public goods** and the **distribution of benefits and incomes** to different groups, as well as technical issues regarding productive efficiency.

7. Differences in the quality of care at a particular point in time are usually dwarfed by changes in the effectiveness of care over time. Hence, a health care system must provide resources and slack to make room for experiments, fostering the technological and organizational changes that bring about **dynamic efficiency**.

8. The health care system is **path dependent** with institutions and organizations embedded in a cultural and financial matrix. This makes progress **slow and inertial, with delayed responses** to changes in the political, economic, and scientific environment.

9. Medical care has not yet experienced the **information technology** revolution or **financial restructuring** that forced many organizations to become more efficient over the last 40 years. In the future, **teamwork** and linked information systems will matter more to medical professions than solo practices and piece-by-piece quality assurance.

10. **Values** ultimately mean more in health economics than the efficacy of medical technology or the estimation of costs. Analysis will increasingly focus on **the economics of caring and information**, not production.

PROBLEMS

1. {*allocation*} Will health care be more efficient or less efficient in 2020? Will people spend more money or less money on health care?

2. {*budget*} Will Medicare go broke by 2020 as some analysts predict? Why or why not? What historical evidence could you give to support your answer?

3. {*distribution*} Which matters more: how healthy we are on average or *who* gets healthy?

4. {*distribution*} Why redistribute health insurance costs and not automobile insurance costs?

5. {*values*} Economists debate the future of Medicare by arguing about which set of numbers best represents reality. Do these numbers represent objective or subjective values?

6. {*economic organization, distribution*} Who will make the decisions regarding medical care in the year 2020? Which of these groups will have more or less power over those decisions in 2020?

   a. Physicians
   b. Nurses
   c. Pharmaceutical companies
   d. Biotechnology investors
   e. U.S. senators
   f. AARP (formerly the American Association of Retired Persons)
   g. Disability advocates
   h. Children
   i. Economists

7. {*productivity*} As medical technology continues to develop, will the marginal productivity of each additional dollar spent on it increase or decrease? What about the average productivity per dollar spent on medical care?

8. {*economic organization, distribution*} Are health care funds spent to maximize health or to maximize the welfare of those who make the decisions?

9. {*distribution*} Which is more representative of the average family income: the median or the mean? Does random variation make distribution of costs more or less of a problem?

10. {*allocation, budget*} Given the ever increasing age of the population and advance of medical technology, why would anyone expect the growth of medical costs to slow down in the future?

ENDNOTES

1. Paul Samuelson and William Nordhaus, *Economics*, 14th ed. (New York: McGraw-Hill, 1992), p. 19.
2. Daniel Kahneman, Paul Slovic, and Amos Tversky, *Judgment Under Uncertainty: Heuristics and Biases* (New York: Cambridge University Press, 1982); this is the classic in the field. See also: Richard H. Thaler and Cass R. Sunstein, *Nudge: Improving Decisions About Health, Wealth and Happiness* (New Haven: Yale University Press, 2008; Richard Frank, "Behavioral Economics and Health Economics," NBER working paper 10881, November 2004; Jeffrey Liebman and Richard Zeckhauser, "Simple Humans, Complex Insurance, Subtle Subsidies," NBER working paper 14330, September 2008; Richard Frank and Karine Lamiraud, "Choice, Price Competition and Complexity in Markets for Health Insurance," NBER working paper 13817, February 2008; Jason Abaluck and Jonathan Gruber, "Choice Inconsistencies Among the Elderly: Evidence from Plan Choice in the Medicare Part D Program," NBER working paper 14759, February 2009; Emmanuel Saez, "Details Matter: The Impact of Presentation and Information on the Take-up of Financial Incentives for Retirement Saving," *American Economic Journal: Economic Policy* 1, no. 1 (2009): 204–228.
3. It is possible to construct a production function that moves up and yet is steeper, with greater average productivity and yet lower marginal productivity for a given set of inputs, but it requires some contortion to do so, and such quirks are unlikely to explain the large and persistent rise in health care spending that has accompanied the twentieth-century advance of health care technology. Some other explanation must be found if the attempt is to remain plausible.
4. Alan Garber and Jonathan Skinner, "Is American Health Care Uniquely Inefficient?" NBER working paper 14257, August 2008; Jonathan Skinner and Douglas Staiger, "Technology Diffusion and Productivity Growth in Health Care," NBER working paper 14865, April 2009.
5. Think about how easy it is to find a site for a needed garbage dump, the popularity of charging for pollution, or the endurance of subsidies for cotton, honey and, yes, even tung oil.
6. William D. Nordhaus, "The Health of Nations: The Contribution of Improved Health to Living Standards," NBER working paper 8818, January 2002.
7. David M. Cutler and Mark McClellan, "Is Technological Change in Medicine Worth It?" *Health Affairs* (September 2001): 11–29.
8. Atul Gawande, "Getting There from Here: How Should Obama Reform Health Care?" *The New Yorker*, 26 January 2009, pp. 26–33.
9. Congressional Budget Office, *The Budget and Economic Outlook: An Update*, p. XII, September 2008; Peter Orzag, "The Long-Term Budget Outlook and Options for Slowing the Growth of Health Care Costs: Testimony for the Senate Finance Committee," Congressional Budget Office, June 17, 2008.
10. The Economist, "Medicine Goes Digital: A Special Report on Health Care and Technology," *The Economist*, 18 pages, April 18, 2009.
11. Randall D. Cebul et al., "Organizational Fragmentation and Care Quality in the U.S. Health Care System," NBER working paper 14212, August 2008.
12. George D. Lundberg, *Severed Trust: Why American Medicine Hasn't Been Fixed* (New York: Basic Books, 2000); R. J. Blendon et al., "Satisfaction with Health Care Systems in Ten Nations," *Health Affairs* 9, no. 2 (Summer 1990): 185–192; R. J. Blendon et al., "Understanding the American Public's Health Priorities: A 2006 Perspective," *Health Affairs* 25, no. 6 (October 2006): w508–w515.
13. Brian K. Bucks, Arthur B. Kennickell, Traci L. Mach and Kevin B. Moore, "Changes in U.S. Family Finances from 2004 to 2007: Evidence from the Survey of Consumer Finances," Federal Reserve Bulletin (2008), pp. A8–38, http://www.federalreserve.gov/pubs/bulletin/.
14. Daniel Polsky and David Grande, "The Burden of Health Care Costs for Working Families—Implications for Reform." *New England Journal of Medicine* 361, no. 5 (July 30, 2009), p.437–439; Didem M. Bernard, Jessica S. Banthin, and William Encinosa, "Wealth, Income and the Affordability for Health Insurance Coverage," *Health Affairs* 28, no. 3 (May 2009): 887–896.

15. Vanessa Fuhrmans and Jane Zhang, "U.S. Reduces Subsidies for Private Medicare," *Wall Street Journal*, 7 April 2009.

16. The exceptions, such as prostitution and hard drugs, are illustrative in themselves of the problems with prohibiting "freedom to spend on whatever you want."

17. Kaiser Family Foundation, *Health Insurance Coverage for Older Adults: Implications of a Medicare Buy-In*, Publication No. 7904 (May 14, 2009), www.kff.org/healthreform/7904.cfm.

18. Ezekiel J. Emmanuel, Victor R. Fuchs, and Alan M. Garber, "Essential Elements of a Technology and Outcomes Assessment Initiative," *Journal of the American Medical Association* 298 (2007): 1323–1325.

19. Morgan Lewis Jr., "No Place Like Home," *Medical Economics* (July 24, 2009) p.14–17.

GLOSSARY

Activities of Daily Living (ADLs) A checklist measure of the extent of disability and functional status.

Actuarially Fair Premium A premium equal to the expected value of the loss, although in practice all premiums must be set higher in order to cover overhead costs.

Actuary Accredited insurance mathematician who calculates premium rates and company reserve requirements using statistical studies.

Administered Prices Prices which are specified by an administrative agency, rather than being set in the market.

Administered Service Only (ASO) A self-insured health plan in which the employer bears all the risk of losses, but hires an administrator to process claims.

Administratively Necessary Days (ANDs) Payment for days when a patient's medical status is such that they should have been discharged from the hospital but were not because no nursing home beds were available.

Adverse Selection A disproportionate share of bad risks. When given a choice, the people who choose to purchase insurance are likely to be a group with higher than average losses.

Agency The process of having one party (the agent) make decisions on behalf of another (the principal).

Aggregation The process of clumping together; the creation of summary measures for a population as a whole; study at the system or group level.

Allocative Efficiency Allowing those who value a good more to consume more. Total consumption value is maximized by allowing the process to continue toward an equilibrium where for each individual, marginal benefit = marginal cost. Also, targeting medical care to those most in need so as to maximize average life expectancy.

American Medical Association (AMA) The professional organization which represents the

interest of MD physicians in the United States and lobbies government agencies on their behalf.

Anti-trust Legal restrictions relating to collusion between firms and market domination.

Arbitrage The process by which the prices of a good selling to different persons or in different markets are brought together by trade. Also, the act of buying and selling in anticipation of price movements—which makes the price adjust more rapidly to information.

Assignment An agreement by a physician to take payment directly from Medicare, and to accept the amount as payment in full (i.e., with no balance billing).

Average Cost The total cost divided by the number of units.

Balance Billing Making the patient pay for the balance of any charges in excess of the amount allowed by the insurance company.

Balanced Budget Act of 1997 An act passed by the U.S. Congress in 1997 that significantly reduced provider payments and expanded the role of managed care in the Medicare Program.

Branded Drugs Drugs whose production and sale are protected by a patent. Also, the brand-name drug produced by the initial firm even after its patent expires and other firms begin to sell competing generic versions.

Cap A limit on the amount that an insurance company will pay. The cap may be an overall maximum, such as a lifetime maximum of $250,000, or may apply to specific services, such as a $500 per year cap on outpatient mental health counseling.

Capitation Paying a fixed amount per enrolled person per month for a defined set of services which does not vary with **utilization**.

Case-Mix Reimbursement Adjustment of reimbursement to account for differences in patient diagnoses, and sometimes for the severity of illness as well.

Certificate of Need (CON) A legal requirement that approval from a state agency to certify need (CON) must be obtained before a health care facility is built or remodeled.

Ceteris Paribus All other factors being held constant.

Charges The amount appearing on the patient's bill.

Chiropractic An alternative form of medical practice which emphasizes spinal manipulation in the treatment of disease, often to the exclusion of drugs and surgery. Although chiropractors are found in most communities, they are often not accepted by the organized medical profession.

Circular Flow of Funds The circulation of money facilitates exchange; it is not used up or consumed. Each dollar spent by a consumer goes to a producer, who in turn gives it to an owner, worker or supplier, who as consumers send those dollars on to another producer, and so on in an unending circular flow.

Clinical Pathways A protocol, or defined standard set of tests and procedures to be used in diagnosing or treating a particular symptom or disease.

Clinical Trials Testing of new drugs or medical technology on humans.

Coase Theorem The hypothesis that the type of economic organization (profit or non-profit, one firm or many, capitalist or socialist) and which party holds ownership rights (e.g., chemical firms or fishermen, homeowners or airport operators) would not matter if there were no transaction costs.

Coinsurance The amount of the bill not paid by insurance, but by the patient. A plan with 15% coinsurance means that the insurance company pays 85% and the person pays 15%.

Community Rating Setting the same premium rate for every person in the community regardless of age, sex or previous illness.

Comparative Statics The study of a system by comparing how the state of equilibrium differs when some set of parameters (incomes, prices, fertility) differs; in contrast to **dynamics** in which the process of change is the focus of study.

Compounding Adding to; the accumulation of growth over time; how a small percentage increase eventually leads, with interest on the interest, to doubling, quadrupling and many-fold increasing.

Concurrent Review Daily checks by an HMO on the status of a patient to monitor, and if necessary, modify or terminate, the provision of services.

Consumer Price Index (CPI) A measure of the average change in price over time in a fixed "market basket" of goods and service purchased either by urban wage earners and clerical workers or by all urban consumers.

Consumer Surplus The difference between what consumers are willing to pay for a product and the market clearing price. As such, consumer surplus is represented by the area under the demand curve but above market price.

Consumption Function The relationship between consumption and income as income changes; the fraction of total income saved as the level or composition of aggregate income changes.

Continuing Care Retirement Communities (CCRCs) Living quarters for elderly persons with provisions for meals, transportation, therapy and other assistance, usually constructed with an adjacent nursing home. Financial risks to the individual are often reduced through prepayment. Also known as lifecare communities.

Copayment A copayment is a specified amount that the patient must pay with each service received, such as the $2 for each prescription that many drug plans make the pharmacist collect, $10 for each day in the hospital under Medicare, $5 for each visit to the doctor under some HMO plans, etc. One of the purposes of copayments is to discourage overutilization. Thus while deductibles and coinsurance may sometimes be covered under a spouse's plan or other insurance, the insured must usually pay the copayment out of pocket.

Cost Reimbursement Retrospective payment for services based upon audited cost reports, often including complex limits and rules for allocation.

Cost Shifting The process of using excess revenues from one set of services or patients to subsidize other services or patient groups.

Cost-Benefit Analysis (CBA) A set of techniques for assisting in the making of decisions, which translates all relevant concerns into market (dollar) terms.

Cost-Effectiveness Analysis (CEA) Comparison of the costs of different ways of achieving an objective (cases prevented, years of life saved). Similar to CBA, except that CEA does not require benefits to be expressed in dollar terms.

Cream Skimming Choosing to provide only the most profitable services, or to insure only the healthiest patients to avoid subsidizing public goods (education, research, indigent care) and to obtain extra profits.

Cross-Sectional Analysis Statistics constructed using observations across different individuals or groups at one point in time, as opposed to **longitudinal** or **time-series** analysis.

Deductible An amount that must be paid by the individual before the insurance company begins to pay. For example, many policies have a $100 per year deductible. This means that if total insured medical bills were $730, the insurance would apply only after the person had paid the first $100, that is, to $630.

Demand A schedule of the amount that will be consumed in the market at varying prices.

Demographic Transition The period of rapidly increasing population which usually occurs during economic development as a poor society with high mortality and high birth rates transitions to a wealthy society with low mortality and low birth rates.

Demographics Age, sex, and other characteristics of populations.

Derived Demand The demand for an input due to the demand for output; demand for a good due to its use, rather than in itself (e.g., the demand for x-ray film is derived from the demand for medical diagnoses, which in turn are derived from a consumer's demand for health).

Detailing Marketing of pharmaceuticals to physicians by drug company representatives (detailers); offers of free samples and advice in order to increase the number of times a drug is prescribed.

Diagnostically Related Grouping (DRG) A system of reimbursement which compensates by the case (rather than per day or per charged item) based on the diagnosis of the patient.

Diminishing Marginal Returns As additional amounts of a variable input are put into the production process, holding constant all other variables, the incremental amount added to total output becomes smaller and smaller.

Discounted FFS Contracts with providers to pay a specified percentage of usual charges.

Discounting Adjustment of valuation for the passage of time, reflecting the fact that the present value of a future good is smaller. Also, adjustments to reflect risk, reductions in the quality of life, and other factors.

Diseconomies of Scale The average cost per unit rises as the quantity produced increases.

Distribution How evenly things are shared, divided or spread out. The amount or frequency in the top 10%, second 10%, and so on. In statistics, the shape of the graph when the number or probability of observations is arranged in order of magnitude (e.g., normal distribution, skewed distribution).

Dynamic Efficiency Use of inputs so as to maximize long-run value over time, taking account of the need for tinkering to bring about technological and organizational advances.

Dynamic Shortage A temporary deficit in supply caused by a sudden increase in demand, or sudden drop in supply.

Dynamics The process of change; the study of how change occurs over time, including the order, timing and strength of interacting forces.

Economies of Scale The average cost per unit decreases as output increases.

Efficacy The ability to actually cure a disease; how well a treatment works in practice.

Elasticity The percentage change in one variable when another variable changes by one percent.

Enrollee A person covered by a health benefits plan.

Entitlements Social insurance payments to which beneficiaries are entitled by law with little regard to actual contributions or premiums, or income qualifications (e.g., Medicare, Social Security).

Entrepreneur The person who undertakes the effort to create an organization and the network of contracts necessary for its success.

Equity In health services research, equity is the extent of equality in health, income, or other resources. In finance, equity refers to the net worth of the organization (assets – liabilities); the capital belonging to the owners. (See **Leverage**.)

ERISA The "Employee Retirement And Income Security Act of 1974" and subsequent amendments which govern most health insurance contracts, and in particular, exempt self-insured plans from most state regulation.

Expected Value The value of an outcome multiplied by its probability of occurring. Also, the probability-weighted average of all possible outcomes.

Experience Rating Setting a group premium based on the actual losses experienced by that group during the prior year or years.

Externalities The effects of a transaction between parties on outsiders; the uncompensated effects of an action (e.g., pollution); side-effects.

Fallacy of Composition The logical error of assuming that what holds true for the individuals within a group must also hold true for the group collectively, or vice-versa.

Fee Schedule A list of approved fees for each service promulgated by an insurance company, government agency, or professional society.

Fee-For-Service (FFS) Payment for health care based on the charges for each service or item used.

FEHBP The Federal Employees Health Benefits Plan (FEHBP) is the system through which all federal employees, including congresspeople and senators, obtain health insurance. In each area, several plans that meet or exceed the specified qualifications are offered, and the government pays an amount equal to the lowest-priced plan premium. The employee must pay the amount by which the plan chosen exceeds that of the lowest-cost plan.

Firm An organization that is responsible for coordinating the transformation of inputs, such as land, labour, capital, and entrepreneurship, into some final output or outputs.

Flexible Budget A budget that is adjusted for changes in the volume of service.

Flexner Report The critique written in 1910 which led to the reform of medical education and established the MD degree as a qualification for licensure.

Flow The amount over a period of time (i.e., income, annual mortality rate).

Food and Drug Administration (FDA) The federal agency with jurisdiction over labeling, manufacture, and sale of food and drugs for human consumption.

Formulary A list of approved drugs for reimbursement with all non-approved drugs paid at a lesser rate or not at all.

Free Rider A person who allows others to produce a public good, and then uses it without paying. For example, most poor country prevention programs are free-riders, dependent upon the research of rich countries to do the research and produce the vaccines needed to control infectious diseases.

Full Time Equivalents (FTE) A measure of the quantity of labor used.

Fundamental Theorem of Exchange Any voluntary exchange between persons must make both of them better off since they willingly agreed to trade.

Gatekeeper A primary physician who manages and approves all services for the patient who enrolls in his practice.

Generic Drugs Drugs which are identical in chemical composition to a brand name pharmaceutical preparation, but produced by competitors after the firm's patent expires.

Global Budget A fixed total budget for all health services.

Grandfathering Approving those who are already in practice to continue even if they do not meet the new standards.

Gross Domestic Product (GDP) The total market value of all production in a nation.

Group Insurance Contract for insurance made with an employer or other entity, called the policyholder, that covers a group of persons as a single unit.

Health Maintenance Organization (HMO) An organization that contracts to provide comprehensive medical services (not reimbursement) for a specified fee each month. The term health maintenance organization arose because doctors under this arrangement have a financial incentive to keep their patients healthy, since they are not paid more for providing more services.

Health Insurance Portability and Accountability Act of 1996 (HIPAA) A legislated set of rules to increase efficiency by standardizing billing and making health care transactions paperless. HIPAA also specified rules governing access to records, privacy, confidentiality, combat fraud, develop medical savings accounts, and other matters.

Homeopathy An alternative form of health practice emphasizing natural remedies used in extremely dilute solutions.

Hospital Privileges The rights of those doctors who have been voted acceptance on the hospital's medical staff to admit patients and perform surgery.

Human Capital Analysis of investments of time, effort, and money in education or health that improve a person's productivity as analogous to investments of financial capital.

Income Distribution The fraction of all income earned by the top 10 percent of the population, the second 10 percent, and so on; the degree of disparity in incomes between the rich and the poor.

Income Elasticity The percentage change in expenditures due to a one percent change in income. Income elasticities below 1.0 mean that although spending on a good rises with income, it rises less than proportionately so that the fraction of total income spent on that good is reduced. With income elasticities greater than 1.0 (luxury goods), spending rises more than proportionately so that the share of total income spent on the good increases as income increases.

Indemnity Benefit A specified dollar amount reimbursed for a particular injury or type of care, such as $15 for each x-ray or $475 for gall bladder removal, is an indemnity benefit. Life insurance, which provides a specified dollar amount in case of death, has an indemnity benefit.

Independent Practice Association (IPA-HMO) An HMO formed by non-exclusive contracts with many providers who operate independently, as opposed to closed group staff HMO where physicians work exclusively for the HMO and are often on salary.

Inflation A measure of the reduction in the real purchasing power of currency over time.

Information Asymmetry The disparity in information between a buyer and a seller in a transaction.

Inpatient Services or goods provided within a hospital or nursing home.

Intensity (of services) The amount of inputs used to provide each unit of service. For example, an urban university hospital will typically provide complex services of high intensity, while a primary care doctor on an emergency call in an isolated rural area will use far fewer resources to treat the same injury.

Investigational New Drug (IND) A designation of FDA approval to begin the testing of a drug.

Kickbacks Surreptitious payments made in order to obtain business.

Leverage The ratio of debt to equity, or the amount of assets per dollar of net capital.

Licensure The establishment of legal restrictions specifying which individuals or firms have the rights to provide services or goods.

Life-Cycle Hypothesis Assertion that individual spending at any point in time is based on their long-run expected income over the life-cycle rather than just current income at that point in time; a common form of the **permanent income** hypothesis.

Loading Factor (or Load) The percentage of total premiums used for administrative costs, profits, and all items other than medical benefits.

Long-Term Care (LTC) Nursing homes, visiting nurses, home I.V. and other services provided to chronically ill or disabled persons.

Longitudinal Analysis Study of a set of individuals or groups tracking how they change over time.

Macroeconomics (from the Greek 'macro' meaning large) The branch of economics that studies how the economy as a whole operates, covering such topics as total output, employment and price levels. See also **Microeconomics**.

Major Medical In order to compete with the Blue Cross service benefits, commercial insurance companies came up with plans with deductibles and coinsurance that could be sold for much less. Often today, major medical is used as a supplement, while some basic services, such as hospital and doctor visits, are covered in full.

Malpractice The legal framework specifying failure to meet professional standards.

Malthusian Hypothesis The expectation that any increase in food supply would eventually lead to a matching increase in the number of people living at a subsistence level, so that on average, living conditions would be no better than before.

Managed Behavioral Health Mental health and substance abuse services managed by an MCO.

Managed Care The use of a manager to control utilization of medical services and control costs. Often associated with HMOs, other forms of managed care include peer review panels, pre-approval procedures for surgery, case management for the chronically ill, formularies limiting pharmacy reimbursement to an approved list, and other contractual provisions.

Managed Care Organization (MCO) An HMO, PPO, or other organization that accepts financial risk and manages care.

Managed Competition A policy of increased reliance on competing HMO's and a fixed limit to tax subsidies so that employees would bear the full marginal cost of their health benefit plans.

Mandated Benefits Specific services (e.g., pregnancy, alcoholism detoxification) for which a state requires all health plans to provide coverage.

Marginal Incremental; a one unit increase.

Marginal Propensity to Consume The fraction of an additional dollar that would be spent on consumption, and thus not invested as savings.

Marginal Productivity The incremental output obtained with one more unit of input.

Marginal Cost The increase in total costs caused by the production of one more unit of output.

Market Failure The inability of the market to arrive at a reasonably efficient equilibrium under certain conditions, notably the existence of public goods and externalities, lack of clear property rights, inability of some consumers to act in their own best interest, natural monopoly due to constantly declining average costs of production, and excessive transaction costs or information asymmetry.

Means Testing Setting a standard of low income in order to qualify for a government benefit, e.g., Medicaid.

Medicaid Combined state/federal program to insure people whose incomes are insufficient to pay for health care; primarily those on welfare or older people in nursing homes.

Medical Savings Account (MSA) A proposal to replace regular health insurance and HMOs by allowing people to place money in a tax-free savings account to be used for medical expenses, in conjunction with the purchase of a catastrophic stop-loss health insurance plan covering expenses in excess of a specified amount such as $3,000.

Medicare A Federal government insurance program that provides hospital benefits (part A), medical benefits (part B) and drug benefits (part D) to persons over age 65 and some qualified widows and disabled.

Medigap A policy designed to pay coinsurance, deductibles, drugs, and other expenses not fully covered by Medicare.

Microeconomics (from the Greek 'micro' meaning small) A field of economics that uses economic theory to study how individual consumers and firms make economic decisions.

Monopoly A market in which there is a single provider(seller).

Monopoly Rents Profits in excess of competitive market returns due to a monopolist's ability to unilaterally increase prices.

Monopsony A market characterized by a single buyer that has the ability to influence market price.

Moral Hazard Any change in behavior due to insurance which increases expected losses, such as the higher utilization of covered medical services by employees or the acceptance of more risky loans by insured banks.

Morbidity Illness or disability, especially when expressed as a rate (e.g.; sick days per year per 1,000 employees).

Mortality Death, usually expressed as a rate per one hundred, thousand, or hundred-thousand.

Need A professional determination of the quantity that should be supplied (as distinct from market demand).

NICE The National Institute for Clinical Effectiveness (NICE) is an independent council operating in the UK to provide independent advice on the costs and benefits of new drugs and therapies, and to make recommendations for the National Health Service regarding their use and reimbursement.

Normative Shortage When too little is supplied according to professional opinion, although not necessarily according to market behavior (e.g., there is a shortage of raw vegetables in the diet of teenagers).

Occupancy Rate The percentage of a hospital's beds filled at a specific time.

Off-Label The use of a prescription drug for diseases other than those for which it has been approved by the FDA.

Opportunity Cost What must be given up in order to do or obtain something; the highest-valued alternative which must be foregone. For example, the opportunity cost of taking the final exam may be missing out on a trip to Bermuda.

Option Demand Willingness to pay for access to a good which may or may not be used, e.g., emergency room, spare tire.

Osteopathy An alternative form of medical practice which emphasizes spinal adjustment as well as surgery and drugs in the treatment of disease. Originally quite distinct from mainstream allopathic medicine, osteopathy is now almost identical so that MDs and DOs usually practice together, although DOs are more likely to be generalists focusing on primary care.

Out-of-Pocket Payments made by individuals or their family, rather than an insurance company, HMO, government, or other third party, for medical care.

Outpatient Services provided in a physicians' office, clinic, or other ambulatory setting.

Over-the-Counter A drug that consumers can purchase without a prescription from a physician.

Patents A legal monopoly for a specified period of years given to a firm which makes a discovery.

Path Dependence The idea that the current situation develops out of the past and cannot be fully understood without considering the steps that led up to it. Also, an observation by social scientists that change in most systems tends to be slow and inertial, depending on people and organizations that are embedded in specific cultures and institutions facing durable legal and financial constraints. In geometry, it is the fact that the area under a curve depends not only on the starting and ending points, but also on the path between these two points.

Per Diem Per day payment for services.

Per Member Per Month (PMPM) The standard form of HMO payment, also known as **capitation**.

Permanent Income Expected long-run average income, as opposed to the transitory income which a person (or group) may have during the current month or year.

Pharmacoeconomics Cost-benefit analysis of drugs; assessment of the market for a drug.

Point of Service Plan (POS) An HMO which offers partial reimbursement for services which a patient chooses to obtain outside of the HMO network.

Population Medicine Analysis and assessment of health care on the basis of the community or group rather than the individual; design of a system with services targeted to those of greatest need; making trade-offs to optimize average health, rather than doing the best possible for one specific individual under treatment.

Practice Variation Differences in the number of medical services provided not explainable by any differences in the population served. Also known as small area variation.

Pre-authorization A requirement that the doctor or the patient obtain approval from the HMO before the service is provided.

Pre-existing Condition An insurance contract may specify that it will not pay for medical problems already diagnosed or under treatment before the policy is purchased, known as pre-existing conditions. A person with AIDS who bought a policy with such a clause would find that it paid for his broken leg, and maybe even to have his tooth drilled, but not for anything related to AIDS. Often the pre-existing condition exclusion will only apply to the first 6 months or year of coverage. This, and other exclusionary clauses, are a major way of reducing adverse selection when medical insurance is marketed to individuals.

Preferred Provider Organization (PPO) A health insurance plan which offers enrollees a discount for using hospitals and physicians within an approved network of contracted providers.

Premiums Payments made in advance to provide medical services or reimbursement in the future.

Price Discrimination Charging different people different prices for the same good.

Price Index A measure of the purchasing power of money, usually set arbitrarily equal to 100 at one specific point in time (or space). The average change in prices weighted by the expenditure on each item.

Primary Care The basic medical attention provided by a physician to a patient seeking care, as distinct from referral services obtained from specialists, or tertiary care provided in technologically sophisticated hospitals.

Progressive A progressive policy is one that redistributes costs and benefits in favor of those toward the bottom. A progressive tax, such as the U.S. income tax, is one that takes a larger percentage from high-income persons or groups. (See **Regressive**.)

Property Rights The right to use, sell, or to derive income from a good.

Prospective Payment Payments set in advance, especially in contrast to retrospective **cost reimbursement**.

Provider Network The set of physicians, hospitals and others with which an MCO has signed a contract to provide care for enrollees.

Public Goods Goods that are consumed or financed collectively (e.g., clean air, national defense, discovery of penicillin) either because it is impossible to include/exclude any consumer who does not pay (see **free rider**), or because once produced, there is no additional cost for additional consumers.

QALYs (Quality Adjusted Life-Years) A way of measuring the value of a medical intervention by the increase in life expectancy, adjusted for difference in disability and timing.

Rationality The notion that consumers will never purposely make themselves worse off and have the ability to rank preferences and allocate income in a fashion that derives the maximum level of utility.

RBRVS The "resource-based relative value system" developed for Medicare to reimburse ambulatory services based on the estimated time, effort, skill, equipment, and other resources needed to provide each service.

RCCAC The "ratio of costs-to-charges applied to charges" methodology used to apportion cost reimbursements.

Redistribution Policies that have the effect of changing the pattern of consumption by different income classes; allowing the poor to consume a larger share of GDP.

Regressive A regressive policy is one that redistributes costs and benefits disproportionately in favor of those at the top. A regressive tax is one that takes a proportionately larger share of income from those at the bottom; for example, cigarette taxes. (See **Progressive**.)

Regulatory Balloon The observation that any regulation pushing costs down on one side is apt to exert pressure pushing costs up in some other direction.

Regulatory Capture The subtle takeover of a regulatory agency by the industry it was meant to regulate, so that it tends to represent the interests of the industry, rather than the public.

Reimbursement The process of paying for the costs incurred, especially through a third party.

Reinsurance Acceptance by a second insurer (the reinsurer) of all or part of the risk undertaken by the first insurer; usually used to cover very large losses and protect against bankruptcy. For example, a reinsurer may agree that if total losses exceed the $5 million in expected claims by more than $1 million, they will, for a price, pick up 90% of the extra losses.

Relative Value Scales A list of point scores for each service to be used in setting reimbursement.

Rents Profits in excess of those necessary in order to call forth the requisite supply of inputs in the market. Compensation above competitive amounts obtained by professionals who are able to control supply.

Retention Ratio Agreement A contract specifying an allowed ratio of premiums to medical expenses with some fraction of any excess underwriting gains to be returned to the firm or used to reduce premiums in the following year.

Retrospective Review Monitoring records after discharge and disallowing (refusing to pay for) any services that do not meet specified standards of medical necessity and timeliness.

Revolving Door Term used to describe staff that leave a regulatory agency to work within the industry which is supposed to be regulated, and vice-versa. Such changes in employment may compromise the agency's objectivity.

Risk The chance or probability that an event will occur.

Risk Adjustment The process of setting the capitation rate for an insurance policy based on the health status and expected medical costs of an individual or group purchasing the plan.

Risk Aversion The extent to which an individual is willing to pay to reduce variation in losses or income due to random events.

Risk Pooling Forming a group so that individual risks can be shared among many people.

Risk Selection Enrollment of healthier-than-average persons into an insured group.

Sanitary Revolution The 19th-century campaign to clean up the environment and change personal behavior to conform to Victorian notions: "cleanliness is next to godliness."

Scarcity Scarcity exists when the quantity of a good or service available is insufficient to satisfy demand at a zero price. An economic good is thus any good or service which is scarce relative to our wants for it.

Selection Bias A disproportionate share of above- or below-average persons in the group.

Self-Insurance A health plan funded and controlled by the firm itself, so that no risk is transferred to an insurance company, although benefits may be administered by an outside party. Self-insurance often enables a firm to avoid regulations governing purchased health insurance.

Service Benefits If the insurance company contracts directly with the doctor or hospital to provide the service rather than setting up some form of financial reimbursement, this is a service benefit. Blue Cross provides service benefits through its contracts with hospitals. An advantage of a service benefit to the insurance company is that they usually get a discount off the price that the patient would have to pay directly for the services rendered. An advantage to the consumer is that they obtain complete medical care as a service, without having to file insurance forms, or pay and wait for reimbursement from the insurance company.

Shared-Income Hypothesis Income becomes more and more important as a determinant of health-care spending as the unit of observation increases in size from the individual to the nation.

Social Insurance Pooling funded through taxes for protection against risks provided by the government for all (or almost all) of the citizens in a society. Social Security in the United States and the National Health Service in England are examples of social insurance plans.

Spend-Down The process of spending or giving away assets by elderly persons so as to qualify for Medicaid reimbursement of long-term care expenses.

Stock The amount at a point in time (i.e., total assets, population).

Stop-Loss A limit on the maximum amount a person would ever have to pay is known as a stop-loss. If a family has a $1,000 stop-loss, then the insurance company will pay everything after the family's out-of-pocket expenses reach $1,000.

Sub-capitation Carving out a specialized service (physical therapy, mental health) and paying the specialized provider on a per-member per-month basis.

Subsistence Having barely enough food and other resources to sustain life.

Tertiary Care Specialized medical care delivered in technologically sophisticated hospitals.

Third-Party Administrator An organization that processes claims for a self-insured firm, but bears no financial risk for losses.

Third-Party Transaction An exchange which is indirect and often pools the funds of many individuals with money collected and disbursed by a third party such as an insurance company, voluntary non-profit organization, or government agency.

Time-Series Analysis Statistics using multiple observations of an individual or group over time; statistical analysis of the dynamics of change.

Trade-off The idea that every individual will voluntarily sacrifice some of one good or service in exchange for a sufficient increase in the amount of some other.

Transaction Costs All costs, monetary and non-monetary, whether counted or not, of carrying on trade.

Triple-Option A complete array of plans consisting of an HMO, a PPO, and an indemnity plan, offered by an insurer as a package. The package as a whole is experience rated, so that any one option may be significantly over- or under-priced to create cross-subsidies between plans.

Two-Party Transaction An exchange between a buyer and seller, usually trading money for goods or services.

Underwriting Gains (Losses) The amount by which premiums received exceed (fall short of) benefits paid out.

Universal Health Insurance A national plan providing health insurance or services to all citizens, or to all residents.

Usual, Customary, and Reasonable (UCR) A method for setting the maximum allowed fee for each service based on usual charges by other physicians in the area, the customary charge by this particular doctor over the preceding year, and "reasonable" adjustments for severity or special conditions.

Utilization The number of services used, often expressed per 1,000 persons per month or year.

Utilization Review (UR) Monitoring of medical records to determine if services are appropriate and should be paid for.

Variability The extent of random changes over time or between persons.

Voluntary Organization A nonprofit organization, such as a hospital or social service agency, governed by a board of concerned citizens rather than owners or elected officials.

Welfare Loss The decline in social welfare (total value of consumption/production) due to monopoly supply restrictions, price controls, rationing, taxes, or other interventions that cause misallocation of resources. Also known as deadweight losses.

Welfare Triangle The reduction in consumer's surplus caused by a reduction in quantity sold due to monopoly supply restrictions, price controls, or other distortion.

Willingness to Pay (WTP) How much a person is willing to give up in order to obtain some item or specified improvement in quality of life.

Withhold A pool of money for providers which is held back and distributed by the HMO only if total expenses for the year end up being at or below acceptable levels.

Workers Compensation A mandatory insurance program covering the costs of medical treatment and disability due to work-related accidents and illness.

Wrap-Around An insurance policy designed to create a more comprehensive set of coverages sold with an underlying base policy.

INDEX

A

Abbreviated New Drug Application (ANDA), 258–259
Abortion, 367–368
Abramson, Leonard, 298–300
Academic medical centers, 18
Access to treatment, 89
Activities of daily living (ADL)
    evaluation form, 235
    long term care and, 234
Actuarially fair premium, 81
Addiction, 368–369
Adjusted charges, 64
Adjustment for risk, cost-benefit analysis and, 51
Administered prices, hospitals and, 219–220
Administered services only (ASO), 116
Administratively necessary days (ANDs), 235–236
Adverse selection, 90–92
Aetna, 300
Agency, 147
Agency issues, 288–289
Aging, 239–240. *See also* Long term care
Agreement on Trade-Related Aspects of Intellectual Property Rights (TRIPS), 259
Agricultural age, 375–380
    civilization, war, and government and, 376–377
    food supply and, 378
    investment and trade and, 376
    Malthusian hypothesis and, 379–380
    plague and, 378
    population declines and, 377
    rise of economics and, 378–379
AIDS. *See* HIV/AIDS
Allegheny bankruptcy, 292
Allocative efficiency, 43
Alzheimer's disease, 228
American Medical Association (AMA)
    chiropractic care and, 160–161
    code of medical ethics, 167
    control over physician supply (1930-1965), 159–161
    substitute providers and, 160–161

Ancillary service abuses, 169
Anesthesia, as medical breakthrough, 158–159
Angioplasty, 29
Annualized employment growth rates, 315
Anti-kickback laws, 169
Anti-substitution laws, 258
Antiseptics, as medical breakthrough, 158–159
Arbitrage, 34
Artificial heart development, 26–27
Aspirin, 29
Asset transfers, 232
Asset valuation, 283–284
Assignment to insurer, 140
Asymmetric information, 147
Audits, 128
Average costs, calculating, 53–54
Average *vs.* marginal value, 28–30
Average wholesale price (AWP), 252

B

Backward-bending supply, 145
Balance billing, 140
Balanced Budget Act of 1997, 220, 321
Bankruptcy, 292
Behavioral economics, 430
Benefit-cost principles, 12–13
Better health as a goal, 62–63
Billable events, physician incomes and, 142
Biologics Control Act of 1902, 256
Birth rates, 374
Block booking, 213
Blue Cross/Blue Shield, 98, 125, 129
Bond of trust, doctors and patients, 146–147
Borrowing, hospitals and, 293
Breast cancer, 29–30, 66
Budget constraints, 11, 312, 322
Budgeting, hospitals and, 209–210, 219–220
Bureau of Indian Affairs, 112

Bureaucratic objectives, government and, 347
Business risk assessment, 285–286

C

Capacity constraints, 322
Capital financing. *See also* Ownership
  business risk assessment and, 285–286
  cash flow perpetuity and, 278
  characteristics of, 275–276
  corporate advantage and, 297–300
  drug companies and, 285
  financial intermediaries and, 289–290
  HMOs and, 293–297
  hospitals and, 290–293
  human capital and, 280–281
  interest rates and, 277–278
  internal rate of return and, 278–280
  medical education as investment,
    280–281
  net present value and, 279–280
  nursing homes and, 285
  present value and, 277–278
  risk and, 281–283
  time value of money and, 276–277
  uncorrelated and correlated risks,
    284–286
  valuing assets and, 283–284
Capitation, hospital financing and, 189–192
Capitation rates, 125–127, 140
Caring, financial compensation and, 3–4
Carter, Jimmy, 321
Case-mix reimbursement systems, 234–235
Cash flow, 278, 283–284
Catastrophic insurance, 115
Centers for Disease Control and Prevention
  (CDC), 355
Certificates of need (CON), 230, 232–233
  effects of, 233–234
  legislation and, 217–219
  Medicaid budgets and, 233
  new construction and, 233
  nursing home profits and, 233
Change, adjustments to, 312–319
Charity
  care funding, 194–195
  financing medical care and, 80–81, 112
  shifting overhead and, 17–18
China, market size in, 401
Chiropractors, 160–161
Choice, benefits *vs.* costs and, 12–13
Circularity, money flow and, 12
Claritin, 32–33, 269
Clinical pathways, 173
Clinical trials, pharmaceutical, 260–261

Clinics
  block booking and, 213
  early formation of, 390
Closed-ended health care financing, 101
Closed-panel HMO, 121
Co-insurance, 140
Coase theorem, 340
Code creep, 141
Code of Hammurabi, 167–168
Competition, pros and cons of, 348–350
Competitive success, hospitals and, 198–199
Compounding, 374
Concentrated benefits, government programs
  and, 346
Concierge practice, 440
Concurrent review, 127
Consistently irrational choices, 430
Consumer directed health plans, 114
Consumption function, 307–309
Continuing care retirement communities,
  242–243
Contracts
  hospitals competing for, 197–198
  timing and risk and, 13–14
Contractual reforms, cost reductions and,
  121–122
Contractual relationships, pharmaceutical firms
  and, 265
Copayments, 139
Corporations
  advantages of, 297–300
  equity and debt and, 288
  U.S. Healthcare example, 298–300
Correlated risks, 284–286
Cost accounting, 64
Cost-benefit analysis, 49–59
  adjustment for risk and, 51
  calculating marginal and average costs, 53–54
  characteristics of, 48
  cumulative benefits of treatment, 57
  defining marginal, 54
  expected value and, 51, 58–59
  intensity margin example, 54–56
  knee injury example, 49–52
  limited perspective of, 72
  making choices and, 49–59
  marginal cost and, 52–53
  opportunity costs and, 55, 57–58
  public goods and, 361–362
  public policy decision making and, 72
  severity margin and, 56–57
  stepwise choices and, 52–53
  time discount and, 52
  willing to pay and, 50

Cost controls, 320–322
Cost measurements, 64–65
  adjusted charges and, 64
  cost accounting and, 64
  extrapolation from comparable services
    and, 64
  follow-up and treatment, 64
  provider time and inconvenience, 65
  secondary treatment costs and, 64–65
  time and pain of patient and family, 65
Cost minimization, 43
Cost reimbursement, hospitals and, 188–189
Cost shifting, 9, 18, 192–196
Cost structure, pharmaceuticals and, 255
Cream skimming, 195
Cumulative benefits of treatment, 57

D

Database profiling, 127
Day care centers, 363
Death rates. *See* Mortality rates
Death while hospitalized, 191
Decision process, efficiency steps in, 42–44
Defensive medicine, 146
Defined contribution health plans, 114
Deinstutionalization, 343
Demand and supply intersection, 38–39
Demand curves, 26–30, 40
  consumer surplus and, 28–30
  demand shifters, 30
  firm demand, 30–31
  individual demand, 30
  law of demand and, 27
  marginal analysis and, 27–28
  marginal revenue and, 31–32
  marginal *vs.* average value of medicine and,
    28–30
  market demand, 30
Demand for health, 42
Demand shifters, 30
Demand *vs.* need, 39–40
Department of Veterans Affairs, 112
Derived demand, 41
Detailing, 264
Determinants of health, 40–41
Diagnostically related groups (DRGs), 101, 189,
  220, 321
Diamonds–water paradox, 27–28
Diffuse costs, 346
Diminishing marginal utility, 15
Direct-to-consumer advertising,
  pharmaceuticals and, 268–269
Disability, 337–338
Discharge planning, 128

Discounted fees, managed care plans and, 140
Discounting over time, 69
Diseconomies of scale, hospitals and, 214–215
Distribution
  costs and benefits and, 71–72
  equity and, 18–19
Distributional crisis, 437
Doctor-patient relationship, 146–147
  agency and, 147
  asymmetric information and, 147
  bond of trust and, 146–147
Doctor visits, value of, 41
Doctor workshops, hospitals as, 145
Doctors of osteopathy (D.O.s), 159–160,
  163–164
Drug prescription overcharging, 168. *See also*
  Pharmaceuticals
Drug Price Competition and Patent Term
  Restoration Act of 1984, 258
Drug testing. *See also* Pharmaceuticals
  average length of, 261
  clinical trials and, 260–261
  new drug applications and, 260, 261
  Phase I testing and, 260
  Phase II testing and, 260
  Phase III testing and, 260–261
  stages of, 260
Dynamic efficiency, 43, 432–434

E

Economic efficiency, 434
Economic growth, health care and, 373–374
Economic modeling, 380
Economic principles, 11–14
  adaptation and evolution, 14
  choice, 12–13
  circularity, 12
  contracts, 13–14
  investment, 13
  maximization, 12
  opportunity cost, 11–12
  scarcity (budget constraints), 11
  trade, 12
  willingness to pay, 12
Economic security, value of, 387–389
Economics
  fundamental theorem of exchange and, 2
  terms of trade and, 2–3
Economies of scale
  group practice and, 165
  hospitals and, 214–215
Education return on investment, 281
Efficiency, decision process and, 42–44
Elasticity, 32

Elderly, difficulties in obtaining insurance, 99
Emergency calls, group practice and, 166
Emotional distress, 65
Employee Retirement and Security Act of 1974 (ERISA), 118
Employer-based group health insurance, 109–111, 440
Employment
    annual percentage change and, 325
    dynamics of, 323–327
    growth rates and, 315
    Medicare effects on, 326–327
    trends and, 325
Entitlement programs, 100–101, 119, 345. *See also* Medicare and Medicaid
Environmental Protection Agency (EPA), 358
Epidemics, 363–364
Equity and distribution, 18–19
European Union, pharmaceutical trade and, 423–424
Evidence-based medicine, 65–66, 173
Expected value, 51, 58–59
Experience rating, 116
Extend Medicare, 439–440
Externalities, cost, 339
Extrapolation from comparable services, 64

F

Family, time and pain of, 65
Family and friends, financing medical care and, 80
Family role, long term care and, 227
FDA Modernization Act of 1997, 259
Federal Employees Health Benefits Plan (FEHBP), 128, 440
Federal grants, 4
Federal Health Board, 440
Fee-for-service payments, 127, 135–136
Financial analysis, timing and risk and, 5
Financial intermediaries, 4, 289–290
Financial reimbursement cycles, 237–239
Financing medical care, 4–5. *See also* Capital financing; Insurance
    charity and, 80–81
    family and friends and, 80
    physician, 135–141
    private market insurance contracts and, 81–83
    savings and, 80
    social insurance and, 82
    sources of, 7–9
    strengths and weakness and, 82–83
Firm demand, 30
Firm demand curve, 31

Firm size, percentage of workers insured and, 111
Fixed budgets, 209
Fixed domestic graduation rates (1980-2008), 162
Fixed premiums, 116–117
Flexible budgets, 209
Flexner Report, 158–159, 164
Food, Drug, and Cosmetics Act of 1938, 257
Food and Drug Administration (FDA), 358
Forecasting health expenditures, 319–320
Foreign medical graduates, 163
Foreign physicians, 161–162
Franchise chains, HMOs and, 296–297
Free-rider problem, 338
Full-time equivalent employees, 165
Fundamental theorem of exchange, 2
Future health care spending, 441
Future trends, 442–443

G

Gatekeeping, managed care plans and, 125
Generic drugs, 249
Generic substitution, 128
Genetics, 19
Geographic practice cost indexes (GPCI), 138
Germany health system, 417–421
    ambulatory *vs.* hospital care, 419
    fee-for-service payments and, 419–420
    hospitals and, 420
    pharmaceutical sector and, 420
    private health insurance and, 419
    risk group categorization and, 418
    sickness funds and, 418–419
    social insurance and, 417
    statutory system and, 417
Global budgets, hospitals and, 188
GMENAC Report, 162
Going public, 288
Government
    business objectives and, 347
    care of poor and, 343–344
    as citizen's agent, 346–348
    disability policy and, 337–338
    entitlement financing and, 334, 345
    fund distribution and, 335
    health financing and, 333–334
    health regulation and, 345
    income group benefits and, 348
    law and order and, 337–338
    market efficiency and, 336
    market failure and, 341–343
    in mixed economy, 337
    natural monopolies and, 341–342

necessity of, 335–336
under perfect competition conditions, 336
political interest groups and, 347
politicians and, 340–341
production of, 345
public goods and externalities and, 338–341
public welfare maximization and, 346
redistribution of wealth and, 343–344
regulation and competition and, 348–350
regulatory capture and, 346–347
roles of, 335–337
subsidies and, 345
transaction costs and property rights, 339–340
varieties of, 345
Grants, hospital financing and, 187
Gross domestic product (GDP), 318–319
Group Health Association, 296–297
Group practice, 165–167
bonus plans and, 169
comparative advantage and, 166
economies of scale and, 165
emergency calls and, 166
full-time equivalent employees and, 165
labor costs and, 165
management time and, 167
net earnings and, 165
physician assistants and, 166
risk sharing and, 165–166
senior-junior doctor partnerships, 167

H

Hansen's disease, 364
Harris-Kefauver Drug Amendments of 1962, 258
Harvard University, 91
Harvey, William, 390
Hassle costs, 65
Hatch-Waxman Act, 258
Health economics. *See also* Health spending; Macroeconomics of medical care
changes in health and, 15
cost-shifting and, 9
differences over time and place, 16
diminishing marginal utility and, 15
dynamic change and, 15–16
flow of funds and, 8–9
funding in United States, 6–8
geographic location and, 17
illness is contingent, urgent, uncertain, 14
individual choices and, 17
patient care and compensation, 3–4
personal tastes and preferences and, 17
pricelessness of health, 15
quality, not quantity and, 16

research and technology and, 15–16
sources of financing, 7–9
spending growth and, 9
terms of trade and, 2–3
Health insurance, 83–88. *See also* Insurance plans; Medicare and Medicaid
adverse selection and, 90–92
benefit determination and, 88
defined contribution health plans, 114
employer-based group health insurance, 109–111
entitlement funding, 100–101
expenditure concentration and, 84
expenditure distributions and, 84
as funding mechanism, 100–101
high-deductible insurance, 115
historical aspects of, 97–99, 389
indemnity insurance plans, 88
insurance contracts, 116–117, 128–129
labor markets and, 96–97
managed care and, 88
moral hazard and, 92–95
popular misconceptions about, 87
premature death and, 92
price competitiveness of, 175–176
risk aversion and, 88–90
self-paid private insurance, 112
State Children's Health Insurance Program, 113
tax benefits and, 95–96
third-party transactions and, 86–87
types of, 108–113
underwriting cycle and, 117–118
uninsured, 112–113
U.S. coverage and, 109
variability and, 85–86
Health insurers, as financial intermediaries, 290
Health maintenance organizations (HMO). *See also* Managed care plans
business risks and, 293–294
capitation rate and, 140
closed-panel HMOs, 121
competition and, 127
contracts and, 120, 197–198
evolution of, 294–296
FFS payments and, 127
franchise chains and, 296–297
Group Health Association example, 296–297
Kaiser Health Plan example, 294–296
medical loss ratios and, 123–124
organizational change and, 122–123
physician incentive under, 141
reduced deductibles and copayments and, 129

Health maintenance organizations
(HMO) (*cont.*)
    referrals and, 121
    withholds and, 127
Health Professions Educational Assistance Acts,
    161–162, 217
Health regulation, governmental, 345
Health reimbursement accounts (HRA), 114
Health risks, public nature of, 17
Health savings accounts (HSA), 114–115
Health spending. *See also* Health economics
    adjusting to changes in, 313–315
    forecasting of, 319–320
    implications of, 404–405
    micro and macro determinants of, 402–404
Heart attacks, 216
Heart transplants, 56
High-cost outliers, hospital financing and, 191
High-income countries, 413–422
    Germany health system, 417–421
    Japanese health system, 413–417
    United States health system, 421–422
Highest risk, targeting diagnosis and treatment
    to, 62
Hill-Burton Act of 1946, 217
History of health insurance, 97–99
History of medicine
    agricultural age and, 375–380
    income and health and, 385–386
    industrial age and, 380–384
    information age and, 384–385
    modern medicine's rise, 389–393
    mortality ratios by social class, 387
    social security and health insurance, 389
    stone age and, 374–375
HIV/AIDS, 118, 364–365
HMO-POS (point of service) plans, 125
Home health care
    financial reimbursement and, 237–239
    growth areas in, 228
    Medicaid and Medicare abuse and, 238
Home health resource groups (HHRG), 238
Homeless, 343
Homosexuality, 367
Hormone replacement therapy, 173
Hospital costs
    accounting *vs.* economic costs, 211–214
    administered prices and, 219–220
    block booking and, 213
    budgetary review and, 219–220
    budgeting uncertainty and, 209–210
    certificate-of-need legislation and, 217–219
    contracting out and, 215
    controlling through regulation, 217–220

cost per patient, 206–207
diagnostically related groups and, 220
diseconomies of scale and, 214–215
economies of scale and, 214–215
efficiency and total spending, 216
fixed budget and, 209
flexible budget and, 209
high-cost outliers and, 191
operating budget and, 209
per patient day, 218–219
price controls and, 219
pro forma financial statements, 209
prospective payment system and, 220
quality and, 215–216
short-run *vs.* long-run cost functions,
    207–208
size-cost relationship, 214–215
specialized units and, 215
strategic budget and, 209
technology and, 215–216
timing and, 211–213
utilization reviews and, 219
variation and, 206–207
Hospital financing
    borrowing, 293
    capital financing and, 290–293
    capitation and, 189–192
    charges by, 188
    competing for contracts and, 197–198
    competing for patients and, 196–197
    competing for physicians and, 197
    cost reimbursement and, 188–189
    cream skimming and, 195
    diagnostically related group payments, 189
    financial management and cost shifting,
        192–196
    global budgets and, 188
    hospital characteristics and, 187
    major types of reimbursement, 187
    managed care contracts and, 192
    measuring competitive success and,
        198–199
    measuring market competitiveness and, 199
    per diem and, 188
    philanthropy and grants, 187
    rates adjusted for special situations,
        190–191
    ratio of cost to charges applied to charges
        (RCCAC), 188–189
    revenue maximization and, 194
    revenue sources and, 186–192
Hospitals
    control of, 199–201
    development of modern hospital, 184–186

as doctor workshops, 145
hospital chains, 293
patients who die in, 191
short-stay outliers and, 190
transfers and readmissions, 190–191
Human capital, 13, 280–281
Human life, valuing, 66–68

I

Illness, contingent/urgent/ and
uncertain, 14
Incentives
insurance plans and, 128–129
physician financing and, 141
Income distribution, 336, 405
Income elasticity, 308
Income groups, government policy
towards, 348
Indemnity plans, 81–82, 88, 121
Independent practice association (IPA)
HMOs, 140
Individual choices, lifestyle and, 17
Individual demand, 30
Individual reimbursement, 140
Industrial age, 380–384
demographic changes during, 382–384
income distribution and, 383–384
Malthus' predictions and, 381–382
middle classes and, 383–384
technological advances and, 381
Infectious disease externalities, 363–366
day care centers and, 363
epidemics and, 363–364
HIV/AIDS, 364–365
sanitary revolution and, 365–366
sexually transmitted diseases and, 363
U.S. Public Health Service and, 366
Inflation, 315–318
Information
consumer ignorance and, 358
public vs. private sector and, 358–359
responsibility for, 357–358
technology and, 436
Information age, 384–385
Insurance. See Health insurance
Insurance companies, pharmaceutical costs
and, 253
Intensity margin, 54–56
Intensive care management, 127
Internal rate of return (IRR), 278–280
International health care
differences among nations, 399–402
health as national luxury good, 402–403
health expenditures and, 399–401

high-income countries, 413–422
low-income countries, 405–409
market size and, 401–402
medical equipment trade and, 423
middle-income countries, 409–413
per capita health expenditures and
income, 403
pharmaceutical trade and, 423–424
service trade and, 423
spending and health improvement,
404–405
International medical graduates, 163
Internet pharmacies, 252
Investigational New Drug (IND) applications,
259–261
Investment, future productivity and, 13

J

Japan health system, 413–417
Elderly Health System, 416
flow of funds in, 415
generalist physicians vs. specialists, 414
large vs. small hospitals, 414
medical fee schedule in, 416–417
pharmaceutical trade, 423–424
universal health insurance, 414–416
Jenner, Edward, 391

K

Kahneman, Daniel, 430
Kaiser Health Plan, 294–296
Kaiser Permanente, 121–123
Kefauver, Estes, 258
Kenya health system, 408–409
government and private sources and,
408–409
National Hospital Insurance Fund, 409
physician private practice and, 409
religious missions and, 409
traditional healers and herbalists, 409
Kickbacks, 167–168
Kircher, Athanasius, 390
Knee injuries, cost-benefit analysis and,
49–52

L

Labor costs, group practice and, 165
Labor-leisure choice, physician, 36, 145
Labor markets, health insurance effects on,
96–97
Laboratory testing, 193–194, 215
Latent demand, 26
Law of demand, 27
Law of diminishing returns, 380

Legal control over physicians, 159
Leprosy, 364
Licensure
   AMA controls (1930–1965), 159–161
   medical care quality and, 151–152
   patient needs and, 148–149
   physician profits and, 149–150
   strong *vs.* weak, 152–153
   supply and demand and, 149
   vs. unlicensed professions, 150–151
Life, value of, 387–389
Life expectancy
   better medical care and, 392–393
   income per capita and, 404–405
Lifestyle, individual choices and, 17
Loading factor, private market insurance
  and, 81
Long-run capital budget, 209
Long-run hospital costs, 207–208
Long term care. *See also* Certificates of need;
  Nursing homes
   activities of daily living and, 234
   administratively necessary days and,
     235–236
   asset transfers and, 232
   case-mix reimbursement and, 234–235
   certificates of need and, 232–234
   continuing care retirement communities,
     242–243
   defining boundaries and, 240–241
   dimensions needed, 227–228
   elderly population and, 225
   financial reimbursement cycles and,
     237–239
   home health care and, 228, 237–239
   insurance and, 241
   market development and, 225–227
   Medicaid and, 229–232
   money and quality and, 232
   rate of institutionalization and, 227
   resource utilization groups and,
     234
   service substitution and, 235–236
   social support and, 228–229
   spending down and, 232
   traditional family role in, 227
   types of care, 227–229
   wealthy elderly and, 242–243
Long term care insurance, 241
Low-benefit treatments, 66
Low-income countries, 405–409
   Kenya health system, 408–409
   resource misallocation and, 406
   starvation in, 406

Sudan health system, 406–408
   women's health in, 406
Luxury good, health as, 402–403

M

Macroeconomics of medical care. *See also*
  Health economics
   adjusting to change and, 312–319
   annualized employment growth rates
     and, 315
   budget constraints and, 312, 322
   capacity constraints and, 322
   central issues and, 305–306
   consumption function and, 307–309
   cost controls and, 320–322
   employment and, 323–327
   forecasting future health expenditures and,
     319–320
   GDP adjustments and, 318–319
   health spending adjustments and, 313–315
   income elasticity and, 308
   inflation adjustments and, 315–318
   macroeconomic shock, 322
   permanent income and, 314–315
   permanent income hypothesis and, 309–310
   physician supply and, 313
   public and private decisions and, 311–312
   recession and, 316
   shared income hypothesis and, 310–311
   spending and, 306–307
   time series analysis and, 318–319
   U.S. health expenditures per capita, 307
   wages and, 327–328
   workforce dynamics and, 323–328
Mail-order pharmacies, 252
Malpractice insurance, 146
Malthus, Thomas, 379
Malthusian hypothesis, 379–380
Managed care organization (MCO), 120
Managed care plans, 119–124. *See also* Health
  maintenance organizations
   capitation rates and, 125–127, 140
   contracting and, 197–198
   contracts with hospitals and, 192
   contractual reforms and, 121–122
   cutting quality of services and, 121
   discounted fees and, 140
   flow of funds with, 120
   gatekeeping and, 125
   impetus behind, 119–120
   management and, 120–121
   negotiated fees and, 140
   pharmaceutical costs and, 253, 264–265
   physician salaries and, 140

price cutting and, 121–122
provider networks and, 124–125
substituting cheaper forms of care, 122
utilization reviews and, 127–128
withholds and, 127
Management time, group practices
and, 167
Mandated benefits, 118–119
Mandatory generic substitution
(MGS), 126
Marcus Welby, M.D., 174
Marginal analysis, 27–28, 55
Marginal benefits, declining, 60
Marginal costs, calculating, 53–54
Marginal productivity, 37
Marginal revenue, 31–34
Marginal *vs.* average value, 28–30
Market competitiveness, hospitals and, 199
Market demand, 30
Market efficiency, 336
Market failure, 336, 341–343
Market size, 401–402
Market supply and demand, 38–39
Maternal and Child Health Bureau, 112
Maternity care, 196
Maximization
average benefits and, 61–62
marginal benefits and, 60
misleading averages and, 61–62
net benefits and, 60–61
optimization and, 60–61
targeting highest risk cases and, 62
Maximum net benefits, 60–61
Mayo Clinic, 167
Meals on Wheels, 228
Medicaid
balance billing and, 140
certificates of need and, 232–234
components of, 112
dependency or right, 343–344
drug discount policy, 264
establishment of, 99
home health care and, 238
hospital cost shifting and, 193
hospital financial picture and, 291
long term care and, 229–232
patient access to physician and, 141
pharmaceuticals and, 253
reducing expenditures and, 101
Medical arms race, 197
Medical care demand, 41
Medical care dissatisfaction, 436
Medical care spending, 306–307
Medical care uncertainty, 148

Medical costs
distributional crisis and, 437
entrenched interests and, 438
falling satisfaction and, 437–438
future reductions and, 63–64
health outcome improvement and, 436
Medical Economic Index, 139
Medical education, 157–158
AMA and licensure (1930–1965), 159–161
cost of, 158
fixed domestic graduation rates
(1980–2008), 162
great medical student expansion
(1970–1980), 161–162
Health Professions Educational Assistance
Act of 1963, 161–162
as investment, 280–281
licensure and, 158–162
original grandfathering of, 159
selection and, 157–158
Medical equipment, international trade and, 423
Medical home concept, 440
Medical loss ratios, 123–124
Medical practice expenses
labor–leisure choice and, 144–145
nonphysician inputs and, 144
physicians, 143–144
practice size and, 143–144
unpaid hospital inputs and, 145–146
Medical practice variations, 171–174
Medical savings accounts (MSA), 114
Medical technology. *See* Research and
technology
Medicare
anti-kickback laws and, 169
balance billing and, 140
Balanced Budget Act of 1997 and, 220, 321
components of, 109
contracts, 99
dependency or right, 343–344
diagnostically related group payments
(DRGs) and, 189
establishment of, 99
extra treatment value and, 56
funding charity care and, 194–195
high-cost outliers and, 191
home health care and, 238
hospital cost shifting and, 193–195
hospital financial picture and, 291
patients who die and, 191
prospective payment system and, 321
RCCAC methodology and, 188
reducing expenditures and, 101

Medicare (*cont.*)
  resource-based relative value scale and, 136–139
  short-stay outliers and, 190
  supplemental market and, 430
  transfers and readmissions and, 190–191
  twelve standard supplement plans, 110
Medicare Advantage plans, 438
Medicare D, 263–264
Medicine as a profession, 3–4
Medigap insurance, 109
Mental illness, 118
Mexico health system, 410–411
  government spending and, 411
  health insurance coverage in, 410
  incentives and, 411
  private providers and, 411
Middle-income countries, 409–413
  disadvantaged populations and, 410
  industrial paternalism and, 409–410
  Mexico health system, 410–411
  Poland health system, 411–413
Mixed economy, 337
Modern medicine, 389–393
  preconditions for change and, 390
  science and technology growth, 390–391
Money, time value of, 276–277
Monopolies, 341–342
Monopoly rents, 341
Monopsony market power, governmental, 264
Moral hazard, 92–95
  price elasticity of demand and, 93–94
  welfare losses due to, 94–95
Mortality rates, 19, 374
Myocardial infarction, 216

N

National Center for Health Statistics (NCHS), 357–358
National Institute for Clinical Effectiveness (NICE), 262
National Institutes of Health (NIH), 357
Natural monopolies, 341
Need *vs.* demand, 39–40
Negotiated fees, managed care plans and, 140
Net present value (NPV)
  internal rate of return and, 279–280
  risky returns and, 282–283
New Drug Application (NDA), 261
New molecular entities (NMEs), 268
Nightingale, Florence, 391
Nixon, Richard, 320
Nixon price controls, 320
Non-M.D. physician growth, 163–164

Nonprofit hospitals, 200–201
Nursing homes. *See also* Long term care
  care level and profit, 235–236
  cost breakdown and, 229
  financial risks and, 285
  long-term care market development and, 225–227
  Medicaid and, 229–232
  private pay patients and, 233
  profits and, 233
  sources and uses of funds, 230
  spending down and, 232
  two-part market and, 231

O

Off-label uses, pharmaceuticals, 264
Open-ended health care financing, 101
Operating budgets, 209
Opportunity costs, 11–12, 55, 57–58
Optimization, maximum net benefits and, 60–61
Organizational change, reducing costs and, 122–123
Over-the-counter (OTC) drugs, 257, 269
Ownership. *See also* Capital financing
  equity and debt, 287–288
  going public and, 288
  independent corporations and, 288
  ownership and agency, 287–290
  partnerships and, 287–288

P

Pain price, 36
Partnerships, 287–288
Patents, drug, 261
Path dependence, 435–439
Pathologists, 145–146
Patient competition, hospitals and, 196–197
Patient time and pain, 65
Payment type, access to physician care and, 141
Per diem payments, 188
Per member per month (PMPM) plans, 125–127
Permanent income hypothesis, 309–310
Perpetuity, 278
Personal tastes, health economics and, 17
Pharmaceuticals, 253–255. *See also* Drug testing
  advertising and promotional activities and, 254
  average wholesale price and, 252
  Claritin example, 269
  contractual relationships and, 265
  cost structure and, 255
  detailing and, 264

direct-to-consumer advertising and, 268
distribution *vs.* marketing and, 266–268
drug manufacturing costs and, 254
drug testing and, 260–261
financial risks and, 285
flow of funds and, 252
government monopsony market power and, 264
group purchasers and, 264
history and regulation of, 255–259
industry structure and competition, 262–270
insurance companies and, 253
international review agencies and, 262
international trade and, 423–424
Internet pharmacies, 252
mail-order pharmacies, 252
major legislation affecting, 257
managed care and, 264–265
market segmentation and, 264
Medicare D and, 263–264
middlemen role and, 266–268
off-label uses, 264
patents and, 261
pharmaceutical firms and, 253–255
pharmacies role and, 268
pharmacoeconomics, 261–262
pharmacy benefit managers and, 250–251, 253
price reductions and, 265
product differentiation and, 265
profits and, 255
reference price and, 262
research and development and, 254–255, 259–261
research productivity and, 268–270
retail pharmacies, 252
sales, research and development, and profits, 250
sources of financing, 249–251
technology assessment and, 261–262
trends and, 270
value and cost and, 265–266
wholesalers and, 253
Pharmacies, retail
carve-outs and, 126
profits and, 268
role of, 252
triple-tier benefits and, 126
Pharmacoeconomics, 261–262
Pharmacy benefit managers (PBMs), 250–251, 253
Philanthropic funding, 187, 193
Physician assistants, 166

Physician expenses
general expenses, 143–144
malpractice and, 146
Physician financial reimbursements
assignment to insurer and, 140
balance billing and, 140
co-insurance and, 140
copayments and, 139
fee-for-service payments and, 135–136
fee schedules and, 136
incomes, 142–143, 164
individual reimbursement and, 140
insurance company payments and, 136
managed care plans and, 140–141
payment type and physician incentives, 141
plan deductibles and, 139–140
reimbursement mechanisms and, 141–142
relative value scales and, 136–139
salaried physicians, 140–141
usual, customary, and reasonable fees and, 136
Physician licensure, 149–150
Physician recruitment, hospitals and, 196–197
Physician supply, 159–161, 313. *See also* Medical education
balancing supply and incomes, 164
earnings potential and, 164
flow of new entrants and, 162–164
growth of non-M.D. physicians, 163–164
immigration of international medical graduates and, 163
Plagues, 378
Plan deductibles, 139–140
Point of service plans, 125
Poland health system, 411–413
capitation payments and, 412–413
mandatory insurance and, 412
overuse of, 412
pharmaceuticals and, 412
primary *vs.* specialty physicians in, 413
private resources and, 412
Political interest groups, 347
Politicians, 340–341
Population growth, 374
Population medicine, 173–174
Pre-admission testing, 127
Pre-certification, 127
Pre-tax spending accounts, 114
Preferred provider organizations (PPO), 120–121, 124–125, 129
Premature death, insurance and, 92
Premiums, private market insurance and, 81

Prescription drug privatization, 355
Prescription Drug User Fee Act of 1993, 261
Preston, Samuel, 392
Price competitiveness, insurance market and,
175–176
Price controls, 219
Price discounts, 126
Price discrimination, 34–35, 169–171
Price elasticity, 32–34
Price reductions, pharmaceutical, 265
Pricelessness of health, 15
Primary care physicians, 125
Private decision making, 311–312
Private demand curves, 360–361
Private market insurance contracts, 81–83
    actuarially fair premium and, 81
    indemnity plans and, 81–82
    premiums and, 81
    risk pooling and, 81
Product differentiation, pharmaceuticals,
265
Production function, 37–38, 43
Production of health, 40–42
Professional standards review organization
(PRSO), 219
Property rights, 339–340
Prospective payment system (PPS),
220, 321
Provider networks, 124–125
Provider time and inconvenience, 65
Provigil, 267
Public decision making, 311–312
Public demand curves, 360–361
Public goods, 336, 338–341
    characteristics of, 354–359
    cost-benefit analysis and, 361–362
    demand for, 360–361
    infectious disease externalities, 363–366
    information and, 357–359
    insurance and, 356
    local conditions and, 355
    privatizing, 355–356
    provision of, 362
    public health in action, 366–370
    purchasing of, 362
    pure public goods theory, 359–362
    social costs and, 356
Public health in action, 366–370
    abortion and, 367–368
    addiction and, 368–369
    sexual behavior and, 366–377
    war and, 369–370
Public policy decision making, cost-benefit
analysis and, 72

Public welfare maximization, 346
Pure public good theory, 359–362

Q

QALY league tables, 69–71
Quality
    hospital competition and, 196
    hospital costs and, 215–216
    measurement of, 16
Quality-adjusted life years (QALY), 68–71
    discounting over time, 69
    factors and, 69
    league tables, 69–71
Quality Care Compensation System
(QCCS), 299
Quality not quantity, 16

R

Radiologists, 145
Ratio of cost to charges applied to charges
(RCCAC), 188–189
Rational choice theory, 21–22, 430
Readmissions, hospital financing and, 190–191
Rebates, 126
Recessions, 316
Recruitment incentives, hospitals and, 196–197
Reference prices, pharmaceutical, 262
Referral fees, 167–168
Regulation
    controlling hospital costs and, 217–220
    government and, 346–347
    pros and cons of, 348–350
Reimbursement mechanisms, physician
financing and, 141–142
Reimbursement system, billable events
and, 142
Reinsurance, 116
Relative value scales, 136
Rents, 340
Research and technology
    benefits to society and, 433
    cutting costs *vs.* enhancing quality, 215–216
    dynamic change and, 15–16
    modern hospital and, 185–186
    pharmaceutical, 259–261
    reimbursements and, 17–18
Research productivity, pharmaceuticals and,
268–270
Resource-based relative value scale (RBRVS),
101, 136–139
    conversion factor and, 139
    fee updates and, 139
    proposed relative value units, 138
    relative value scale, 137–138

Resource misallocation, low-income countries and, 406
Resource utilization groups (RUGS), 234
Retail pharmacies, 252
Retention ratio agreement, 116
Retrospective reviews, 128
Revenue maximization, hospitals and, 194
Risk
    aversion to and medical insurance, 88–90
    business risk assessment, 285–286
    capital financing and, 281–283
    correlated and uncorrelated, 284–286
    group practice and, 165–166
    pooling, 81, 438
    risk reduction value, 388–389

S

Salaries, physician, 140
Samuelson, Paul, 429
Sanitary revolution, 365–366
Savings, financing medical care and, 80
Scarcity (budget constraints), 11
Second opinions, 127
Secondary treatment costs, 64–65
Selective reporting, 66
Self-insurance, 116–117
Self-paid private insurance, 112
Senior-junior doctor partnerships, 167
Service substitution, long term care and, 235–236
Severity or risk margin, 54, 56–57
Sexual preferences, 367
Sexually transmitted diseases, 363
Shared income hypothesis, 310–311
Shifting demand and supply curves, 38–39
Short-run hospital costs, 207–208
Short-stay outliers, hospital costs and, 190
Small area variations, 171–174
Small hospitals, costs per day and, 214
Smith, Adam, 28
Smoke detector study, 67–68
Smoke-free workplace, 21
Smoking, as personal choice, 20–21
Social class, mortality ratios by, 387
Social insurance, 82
Social Security, historical aspects of, 389
Social Security Act of 1965, 99
Social support, long term care and, 228–229
Special situations, hospital rates and, 190–191
Specialized units, hospital costs and, 215
Specialties, physician income by, 142
Stark law, 169
Starvation, low-income countries and, 406

State Children's Health Insurance Program (SCHIP), 113
State taxes, self-insurance and, 118–119
Statistics, 391
Stepwise choice, cost-benefit analysis and, 52–53
Stone age, 374–375
Strategic budgets, 209
Subsidies, government and, 345
Substance Abuse and Mental Health Services Administration, 112
Substitute providers, organized medicine response to, 160–161
Substituting cheaper forms of care, 122
Substitution, pharmacy costs and, 126
Sudan health system, 406–408
    economic retrenchments and natural disasters and, 407
    financing sources and, 407
    government spending and, 407
    private funds and, 407–408
    private sector and, 407
Supply curves, 30–32, 37
Surgical techniques, modern, 391

T

Targeting diagnosis and treatment, 62
Tax benefits, 95–96
Taxpayer support, new innovations and, 4
Teaching, shifting overhead and, 17–18
Teamwork, 436
Technology. *See* Research and technology
Terms of trade, 2–3
The Jungle (Sinclair), 256
Third party payments, 9
Tiered pharmacy benefit plans, 126
Time and pain, patients and family and, 65
Time discount, cost-benefit analysis and, 52
Time price, 36
Timing and risk, 5
Tonsillectomy, 171–172
Transaction costs, 43, 336, 339–340
Transfers, hospital financing and, 190–191
Triaging patients, 215
Triple-option plans, 125
Triple-tier drug benefit plans, 126
Trust, doctor-patient relationship and, 146–147
Tversky, Amos, 430

U

Uncertainty in medical care, 30, 148
Uncorrelated risks, 284–286
Unequal health distribution, 431–432
Uninsured, 112–113
Union benefit, medical coverage as, 98

United Nations Children's Fund (UNICEF), 407
Universal health insurance coverage, 129, 414–415, 438–439
University hospitals costs, 194
U.S. Healthcare, 298–300
U.S. Public Health Service, 366
Usual, customary and reasonable (UCR) fee schedules, 136
Utilization reviews, 127–128, 192, 219

V

Value of economic security, 387–389
Value of health, 432
Value of life, 66–68, 387–388
Value of risk reduction, 388–389
Variability, insured groups and, 85–86
Visiting nursing services, 227
Voluntary regulation, 321

Voluntary sector, 345
von Leewenhoek, Anton, 390

W

Wage dynamics, 327–328
War, 369–370
Water–water paradox, 29–30
Wealthy elderly, long term care and, 242–243
Welfare losses, 94
Welfare triangle, 94
Wholesalers, pharmaceutical, 253, 266–267
Willingness to pay, 12, 50
Withholds, 127
Women's health, low-income countries and, 406
Workforce dynamics, 323–328
    employment and, 323–327
    wages and, 327–328
World Health Organization (WHO), 407
World Trade Organization (WTO), 259